Cystic Fibrosis Lung Disease: Mechanisms, Targets and Therapeutics

Cystic Fibrosis Lung Disease: Mechanisms, Targets and Therapeutics

Editor: Ryan Payne

AMERICAN
MEDICAL PUBLISHERS
www.americanmedicalpublishers.com

AMERICAN
MEDICAL PUBLISHERS
www.americanmedicalpublishers.com

Cataloging-in-Publication Data

Cystic fibrosis lung disease : mechanisms, targets and therapeutics / edited by Ryan Payne.
p. cm.
Includes bibliographical references and index.
ISBN 979-8-88740-583-4
1. Cystic fibrosis. 2. Cystic fibrosis --Diagnosis. 3. Cystic fibrosis --Treatment. 4. Genetic disorders. I. Payne, Ryan.
RC858 .C97 2023
616.37--dc23

American Medical Publishers,
41 Flatbush Avenue,
1st Floor, New York,
NY 11217, USA

ISBN 979-8-88740-583-4 (Hardback)

Contents

Preface

The purpose of the book is to provide a glimpse into the dynamics and to present opinions and studies of some of the scientists engaged in the development of new ideas in the field from very different standpoints. This book will prove useful to students and researchers owing to its high content quality.

Cystic fibrosis (CF) refers to a type of genetic disease that affects the lungs, digestive system and other organs. This disease occurs when the protein that generates mucus fails to function normally. Respiratory symptoms caused by CF include persistent coughing, wheezing and shortness of breath, along with other difficulties in breathing. Patients with CF display lung disease that is consistent with the breakdown of innate airway defense mechanisms. The diagnosis of CF is done by performing a sweat test, which determines the amount of salt present in the patient's body. CF has no known treatment options, but antibiotics that can be administered intravenously, breathed, or taken orally are used to manage this disease. A lung transplant may eventually be required, in case the lungs have suffered severe damage. This book provides comprehensive insights into cystic fibrosis. It will prove to be immensely beneficial to students and researchers in this field. Most of the topics introduced in this book cover mechanisms, targets and therapeutics for this lung disease.

At the end, I would like to appreciate all the efforts made by the authors in completing their chapters professionally. I express my deepest gratitude to all of them for contributing to this book by sharing their valuable works. A special thanks to my family and friends for their constant support in this journey.

Editor

1

The Role of Specialized Pro-Resolving Mediators in Cystic Fibrosis Airways Disease

Maelle Briottet, Mickael Shum and Valerie Urbach*

Institut national de la santé et de la recherche médicale (Inserm) U955, Institut Mondor de Recherche Biomédicale (IMRB), Créteil, France

***Correspondence:**
Valerie Urbach
valerie.urbach@inserm.fr

Cystic Fibrosis (CF) is a recessive genetic disease due to mutations of the Cystic Fibrosis Transmembrane Conductance Regulator (*CFTR*) gene encoding the CFTR chloride channel. The ion transport abnormalities related to *CFTR* mutation generate a dehydrated airway surface liquid (ASL) layer, which is responsible for an altered mucociliary clearance, favors infections and persistent inflammation that lead to progressive lung destruction and respiratory failure. The inflammatory response is normally followed by an active resolution phase to return to tissue homeostasis, which involves specialized pro-resolving mediators (SPMs). SPMs promote resolution of inflammation, clearance of microbes, tissue regeneration and reduce pain, but do not evoke unwanted immunosuppression. The airways of CF patients showed a decreased production of SPMs even in the absence of pathogens. SPMs levels in the airway correlated with CF patients' lung function. The prognosis for CF has greatly improved but there remains a critical need for more effective treatments that prevent excessive inflammation, lung damage, and declining pulmonary function for all CF patients. This review aims to highlight the recent understanding of CF airway inflammation and the possible impact of SPMs on functions that are altered in CF airways.

Keywords: cystic fibrosis, CF airway inflammation, specialized pro-resolving lipid mediators, bioactive lipids, lipoxin, resolvin

INTRODUCTION

CF is a multisystemic disorder with the lung disease being the main cause of morbidity and mortality. It is commonly acknowledged that the reduced ASL height in CF, is responsible for an altered mucociliary clearance which favors infections and persistent inflammation, leading to progressive lung destruction and respiratory failure (Davis, 2006). However, CF airway inflammation is excessive and ineffective against pathogens, can occur very early in the development of the disease and in some cases without any sign of infection (Balough et al., 1995; Khan et al., 1995; Armstrong et al., 1997; Balázs and Mall, 2019).

While acute inflammation is protective, excessive swarming of polymorphonuclear neutrophils (PMN) amplifies inflammation with collateral tissue damage. Therefore, the inflammatory response is normally followed by an active resolution phase to return to tissue homeostasis in which among other mediators (cytokines, chemokines, immune cells), bioactive lipids might play a crucial role.

Prostaglandins and leukotrienes stimulate the initiation and propagation phases of inflammation (Samuelsson et al., 1987; Funk, 2001) and the role of other lipid mediators called specialized pro-resolving mediators (SPMs) such as lipoxins, resolvins, protectins, and maresins has been demonstrated in the resolution phase (for recent review (Serhan and Levy, 2018)). SPMs promote resolution of inflammation, clearance of microbes, tissue regeneration and reduce pain, but do not evoke unwanted immunosuppression.

Abnormal SPM production or function have been related to widely occurring disorders, including CF airway disease. The airways of CF patients showed a decreased production of SPMs even in the absence of pathogens, which is consistent with other reports showing that inflammation in CF might not only be a consequence of chronic infection but could be related to intrinsic abnormalities of the inflammatory response (Muhlebach et al., 1999; Muhlebach and Noah, 2002; Karp et al., 2004; Ringholz et al., 2014; Bartlett et al., 2016; Isopi et al., 2020). The two SPMs, lipoxin A4 (LXA4) and resolvin D1 (RvD1), have the unique ability to restore the airway surface hydration, to damp the pro-inflammatory program and to fight infection in CF airways circumventing the most difficult aspects of CF pathophysiology (Karp et al., 2004; Grumbach et al., 2009; Verrière et al., 2012; Buchanan et al., 2013; Al-Alawi et al., 2014; Higgins et al., 2014; Higgins et al., 2016; Codagnone et al., 2017; Ringholz et al., 2018; Isopi et al., 2020). Furthermore, SPM levels in the airway correlate with CF patients lung function (Chiron et al., 2008; Eickmeier et al., 2017).

The prognosis for CF has greatly improved but it remains a severe and lethal disease. One promising therapy recently emerged, with small molecule correctors of mutated CFTR, which improve CFTR function and trafficking to the plasma-membrane [for recent review, see (Lopes-Pacheco, 2019)]. However, these therapies are gene mutation specific and their long-term impact on airway inflammation is still controversial (Jarosz-Griffiths et al., 2020; Volkova et al., 2020). To date there remains a critical need for more effective treatments that prevent excessive inflammation, lung damage, and declining pulmonary function for all CF patients.

This review highlights the current understanding of CF airway inflammation in the context of the recently described role of SPMs in chronic inflammation and the possible benefits of exogenous SPMs treatment in CF airways.

ACUTE INFLAMMATION AND SPECIALIZED PRO-RESOLVING MEDIATORS

Specialized Pro-resolving Mediators (SPMs) are a new family of lipid mediators involved in the acute inflammatory process.

Excessive inflammation is considered a common component of a vast range of chronic diseases including vascular diseases, metabolic syndrome, cancer, and neurological and airway diseases. Chronic inflammation is a pathological condition characterized by a persistent inflammatory process which ultimately leads to tissue degradation and/or remodeling (Kotas and Medzhitov, 2015; Uluçkan and Wagner, 2017). Either innate or adaptive immune responses can be involved in chronic inflammation. Chronic inflammation stems from a failure to eliminate the excessive pathogen load and/or from a dysfunctional immune system including failure to resolve inflammation (Nathan, 2002; Nathan and Ding, 2010).

In contrast, acute inflammation is a protective immune response against microbial pathogens, tissue injury or other harmful stimuli which evolved to eliminate invading organisms and to enhance tissue repair (Germolec et al., 2018). The inflammatory process is thus normally self-limited without progressing to chronic inflammation and fibrosis, leading to a return to tissue homeostasis. Resolution was considered a passive process in which the mediators involved in generating the inflammatory response would just dilute and dissipate. With identification of the family of bioactive lipid mediators SPMs, Serhan's team provided evidence that resolution of inflammation is an active, programmed response and not simply a process of diluting chemoattractant gradients (Samuelsson et al., 1987; Brady et al., 1995; Nathan, 2002; Serhan and Levy, 2018).

Therefore, inflammatory response is currently described as a physiological process divided into initiation and resolution phases, where lipid mediators, namely prostaglandins (PG), leukotrienes (LT), and SPMs play pivotal roles (Samuelsson et al., 1980; Funk, 2001). PGE_2 and PGI_2 induce vascular dilatation and permeability allowing PMN trafficking from blood circulation to enter the site of inflammation (Ley et al., 2007). LTB4 plays a role as a main chemoattractant driving PMNs to the inflammatory site to phagocytose pathogens. The resolution phase, orchestrated by SPMs in concert with other mediators, starts with cessation of PMN influx (**Figures 1A, B**) (Serhan et al., 2018). The families of SPMs identified to date are lipoxins (LX), resolvins (Rv), protectins (PD), and maresins (MaR). Their roles have been described in microbial defense, pain, organ protection and tissue regeneration, wound healing, cancer, reproduction, and neurobiology-cognition. SPMs play a crucial role in inhibiting the nuclear factor κB (NF-κB) (Chiang et al., 2006; Liao et al., 2012) and the synthesis of pro-inflammatory cytokines (Schwab et al., 2007; Krishnamoorthy et al., 2010; Chiang et al., 2012). SPMs also inhibit leukocyte chemotaxis and migration (Lee et al., 1989; Soyombo et al., 1994; Serhan et al., 1995; Papayianni et al., 1996; Sun et al., 2007; Isobe et al., 2012) (**Figures 1A, B**) as well as enhance innate microbial killing and clearance by stimulating leukocytes' phagocytosis of bacteria (Chiang et al., 2012; Chiang et al., 2015; Codagnone et al., 2018). They enhance macrophages' efferocytosis of apoptotic immune cells and cell debris (Godson et al., 2000; Schwab et al., 2007; Dalli and Serhan, 2012; Rogerio et al., 2012; Grabiec and Hussell, 2016) (**Figure 1C**). The repair of tissue damages generated by the inflammatory process also involves SPMs in promoting tissue regeneration (Dalli et al., 2014; Dalli et al., 2016) (**Figure 1D**). Beyond innate phagocyte responses to resolve acute inflammation, SPMs appear to play critical roles in regulating adaptive immunity (Barnig et al., 2013; Krishnamoorthy et al., 2015; Chiurchiù et al., 2016).

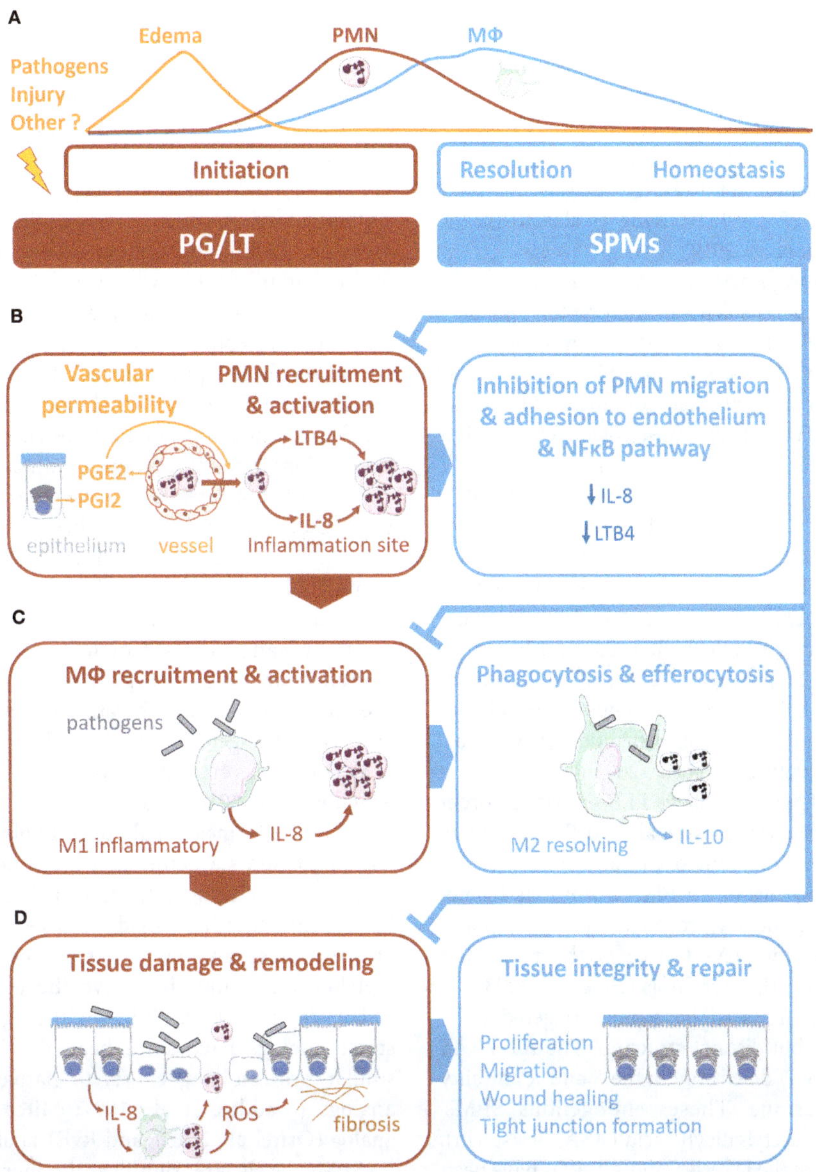

FIGURE 1 | Illustration of specialized pro-resolving mediators' (SPMs) multiple functions in the acute resolution of inflammation. **(A)** Acute inflammation evolved as a sequence of initiation and resolution phases that aim to drive back tissues toward homeostasis. The role of lipid mediators, prostaglandins (PG), leukotriene (LT), and SPMs can be related to each phase. **(B)** PGE2 and PGE2 and LTB4 play pivotal roles in the vascular response and leukocyte trafficking during the initiation phase. The SPMs, lipoxins, resolvins, protectins, and maresins produced at the inflammation, stimulate the cellular events that counter-regulate pro-inflammatory mediators and regulate polymorphonuclear (PMN) chemotaxis and migration, inhibiting LTB4 and pro-inflammatory cytokines synthesis (IL-8). **(C)** SPMs regulate monocyte and macrophage (MΦ) response. SPMs drive differentiation from inflammatory MΦ (M1) to resolving MΦ (M2), inhibit pro-inflammatory cytokine production (IL-8) induced by bacteria, stimulate anti-inflammatory cytokines synthesis (IL-10), enhance MΦ phagocytic function and efferocytosis of apoptotic PMN. **(D)** SPMs promote regeneration of tissue damaged by the inflammatory process.

SPMs exert their multiple actions through different cellular pathways involving diverse receptors (Chiang and Serhan, 2017). The first SPM receptor to be described is the N-formyl peptide receptor 2 (FPR2), a G protein-coupled receptor (GPCR) expressed in PMNs (Fiore et al., 1992) and other leukocytes (Chiang et al., 2006) as well as epithelial cells with high affinity for LXA4 (Fiore et al., 1994; Maddox et al., 1997; Chiang et al., 2003). Besides LXA4 and Aspirin-triggered 15-epi-LXA4 (AT-LXA4), FPR2 is also activated by Annexin A1 (ANXA1) (Perretti et al., 2002a; Bena et al., 2012). To date, five other specific SPM GPCRs have been identified in human and murine cells: GPR32, ChemR23, GPR18, GPR37, and GPR148. FPR2 and GPR32 mediate the RvD1, RvD3, and RvD5 immuno resolving actions (Krishnamoorthy et al., 2010; Hellmann et al., 2011; Recchiuti et al., 2011; Chiang et al., 2012; Gavins et al., 2012; Barnig et al., 2013; Buchanan et al., 2013; Dalli et al., 2013b; Lee and Surh, 2013; Recchiuti et al., 2014; Norling et al., 2016). Human GPR32 is mostly expressed in PMNs, monocytes, macrophages, and endothelial cells (Krishnamoorthy et al., 2010). Of note, RvD1 contributes to resolving inflammation by regulating a set of microRNAs specific to each receptor, FPR2 and GPR32 (Krishnamoorthy et al., 2010; Recchiuti et al., 2011). RvE1 and RvE2 exert potent and cell-specific actions on leukocytes *via* Chem32 (Tjonahen et al., 2006; Oh et al., 2012). GPR18 has been identified as the receptor for RvD2 (Chiang et al., 2015; Chiang et al., 2017), GPR37 for PD1 (Bang et al., 2018), and GPR148 for MaR1 (Chiang et al., 2019).

The cell signaling pathways activated by SPMs appear to be cell specific and do not depend solely on the receptor they bind to. In human epithelial cells, LXA4, and Mar1 stimulate a large increase in intracellular calcium promoting ASL height increase and epithelial repair in airway epithelia, and mucin secretion in conjunctival goblet cells (Lee et al., 1989; Nigam et al., 1990; Romano et al., 1996; Bonnans et al., 2003; Grumbach et al., 2009; Buchanan et al., 2013; Higgins et al., 2014; Hodges et al., 2017; Ringholz et al., 2018; Olsen et al., 2020). In contrast, in PMNs, LXA4 only induces a small increase in calcium and inhibits intracellular calcium mobilization induced by LTB4 in a context of PMN migration (Lee et al., 1989; Nigam et al., 1990; Romano et al., 1996; Grumbach et al., 2009; Buchanan et al., 2013; Higgins et al., 2014; Hodges et al., 2017; Ringholz et al., 2018). In human PMNs, stimulation of the LXA4 receptor inhibits phospholipase D (PLD) activity and superoxide anion generation (Levy et al., 1999; Levy and Serhan, 2000; Levy et al., 2005b), while in rat conjunctival goblet cells, LXA4 stimulates PLD activity in order to increase mucin secretion (Hodges et al., 2017). Binding to FPR2 can mediate both pro-inflammatory or anti-inflammatory responses depending on its ligand. In PMNs, while its ligand, serum amyloid A (SAA) induces a pro-inflammatory response with increased IL-8 secretion, LXA4 triggers the resolution characterized by a decreased IL-8 synthesis (He et al., 2003).

A distinct category of SPMs is the aspirin-triggered (AT) SPMs, which have a close but distinct structure. The AT-LXA4 and AT-LXB4 (15-epi-LXB4) differ only in the *S* and *R* chirality of their 15-hydroxyl residue. Theses endogenous SPMs' biosynthesis is induced by acetylsalicylic acid (ASA, or aspirin). To date, AT-LXs, AT-Rvs of the D series, and AT-PDs have been identified (Clària and Serhan, 1995; Chiang and Serhan, 2004; Serhan et al., 2004). They exert similar pro-resolving properties (Eickmeier et al., 2013; Wang et al., 2017; Liu et al., 2018; Hu et al., 2019).

Other mediators have been shown to play a role in the resolution of inflammation [for recent reviews, see (Perretti and D'Acquisto, 2009; Wallace et al., 2015; Schett and Neurath, 2018)]. ANXA1 and its derived peptides display a wide range of pro-resolving actions, among which inhibition of neutrophil recruitment, neutrophil/endothelium interaction and efferocytosis enhancement (Perretti et al., 2002b; Hayhoe et al., 2006; Scannell et al., 2007; D'Acquisto et al., 2008; Dalli et al., 2013a). In macrophages, the purine nucleoside adenosine promotes macrophage polarization toward resolution phenotype (M2), inhibits production of pro-inflammatory cytokines, and increases VEGF (Pinhal-Enfield et al., 2003; Csóka et al., 2012). Gaseous mediators such as carbon monoxide (CO), hydrogen sulfide (H_2S), and nitric oxide (NO) also display anti-inflammatory and pro-resolving properties. Among them, NO possesses pro-apoptotic qualities, H2S reduces leukocyte-endothelium interaction through activation of K_{ATP} channels, CO inhibits NF-κB activation and proinflammatory cytokines secretion in colonic epithelial cells. However, NO and adenosine, can also display pro-inflammatory effects depending on the concentration, localization, receptors involved, and timing in the inflammatory response [reviewed in (Brüne, 2005; Vass and Horvath, 2008)]. In addition, these mediators share common anti-inflammatory pathways with SPM signaling pathways. The ANXA1's anti-inflammatory actions rely on its ligation to the ALX/FPR2 receptor (Perretti et al., 2002b). Adenosine mediates Cl^- secretion in epithelial cells through intracellular calcium signaling in CF airway epithelium (Chao et al., 1994). The pro-resolution neuromodulator netrin-1 contributes to SPM production in mice peritoneal inflammation (Mirakaj et al., 2014). CO stimulates SPM biosynthesis through the regulation of 15LO1 *in vivo* in mice and baboons as well as *in vitro* in human cells (Chiang et al., 2013; Dalli et al., 2015). Physiologic hypoxia also stimulates SPMs synthesis by M2 macrophages-neutrophils interaction (Norris et al., 2019).

In humans, SPMs which are rapidly metabolized and degraded are found at pico to nanogram levels in blood, breastmilk, the airways (breath condensate and sputum), urine, and tears (Gangemi et al., 2003; Levy et al., 2007; Psychogios et al., 2011; Mas et al., 2012; Weiss et al., 2013; Colas et al., 2014; Ringholz et al., 2014; Sasaki et al., 2015; Barden et al., 2016; Dalli et al., 2017; Eickmeier et al., 2017; English et al., 2017). The short half-life of SPMs, whether they are endogenous or synthetic, led to the manufacturing of the first analogs of LXA4 by Serhan and his collaborators have made it easier to study their biological effects. These analogs differ structurally to prevent their metabolization and thus have the advantage of being more stable (Serhan et al., 1995). Other generations of synthetic stable analogs have since been developed and have shown similar pro-resolving effects to native SPMs, such as LXA4 analogs (Maddox et al., 1997; Mitchell et al., 2002), RvD1 analog (Orr et al., 2015), and RvE1 analog (Arita et al., 2006).

SPMs levels are significantly increased in inflammatory exudates in rheumatoid arthritis, skin blisters, bronchoalveolar lavage (BAL) fluids from patients with airway diseases (Lee et al., 1990; Karp et al., 2004; Planagumà et al., 2008; Morris et al., 2009; Ringholz et al., 2014; Norling et al., 2016; Motwani et al., 2018a; Motwani et al., 2018b). However, SPMs levels are shown to be decreased and unbalanced compared to pro-inflammatory eicosanoids in patients with chronic conditions including airway diseases. Lower LXA4 and LXB4 levels in sputum, BAL, and blood correlate with a more severe asthma phenotype. LXA4 levels have been found to be reduced in the sputum of Chronic Obstructive Pulmonary Disease (COPD) patients during exacerbation (Levy et al., 2005a; Vachier et al., 2005; Levy et al., 2007, 1; Schwab et al., 2007; Planagumà et al., 2008; Balode et al., 2012; Liao et al., 2012; Karra et al., 2015; Codagnone et al., 2018; Serhan et al., 2018). Altogether, SPMs, which are conserved structures, are now strong candidates for the role of main actors of the resolution phase of acute inflammation. Reports of decreased SPM biosynthesis or function in inflammatory chronic diseases suggest the involvement of SPMs in their pathogenesis. From these observations, additional fundamental studies aim to shed more light on the precise role of SPMs in these conditions. The next chapter will tackle the known alterations in lipid metabolism and SPMs biosynthesis in CF.

ABNORMAL LIPID METABOLISM AND SPMs BIOSYNTHESIS IN CF

Along with ANXA1 and NO, an abnormal SPMs biosynthesis was reported in CF (Karp et al., 2004; Dalli et al., 2010; Ringholz et al., 2014; Güney et al., 2019).

SPMs biosynthesis results from the interaction of enzymes called lipoxygenases (LOX) and cyclooxygenases (COX) to metabolize essential n-3 (omega 3) and n-6 (omega 6) polyunsaturated fatty acids (PUFA). The main PUFA substrates are arachidonic acid (AA, n-6), eicosapentaenoic acid (EPA, n-3), and docosahexaenoic acid (DHA, n-3) (Serhan et al., 1984; Samuelsson et al., 1987). Different cell types that differentially express LOX and COX enzymes cooperate by exchanging intermediates to produce the final active metabolites (Papayianni et al., 1996; Folco and Murphy, 2006; Sala et al., 2010). While free AA gives rise to the lipoxin family of SPMs, it is also the precursor of pro-inflammatory mediators PG and LT depending on which metabolic enzyme is involved (Samuelsson et al., 1987; Folco and Murphy, 2006). The DHA and EPA metabolites resolvins, protectins, and maresins exert mainly resolving actions (**Figure 2**).

Acute inflammation is the result of a temporal eicosanoids class switching where COX-derived prostaglandins precede biosynthesis of lipoxins. This eicosanoids class switching, characterized by an increased biosynthesis of SPMs and a decrease of eicosanoids involved in the initiation of inflammation, results from the coordinated action of enzymes such as the different isoforms of lipoxygenases (15LO, 5LO, and 12LO), of COX (COX1 and COX2), as well as the leukotriene A4 hydrolase (LT4H) (**Figure 3**). These enzymes are selectively expressed in the cell types involved in the inflammatory process. The 15LO expressed in airway epithelial cells and macrophages and the 12LO in platelets play a central role in the class-switching from the pro-inflammatory lipid mediator LTB4 toward SPMs. Isolated PMNs exposed to PGE2 (to mimic exudates) switched eicosanoid biosynthesis from predominantly LTB4 and 5LO-initiated pathways to LXA4, which is a 15LO product that stops PMN infiltration (Levy et al., 2001). Indeed, the activity of 15LO favors LXA4 synthesis at the expense of LTB4 synthesis that involves LTA4H activity (Haeggström and Funk, 2011) (**Figure 3**). The cellular location of 5LO also plays a crucial role in the LTB4/SPM ratio. Inhibition of

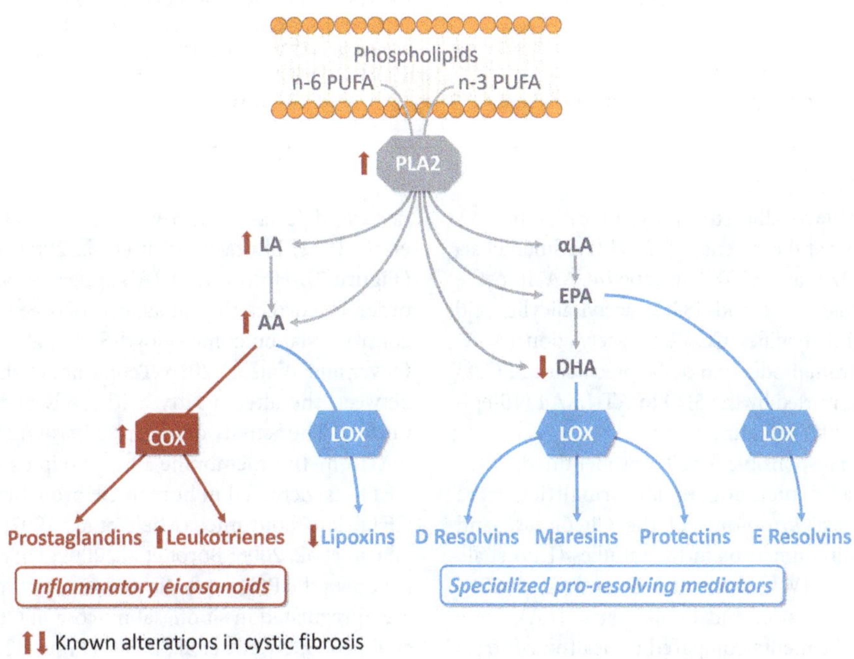

FIGURE 2 | Altered lipid metabolism in cystic fibrosis. The activity of phospholipase A2 (PLA2), which releases essential fatty acid (n-6 and n-3 polyunsaturated fatty acids, PUFA) from phospholipids, is increased in CF bronchial epithelial cells. Free arachidonic acid (AA) which can be released from phospholipids or metabolized from n-6 linoleic acid (LA), is the precursor of prostaglandins and leukotrienes via cyclooxygenase activity (COX), which is increased in CF. AA is also a substrate for lipoxygenases (LOX) to produce lipoxins, found reduced in CF. The n-3 PUFA, α-linoleic acid (α-LA) is metabolized to ecosapentanoic acid (EPA) and docosahexaenoic acid (DHA), found decreased in CF. EPA and DHA are the precursors of resolvins, protectins, and maresins. The pathways involved in the biosynthesis of pro-inflammatory eicosanoids are illustrated in red, the pathways involved in the biosynthesis of specialized pro-resolving mediators in blue.

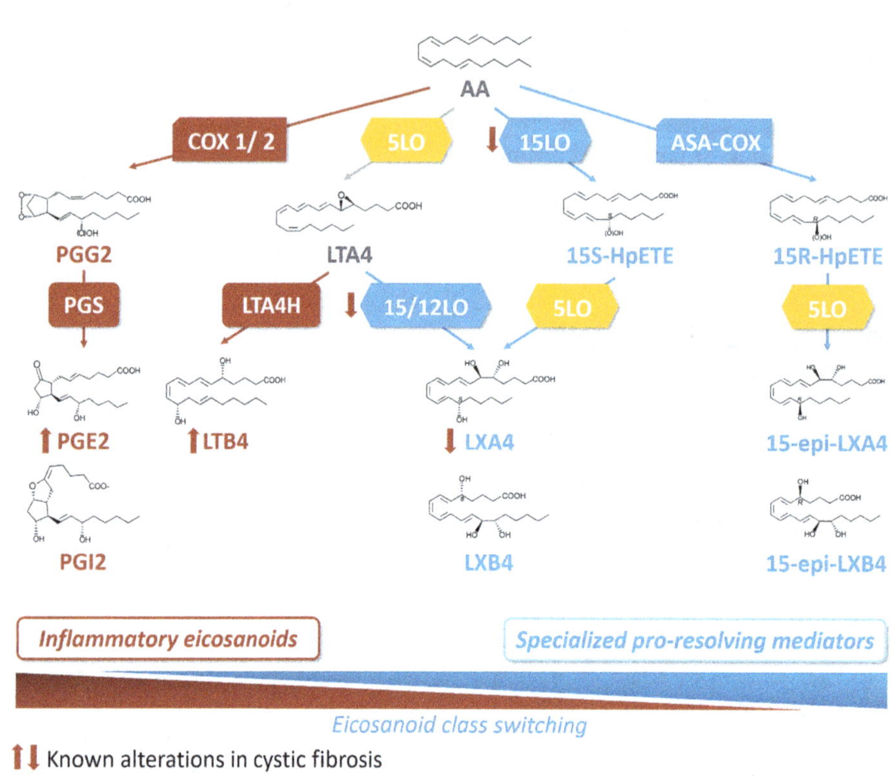

FIGURE 3 | Arachidonic acid (AA) metabolome and abnormal class switching in CF. Arachidonic acid (AA) is metabolized by cyclooxygenase 1 and 2 (COX1/2) and prostaglandin synthase (PGS) into the inflammatory eicosanoids, prostaglandins (PGE2 and PGI2). AA is also a substrate for 5LO to produce leukotriene A4 (LTA4). The 15 lipoxygenase (15LO) activity drives then the SPM, lipoxin A4 (LXA4) synthesis (from LTA4) at the expense of the production of the inflammatory lipid, leukotriene B4 (LTB4) that involves leukotriene A4 hydrolase (LTA4H) activity. The sequential activities of 15LO and 5LO drive the biosynthesis of LXA4, with an intermediate product, 15S hydroperoxyeicosatetraenoic (15S-HpETE). Acetylsalicylic acid inhibited COX (ASA-COX) leads to the production of 15R hydroperoxyeicosatetraenoic acid (15-R-HpETE) which is converted by the 5LO to the SPM, 15-epi-LXA4. In CF, the abnormal class switching from inflammatory biosynthetic pathway to the pro-resolving pathway results into an increased LTB4 and decreased LXA4 biosynthesis in the airway which are responsible for the sustained inflammation.

the CaM kinases by RvD1 favors the extra-nuclear location of 5LO, and the LXA4 biosynthesis at the expense of LTB4 (Fredman et al., 2014). Finally, while COX1 and COX2 metabolize AA into the inflammatory eicosanoids PGE2 and PGI2, acetylsalicylic acid (ASA) inhibits COX1 and modifies COX2 by acetylation (ASA-COX), leading to a shift from production of the precursor of PG, to 15-R-HpETE which is converted by the 5LO to AT-LXA4 (15-epi-LXA4) (Birnbaum et al., 2007) (**Figure 3**).

Before the gene defect responsible for CF was identified, it was suggested that fatty acid metabolism abnormalities were responsible for the clinical symptoms of the CF disease and this has been confirmed in numerous further studies (Kuo et al., 1962) [for recent review, (Wheelock and Strandvik, 2020)]. Lower levels of palmitic, stearic, and linoleic acid (LA), were reported in plasma of CF patients compared to healthy controls (Hubbard et al., 1977; Gibson et al., 1986; Thompson, 1989; Roulet et al., 1997; Strandvik et al., 2001; Al-Turkmani et al., 2007). Initially thought as the result of malabsorption by CF patients (Hubbard et al., 1977), an abnormal lipid metabolism related to CFTR dysfunction was further demonstrated. An imbalance of PUFAs with increased release of AA and decreased levels of DHA in CF was established (Underwood et al., 1972; Bhura-Bandali et al., 2000; Freedman et al., 2004) (**Figure 2**). However, DHA supplementation in CF patients, in order to correct the imbalance between AA and DHA gave a controversial outcome (Lloyd-Still et al., 2006; Coste et al., 2007; Oliver and Watson, 2016; Teopompi et al., 2019). The direct link between the altered fatty acid levels and CFTR dysfunction is unclear. The activity of phospholipase A2 (PLA2), which releases AA from the membrane phospholipids and can interact with CFTR, is increased in human CF bronchial epithelial cells and in CFTR-knockout mice (Miele et al., 1997; Six and Dennis, 2000; Ghosh et al., 2006; Borot et al., 2009; Dif et al., 2010). Free AA is led down the PG metabolic pathway by the COX enzymes, which are upregulated in sinonasal mucosa of CF patients (Roca-Ferrer et al., 2006; Owens et al., 2008) (**Figure 2**). Consistent with this, polymorphisms downregulating COX1 and COX2 expression in CF patients are associated with a better clinical outcome (Czerska et al., 2010). The first studies focused on LXA4 levels and LXA4 to PMN ratio measured in BAL fluids of CF subjects compared to non-CF subjects and suggested a relative decrease of LXA4 to PMN concentrations (Karp et al., 2004). In contrast,

Starosta et al. observed no differences in the absolute LXA4 BAL fluids concentrations between CF patients and controls with a similar degree of neutrophilic airway inflammation. Concentrations were also similar in CF patients with mild versus more severe airway inflammation (Starosta et al., 2006). Another study showed that CFTR defects dampen LXA4 biosynthesis during platelets-PMN interaction (Mattoscio et al., 2010). The ratio of SPMs to the pro-inflammatory eicosanoid LTB4 has also been evaluated by Ringholz et al. in BAL fluid samples from children with CF. An imbalance between resolving (LXA4) and pro-inflammatory eicosanoids (LTB4) was found, suggesting a defect in eicosanoid class switching (Ringholz et al., 2014). Furthermore, a reduced expression of the 12/15LO in the airway of a CF mice model as well as a reduced 15LO2 isoform level in the BAL fluid of patients with F508del mutation (Karp et al., 2004; Ringholz et al., 2014). Similarly, 15LO2 expression has been shown to be decreased by 50% in the nasal polyps of CF patients compared to non-CF (Jeanson et al., 2014) (**Figure 3**). A defective activity of 12LO, another lipoxygenase expressed in platelets, has been shown when inhibiting CFTR (Mattoscio et al., 2010). Although the cellular mechanism by which CFTR could affect LOX levels and/or activities remains unclear, these data are consistent with an abnormal SPMs biosynthesis in CF.

Taken together, the altered lipid metabolism that could result in an imbalance of eicosanoids with higher pro-inflammatory mediators as compared to SPMs would be coherent with the observations of the sustained and inefficient CF airway inflammation as detailed below.

INFLAMMATION IN CF AIRWAY

CF is a recessive monogenic disease due to mutations in the Cystic Fibrosis Transmembrane conductance Regulator (*CFTR*) gene (Kerem et al., 1989; Riordan et al., 1989; Rommens et al., 1989). Over 2,000 mutations of *CFTR* are known, although around two thirds of patients have at least one copy of the F508del mutation (Cystic Fibrosis Mutation Database; Bobadilla et al., 2002). While CFTR dysfunction may affect many organs, the inflammatory airway disease leading to progressive lung damage is the main cause of morbidity and mortality of CF patients (Davis, 2006). Multiple pathways involved in CF airway inflammation have been described.

Ion Transport and Airway Surface Liquid Abnormalities

The dehydrated airway surface liquid (ASL) resulting from ion transport abnormalities is a critical feature of the CF airway pathogenesis (Boucher, 2007). The main CFTR function is to transport chloride from the cytosol to the lumen (Anderson et al., 1991; Linsdell, 2017). CFTR also regulates other epithelial functions (Stutts et al., 1995; Greger et al., 1996), including the activity of the sodium channel (ENaC) located in the same membrane (Hanukoglu and Hanukoglu, 2016). Although several reports suggested no change in ENaC activity associated with CFTR dysfunction (Chen et al., 2010; Itani et al., 2011; Collawn et al., 2012; Fisher et al., 2013; Sun et al., 2014; Tuggle et al., 2014), other functional studies have brought evidence supporting CFTR role in inhibiting sodium absorption by ENaC (Kunzelmann et al., 1995; Ismailov et al., 1996; Kunzelmann et al., 2000; König et al., 2001; Kunzelmann, 2003; Gentzsch et al., 2010; Lazrak et al., 2011). At the expression level, while the α- and β-ENaC subunit amount was reported to be increased in CF nasal epithelium the γ-ENaC was decreased (Bangel et al., 2008). Consistent with a role for ENaC in CF, similar features of human CF lung disease have been reproduced when ENaC is overexpressed in mice (Mall et al., 2004).

Both transepithelial chloride secretion involving chloride channels such as CFTR and the transepithelial sodium absorption *via* ENaC, finely regulate cellular and paracellular water movements generating the ASL layer (Tarran et al., 2001; Tarran, 2004). The ASL constitutes the first line of innate defense in controlling the mucociliary clearance process, trapping and neutralizing inhaled foreign particles in the mucus layer that are then removed from the airways by the ciliated cells (Knowles and Boucher, 2002; Button et al., 2012; Shei et al., 2018). In CF, ion transport abnormalities lead to a reduced ASL height (Boucher, 2007) and result in an impaired ciliary beating, favors mucus plugging in the airways, which constitutes a viscous and nutritive medium for pathogens proliferation in the respiratory tract, especially bacteria.

The content of the ASL layer of CF patients is also affected by dysregulation of bicarbonate transport. Firstly observed in pancreas, decreased bicarbonate secretion has been related to abnormal chloride secretion (Marino et al., 1991). CFTR has been shown to regulate bicarbonate secretion; either directly by being permeant (Poulsen et al., 1994; Illek et al., 1997; Kim et al., 2014), or by interacting with other transporters, such as the chloride/bicarbonate exchangers, SLC26A4 also named pendrin, and/or the ATP12A, a non-gastric form of H^+/K^+-ATPase expressed at the apical side of airway epithelia (Garnett et al., 2011; Scudieri et al., 2018). Indeed, H^+-K^+-ATPase and CFTR-dependent bicarbonate secretion regulate extracellular pH (Coakley et al., 2003). The lack of bicarbonate secretion due to altered CFTR activity or ATP12A increased expression in CF human airways secondary to inflammation and infection are consistent with a more acidic ASL pH in CF (Song et al., 2006; Cho et al., 2011; Scudieri et al., 2018). Furthermore, ASL acidification in CF bronchial epithelial cells can be driven by hyperglycemia and *P. aeruginosa*-related lactate secretion which monitors H^+ secretion (Garnett et al., 2016). Although ASL pH is difficult to measure and ASL pH decrease in CF is still controverted (McShane et al., 2003; Schultz et al., 2017), more acidic ASL could explain some aspect of the pathogenesis of the disease. Indeed, an acidified environment is beneficial for bacteria survival. *In vivo* studies on CF newborn pigs and *in vitro* data obtained on human airway epithelial cells have demonstrated that bacterial killing is impaired in CF due to more acidic ASL pH (Pezzulo et al., 2012; Simonin et al., 2019).

Chronic Airway Infection and Inflammation

In CF, the lung function decline correlates with the chronic colonization by pathogens, including the bacteria *Pseudomonas aeruginosa* (Nixon et al., 2001; Emerson et al., 2002; Konstan et al., 2007) which are potent triggers of PMN response. However, in CF airways challenged by bacteria or viruses, inflammation appears disproportionate to the degree of infection, with a high PMN infiltration and release of pro-inflammatory molecules, such as TNF-α, IL-8, IL-6, IL-1β, proteases, oxidants, PG, and LT, together leading to bronchiectasis and fibrosis (Konstan et al., 1993; Balough et al., 1995; Bonfield et al., 1995; Khan et al., 1995; Noah et al., 1997; Muhlebach et al., 1999; Tirouvanziam et al., 2000; Muhlebach and Noah, 2002). As the first line of defense against microbial agents, macrophages can induce inflammation by stimulating the immune system but they also contribute to ending the inflammation process and to the return to tissue homeostasis, by clearing microbes and dead PMNs for instance. These polar roles define two macrophage subtypes with distinct gene signatures, a pro-inflammatory subtype (M1) and a pro-resolving one (M2) (Mills et al., 2000). M1 cells produce high levels of the pro-inflammatory TNFα, IL-1β, IL-6, and IL-12, while M2 cells secrete high levels of immune-resolving IL-10 and TGFβ1 compared with M1 cells (Bystrom et al., 2008). It has been suggested that altered macrophage function contributes to the sustained inflammation in CF airways (Bruscia and Bonfield, 2016). CF macrophages are hyper-responsive, producing a high amount of pro-inflammatory cytokines when exposed to bacterial stimuli (Bruscia et al., 2009; Bruscia et al., 2011) but showed a defective ability to clear bacteria (Di et al., 2006; Deriy et al., 2009; Porto et al., 2011). There have been reports of CF macrophages failing to polarize into anti-inflammatory M2 and M1 macrophages displaying a hypermetabolic state (Tarique et al., 2017; Lara-Reyna et al., 2019).

Early reports indicated signs of inflammation in the airways of young CF patients even in the absence of infection and questioned the nature of the relationship between infection and inflammation in the CF airways (Balough et al., 1995; Khan et al., 1995; Armstrong et al., 1997). Thanks to systematic newborn screening and methodical, precise phenotyping from longitudinal studies, the early lung disease onset and progression in CF has been better characterized. As early as infancy, CF patients' lower airways show signs of mucus plugging and altered lung structure (Martínez et al., 2005; Stick et al., 2009). Furthermore, BAL fluid samples collected from infants bear evidence of active inflammation with high PMN counts and neutrophil elastase and pro-inflammatory cytokine levels, even before patients encounter their first infection by the conventional CF pathogens (Pillarisetti et al., 2011; Montgomery et al., 2017; Ranganathan et al., 2017; Balázs and Mall, 2019). The presence of sterile inflammation has also been observed in animal models, notably in CFTR-knockout ferrets that show signs of neutrophil-mediated inflammation despite being infection-free (Keiser et al., 2015; Rosen et al., 2018).

Despite the identification of the CFTR gene and the growing mutation database, establishing a correlation between CF genotype and clinical phenotype remains difficult, considering the vastly different disease courses between patients, even between twin siblings sharing the same CFTR mutations (Kerem et al., 1990; Mekus et al., 2000). Genome-wide association studies with large patient cohorts have identified genetic variants of specific loci associated with disease severity, called CF modifier genes, that contribute to phenotypic variability [see recent reviews (Lim et al., 2018; Shanthikumar et al., 2019)]. Among the proteins encoded by the CF modifier genes, some have direct protein-protein interaction with CFTR and/or are involved in immune response (Tugores et al., 2001; Wright et al., 2011; Stanke et al., 2014; Corvol et al., 2015). The trachea of CF and non-CF newborn pigs when challenged by an inflammatory stimulus revealed differential transcriptomes (Bartlett et al., 2016). Therefore, beyond ion transport abnormalities, intrinsic immune abnormalities related to CFTR dysfunction could be involved in the pathogenesis of the CF airway disease.

Dysregulated Calcium Homeostasis

Calcium is a major intracellular second messenger playing a key role in immune functions, among which cytokines secretion and PMN recruitment (Berridge et al., 2003; Immler et al., 2018). Calcium homeostasis has long been known to be dysregulated in CF (Katz et al., 1984; Cabrini and De Togni, 1985).

Initial studies supported the hypothesis of an acquired response from the airway epithelial cells to exogenous pathogens such as *P. aeruginosa* leading to calcium mobilization and hyperinflammation (Denning et al., 1998; Hybiske et al., 2007). Further studies demonstrated that the endoplasmic reticulum (ER), a major intracellular calcium storage compartment, undergoes stress and expansion in CF airway epithelial cells as the result of chronic infection and inflammation (Ribeiro et al., 2005a; Ribeiro et al., 2005b; Ribeiro, 2006). Other studies have suggested that ER stress, NF-κB activation, and IL-8 related expressions are closely linked to CFTR channel mistrafficking and its retention in the ER of different CF models (Weber et al., 2001; Knorre et al., 2002; Antigny et al., 2008a). The ER stress normally results in unfolded protein response (UPR) mediated by proteins located in the ER membrane. However, atypical UPR activation fails to resolve the ER stress in CF and sensitizes the innate immune system to respond more vigorously to microbial challenge (Ribeiro et al., 2005b; Ribeiro, 2006; Kerbiriou et al., 2007; Lin et al., 2008; Blohmke et al., 2012). Finally, calcium transporters are also reported to be altered in CF. In the ER, the retention of the F508del CFTR protein leads to impaired activity of SERCA pump and IP3 receptor, altering calcium exchange between the ER and with the cytosol (Antigny et al., 2008a; Antigny et al., 2008b; Philippe et al., 2015). Calcium influx and efflux at the plasma-membrane have been shown to be impaired by dysfunctional coupling of mutated CFTR with transient receptor potential canonical channels 6 (TRPC6), altered plasma-membrane calcium pump and upregulated complex Orai1/STIM1 formation that increases IL-8 secretion (Antigny et al., 2011; Balghi et al., 2011; Philippe et al., 2015).

Mucus

Mucus was for long observed to be more viscous and thick, in CF airways in *in vitro* and *in situ* studies (Derichs et al., 2011). In addition to altered ion and fluid transport that result in a dehydrated mucous layer, the CF airways are characterized by goblet cell and glandular hyperplasia and subsequent overproduction of the two secreted mucins MUC5B and MUC5AC, which has been reported in both CF patients and CF model systems (Henderson et al., 2014; Esther et al., 2019). Furthermore, structural mucus abnormalities have been described in CF. Analysis of airway mucins from newborn CF pigs' freshly excised airways revealed that MUC5B strands remained attached to submucosal glands and MUC5AC, secreted by goblet cells, is more present and forms sheets that cover MUC5B strands (Ostedgaard et al., 2017). The early work of Inglis, Ballard et al. on excised porcine distal bronchi enlightened the role of chloride and water transport on mucus rheological properties (Inglis et al., 1997; Inglis et al., 1998; Inglis et al., 1999; Ballard et al., 2002). In addition, Perez-Vilar suggested that lower pH would favor interchain disulfide bonds and the ASL volume depletion may increase MUC5B and MUC5AC concentrations and favor interactions (Perez-Vilar and Boucher, 2004). Other studies suggested that mucus swelling and hydration is driven by the Donnan effects (unbalanced repartition of charged particles over a porous barrier) and that HCO_3^- plays a key role in the swelling of the mucins favoring a decrease content of calcium associated mucins (Quinton, 2008; Chen et al., 2010). From the new-born CF piglets and human bronchial epithelium studies, the impaired mucocilliary clearance and rheological properties of mucus appeared dependent on both chloride and pH (Hoegger et al., 2014; Gorrieri et al., 2016; Hill et al., 2018; Hughes et al., 2019). Finally, a pilot study realized on 12 CF volunteers supported that nebulized $NaHCO_3$ was safe and well tolerated and it permit to increase ASL pH and change the rheology of the sputum (Gomez et al., 2020).

Oxidative Stress

Oxidative stress which arises from the loss of the oxidant/antioxidant balance shifted toward oxidant production is described in many airway diseases including CF and triggers lung injuries (Brown et al., 1996) and pro-inflammatory mechanisms (Brown et al., 1996; MacNee, 2001; Boncoeur et al., 2008; Chen et al., 2008; Bartling and Drumm, 2009; Park et al., 2009; Kelly-Aubert et al., 2011; Pongnimitprasert et al., 2012). Increased levels of reactive oxygen species (ROS), such as superoxide anion, and involvement of its main producer, the NADPH oxidase (NOX) enzyme, have been demonstrated in CF mice models and human cell lines (Esposito et al., 1999; Velsor et al., 2006; Pongnimitprasert et al., 2012). In CF airway epithelial cells, the morphology and functions of mitochondria, the main cellular component involved in ROS production (Favia et al., 2019) are altered (Feigal et al., 1982; Von Ruecker et al., 1984; Antigny et al., 2009) and restored by correction of F508del CFTR mutation (Valdivieso et al., 2007; Taminelli et al., 2008; Valdivieso et al., 2012; Atlante et al., 2016). Furthermore, *P. aeruginosa* infection and inflammation-related production of ROS by PMNs and macrophages exacerbate alterations of mitochondrial functions, DNA, and morphology in normal lung epithelial cells. All of these mitochondrial alterations contribute to the establishment of oxidative stress in the airways (Maurice et al., 2019; Causer et al., 2020). Studies from CF mice model, human cell lines, or BAL fluids have shown a reduced uptake, synthesis or activity of antioxidant defenses, such as superoxide dismutase, peroxidases, catalases, and reduced glutathione (GSH) which further enhances oxidative stress (Farrell et al., 1977; Roum et al., 1993; Velsor et al., 2006; Schwarzer et al., 2007; Rottner et al., 2011). In addition to CFTR permeability for GSH, polymorphisms in regulatory genes of the metabolic pathway of GSH were associated with different phenotypes of CF and its severity (Linsdell and Hanrahan, 1998; Hudson, 2001; Jungas et al., 2002; Marson et al., 2013; Marson et al., 2014). Finally, low levels of GSH in BAL could also result from its oxidation by pro-inflammatory products, such as hypochlorous acid, coming from infection-activated PMNs (Kettle et al., 2014).

Abnormal Epithelial Repair

In CF, impaired mucociliary clearance, long-term infection, ineffective inflammation, increased ROS secretion and PMN products contribute to epithelial injury, amplifying airway inflammation (Chmiel and Davis, 2003). Altered CF airway epithelia repair has been more directly related to CFTR dysfunction and expression (Schiller et al., 2010; Itokazu et al., 2014). While CFTR pharmacologic inhibition, repression or mutation affect epithelial cell proliferation and migration and wound healing, CFTR rescue with transfection or CFTR modulators (correctors, potentiators) improves epithelial repair in airway epithelial cultures from patients with the most common mutations (Trinh et al., 2012; Dong et al., 2015; Adam et al., 2018). Other ion channels are also involved in the altered repair processes in CF. Indeed, epidermal growth factor (EGF) and its receptor EGFR signaling, along with potassium channel function are impaired in CF and contribute to reduced cell migration and proliferation (Trinh et al., 2008). The activity and expression of the calcium activated chloride channel, Anoctamin 1 (ANO1), shown to be reduced in human and mice CF airway epithelial cells, could also delay CF airway epithelial cell proliferation and migration (Ruffin et al., 2013).

Dysregulated MicroRNA

MicroRNAs have emerged as important regulators in human physiological and pathological cell processes including the immune system, providing negative feedback regulation of inflammation and ion transport. In CF, microRNA profiling studies have shown that miR155, miR145, miR223, miR494, miR99b, let-7e, miR181b, and miR125a are increased in CF airway epithelial cell lines, CF bronchial brushing samples, and macrophages, compared to non-CF controls (McKiernan and Greene, 2015; Pierdomenico et al., 2017). In contrast, miR126, miR31, miR17 expression is decreased in CF airway epithelial cells. Decreased levels of miR126 correlate with up-regulation of TOM1, a negative regulator of pro-inflammatory cytokines. Decrease of miR31 in CF airways contributes to increased pulmonary cathepsin S production that activates the epithelial sodium channel and inactivates antimicrobial proteins (McKiernan and Greene, 2015). CFTR expression is under control of miR101 (Viart et al., 2015). Therefore, dysregulated microRNAs as critical regulators of epithelial immune responses can play a role in the intrinsic abnormalities of airway inflammation in CF.

IMPACT OF SPMs DEMONSTRATED IN CF MODELS

Abnormal epithelial ion transport, excessive and non-resolving inflammation, chronic bacterial infection, and progressive lung destruction are the main features of CF airway disease, whether they are directly or indirectly related to CFTR misexpression or malfunction. Among the multiple cellular and molecular pathways involved in CF airway pathogenesis, the abnormal SPMs biosynthesis could play a central role. Indeed, SPMs have been demonstrated to regulate several distinct dysfunctions of CF airways that result in excessive and sustained inflammation (**Table 1**, **Figure 4**). Unless specified otherwise, the SPMs used in the studies described from this point on are synthetic exogenous SPMs which have the same chemical structure and half-life as their endogenous counterpart.

Epithelial Ion Transport, ASL and Calcium

Several *in vivo* and *in vitro* studies have provided evidence for SPMs' involvement in regulating airway epithelial ionic transports and ASL layer height in models of airway epithelial diseases, including CF. In a rat model of acute lung injury (ALI), LXA4, RvD1, Mar1 enhance the expression of CFTR, ENaC (ENaC-α and ENaC-γ subunits), Na,K-ATPase (β1 subunit), and aquaporins leading to the stimulation of alveolar fluid clearance (AFC) (Yang et al., 2013; Wang Q. et al., 2014; Zhang et al., 2017) (**Table 2**).

In vitro studies of ion transport in CF airway epithelial cells. In human CF bronchial epithelial cells, LXA4 and RvD1 stimulate an increase of the ASL to a normal height (7 μm) (Verrière et al., 2012; Al-Alawi et al., 2014; Higgins et al., 2014; Ringholz et al., 2018). Stimulation of the surface airway hydration by these SPMs can be inhibited by the FPR2 receptor antagonist, BOC-2 and by BAPTA-AM, indicating this process to be mediated by the FPR2 receptor and highly dependent on intracellular calcium. Furthermore, LXA4 induces a large and sustained intracellular calcium increase in CF airway epithelial cells involving the stimulation of an apical ATP secretion by pannexin channels (PANX1). The subsequent activation of purino-receptors localized in these cells' apical membrane generate calcium entry and calcium release from intracellular stores. A role for the P2Y11, a GPCR purino-receptor leading to a rise in both intracellular cAMP (stimulation of adenylate cyclase [AC]) and calcium mobilization (increased inositol 3 phosphate [IP3]) has been demonstrated upon exposure of CF airway epithelia cells to LXA4 (**Figure 5**) (Bonnans et al., 2003; Verrière et al., 2012; Higgins et al., 2014). In human CF airway epithelial cells, patch-clamp studies have demonstrated that LXA4 stimulates a calcium-activated chloride secretion (Verrière et al., 2012). Another study reported that the LXA4 effect in restoring the ASL height in CF airway epithelial cells also implicates ENaC inhibition (Al-Alawi et al., 2014) (**Figure 5**, **Table 1**).

In vivo *studies of ion transport in CF airway epithelial cells.* The role of LXA4 and RvD1 on chloride secretion and sodium absorption was further confirmed *in vivo* by the recovery of nasal transepithelial potential difference in homozygous F508del CFTR mice (Ringholz et al., 2018) (**Table 1**).

Cytokine Production and Release

As part of the inflammatory response, the role of SPMs in inhibiting pro-inflammatory cytokines production (e.g.: IL-6, IL-8, IL-1β, and TNFα, IL-13) and stimulating anti-inflammatory cytokines (IL-4, IL-10) as well as inhibiting leukocyte chemotaxis and migration has been demonstrated in many chronic diseases. Their role has been established in models of acute lung injury, asthma, and COPD (Lee et al., 1989; Serhan et al., 1995; Papayianni et al., 1996; Hachicha et al., 1999; Bonnans et al., 2002; Vachier et al., 2005; Bonnans et al., 2006; Sun et al., 2007; Aoki et al., 2008; Isobe et al., 2012; Yang et al., 2013; Croasdell et al., 2015; Codagnone et al., 2018) as well as cellular models of viral and bacterial inflammation, or oxidative stress (Chiang et al., 2012; Hsiao et al., 2014; Wang L. et al., 2014; Wang Q. et al., 2014; Cox et al., 2015) and cigarette smoke-induced inflammation (Takamiya et al., 2012; Jiajia et al., 2014) (**Table 3**). The pathways involved in SPM's regulation of inflammation are presented in **Figure 6**.

In vitro *studies in CF.* In CF airway epithelial cells, LXA4 and RvD1 inhibit IL-8 synthesis by preventing IκB degradation induced by TNFα, thus resulting in NF-κB (Ringholz et al., 2018). RvD1 regulates specific genes and proteins involved in leukocyte chemotaxis and infiltration (e.g. CXCL1 [the mice IL-8]) in lung macrophages isolated from mice infected with *P. aeruginosa* (Codagnone et al., 2018; Isopi et al., 2020) (**Table 1**).

In vivo studies in *P. aeruginosa infected mice.* AT-LXA4 stable analog, reduces IL-8 levels and PMN recruitment in a murine model of short-term *P. aeruginosa* lung infection (Karp et al., 2004). RvD1 treatment also produces a significant decrease in PMN, IL-1β, and CXCL1 levels *in vivo* in the lungs of mice infected with *P. aeruginosa* (Codagnone et al., 2018) (**Table 1**).

Human studies in CF. Although, not a direct demonstration of SPMs' impact on cytokine secretion, it is worth noting that human studies reveal that the levels of pro-inflammatory cytokines (IL-6 and IL-8) are inversely correlated with LXA4 and RvD1 in the sputum of patients with CF (Chiron et al., 2008; Ringholz et al., 2014; Eickmeier et al., 2017; Isopi et al., 2020).

Infection

Many actions exerted by SPMs to limit infection have been described in non-CF cells isolated from human and mice macrophages, (Chiang et al., 2012; Colas et al., 2016; Pierdomenico et al., 2017; Codagnone et al., 2018) (**Table 3**). In addition, SPMs (PDn-3DPA, RvD1, and RvD2) stimulate macrophage differentiation from a pro-inflammatory (M1) to a pro-resolutive phenotype (M2) in non-CF models (Dalli and Serhan, 2012; Recchiuti et al., 2014; Croasdell et al., 2015; Pistorius et al., 2018) and enhance the expression of surface receptors involved in the uptake of apoptotic cells (Matte et al., 2019) (**Table 3**). RvD2 also reduces polymicrobial sepsis severity

TABLE 1 | Bioactions of SPMs demonstrated in cystic fibrosis models.

	In vitro studies			
	SPMs	**Models**	**Bioactions**	**References**
Inflammation & infection	LXA4	Human CF and non-CF bronchial epithelial cells (primary, NuLi-1 and CuFi-1) + *P. aeruginosa*	Delays *P. aeruginosa* invasion and migration	Higgins et al., 2016
	LXA4	Human CF peripheral blood human macrophages	Stimulates phagocytosis of zymosan particles and *P. aeruginosa*	Pierdomenico et al., 2017
	AT-LXA4 analog	Human primary bronchial epithelial cells + Short-term *P. aeruginosa*	Inhibits IL-8 secretion	Karp et al., 2004
	RvD1	Murine RAW-264.1 macrophage, Human peripheral blood macrophage, PMN and artery pulmonary endothelial cells + Long-term *P. aeruginosa*	Reduces *P. aeruginosa* bacterial burden Reduces PMNs infiltration by decreasing ICAM-1 expression and increasing vascular permeability	Codagnone et al., 2018
		Human primary CF alveolar macrophages Human bronchial epithelial cells (CuFi-1)	Enhances phagocytosis of *P. aeruginosa* Reduces IL-8 secretion	Ringholz et al., 2018
		Human primary CF leukocytes and epithelial cells	Increases *P. aeruginosa* phagocytosis Reduces genes and protein associated to NF-kB activation and leukocyte infiltration	Isopi et al., 2020
Ion transport & hydration	LXA4	Human CF and non-CF bronchial epithelial cells (primary and NuLi-1, CuFi-1/3/4)	Restores ASL height by increasing calcium activated Cl^- secretion and inhibiting ENaC activity	Verrière et al., 2012 Higgins et al., 2014 Al-Alawi et al., 2014
	RvD1	Human CF and non-CF bronchial epithelial cells (primary and NuLi-1 and CuFi-1)	Restores ASL height	Ringholz et al., 2018
Epithelial structure	LXA4	Human CF and non-CF bronchial epithelial cells (primary and Nu-Li and CuFi-1) + *P. aeruginosa*	Stimulates tight junction formation and ZO-1 expression and trafficking	Higgins et al., 2016
	LXA4	Human CF and non-CF bronchial epithelial cells (primary and Nu-Li and CuFi-1)	Stimulates cell proliferation, migration and wound repair in CF and non-CF cells	Buchanan et al., 2013 Higgins et al., 2014
	In vivo studies			
	SPMs	**Models**	**Bioactions**	**References**
Inflammation & infection	AT-LXA4 analog	C57BL/6 mice + Short-term *P. aeruginosa*	Reduces bacterial burden and PMN infiltration	Karp et al., 2004
	RvD1	C57Bl6/N mice + Long-term *P. aeruginosa*	Reduces *P. aeruginosa* bacterial burden Reduces PMN infiltration Reduces CCL5, CXCL10, CXCL1, IL-1β, IL-17, VEGF Reduces mucous metaplasia Increases miR-21 and miR-155(cytokine secretion) and miR-21 (pathogen recognition)	Codagnone et al., 2018
		CFTR-KO mice (FABP-CFTR)	Reduces *P. aeruginosa* bacterial burden Reduces PMN infiltration Reduces histological signs of lung pathology Increases bacterial and leukocyte clearance by macrophages Improves clinical disease score	Isopi et al., 2020
Ion transport & hydration	RvD1	Homozygous F508del-CFTR mice (FVB/N)	Restores nasal transepithelial potential difference in CF mice	Ringholz et al., 2018

in mice (Spite et al., 2009) and MaR1 and RvD3 enhance *E. coli* phagocytosis by macrophages (Colas et al., 2016) (**Table 3**).

In vitro *studies in CF model of infection.* The role of SPMs in regulating infection was also demonstrated in CF. RvD1 enhances phagocytosis of *P. aeruginosa* by human CF alveolar macrophages (Ringholz et al., 2018). LXA4 also stimulates CF bronchial epithelial cells' protective functions by delaying *P. aeruginosa* invasion and migration (Higgins et al., 2016) (**Table 1**).

In vivo *studies in CF model of infection.* During *P. aeruginosa* lung infection in mice, exogenous administration of SPMs significantly decreases bacterial load, and improves clinical outcome. An AT-LXA4 stable analog, reduces bacterial burden in a murine model of short-term *P. aeruginosa* lung infection (Karp et al., 2004). RvD1 significantly diminishes bacterial growth, mucus metaplasia and lung inflammation resulting from long term exposure of mice to *P. aeruginosa* (Codagnone et al., 2018) (**Table 1**).

Epithelial Repair

In vitro studies have shown that SPMs (LXA4, RvD1, AT-RvD1 RvD2, and RvE1) protect tissues from lung injury in numerous models including CF airway epithelium (Zhang et al., 2010; Kenchegowda et al., 2011; Kakazu et al., 2012; Odusanwo et al.,

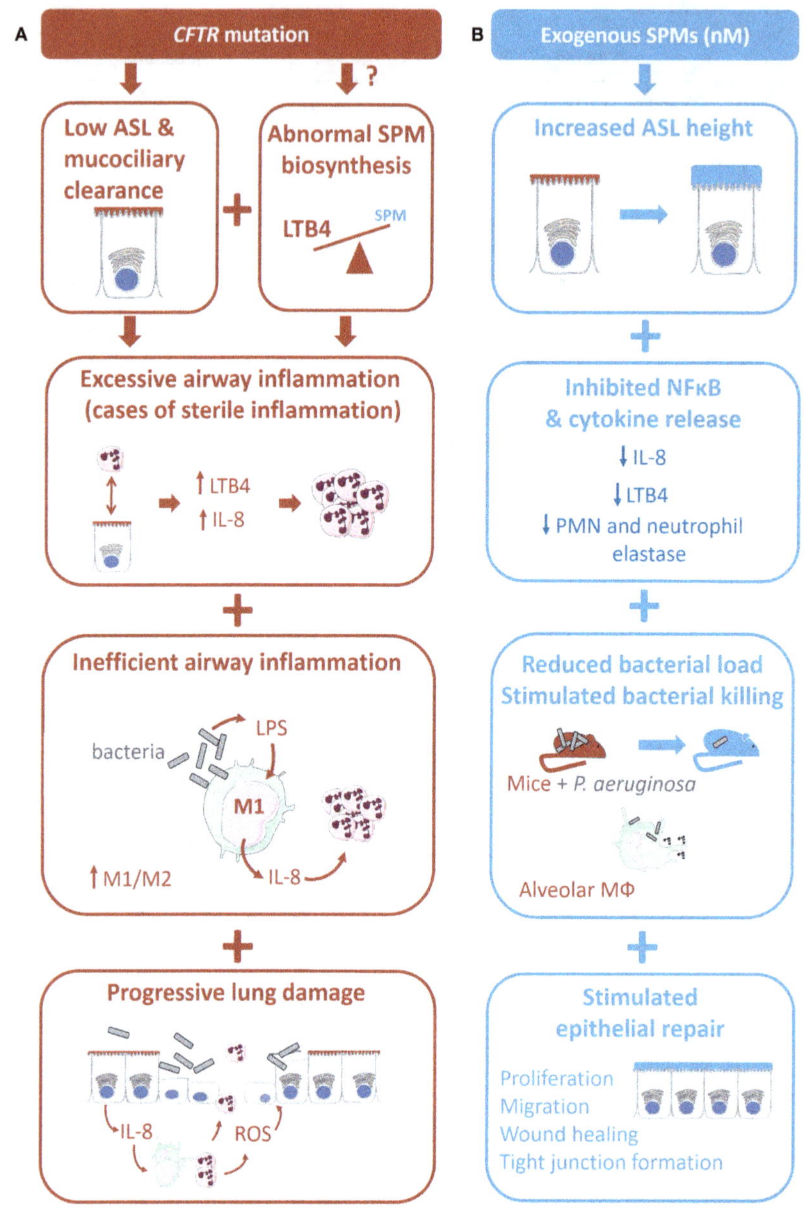

FIGURE 4 | Proposed model for CF airway disease and beneficial impact of exogenous SPM exposure. **(A)** CF is due to the CFTR gene mutation leading to a reduced airway surface liquid layer (ASL) height and abnormal SPM biosynthesis. CF is characterized by an excessive airway inflammation with high amount of PMN and release of pro-inflammatory mediators (cytokines and LTB4). Inflammation in CF is inefficient to clear bacteria due to altered differentiation from M1 proinflammatory macrophages to M2 pro-resolving. Chronic inflammation and sustained inflammation, including oxidative stress (ROS) lead to progressive lung damage and respiratory failure. **(B)** The benefit of SPMs exposure at nM concentration is reported in different models of the CF airway disease. SPMs enhance the ASL height increase in CF bronchial epithelial cells. SPM treatment inhibits IL-8 release induced by TNF in CF airway epithelial cells. SPMs reduce bacterial load in mice models of P. aeruginosa infection and stimulate phagocytosis and bacterial killing in isolated CF alveolar macrophages. SPMs enhance tight junction formation and wound healing by stimulating CF airway epithelial proliferation and migration.

2012; Buchanan et al., 2013; Higgins et al., 2014: Cheng et al., 2016; Higgins et al., 2016; Zhang et al., 2018; Zheng et al., 2018). LXA4 stimulated wound healing by enhancing cell proliferation, migration in human CF bronchial epithelial cells (Buchanan et al., 2013; Higgins et al., 2014) through stimulation of the ALX/FPR2 receptor, intracellular calcium mobilization, KATP potassium channel activation, and the mitogen-activated protein kinase ERK1/2 phosphorylation (Buchanan et al., 2013; Higgins et al., 2014). Moreover, LXA4 restores transepithelial resistance in CF airway epithelial cells by enhancing tight junction formation *via* upregulation of expression of the proteins ZO-1, occludin, claudin-1 during bacterial infection by *P. aeruginosa* (Grumbach et al., 2009; Higgins et al., 2016) (**Figure 7**) (**Table 1**). In corneal epithelium, the role of mitogen-

TABLE 2 | Bioactions of SPMs on ion transport and mucus secretion, demonstrated in non-CF models.

Ion transport and hydration				
Conditions	**SPMs**	**Models**	**Bioactions**	**References**
		***In vitro* studies**		
Other	LXA4	Human bronchial epithelial cells (primary and 16HBE14o-)	Stimulates Ca^{2+} -dependent Cl^- secretion	Bonnans et al., 2003
Acute lung injury	LXA4	Rat primary alveolar type II cells	Stimulates expression of CFTR	Yang et al., 2013
	Mar1		Stimulates expression of ENaC α, β and Na-K-ATPase α1, β1	Zhang et al., 2017
		***In vivo* studies**		
Acute lung injury	LXA4	Sprague-Dawley rat	Stimulate airway fluid clearance	Yang et al., 2013
	RvD1			Wang Q. et al., 2014
	Mar1			Zhang et al., 2017

Mucus secretion				
Conditions	**SPMs**	**Models**	**Bioactions**	**References**
		***In vitro* studies**		
Other	LXA4	Sprague-Dawley Rat primary conjunctival goblet cells	Increases glycoconjugate secretion	Hodges et al., 2017
	RvD1			Lippestad et al., 2017
	RvD2			Botten et al., 2019
	RvE1			Lippestad et al., 2017
	Mar1		Increases glycoconjugate secretion Counter-regulates histamine-induced secretion	Olsen et al., 2020
	RvD1 & RvE1	Sprague-Dawley Rat and Human primary conjunctival goblet cells	Inhibits leukotriene-induced glycoconjugate secretion	Dartt et al., 2011
	RvD1 & AT-RvD1		Counter-regulates histamine-induced secretion	Li et al., 2013
		***In vivo* studies**		
Asthma	RvE1	BALB/c mice	Lowers mucus score	Aoki et al., 2008

activated protein kinase has also been reported to mediate the epithelial repair induced SPMs. The serine/threonine kinase Akt and NrF2 signaling pathways have been described in mediating the response to SPMs in corneal and other epithelial models (Zhang et al., 2010; Kenchegowda et al., 2011; Odusanwo et al., 2012; Wang L. et al., 2014; Posso et al., 2018; Zhang et al., 2018) (**Table 4**).

OTHER POSSIBLE IMPACTS OF SPMs ON ALTERED AIRWAY FUNCTIONS IN CF

Although not demonstrated in CF, the role of SPMs on airway functions altered in CF but demonstrated in other disease models can be pointed out (**Tables 2–5**).

Oxidative Stress

Antibiotics, despite their beneficial action on pulmonary function during acute infections, do not treat oxidative stress (Wood et al., 2002). Although not demonstrated in CF, SPMs have been found to help reduce oxidative stress by restoring oxidant/antioxidant balance through the nuclear erythroid 2-related transcription factor 2 (Nrf2) pathway, which is defective in CF (Posso et al., 2018; Zhang et al., 2018). In the murine model of cigarette smoke- and LPS-induced lung injury, or type 1-diabetes, RvD1 reduces ROS levels and increases antioxidant defense (Wang L. et al., 2014; Posso et al., 2018; Zhang et al., 2018). In corneal epithelium of type 1-diabetic mice, RvD1 increases the amount of the antioxidant GSH (Zhang et al., 2018). *In vitro*, following induced-efferocytosis, RvD1 inactivates NOX in murine macrophages (Lee and Surh, 2013). In human macrophages and bronchial epithelial cells undergoing cigarette-induced oxidative stress, RvD1 and RvD2 decrease protein oxidation (Croasdell et al., 2015) and decrease extracellular H_2O_2 production (Jiajia et al., 2014) (**Table 4**).

Mucus Secretion

Recent studies reveal the impact of SPMs on mucus secretion. Although not studied in CF, RvD1, LXA4, and Mar1 mediated an increase in glycoconjugate and mucin secretion in conjunctival cells (Hodges et al., 2017; Lippestad et al., 2017; Olsen et al., 2020). However, Mar1, RvD1, RvE1, and AT-RvD1 are able to block conjunctival goblet cell secretion when triggered by histamine or leukotriene (Dartt et al., 2011; Li et al., 2013; Olsen et al., 2020). In asthma, RvE1 reduced mucus score (Aoki et al., 2008) and RvD1 lowered mucous metaplasia in infected mice (Codagnone et al., 2018) (**Table 2**).

Regulation of MicroRNA

The microRNA signature of resolution of inflammation has recently started to be reported. Studies at basal state or during

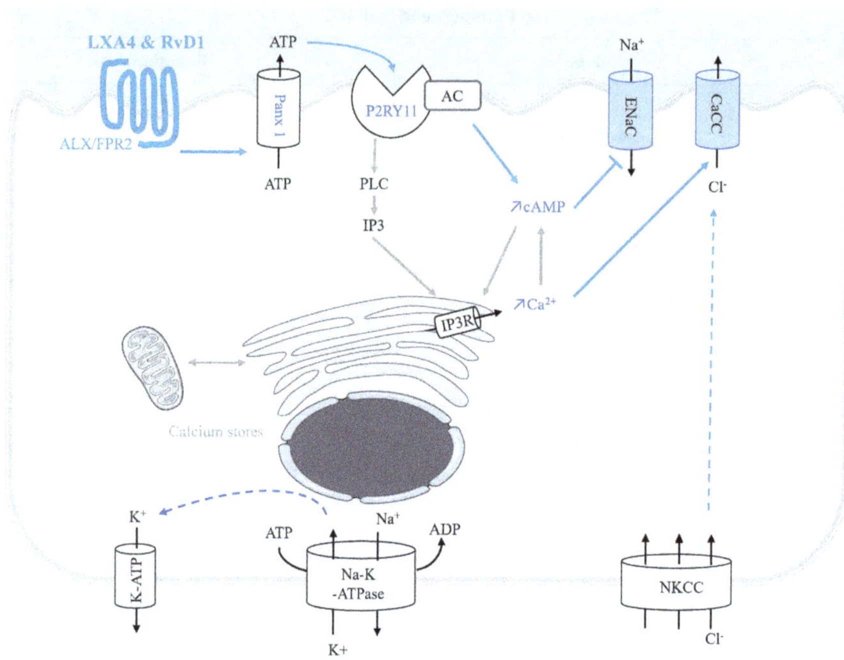

FIGURE 5 | Model of ion transport regulation by LXA4 and RvD1 enabling the restoration of ASL height in CF human bronchial epithelial cells. LXA4 and RvD1 induce a calcium-dependent airway surface liquid (ASL) layer height increase in human CF bronchial epithelial cell lines and primary cultures (Bonnans et al., 2003; Al-Alawi et al., 2014; Higgins et al., 2014; Ringholz et al., 2018; Philippe and Urbach, 2018). This effect involves binding to the FPR2 receptor, stimulation of an ATP secretion into the airway lumen via pannexin 1 channels (Panx1), and subsequent activation of P2Yx purino-receptors, including P2Y11 which leads to a rise in both intracellular cAMP and calcium mobilization by stimulation of adenylate cyclase (AC) activity and inositol 3 phosphate (IP3) signaling pathway. Intracellular calcium and cAMP increases induce stimulation of calcium-activated chloride channel and inhibition of ENaC channel inhibition.

inflammation in mice and human leukocytes have revealed the capacity of resolvins (RvD1/D2, RvD1 stable analog, PD1 and RvE1) to regulate miRNAs that influence NF-κB activity and cytokine production (miR21, miR146b, miR208a, miR155), endothelial integrity (miR-126), leukotriene production (miR219), and pathogen recognition (miR21) (Recchiuti et al., 2011; Fredman et al., 2012; Codagnone et al., 2017; Codagnone et al., 2018). LXA4 also attenuates renal fibrosis by inducing let-7c (Brennan et al., 2013). Furthermore, miR-181b which is overexpressed in CF macrophages and airway epithelial cells, down-regulates the expression of the FPR2 receptor and the pro-resolution signaling pathways (Pierdomenico et al., 2015; Pierdomenico et al., 2017) (**Table 5**).

Adaptative Immunity

SPMs might also play a role in the mediation of the adaptive response. RvD1, RvD2, and Mar1 modulate adaptive immune responses in human peripheral blood lymphocytes. These SPMs prevent naïve $CD4^+$ T cell differentiation into T_H1 and T_H17 in a mechanism mediated by the GPR32 and the FPR2 receptors (Chiurchiù et al., 2016). This role of SPMs in adaptive immunity might be of interest for CF. Indeed, some reports suggested T lymphocytes and activated eosinophils in airway mucosa in CF (Azzawi et al., 2012) and intrinsic impairment of T cell differentiation may contribute to the greater severity and more rapid progression of CF lung disease (Kushwah et al., 2014).

CF AIRWAY DISEASE TREATMENTS AND INFLAMMATION

Antibiotics

Until recently, antibiotics have been the only therapeutic agents that could be used to treat airways inflammation in CF. Antibiotics can work in synergy with the host immunity to kill bacteria with great efficiency. Antibiotics influence immune responses in various ways beyond merely eliminating the source of inflammation, depending on how they are used and how effective they are. Indeed, antibiotics that induce bacteria lysis can lead to the release of highly inflammatory molecules, pathogen-associated molecular patterns (PAMPs), such as lipopolysaccharide (LPS) and therefore augment inflammation (Raetz and Whitfield, 2002).

In contrast, some antibiotics have shown immunomodulatory properties (Ruh et al., 2017) such as macrolides which suppress inflammatory cytokines (Hoyt and Robbins, 2001; Amsden, 2005). Azithromycin has been particularly studied in CF and is routinely used for its immunomodulating effects, having shown to reduce exacerbation frequency and slightly improve lung function when taken continuously (Bush and Rubin, 2003; Southern and Barker, 2004; Olveira et al., 2017). Of interest, while PMN counts and IL-8 levels decrease in CF patients' sputum after antibiotic therapy, LXA4 levels significantly increase and are inversely correlated with IL-8 levels (Chiron et al., 2008).

TABLE 3 | Bioactions of SPMs on cytokine secretion and leukocytes activity, demonstrated in non-CF models.

Cytokines synthesis /Leukocytes activity				
Conditions	**SPMs**	**Models**	**Bioactions**	**References**
		***In vitro* studies**		
TNF-α treatment	LXA4	Human umbilical vein endothelial cells	Up-regulates miR-126-5p (related to endothelial repair and VCAM-1 expression)	Codagnone et al., 2017
	LXA4 and AT-LXA4 analog	Human peripheral blood PMNs	Inhibit TNF-α-initiated neutrophil migration, superoxide generation and IL-1β release	Hachicha et al., 1999
TGF-β1-induced fibrosis	LXA4	Human renal epithelial HK-2 cell line Human mesangial cells Rat renal fibroblast cells (NRK49F)	Up-regulates miR let-7c (reduces renal fibrosis) in human cells Decreases miR let-7c level in rat cells	Brennan et al., 2013
Intestinal *Salmonella Typhimurium*	LXA4 analog	Human intestinal epithelium T84 cell line	Inhibits IL-8 secretion	Gewirtz et al., 1998
Airway *P. aeruginosa*	AT-LXA4 analog	Human primary bronchial epithelial cells	Inhibits IL-8 secretion	Karp et al., 2004
Chemoattractant	LXA4	Human peripheral blood PMNs	Inhibits LTB4/FMLP-induced PMN chemotaxis and migration	Lee et al., 1989
	LXA4, LXB4	Human peripheral blood PMNs, HUVEC	Inhibit LTB4-induced PMN adhesion to endothelial cells and migration across endothelial cell monolayers	Papayianni et al., 1996
	LXA4 analog	Human peripheral blood PMNs, HL-60 cells, HUVEC	Inhibit PMN transendothelial migration and endothelial adhesion	Serhan et al., 1995
	RvD1, AT-RvD1	Human peripheral blood PMNs and microvascular endothelial cells (HMEC-1)	Inhibit PMN transendothelial migration	Sun et al., 2007
	RvE3	Human peripheral blood PMNs	Inhibits PMN chemotaxis	Isobe et al., 2012
Acid lung injury	LXA4	Human bronchial epithelial (HBE) and type II alveolar (A549) cell lines	Inhibits IL-6 release and PMN transendothelial migration	Bonnans et al., 2006
Asthma	LXA4, LXB4	Human asthmatic peripheral blood mononuclear cells	Inhibit IL-8 release	Bonnans et al., 2002
Cigarette smoke	RvD1, RvD2	Human peripheral blood monocytes and alveolar macrophages	Decrease release of pro-inflammatory cytokines (IL-6, IL-8 and TNF-α) and increase release of IL-10 and TGF-β Stimulate phagocytosis and M2 state Decrease levels of protein carbonylation after 24h	Croasdell et al., 2015
	RvE1	Murine macrophage RAW264.7cell line	Stimulates phagocytic activity and reduces cell death	Takamiya et al., 2012
	RvD1	Human bronchial epithelial 16HBE cell line	Reduces IL8 synthesis	Jiajia et al., 2014
	AT-RvD1	Human THP1 macrophages and alveolar epithelial A549 cell lines	Reduces IL-1β secretion in macrophages and IL-6 and IL-8 secretion in alveolar cells	Cox et al., 2015
Polyinosinic-polycytidylic acid	RvD1	Human primary lung epithelial cells	Inhibits IL-6 and IL-8 release	Hsiao et al., 2014
Microbial sepsis	RvD2 analog	Human primary PMNs and HUVEC	Stimulates NO production in HUVEC Reduces L-selectin and CD-18 surface expression Stimulates phagocytosis of *E. Coli* Increases intracellular ROS	Spite et al., 2009
E. Coli	RvD1 analog, RvD5 analog, PD1	Human peripheral blood monocyte and PMN	Increase phagocytosis of *E. Coli* (RvD1,RvD5, PD1) Regulate inflammatory genes (RvD1, RvD5)	Chiang et al., 2012
	Mar1, 22-OH-MaR1, 14-oxo-MaR1	Human primary peripheral blood macrophages	Increase macrophage phagocytosis	Colas et al., 2016
PMA/Ionomycin	RvD1, RvD2, AT-RvD3 MaR1	Human peripheral blood CD8+ and CD4+ T cells	Inhibit TNF-α, IFN-γ, IL-2 production Favor CD+4 T cells differentiation into regulatory T cells Inhibit naive CD+4 T cells differentiation into TH1 and TH17 cells	Chiurchiù et al., 2016

(Continued)

TABLE 3 | Continued

Cytokines synthesis /Leukocytes activity				
Conditions	**SPMs**	**Models**	**Bioactions**	**References**
Other	RvE1, RvD1, RVD2, PD1	Human peripheral blood mononuclear cells	RvD1 regulates miR-146b, miR-21, miR-208 and miR-219-5p RvE1 regulates miR-219-5p and miR-21 but not miR146b RvD2 and PD1 regulate miR-146b and miR-21 but not miR-219-5p	Fredman et al., 2012
	PDn-3 DPA	Human peripheral blood macrophages	Regulates monocyte-to-macrophage differentiation	Pistorius et al., 2018
Sickle-cell disease (SCD)	AT-RvD1 and RvD1	Human endothelial cell line, human SCD blood PMN and erythrocytes	Inhibit neutrophil recruitment Stimulate erythrocytes and PMN efferocytosis	Matte et al., 2019
		***In vivo* studies**		
TNF-α	LXA4 and AT-LXA4 analog	BALB/c mice	Inhibit leukocyte infiltration	Hachicha et al., 1999
Chronic renal fibrosis	LXA4	Male wistar rats	Up-regulates miR let-7c (reduces renal fibrosis)	Brennan et al., 2013
LPS-induced lung injury	LXA4, RvD1	Male Sprague-Dawley rats (BAL)	Reduce TNF-α, IL-6 and IL-1β secretion Increase IL-10 secretion	Wang Q. et al., 2014, Yang et al., 2013
Acute peritonitis	RvD1, AT-RvD1	Male FVB mice	Reduce leukocyte infiltration	Sun et al., 2007
	RvD1	C57Bl/6N mice	Reduces leukocytes infiltration Stimulates M2 differentiation and activity Regulates corresponding genes	Recchiuti et al., 2014
	RvD1 analog	Male FVB mice	Temporally controls miRNAs: at 12h, increases miR21 and miR146b, decreases miR208a (NF-kB signaling) and miR219 (LTB4 production)	Recchiuti et al., 2011
	RvE3	Male FVB mice	Inhibits PMN infiltration	Isobe et al., 2012
Asthma	RvE1	Female BALB/c mice	Lowers mucus score	Aoki et al., 2008
Microbial sepsis	RvD2 analog	Male FVB mice, eNOS-/- & wild type (C57BL/6J) mice	Reduces neutrophils recruitment, leukocyte-endothelial interactions (NO-dependent) Reduces local and systemic bacterial burden Increases peritoneal mononuclear cells Increases survival Reduces IL-6, IL-1β, IL-23, TNF-α	Spite et al., 2009
Peritoneal *E. Coli* & Skin *S. aureus*	RvD1 analog, RvD5 analog, PD1	Male FVB mice, C57BL/6J male mice	Reduces bacterial burden in blood and exudates (RvD1, RvD5) Increase survival (RvD1, RvD5) Amplify antimicrobial response of ciprofloxacin Increase clearance of *S. aureus* with vancomycin Reduce IL-1β, IL-6 and increase IL-10 secretion (RvD1) Reduce KC and TNF-α secretion (RvD5)	Chiang et al., 2012
Peritoneal *E. Coli*	PDn-3 DPA	Male C57Bl/6N mice	Increases macrophages' efferocytosis and bacterial phagocytosis	Pistorius et al., 2018
Sickle-cell disease (SCD)	AT-RvD1	SCD and healthy ($Hba^{tm1(HBA)Tow}$ $Hbb^{tm3(HBG1, HBB)Tow}$) mice	Reduces neutrophils adhesion & transmigration Reduces lung and kidney injury Reduces proinflammatory cytokine	Matte et al., 2019

However, despite its beneficial effects in CF patients, said effects are marginal, especially when taking into account the list of oral treatments patients already contend with on a daily basis, without mentioning the long half-life of this antibiotic and the potential risk of selecting resistant bacteria strains and altering microbiota.

CFTR Modulators

High-throughput screening has allowed to identify small molecules, such as lumacaftor (VX809) tezacaftor (VX661), and elexacaftor (VX-445) to modulate processing and trafficking of CFTR (CFTR correctors) and ivacaftor (VX770) to potentiate its activity as a chloride channel (CFTR potentiator) providing the first drugs to specifically target the CFTR protein defect. Associations of these molecules, the first ones being currently prescribed in routine since the mid-2010s, restore chloride transport and normalizing sweat test results (Lopes-Pacheco, 2019). Beside their main action on epithelial chloride transport and encouraging results on disease progression, their impact on inflammatory cytokine production are controversial and their long term immunomodulatory effects are still discussed (Jarosz-Griffiths et al., 2020; Volkova et al., 2020).

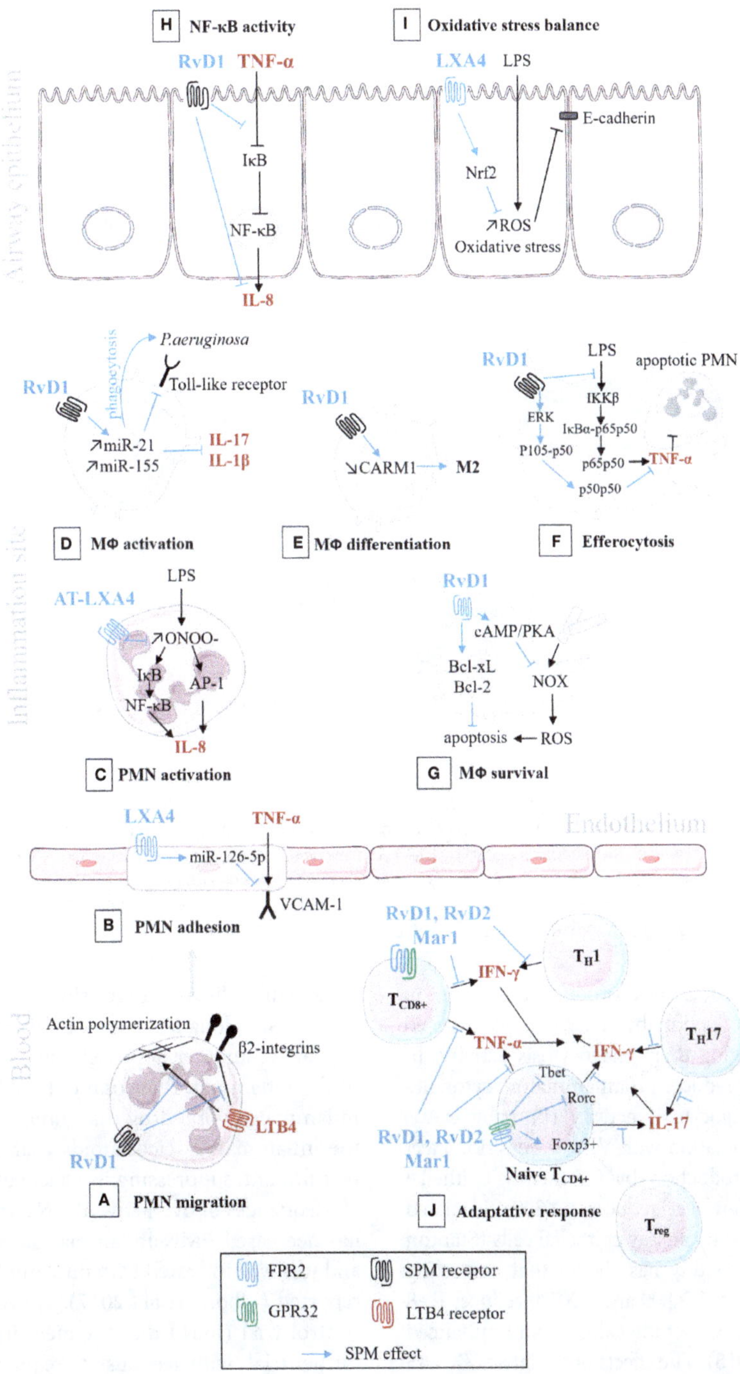

FIGURE 6 | Schematic illustration of SPMs cellular pathways involved in the resolution of inflammation/infection. In black: pro-inflammatory pathways; In blue: bioactions of SPM. **(A)** RvD1 analog down-regulates the migration of PMNs isolated from human peripheral blood, by decreasing actin polymerization, and blocking LTB4-regulated adhesion molecules, 2 integrins. (Krishnamoorthy et al., 2010); **(B)** LXA4 down-regulates VCAM-1 receptor and PMN adhesion to human endothelial cells (Codagnone et al., 2017); **(C)** AT-LXA4 (15-epi-LXA4) down-regulates IL-8 synthesis and secretion, in human PMNs isolated from venous blood (Jozsef et al., 2002); **(D)** RvD1 down-regulates toll-like receptor (TLR), cytokines synthesis and enhances phagocytosis of murine lung macrophage (Codagnone et al., 2018); and enhances phagocytosis and bacterial killing in human CF alveolar macrophage (Ringholz et al., 2018); **(E)** RvD1 stimulates murine macrophage differentiation from M1 to M2 state (Recchiuti et al., 2014); **(F)** RvD1 stimulates efferocytosis of apoptotic PMNs, through the regulation of NF-κB pathways, in murine macrophage (Lee et al., 2013); **(G)** RvD1 inhibits ROS production and increases murine macrophage survival after efferocytosis (Lee and Surh, 2013); **(H)** RvD1 inhibits cytokines secretion by preventing IκB degradation in CF human airway epithelial cell (Ringholz et al., 2018); **(I)** LXA4 inhibits oxidative stress and protects E-cadherin, in human airway epithelial cell (Cheng et al., 2016); **(J)** RvD1, RvD2, and Mar1 regulate the adaptive response, enhance the differentiation to T_{reg} rather than T_H1 and T_H17, in human peripheral blood lymphocytes (Chiurchiù et al., 2016).

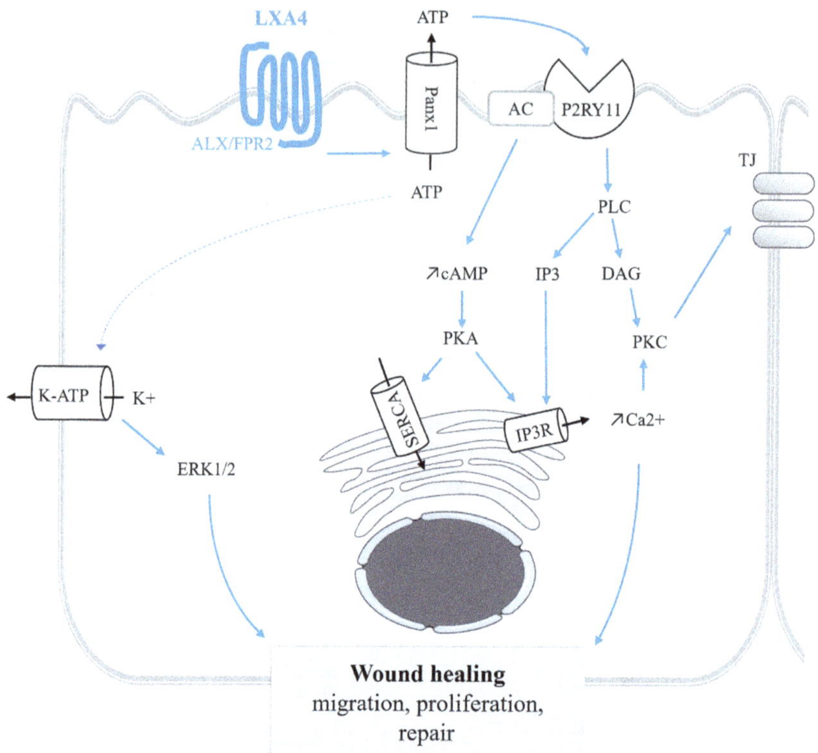

FIGURE 7 | Epithelial repair mediated by LXA4 in bronchial epithelium. LXA4 stimulates wound healing by enhancing cell proliferation, migration of human CF bronchial epithelial cells. This mechanism is mediated by the FPR2 receptor, an apical ATP release and the subsequent stimulation of P2Yx receptors leading to intracellular calcium mobilization. The CF airway epithelial repair induced by LXA4 also involves ERK1/2 phosphorylation and KATP channel stimulation (Buchanan et al., 2013; Higgins et al., 2014). LXA4 maintains airway epithelial structure by stimulating tight junction (TJ) proteins synthesis and trafficking to the apical membrane leading to an increase of transepithelial electrical resistance (Grumbach et al., 2009). SPMs stimulation of the ERK pathway has also been demonstrated in corneal epithelial repair (Xu et al., 2009; Zhang et al., 2010; Kenchegowda et al., 2011; Zhang et al., 2018).

Indeed, the corrector VX809 does not produce an effect on proinflammatory cytokines production by macrophages exposed to *P. aeruginosa* while stimulating their phagocytosis activity. In contrast, the potentiator VX770 reduces proinflammatory cytokines but inhibits macrophages' phagocytosis activity (Barnaby et al., 2018). VX809 alone or in combination with VX770 does not affect pro-inflammatory cytokines production by CF airway epithelial cells. *P. aeruginosa* exposure however reduces VX809-stimulated F508del-CFTR chloride secretion by airway epithelial cells (Stanton et al., 2015). However, another study has shown that correcting CFTR activity by a combination of VX809 and VX770 reduces IL-8 production by CF (F508del) airway epithelial cells and enhanced epithelial repair (Ruffin et al., 2018). The effects of the latest VX-445 on inflammation have yet to be assessed. Although these small molecules have considerably changed the quality of life for many patients, not all CF genotypes can benefit from such therapy. Moreover, the clinical response within an identical genotype is variable and lung function still declines over time when bronchiectasis is established.

Novel Anti-Inflammatory Molecules

To combat inflammation, non-steroid anti-inflammatory drugs (NSAID) have been studied; especially Ibuprofen, which seems to slow lung disease progression (Lands and Stanojevic, 2013) but at the cost of long term usage at high doses and the entailing risks.

Taking another approach and directly targeting biosynthesis of the inflammatory eicosanoid LTB4, acebilustat is a new anti-inflammatory oral drug that inhibits LTA4H. As LTB4 is one of the inflammatory eicosanoids that initiate and amplify PMNs' recruitment, suppressing its effect could diminish the pulmonary consequences of overactive PMNs. In a phase I study, acebilustat has decreased PMN inflammation biomarkers levels in sputum and was well tolerated with only mild to moderate adverse events reported (Elborn et al., 2017). However, a phase II randomized control trial (RCT) did not meet its primary endpoint and no further trials with acebilustat are planned (Elborn et al., 2018). In addition, these anti-inflammatory molecules clearly have a different mechanism of action than immuno-resolvents.

Lenabasum, formerly called JBT-101, is another oral drug under investigation for autoimmune diseases and CF. A first phase II trial conducted with 83 patients has established the safety and tolerance of this drug in CF patients. Another phase II multi-center RCT is ongoing for CF patients with pulmonary exacerbations as the primary outcome. Lenabasum is an endocannabinoid-mimetic that selectively binds to cannabinoid receptor 2 expressed by immune cells, reducing alveolar macrophage secretion of IL-6 and

TABLE 4 | Bioactions of SPMs on epithelial repair and oxidative stress, demonstrated in non-CF models.

Epithelial repair/Oxidative stress				
Conditions	**SPMs**	**Models**	**Bioactions**	**References**
		***In vitro* studies**		
Corneal injury	LXA4	Rabbit corneal epithelial cells	Increases cell proliferation and migration	Kenchegowda et al., 2011
	RvE1	Human corneal epithelial cell line	Stimulates migration	Zhang et al., 2010
Acute lung injury	LXA4	Human bronchial epithelial 16HBE cell line	Protects airway epithelial through inhibition of LPS-induced ROS production. Preserves E-cadherin expression	Cheng et al., 2016
	RvD1	Human primary alveolar type II epithelial cell Human primary lung fibroblast	Enhances cell wound repair and proliferation, differentiation. Reduces apoptosis. Inhibits TGF-Beta-induced epithelial-mesenchymal transition. Inhibits fibroproliferation and myofibroblast differentiation of human lung fibroblasts	Zheng et al., 2018
TNF-α treatment	RvD1	Rat parotid Par-C10 cell line	Inhibits tight junction and cytoskeletal disruption Stimulates cell migration and polarity	Odusanwo et al., 2012
Cigarette smoke	RvD1, RvD2	Human primary peripheral blood monocytes and macrophages, and alveolar macrophages	Decrease levels of protein carbonylation after 24h	Croasdell et al., 2015
	RvD1	Human bronchial epithelial 16HBE cell line	Reduces the production of extracellular H2O2	Jiajia et al., 2014
	AT-RvD1	Male C57BL/6 mice (lung)	Reduces oxidative stress markers and ROS in BAL Restores elastic fibers Reduces alveolar enlargement	Posso et al., 2018
Microbial sepsis	RvD2 analog	Primary human PMNs; primary human umbilical vein endothelial cell *(HUVEC)*	Inhibits extracellular superoxide generation	Spite et al., 2009
Other	LXA4	Human bronchial epithelial 16HBE14o- cell line	Stimulates formation of tight junction through ZO-1, occludin, claudin-1 expression	Grumbach et al., 2009
	RvD1	Murine macrophages RAW264.7 cell line	Inactivates NADPH oxidase (NOX). Increases anti-apoptotic proteins	Lee and Surh, 2013
		***In vivo* studies**		
Corneal injury	LXA4	C57BL/6 mice	Reduces surface area of injury	Kakazu et al., 2012
	RvD1	Diabetic C57BL/6 mice	Stimulates regeneration of the corneal epithelium Diminishes ROS accumulation by increasing GSH synthesis and decreasing NOX expression	Zhang et al., 2018
Acute lung injury	LXA4	BALB/c mice	Protects airway epithelial through inhibition of LPS-induced ROS production. Preserves E-cadherin expression	Cheng et al., 2016
	RvD1		Reduces production of lipid peroxidation malondialdehyde. Increases expression of SOD and HO-1 mRNA	Wang Q. et al., 2014

TNFα in preclinical studies (Ribeiro et al., 2017). Those immunomodulatory effects can be explained by lenabasum's potential to induce SPMs production in animal models (Zurier et al., 2009) and healthy human subjects (Motwani et al., 2018a). This last example showcases how treating chronic inflammation by mobilizing the body's endogenous pro-resolving system rather than trying to stop one of the many triggers of an established and thriving inflammatory process may be the most inclusive and efficient way to treat inflammatory diseases in the future.

CONCLUSION

Nearly 30 years after the discovery of the CFTR gene, many aspects of the pathophysiology of CF remain unclear. The combination of advanced knowledge in the field of the regulation of innate immunity and the current description of CF airway disease revealed novel cellular and molecular mechanisms involved in the abnormal resolution of inflammation in CF. This review highlighted evidence for a role of SPMs to overcome the absence of functional CFTR by stimulating chloride secretion through calcium-dependent channels, while limiting unwanted persistence of inflammation, infection, and tissue damage, and accelerating the return to homeostasis by acting on multiple cells and molecular targets (**Figure 4**).

Even in the age of CFTR modulators, anti-inflammatory therapy remains an area of intense research in CF. The therapeutic use of SPMs might constitute a promising avenue to treat chronic inflammation and infection in all CF patients. However, the therapeutic use of SPMs is greatly limited by their rapid metabolic

TABLE 5 | Bioactions of SPMs on micro-RNA regulation, demonstrated in non-CF models.

micro-RNA				
Conditions	**SPMs**	**Models**	**Bioactions**	**References**
		***In vitro* studies**		
TNF-α treatment	LXA4	Human umbilical vein endothelial cells	Up-regulates miR-126-5p (related to endothelial repair and VCAM-1 expression)	Codagnone et al., 2017
TGF-β-induced fibrosis	LXA4	Human renal epithelial HK-2 cells Human mesangial cells Rat renal NRK49F fibroblasts	Up-regulates miR let-7c and reduces human renal fibrosis Decreases miR let-7c level in rat fibroblasts	Brennan et al., 2013
Other	RvD1 RvE1 RVD2 & PD1	Human peripheral blood mononuclear cells	Regulates miR-146b, miR-21, miR-208 and miR-219-5p Regulates miR-219-5p and miR-21 but not miR146b Regulate miR-146b and miR-21 but not miR-219-5p	Fredman et al., 2012
		***In vivo* studies**		
Chronic renal fibrosis	LXA4	Male wistar rats	Up-regulates miR let-7c and reduces renal fibrosis	Brennan et al., 2013
Acute peritonitis	RvD1 analog	Male FVB mice	Temporally controls miRNAs, increases miR21 and miR146b, decreases miR208a (NF-kB signaling) and miR219 (LTB4 production)	Recchiuti et al., 2011

inactivation before they can reach the site of inflammation. An RvE1 stable analog for dry eye inflammation (NCT00799552), ocular inflammation and pain in cataract surgery (NCT02329743), and allergic conjunctivitis (NCT01639846), and a LXA4 stable analog for periodontal inflammation (NCT0234269) are under clinical trials. The use of SPMs stable analog incorporated in nanoparticles also provides a new possibility for local delivery at the site of inflammation (Van Dyke et al., 2015; Lance et al., 2017). Although promising results have been obtained in animal studies, the efficacy of this experimental data must be established in human clinical trials. Indeed, using analogs with a much longer half-life than native SPMs does raise the question of the potential adverse effects. Long-term exposure to stable SPM analogs with prolonged and enhanced activity might prevent the initiation of further inflammatory responses. Another approach would be to understand more precisely the mechanism by which CFTR dysfunction is related to an abnormal SPMs biosynthesis and potentially reveal new therapeutic targets to treat a wide range of CF mutations. Furthermore, the presentation of CF is very heterogeneous in terms of severity and response to actual treatments; therefore, exploring the correlation at the individual level between SPMs biosynthesis, CF genotype, and the severity of the airway disease could lead to new diagnostic and therapeutic tools as personalized care.

AUTHOR CONTRIBUTIONS

MB wrote the first draft on the impact of SPMs on airway functions altered in CF. MS wrote the first draft of the abnormal lipid metabolism and SPMs biosynthesis in CF. All authors contributed to the article and approved the submitted version.

ACKNOWLEDGMENTS

We thank the Institut National de la Santé Et de la Recherche Médicale (INSERM), the French CF patients association (Vaincre la Mucoviscidose, RF20190502472), the Chancellerie des Universités de Paris (Legs Poix 2020), the Institut Mondor de Recherche Biomédicale (AO inter équipes 2020), the Agence Régionale de Santé Normandie which currently support the authors activity on the role of SPMs in Cystic Fibrosis.

REFERENCES

Adam, D., Bilodeau, C., Sognigbé, L., Maillé, É., Ruffin, M., and Brochiero, E. (2018). CFTR rescue with VX-809 and VX-770 favors the repair of primary airway epithelial cell cultures from patients with class II mutations in the presence of Pseudomonas aeruginosa exoproducts. *J. Cyst. Fibros.* 17, 705–714. doi: 10.1016/j.jcf.2018.03.010

Al-Alawi, M., Buchanan, P., Verriere, V., Higgins, G., McCabe, O., Costello, R. W., et al. (2014). Physiological levels of lipoxin A4 inhibit ENaC and restore airway surface liquid height in cystic fibrosis bronchial epithelium. *Physiol. Rep.* 2, e12093. doi: 10.14814/phy2.12093

Al-Turkmani, M. R., Freedman, S. D., and Laposata, M. (2007). Fatty acid alterations and n-3 fatty acid supplementation in cystic fibrosis. *Prostaglandins Leukot. Essent. Fatty Acids* 77, 309–318. doi: 10.1016/j.plefa.2007.10.009

Amsden, G. W. (2005). Anti-inflammatory effects of macrolides–an underappreciated benefit in the treatment of community-acquired respiratory tract infections and chronic inflammatory pulmonary conditions? *J. Antimicrob. Chemother.* 55, 10–21. doi: 10.1093/jac/dkh519

Anderson, M. P., Gregory, R. J., Thompson, S., Souza, D. W., Paul, S., Mulligan, R. C., et al. (1991). Demonstration that CFTR is a chloride channel by alteration of its anion selectivity. *Science* 253, 202–205. doi: 10.1126/science.1712984

Antigny, F., Norez, C., Becq, F., and Vandebrouck, C. (2008a). Calcium homeostasis is abnormal in cystic fibrosis airway epithelial cells but is normalized after rescue of F508del-CFTR. *Cell Calcium* 43, 175–183. doi: 10.1016/j.ceca.2007.05.002

Antigny, F., Norez, C., Cantereau, A., Becq, F., and Vandebrouck, C. (2008b). Abnormal spatial diffusion of Ca2+ in F508del-CFTR airway epithelial cells. *Respir. Res.* 9, 70. doi: 10.1186/1465-9921-9-70

Antigny, F., Girardin, N., Raveau, D., Frieden, M., Becq, F., and Vandebrouck, C. (2009). Dysfunction of mitochondria Ca2+ uptake in cystic fibrosis airway epithelial cells. *Mitochondrion* 9, 232–241. doi: 10.1016/j.mito.2009.02.003

Antigny, F., Norez, C., Dannhoffer, L., Bertrand, J., Raveau, D., Corbi, P., et al. (2011). Transient Receptor Potential Canonical Channel 6 Links Ca2+ Mishandling to Cystic Fibrosis Transmembrane Conductance Regulator Channel Dysfunction in Cystic Fibrosis. *Am. J. Respir. Cell Mol. Biol.* 44, 83–90. doi: 10.1165/rcmb.2009-0347OC

Aoki, H., Hisada, T., Ishizuka, T., Utsugi, M., Kawata, T., Shimizu, Y., et al. (2008). Resolvin E1 dampens airway inflammation and hyperresponsiveness in a murine model of asthma. *Biochem. Biophys. Res. Commun.* 367, 509–515. doi: 10.1016/j.bbrc.2008.01.012

Arita, M., Oh, S. F., Chonan, T., Hong, S., Elangovan, S., Sun, Y. P., et al. (2006). Metabolic inactivation of resolvin E1 and stabilization of its anti-inflammatory actions. *J. Biol. Chem.* 281, 22847–22854. doi: 10.1074/jbc.M603766200

Armstrong, D. S., Grimwood, K., Carlin, J. B., Carzino, R., Gutièrrez, J. P., Hull, J., et al. (1997). Lower airway inflammation in infants and young children with cystic fibrosis. *Am. J. Respir. Crit. Care Med.* 156, 1197–1204. doi: 10.1164/ajrccm.156.4.96-11058

Atlante, A., Favia, M., Bobba, A., Guerra, L., Casavola, V., and Reshkin, S. J. (2016). Characterization of mitochondrial function in cells with impaired cystic fibrosis transmembrane conductance regulator (CFTR) function. *J. Bioenerg. Biomembr.* 48, 197–210. doi: 10.1007/s10863-016-9663-y

Azzawi, M., Johnston, P. W., Majumdar, S., Kay, A. B., and Jeffery, P. K. (2012). T Lymphocytes and Activated Eosinophils in Airway Mucosa in Fatal Asthma and Cystic Fibrosis. *Am. Rev. Respir. Dis.* 145 (6), 1477–1482. doi: 10.1164/ajrccm/145.6.1477

Balázs, A., and Mall, M. A. (2019). Mucus obstruction and inflammation in early cystic fibrosis lung disease: Emerging role of the IL-1 signaling pathway. *Pediatr. Pulmonol.* 54(Suppl 3), S5–S12. doi: 10.1002/ppul.24462

Balghi, H., Robert, R., Rappaz, B., Zhang, X., Wohlhuter-Haddad, A., Evagelidis, A., et al. (2011). Enhanced Ca2+ entry due to Orai1 plasma membrane insertion increases IL-8 secretion by cystic fibrosis airways. *FASEB J.* 25, 4274–4291. doi: 10.1096/fj.11-187682

Ballard, S. T., Trout, L., Mehta, A., and Inglis, S. K. (2002). Liquid secretion inhibitors reduce mucociliary transport in glandular airways. *Am. J. Physiol.-Lung Cell. Mol. Physiol.* 283, L329–L335. doi: 10.1152/ajplung.00277.2001

Balode, L., Strazda, G., Jurka, N., Kopeika, U., Kislina, A., Bukovskis, M., et al. (2012). Lipoxygenase-derived arachidonic acid metabolites in chronic obstructive pulmonary disease. *Medicina (Kaunas)* 48 (6), 292–298.

Balough, K., McCubbin, M., Weinberger, M., Smits, W., Ahrens, R., and Fick, R. (1995). The relationship between infection and inflammation in the early stages of lung disease from cystic fibrosis. *Pediatr. Pulmonol* 20, 63–70. doi: 10.1002/ppul.1950200203

Bang, S., Xie, Y.-K., Zhang, Z.-J., Wang, Z., Xu, Z.-Z., and Ji, R.-R. (2018). GPR37 regulates macrophage phagocytosis and resolution of inflammatory pain. *J. Clin. Invest.* 128, 3568–3582. doi: 10.1172/JCI99888

Bangel, N., Dahlhoff, C., Sobczak, K., Weber, W.-M., and Kusche-Vihrog, K. (2008). Upregulated expression of ENaC in human CF nasal epithelium. *J. Cyst. Fibros.* 7, 197–205. doi: 10.1016/j.jcf.2007.07.012

Barden, A. E., Mas, E., and Mori, T. A. (2016). n-3 Fatty acid supplementation and proresolving mediators of inflammation. *Curr. Opin. Lipidol.* 27, 26–32. doi: 10.1097/MOL.0000000000000262

Barnaby, R., Koeppen, K., Nymon, A., Hampton, T. H., Berwin, B., Ashare, A., et al. (2018). Lumacaftor (VX-809) restores the ability of CF macrophages to phagocytose and kill Pseudomonas aeruginosa. *Am. J. Physiol. Lung Cell. Mol. Physiol.* 314, L432–L438. doi: 10.1152/ajplung.00461.2017

Barnig, C., Cernadas, M., Dutile, S., Liu, X., Perrella, M. A., Kazani, S., et al. (2013). Lipoxin A4 regulates natural killer cell and type 2 innate lymphoid cell activation in asthma. *Sci. Transl. Med.* 5, 174ra26. doi: 10.1126/scitranslmed.3004812

Bartlett, J. A., Ramachandran, S., Wohlford-Lenane, C. L., Barker, C. K., Pezzulo, A. A., Zabner, J., et al. (2016). Newborn Cystic Fibrosis Pigs Have a Blunted Early Response to an Inflammatory Stimulus. *Am. J. Respir. Crit. Care Med.* 194, 845–854. doi: 10.1164/rccm.201510-2112OC

Bartling, T. R., and Drumm, M. L. (2009). Oxidative Stress Causes IL8 Promoter Hyperacetylation in Cystic Fibrosis Airway Cell Models. *Am. J. Respir. Cell Mol. Biol.* 40, 58–65. doi: 10.1165/rcmb.2007-0464OC

Bena, S., Brancaleone, V., Wang, J. M., Perretti, M., and Flower, R. J. (2012). Annexin A1 interaction with the FPR2/ALX receptor: identification of distinct domains and downstream associated signaling. *J. Biol. Chem.* 287, 24690–24697. doi: 10.1074/jbc.M112.377101

Berridge, M. J., Bootman, M. D., and Roderick, H. L. (2003). Calcium signalling: dynamics, homeostasis and remodelling. *Nat. Rev. Mol. Cell Biol.* 4, 517–529. doi: 10.1038/nrm1155

Bhura-Bandali, F. N., Suh, M., Man, S. F., and Clandinin, M. T. (2000). The deltaF508 mutation in the cystic fibrosis transmembrane conductance regulator alters control of essential fatty acid utilization in epithelial cells. *J. Nutr.* 130, 2870–2875. doi: 10.1093/jn/130.12.2870

Birnbaum, Y., Ye, Y., Lin, Y., Freeberg, S. Y., Huang, M.-H., Perez-Polo, J. R., et al. (2007). Aspirin augments 15-epi-lipoxin A4 production by lipopolysaccharide, but blocks the pioglitazone and atorvastatin induction of 15-epi-lipoxin A4 in the rat heart. *Prostaglandins Other Lipid Mediat.* 83, 89–98. doi: 10.1016/j.prostaglandins.2006.10.003

Blohmke, C. J., Mayer, M. L., Tang, A. C., Hirschfeld, A. F., Fjell, C. D., Sze, M. A., et al. (2012). Atypical Activation of the Unfolded Protein Response in Cystic Fibrosis Airway Cells Contributes to p38 MAPK-Mediated Innate Immune Responses. *J. Immunol.* 189, 5467–5475. doi: 10.4049/jimmunol.1103661

Bobadilla, J. L., Macek, M., Fine, J. P., and Farrell, P. M. (2002). Cystic fibrosis: a worldwide analysis of CFTR mutations–correlation with incidence data and application to screening. *Hum. Mutat.* 19, 575–606. doi: 10.1002/humu.10041

Boncoeur, E., Criq, V. S., Bonvin, E., Roque, T., Henrion-Caude, A., Gruenert, D. C., et al. (2008). Oxidative stress induces extracellular signal-regulated kinase 1/2 mitogen-activated protein kinase in cystic fibrosis lung epithelial cells: Potential mechanism for excessive IL-8 expression. *Int. J. Biochem. Cell Biol.* 40, 432–446. doi: 10.1016/j.biocel.2007.08.013

Bonfield, T. L., Panuska, J. R., Konstan, M. W., Hilliard, K. A., Hilliard, J. B., Ghnaim, H., et al. (1995). Inflammatory cytokines in cystic fibrosis lungs. *Am. J. Respir. Crit. Care Med.* 152, 2111–2118. doi: 10.1164/ajrccm.152.6.8520783

Bonnans, C., Vachier, I., Chavis, C., Godard, P., Bousquet, J., and Chanez, P. (2002). Lipoxins are potential endogenous antiinflammatory mediators in asthma. *Am. J. Respir. Crit. Care Med.* 165, 1531–1535. doi: 10.1164/rccm.200201-053OC

Bonnans, C., Mainprice, B., Chanez, P., Bousquet, J., and Urbach, V. (2003). Lipoxin A4 stimulates a cytosolic Ca2+ increase in human bronchial epithelium. *J. Biol. Chem.* 278, 10879–10884. doi: 10.1074/jbc.M210294200

Bonnans, C., Fukunaga, K., Levy, M. A., and Levy, B. D. (2006). Lipoxin A4 Regulates Bronchial Epithelial Cell Responses to Acid Injury. *Am. J. Pathol.* 168, 1064–1072. doi: 10.2353/ajpath.2006.051056

Borot, F., Vieu, D.-L., Faure, G., Fritsch, J., Colas, J., Moriceau, S., et al. (2009). Eicosanoid release is increased by membrane destabilization and CFTR inhibition in Calu-3 cells. *PLoS One* 4, e7116. doi: 10.1371/journal.pone.0007116

Botten, N., Hodges, R. R., Li, D., Bair, J. A., Shatos, M. A., Utheim, T. P., et al. (2019). Resolvin D2 elevates cAMP to increase intracellular [Ca2+] and stimulate secretion from conjunctival goblet cells. *FASEB J.* 33, 8468–8478. doi: 10.1096/fj.201802467R

Boucher, R. C. (2007). Evidence for airway surface dehydration as the initiating event in CF airway disease. *J. Intern. Med.* 261, 5–16. doi: 10.1111/j.1365-2796.2006.01744.x

Brady, H. R., Papayianni, A., and Serhan, C. N. (1995). Potential vascular roles for lipoxins in the "stop programs" of host defense and inflammation. *Trends Cardiovasc. Med.* 5, 186–192. doi: 10.1016/1050-1738(95)00055-E

Brennan, E. P., Nolan, K. A., Börgeson, E., Gough, O. S., McEvoy, C. M., Docherty, N. G., et al. (2013). Lipoxins Attenuate Renal Fibrosis by Inducing let-7c and Suppressing TGF β R1. *J. Am. Soc Nephrol.* 24, 627–637. doi: 10.1681/ASN.2012060550

Brown, R. K., Wyatt, H., Price, J. F., and Kelly, F. J. (1996). Pulmonary dysfunction in cystic fibrosis is associated with oxidative stress. *Eur. Respir. J.* 9, 334–339. doi: 10.1183/09031936.96.09020334

Brüne, B. (2005). The Intimate Relation Between Nitric Oxide and Superoxide in Apoptosis and Cell Survival. *Antioxid. Redox Signal.* 7, 497–507. doi: 10.1089/ars.2005.7.497

Bruscia, E. M., and Bonfield, T. L. (2016). Cystic Fibrosis Lung Immunity: The Role of the Macrophage. *J. Innate Immun.* 8, 550–563. doi: 10.1159/000446825

Bruscia, E. M., Zhang, P.-X., Ferreira, E., Caputo, C., Emerson, J. W., Tuck, D., et al. (2009). Macrophages Directly Contribute to the Exaggerated Inflammatory Response in Cystic Fibrosis Transmembrane Conductance Regulator-/- Mice. *Am. J. Respir. Cell Mol. Biol.* 40, 295–304. doi: 10.1165/rcmb.2008-0170OC

Bruscia, E. M., Zhang, P.-X., Satoh, A., Caputo, C., Medzhitov, R., Shenoy, A., et al. (2011). Abnormal trafficking and degradation of TLR4 underlie the elevated inflammatory response in cystic fibrosis. *J. Immunol. Baltim. Md 1950* 186, 6990–6998. doi: 10.4049/jimmunol.1100396

Buchanan, P. J., McNally, P., Harvey, B. J., and Urbach, V. (2013). Lipoxin A_4;-mediated KATP potassium channel activation results in cystic fibrosis airway epithelial repair. *Am. J. Physiol. Lung Cell. Mol. Physiol.* 305, L193–L201. doi: 10.1152/ajplung.00058.2013

Bush, A., and Rubin, B. K. (2003). Macrolides as Biological Response Modifiers in Cystic Fibrosis and Bronchiectasis. *Semin. Respir. Crit. Care Med.* 24, 737–748. doi: 10.1055/s-2004-815669

Button, B., Cai, L.-H., Ehre, C., Kesimer, M., Hill, D. B., Sheehan, J. K., et al. (2012). Periciliary Brush Promotes the Lung Health by Separating the Mucus Layer from Airway Epithelia. *Science* 337, 937–941. doi: 10.1126/science.1223012

Bystrom, J., Evans, I., Newson, J., Stables, M., Toor, I., van Rooijen, N., et al. (2008). Resolution-phase macrophages possess a unique inflammatory phenotype that is controlled by cAMP. *Blood* 112, 4117–4127. doi: 10.1182/blood-2007-12-129767

Cabrini, G., and De Togni, P. (1985). Increased cytosolic calcium in cystic fibrosis neutrophils effect on stimulus - secretion coupling. *Life Sci.* 36, 1561–1567. doi: 10.1016/0024-3205(85)90380-7

Causer, A. J., Shute, J. K., Cummings, M. H., Shepherd, A.II, Gruet, M., Costello, J. T., et al. (2020). Circulating biomarkers of antioxidant status and oxidative stress in people with cystic fibrosis: A systematic review and meta-analysis. *Redox Biol.* 32, 101436. doi: 10.1016/j.redox.2020.101436

Chao, A. C., Zifferblatt, J. B., Wagner, J. A., Dong, Y.-J., Gruenert, D. C., and Gardner, P. (1994). Stimulation of chloride secretion by P1 purinoceptor agonists in cystic fibrosis phenotype airway epithelial cell line CFPEo-. *Br. J. Pharmacol.* 112, 169–175. doi: 10.1111/j.1476-5381.1994.tb13047.x

Chen, J., Kinter, M., Shank, S., Cotton, C., Kelley, T. J., and Ziady, A. G. (2008). Dysfunction of Nrf-2 in CF Epithelia Leads to Excess Intracellular H2O2 and Inflammatory Cytokine Production. *PLoS One* 3, e3367. doi: 10.1371/journal.pone.0003367

Chen, J.-H., Stoltz, D. A., Karp, P. H., Ernst, S. E., Pezzulo, A. A., Moninger, T. O., et al. (2010). Loss of anion transport without increased sodium absorption characterizes newborn porcine cystic fibrosis airway epithelia. *Cell* 143, 911–923. doi: 10.1016/j.cell.2010.11.029

Cheng, X., He, S., Yuan, J., Miao, S., Gao, H., Zhang, J., et al. (2016). Lipoxin A4 attenuates LPS-induced mouse acute lung injury via Nrf2-mediated E-cadherin expression in airway epithelial cells. *Free Radic. Biol. Med.* 93, 52–66. doi: 10.1016/j.freeradbiomed.2016.01.026

Chiang, N., and Serhan, C. N. (2004). Aspirin triggers formation of anti-inflammatory mediators: New mechanism for an old drug. *Discov. Med.* 4, 470–475. doi: 10.1038/ncb1456

Chiang, N., and Serhan, C. N. (2017). Structural elucidation and physiologic functions of specialized pro-resolving mediators and their receptors. *Mol. Aspects Med.* 58, 114–129. doi: 10.1016/j.mam.2017.03.005

Chiang, N., Takano, T., Arita, M., Watanabe, S., and Serhan, C. N. (2003). A novel rat lipoxin A4 receptor that is conserved in structure and function. *Br. J. Pharmacol.* 139, 89–98. doi: 10.1038/sj.bjp.0705220

Chiang, N., Serhan, C. N., Dahlén, S.-E., Drazen, J. M., Hay, D. W. P., Rovati, G. E., et al. (2006). The lipoxin receptor ALX: potent ligand-specific and stereoselective actions in vivo. *Pharmacol. Rev.* 58, 463–487. doi: 10.1124/pr.58.3.4

Chiang, N., Fredman, G., Bäckhed, F., Oh, S. F., Vickery, T., Schmidt, B. A., et al. (2012). Infection regulates pro-resolving mediators that lower antibiotic requirements. *Nature* 484, 524–528. doi: 10.1038/nature11042

Chiang, N., Shinohara, M., Dalli, J., Mirakaj, V., Kibi, M., Choi, A. M. K., et al. (2013). Inhaled Carbon Monoxide Accelerates Resolution of Inflammation via Unique Proresolving Mediator–Heme Oxygenase-1 Circuits. *J. Immunol.* 190, 6378–6388. doi: 10.4049/jimmunol.1202969

Chiang, N., Dalli, J., Colas, R. A., and Serhan, C. N. (2015). Identification of resolvin D2 receptor mediating resolution of infections and organ protection. *J. Exp. Med.* 212, 1203–1217. doi: 10.1084/jem.20150225

Chiang, N., de la Rosa, X., Libreros, S., and Serhan, C. N. (2017). Novel Resolvin D2 Receptor Axis in Infectious Inflammation. *J. Immunol. Baltim. Md 1950* 198, 842–851. doi: 10.4049/jimmunol.1601650

Chiang, N., Libreros, S., Norris, P. C., de la Rosa, X., and Serhan, C. N. (2019). Maresin 1 activates LGR6 receptor promoting phagocyte immunoresolvent functions. *J. Clin. Invest.* 129, 5294–5311. doi: 10.1172/JCI129448

Chiron, R., Grumbach, Y. Y., Quynh, N. V., Verriere, V., and Urbach, V. (2008). Lipoxin A(4) and interleukin-8 levels in cystic fibrosis sputum after antibiotherapy. *J. Cyst Fibros* 7, 463–468. doi: 10.1016/j.jcf.2008.04.002

Chiurchiù, V., Leuti, A., Dalli, J., Jacobsson, A., Battistini, L., Maccarrone, M., et al. (2016). Proresolving lipid mediators resolvin D1, resolvin D2, and maresin 1 are critical in modulating T cell responses. *Sci. Transl. Med.* 8, 353ra111-353ra111. doi: 10.1126/scitranslmed.aaf7483

Chmiel, J. F., and Davis, P. B. (2003). State of the Art: Why do the lungs of patients with cystic fibrosis become infected and why can't they clear the infection? *Respir. Res.* 4:8. doi: 10.1186/1465-9921-4-8

Cho, D.-Y., Hwang, P. H., Illek, B., and Fischer, H. (2011). Acid and base secretion in freshly excised nasal tissue from cystic fibrosis patients with ΔF508 mutation. *Int. Forum Allergy Rhinol.* 1, 123–127. doi: 10.1002/alr.20028

Clària, J., and Serhan, C. N. (1995). Aspirin triggers previously undescribed bioactive eicosanoids by human endothelial cell-leukocyte interactions. *Proc. Natl. Acad. Sci. U. S. A.* 92, 9475–9479. doi: 10.1073/pnas.92.21.9475

Coakley, R. D., Grubb, B. R., Paradiso, A. M., Gatzy, J. T., Johnson, L. G., Kreda, S. M., et al. (2003). Abnormal surface liquid pH regulation by cultured cystic fibrosis bronchial epithelium. *Proc. Natl. Acad. Sci.* 100, 16083–16088. doi: 10.1073/pnas.2634339100

Codagnone, M., Recchiuti, A., Lanuti, P., Pierdomenico, A. M., Cianci, E., Patruno, S., et al. (2017). Lipoxin A4 stimulates endothelial miR-126–5p expression and its transfer via microvesicles. *FASEB J.* 31, 1856–1866. doi: 10.1096/fj.201600952R

Codagnone, M., Cianci, E., Lamolinara, A., Mari, V. C., Nespoli, A., Isopi, E., et al. (2018). Resolvin D1 enhances the resolution of lung inflammation caused by long-term Pseudomonas aeruginosa infection. *Mucosal Immunol.* 11, 35–49. doi: 10.1038/mi.2017.36

Colas, R. A., Shinohara, M., Dalli, J., Chiang, N., and Serhan, C. N. (2014). Identification and signature profiles for pro-resolving and inflammatory lipid mediators in human tissue. *Am. J. Physiol. Cell Physiol.* 307, C39–C54. doi: 10.1152/ajpcell.00024.2014

Colas, R. A., Dalli, J., Chiang, N., Vlasakov, I., Sanger, J. M., Riley, I. R., et al. (2016). Identification and Actions of the Maresin 1 Metabolome in Infectious Inflammation. *J. Immunol.* 197, 4444–4452. doi: 10.4049/jimmunol.1600837

Collawn, J. F., Lazrak, A., Bebok, Z., and Matalon, S. (2012). The CFTR and ENaC debate: how important is ENaC in CF lung disease? *Am. J. Physiol. Lung Cell. Mol. Physiol.* 302, L1141–L1146. doi: 10.1152/ajplung.00036.2012

Corvol, H., Blackman, S. M., Boëlle, P.-Y., Gallins, P. J., Pace, R. G., Stonebraker, J. R., et al. (2015). Genome-wide association meta-analysis identifies five modifier loci of lung disease severity in cystic fibrosis. *Nat. Commun.* 6, 1–8. doi: 10.1038/ncomms9382

Coste, T. C., Armand, M., Lebacq, J., Lebecque, P., Wallemacq, P., and Leal, T. (2007). An overview of monitoring and supplementation of omega 3 fatty acids in cystic fibrosis. *Clin. Biochem.* 40, 511–520. doi: 10.1016/j.clinbiochem.2007.01.002

Cox, R., Phillips, O., Fukumoto, J., Fukumoto, I., Tamarapu Parthasarathy, P., Mandry, M., et al. (2015). Resolvins Decrease Oxidative Stress Mediated Macrophage and Epithelial Cell Interaction through Decreased Cytokine Secretion. *PLoS One* 10, e0136755. doi: 10.1371/journal.pone.0136755

Croasdell, A., Thatcher, T. H., Kottmann, R. M., Colas, R. A., Dalli, J., Serhan, C. N., et al. (2015). Resolvins attenuate inflammation and promote resolution in cigarette smoke-exposed human macrophages. *Am. J. Physiol.-Lung Cell. Mol. Physiol.* 309, L888–L901. doi: 10.1152/ajplung.00125.2015

Csóka, B., Selmeczy, Z., Koscsó, B., Németh, Z. H., Pacher, P., Murray, P. J., et al. (2012). Adenosine promotes alternative macrophage activation via A2A and A2B receptors. *FASEB J.* 26, 376–386. doi: 10.1096/fj.11-190934

Cystic Fibrosis Mutation Database, Available at: http://www.genet.sickkids.on.ca/cftr/ (Accessed March 23, 2020).

Czerska, K., Sobczynska-Tomaszewska, A., Sands, D., Nowakowska, A., Bak, D., Wertheim, K., et al. (2010). Prostaglandin-endoperoxide synthase genes COX1 and COX2 - novel modifiers of disease severity in cystic fibrosis patients. *J. Appl. Genet.* 51, 323–330. doi: 10.1007/BF03208862

Dalli, J., and Serhan, C. N. (2012). Specific lipid mediator signatures of human phagocytes: microparticles stimulate macrophage efferocytosis and pro-resolving mediators. *Blood* 120, e60–e72. doi: 10.1182/blood-2012-04-423525

Dalli, J., Rosignoli, G., Hayhoe, R. P., Edelman, A., and Perretti, M. (2010). CFTR inhibition provokes an inflammatory response associated with an imbalance of the annexin A1 pathway. *Am. J. Pathol.* 177, 176–186. doi: 10.2353/ajpath.2010.091149

Dalli, J., Consalvo, A. P., Ray, V., Di Filippo, C., D'Amico, M., Mehta, N., et al. (2013a). Proresolving and Tissue-Protective Actions of Annexin A1–Based Cleavage-Resistant Peptides Are Mediated by Formyl Peptide Receptor 2/Lipoxin A_4 Receptor. *J. Immunol.* 190, 6478–6487. doi: 10.4049/jimmunol.1203000

Dalli, J., Consalvo, A. P., Ray, V., Filippo, C. D., D'Amico, M., Mehta, N., et al. (2013b). Proresolving and Tissue-Protective Actions of Annexin A1–Based Cleavage-Resistant Peptides Are Mediated by Formyl Peptide Receptor 2/Lipoxin A4 Receptor. *J. Immunol.* 190, 6478–6487. doi: 10.4049/jimmunol.1203000

Dalli, J., Chiang, N., and Serhan, C. N. (2014). Identification of 14-series sulfido-conjugated mediators that promote resolution of infection and organ protection. *Proc. Natl. Acad. Sci. U. S. A.* 111, E4753–E4761. doi: 10.1073/pnas.1415006111

Dalli, J., Kraft, B. D., Colas, R. A., Shinohara, M., Fredenburgh, L. E., Hess, D. R., et al. (2015). The Regulation of Proresolving Lipid Mediator Profiles in Baboon Pneumonia by Inhaled Carbon Monoxide. *Am. J. Respir. Cell Mol. Biol.* 53, 314–325. doi: 10.1165/rcmb.2014-0299OC

Dalli, J., Vlasakov, I., Riley, I. R., Rodriguez, A. R., Spur, B. W., Petasis, N. A., et al. (2016). Maresin conjugates in tissue regeneration biosynthesis enzymes in human macrophages. *Proc. Natl. Acad. Sci. U. S. A.* 113, 12232–12237. doi: 10.1073/pnas.1607003113

Dalli, J., Colas, R. A., Arnardottir, H., and Serhan, C. N. (2017). Vagal regulation of Group 3 innate lymphoid cells and the immunoresolvent PCTR1 controls infection resolution. *Immunity* 46, 92–105. doi: 10.1016/j.immuni.2016.12.009

Dartt, D. A., Hodges, R. R., Li, D., Shatos, M. A., Lashkari, K., and Serhan, C. N. (2011). Conjunctival Goblet Cell Secretion Stimulated by Leukotrienes Is Reduced by Resolvins D1 and E1 To Promote Resolution of Inflammation. *J. Immunol. Baltim. Md 1950* 186, 4455–4466. doi: 10.4049/jimmunol.1000833

Davis, P. B. (2006). Cystic fibrosis since 1938. *Am. J. Respir. Crit. Care Med.* 173, 475–482. doi: 10.1164/rccm.200505-840OE

Denning, G. M., Railsback, M. A., Rasmussen, G. T., Cox, C. D., and Britigan, B. E. (1998). Pseudomonas pyocyanine alters calcium signaling in human airway epithelial cells. *Am. J. Physiol.-Lung Cell. Mol. Physiol.* 274, L893–L900. doi: 10.1152/ajplung.1998.274.6.L893

Derichs, N., Jin, B., Song, Y., Finkbeiner, W. E., and Verkman, A. S. (2011). Hyperviscous airway periciliary and mucous liquid layers in cystic fibrosis measured by confocal fluorescence photobleaching. *FASEB J.* 25, 2325–2332. doi: 10.1096/fj.10-179549

Deriy, L. V., Gomez, E. A., Zhang, G., Beacham, D. W., Hopson, J. A., Gallan, A. J., et al. (2009). Disease-causing Mutations in the Cystic Fibrosis Transmembrane Conductance Regulator Determine the Functional Responses of Alveolar Macrophages. *J. Biol. Chem.* 284, 35926–35938. doi: 10.1074/jbc.M109.057372

Di, A., Brown, M. E., Deriy, L. V., Li, C., Szeto, F. L., Chen, Y., et al. (2006). CFTR regulates phagosome acidification in macrophages and alters bactericidal activity. *Nat. Cell Biol.* 8, 933–944.

Dif, F., Wu, Y.-Z., Burgel, P.-R., Ollero, M., Leduc, D., Aarbiou, J., et al. (2010). Critical role of cytosolic phospholipase A2{alpha} in bronchial mucus hypersecretion in CFTR-deficient mice. *Eur. Respir. J.* 36, 1120–1130. doi: 10.1183/09031936.00183409

Dong, J., Jiang, X., Zhang, X., Liu, K. S., Zhang, J., Chen, J., et al. (2015). Dynamically Regulated CFTR Expression and Its Functional Role in Cutaneous Wound Healing: CFTR IN CUTANEOUS WOUND HEALING. *J. Cell. Physiol.* 230, 2049–2058. doi: 10.1002/jcp.24931

D'Acquisto, F., Perretti, M., and Flower, R. J. (2008). Annexin-A1: a pivotal regulator of the innate and adaptive immune systems. *Br. J. Pharmacol.* 155, 152–169. doi: 10.1038/bjp.2008.252

Eickmeier, O., Seki, H., Haworth, O., Hilberath, J. N., Gao, F., Uddin, M., et al. (2013). Aspirin-triggered resolvin D1 reduces mucosal inflammation and promotes resolution in a murine model of acute lung injury. *Mucosal Immunol.* 6, 256–266. doi: 10.1038/mi.2012.66

Eickmeier, O., Fussbroich, D., Mueller, K., Serve, F., Smaczny, C., Zielen, S., et al. (2017). Pro-resolving lipid mediator Resolvin D1 serves as a marker of lung disease in cystic fibrosis. *PLoS One* 12, e0171249. doi: 10.1371/journal.pone.0171249

Elborn, J., Horsley, A., MacGregor, G., Bilton, D., Grosswald, R., Ahuja, S., et al. (2017). Phase I Studies of Acebilustat: Biomarker Response and Safety in Patients with Cystic Fibrosis: Acebilustat Phase I Biomarkers in Patients with Cystic Fibrosis. *Clin. Transl. Sci.* 10, 28–34. doi: 10.1111/cts.12428

Elborn, J. S., Ahuja, S., Springman, E., Mershon, J., Grosswald, R., and Rowe, S. M. (2018). EMPIRE-CF: A phase II randomized placebo-controlled trial of once-daily, oral acebilustat in adult patients with cystic fibrosis – Study design and patient demographics. *Contemp. Clin. Trials* 72, 86–94. doi: 10.1016/j.cct.2018.07.014

Emerson, J., Rosenfeld, M., McNamara, S., Ramsey, B., and Gibson, R. L. (2002). Pseudomonas aeruginosa and other predictors of mortality and morbidity in young children with cystic fibrosis. *Pediatr. Pulmonol.* 34, 91–100. doi: 10.1002/ppul.10127

English, J. T., Norris, P. C., Hodges, R. R., Dartt, D. A., and Serhan, C. N. (2017). Identification and Profiling of Specialized Pro-Resolving Mediators in Human Tears by Lipid Mediator Metabolomics. *Prostaglandins Leukot Essent Fat. Acids* 117, 17–27. doi: 10.1016/j.plefa.2017.01.004

Esposito, L. A., Melov, S., Panov, A., Cottrell, B. A., and Wallace, D. C. (1999). Mitochondrial disease in mouse results in increased oxidative stress. *Proc. Natl. Acad. Sci.* 96, 4820–4825. doi: 10.1073/pnas.96.9.4820

Esther, C. R., Muhlebach, M. S., Ehre, C., Hill, D. B., Wolfgang, M. C., Kesimer, M., et al. (2019). Mucus accumulation in the lungs precedes structural changes and infection in children with cystic fibrosis. *Sci. Transl. Med.* 11 (486), eaav3488. doi: 10.1126/scitranslmed.aav3488

Farrell, P. M., Bieri, J. G., Fratantoni, J. F., Wood, R. E., and di Sant'Agnese, P. A. (1977). The Occurrence and Effects of Human Vitamin E Deficiency. *J. Clin. Invest.* 60, 233–241. doi: 10.1172/JCI108760

Favia, M., de Bari, L., Bobba, A., and Atlante, A. (2019). An Intriguing Involvement of Mitochondria in Cystic Fibrosis. *J. Clin. Med.* 8:1890. doi: 10.3390/jcm8111890

Feigal, R. J., Tomczyk, M. S., and Shapiro, B. L. (1982). The calcium abnormality in cystic fibrosis mitochondria: Relative role of respiration and ATP hydrolysis. *Life Sci.* 30, 93–98. doi: 10.1016/0024-3205(82)90640-3

Fiore, S., Ryeom, S. W., Weller, P. F., and Serhan, C. N. (1992). Lipoxin recognition sites. Specific binding of labeled lipoxin A4 with human neutrophils. *J. Biol. Chem.* 267, 16168–16176. doi: 10.1084/jem.180.1.253

Fiore, S., Maddox, J. F., Perez, H. D., and Serhan, C. N. (1994). Identification of a human cDNA encoding a functional high affinity lipoxin A4 receptor. *J. Exp. Med.* 180, 253–260.

Fisher, J. T., Tyler, S. R., Zhang, Y., Lee, B. J., Liu, X., Sun, X., et al. (2013). Bioelectric Characterization of Epithelia from Neonatal CFTR Knockout Ferrets. *Am. J. Respir. Cell Mol. Biol.* 49, 837–844. doi: 10.1165/rcmb.2012-0433OC

Folco, G., and Murphy, R. C. (2006). Eicosanoid transcellular biosynthesis: from cell-cell interactions to in vivo tissue responses. *Pharmacol. Rev.* 58, 375–388. doi: 10.1124/pr.58.3.8

Fredman, G., Li, Y., Dalli, J., Chiang, N., and Serhan, C. N. (2012). Self-Limited versus Delayed Resolution of Acute Inflammation: Temporal Regulation of Pro-Resolving Mediators and MicroRNA. *Sci. Rep.* 2, 639. doi: 10.1038/srep00639

Fredman, G., Ozcan, L., Spolitu, S., Hellmann, J., Spite, M., Backs, J., et al. (2014). Resolvin D1 limits 5-lipoxygenase nuclear localization and leukotriene B4 synthesis by inhibiting a calcium-activated kinase pathway. *Proc. Natl. Acad. Sci. U. S. A.* 111, 14530–14535. doi: 10.1073/pnas.1410851111

Freedman, S. D., Blanco, P. G., Zaman, M. M., Shea, J. C., Ollero, M., Hopper, I. K., et al. (2004). Association of cystic fibrosis with abnormalities in fatty acid metabolism. *N. Engl. J. Med.* 350, 560–569. doi: 10.1056/NEJMoa021218

Funk, C. D. (2001). Prostaglandins and Leukotrienes: Advances in Eicosanoid Biology. *Science* 294, 1871–1875. doi: 10.1126/science.294.5548.1871

Gangemi, S., Luciotti, G., D'Urbano, E., Mallamace, A., Santoro, D., Bellinghieri, G., et al. (2003). Physical exercise increases urinary excretion of lipoxin A4 and related compounds. *J. Appl. Physiol. Bethesda Md 1985* 94, 2237–2240. doi: 10.1152/japplphysiol.01004.2002

Garnett, J. P., Hickman, E., Burrows, R., Hegyi, P., Tiszlavicz, L., Cuthbert, A. W., et al. (2011). Novel Role for Pendrin in Orchestrating Bicarbonate Secretion in Cystic Fibrosis Transmembrane Conductance Regulator (CFTR)-expressing Airway Serous Cells. *J. Biol. Chem.* 286, 41069–41082. doi: 10.1074/jbc.M111.266734

Garnett, J. P., Kalsi, K. K., Sobotta, M., Bearham, J., Carr, G., Powell, J., et al. (2016). Hyperglycaemia and Pseudomonas aeruginosa acidify cystic fibrosis airway surface liquid by elevating epithelial monocarboxylate transporter 2 dependent lactate-H+ secretion. *Sci. Rep.* 6, 37955. doi: 10.1038/srep37955

Gavins, F. N. E., Hughes, E. L., Buss, N. A. P. S., Holloway, P. M., Getting, S. J., and Buckingham, J. C. (2012). Leukocyte recruitment in the brain in sepsis: involvement of the annexin 1-FPR2/ALX anti-inflammatory system. *FASEB J.* 26, 4977–4989. doi: 10.1096/fj.12-205971

Gentzsch, M., Dang, H., Dang, Y., Garcia-Caballero, A., Suchindran, H., Boucher, R. C., et al. (2010). The cystic fibrosis transmembrane conductance regulator impedes proteolytic stimulation of the epithelial Na+ channel. *J. Biol. Chem.* 285, 32227–32232. doi: 10.1074/jbc.M110.155259

Germolec, D. R., Shipkowski, K. A., Frawley, R. P., and Evans, E. (2018). "Markers of Inflammation," in *Immunotoxicity Testing: Methods and Protocols Methods in Molecular Biology*. Eds. J. C. DeWitt, C. E. Rockwell and C. C. Bowman (New York, NY: Springer), 57–79. doi: 10.1007/978-1-4939-8549-4_5

Gewirtz, A. T., McCormick, B., Neish, A. S., Petasis, N. A., Gronert, K., Serhan, C. N., et al. (1998). Pathogen-induced chemokine secretion from model intestinal epithelium is inhibited by lipoxin A4 analogs. *J. Clin. Invest.* 101, 1860–1869. doi: 10.1172/JCI1339

Ghosh, M., Tucker, D. E., Burchett, S. A., and Leslie, C. C. (2006). Properties of the Group IV phospholipase A2 family. *Prog. Lipid Res.* 45, 487–510. doi: 10.1016/j.plipres.2006.05.003

Gibson, R. A., Teubner, J. K., Haines, K., Cooper, D. M., and Davidson, G. P. (1986). Relationships between pulmonary function and plasma fatty acid levels in cystic fibrosis patients. *J. Pediatr. Gastroenterol. Nutr.* 5, 408–415. doi: 10.1097/00005176-198605000-00013

Godson, C., Mitchell, S., Harvey, K., Petasis, N. A., Hogg, N., and Brady, H. R. (2000). Cutting edge: lipoxins rapidly stimulate nonphlogistic phagocytosis of apoptotic neutrophils by monocyte-derived macrophages. *J. Immunol. Baltim. Md 1950* 164, 1663–1667. doi: 10.4049/jimmunol.164.4.1663

Gomez, C. C. S., Parazzi, P. L. F., Clinckspoor, K. J., Mauch, R. M., Pessine, F. B. T., Levy, C. E., et al. (2020). Safety, Tolerability, and Effects of Sodium Bicarbonate Inhalation in Cystic Fibrosis. *Clin. Drug Investig.* 40, 105–117. doi: 10.1007/s40261-019-00861-x

Gorrieri, G., Scudieri, P., Caci, E., Schiavon, M., Tomati, V., Sirci, F., et al. (2016). Goblet Cell Hyperplasia Requires High Bicarbonate Transport To Support Mucin Release. *Sci. Rep.* 6, 36016. doi: 10.1038/srep36016

Grabiec, A. M., and Hussell, T. (2016). The role of airway macrophages in apoptotic cell clearance following acute and chronic lung inflammation. *Semin. Immunopathol.* 38, 409–423. doi: 10.1007/s00281-016-0555-3

Greger, R., Mall, M., Bleich, M., Ecke, D., Warth, R., Riedemann, N., et al. (1996). Regulation of epithelial ion channels by the cystic fibrosis transmembrane conductance regulator. *J. Mol. Med. Berl. Ger.* 74, 527–534. doi: 10.1007/bf00204979

Grumbach, Y., Quynh, N. V. T., Chiron, R., and Urbach, V. (2009). LXA4 stimulates ZO-1 expression and transepithelial electrical resistance in human airway epithelial (16HBE14o-) cells. *Am. J. Physiol. Lung Cell. Mol. Physiol.* 296, L101–L108. doi: 10.1152/ajplung.00018.2008

Güney, E., Emiralioğlu, N., Cinel, G., Yalçın, E., Doğru, D., Kiper, N., et al. (2019). Nasal nitric oxide levels in primary ciliary dyskinesia, cystic fibrosis and healthy children. *Turk. J. Pediatr.* 61:20. doi: 10.24953/turkjped.2019.01.004

Hachicha, M., Pouliot, M., Petasis, N. A., and Serhan, C. N. (1999). Lipoxin (LX) A4 and aspirin-triggered 15-epi-LXA4 inhibit tumor necrosis factor 1alpha-initiated neutrophil responses and trafficking: regulators of a cytokine-chemokine axis. *J. Exp. Med.* 189, 1923–1930. doi: 10.1084/jem.189.12.1923

Haeggström, J. Z., and Funk, C. D. (2011). Lipoxygenase and leukotriene pathways: biochemistry, biology, and roles in disease. *Chem. Rev.* 111, 5866–5898. doi: 10.1021/cr200246d

Hanukoglu, I., and Hanukoglu, A. (2016). Epithelial sodium channel (ENaC) family: Phylogeny, structure-function, tissue distribution, and associated inherited diseases. *Gene* 579, 95–132. doi: 10.1016/j.gene.2015.12.061

Hayhoe, R. P. G., Kamal, A. M., Solito, E., Flower, R. J., Cooper, D., and Perretti, M. (2006). Annexin 1 and its bioactive peptide inhibit neutrophil-endothelium interactions under flow: indication of distinct receptor involvement. *Blood* 107, 2123–2130. doi: 10.1182/blood-2005-08-3099

He, R., Sang, H., and Ye, R. D. (2003). Serum amyloid A induces IL-8 secretion through a G protein-coupled receptor, FPRL1/LXA4R. *Blood* 101, 1572–1581. doi: 10.1182/blood-2002-05-1431

Hellmann, J., Tang, Y., Kosuri, M., Bhatnagar, A., and Spite, M. (2011). Resolvin D1 decreases adipose tissue macrophage accumulation and improves insulin sensitivity in obese-diabetic mice. *FASEB J.* 25, 2399–2407. doi: 10.1096/fj.10-178657

Henderson, A. G., Ehre, C., Button, B., Abdullah, L. H., Cai, L.-H., Leigh, M. W., et al. (2014). Cystic fibrosis airway secretions exhibit mucin hyperconcentration and increased osmotic pressure. *J. Clin. Invest.* 124, 3047–3060. doi: 10.1172/JCI73469

Higgins, G., Buchanan, P., Perriere, M., Al-Alawi, M., Costello, R. W., Verriere, V., et al. (2014). Activation of P2RY11 and ATP release by lipoxin A4 restores the airway surface liquid layer and epithelial repair in cystic fibrosis. *Am. J. Respir. Cell Mol. Biol.* 51, 178–190. doi: 10.1165/rcmb.2012-0424OC

Higgins, G., Fustero Torre, C., Tyrrell, J., McNally, P., Harvey, B. J., and Urbach, V. (2016). Lipoxin A 4 prevents tight junction disruption and delays the colonization of cystic fibrosis bronchial epithelial cells by Pseudomonas aeruginosa. *Am. J. Physiol.-Lung Cell. Mol. Physiol.* 310, L1053–L1061. doi: 10.1152/ajplung.00368.2015

Hill, D. B., Long, R. F., Kissner, W. J., Atieh, E., Garbarine, I. C., Markovetz, M. R., et al. (2018). Pathological mucus and impaired mucus clearance in cystic fibrosis patients result from increased concentration, not altered pH. *Eur. Respir. J.* 52, 1801297. doi: 10.1183/13993003.01297-2018

Hodges, R. R., Li, D., Shatos, M. A., Bair, J. A., Lippestad, M., Serhan, C. N., et al. (2017). Lipoxin A4 activates ALX/FPR2 Receptor to Regulate Conjunctival Goblet Cell Secretion. *Mucosal Immunol.* 10, 46–57. doi: 10.1038/mi.2016.33

Hoegger, M. J., Fischer, A. J., McMenimen, J. D., Ostedgaard, L. S., Tucker, A. J., Awadalla, M. A., et al. (2014). Impaired mucus detachment disrupts mucociliary transport in a piglet model of cystic fibrosis. *Science* 345, 818–822. doi: 10.1126/science.1255825

Hoyt, J. C., and Robbins, R. A. (2001). Macrolide antibiotics and pulmonary inflammation. *FEMS Microbiol. Lett.* 205, 1–7. doi: 10.1111/j.1574-6968.2001.tb10917.x

Hsiao, H.-M., Thatcher, T. H., Levy, E. P., Fulton, R. A., Owens, K. M., Phipps, R. P., et al. (2014). Resolvin D1 Attenuates Polyinosinic-Polycytidylic Acid–Induced Inflammatory Signaling in Human Airway Epithelial Cells via TAK1. *J. Immunol.* 193, 4980–4987. doi: 10.4049/jimmunol.1400313

Hu, X., Shen, H., Wang, Y., Zhang, L., and Zhao, M. (2019). Aspirin-triggered resolvin D1 alleviates paraquat-induced acute lung injury in mice. *Life Sci.* 218, 38–46. doi: 10.1016/j.lfs.2018.12.028

Hubbard, V. S., Dunn, G. D., and di Sant'Agnese, P. A. (1977). Abnormal fatty-acid composition of plasma-lipids in cystic fibrosis. A primary or a secondary defect? *Lancet Lond. Engl.* 2, 1302–1304. doi: 10.1016/s0140-6736(77)90359-2

Hudson, V. M. (2001). Rethinking cystic fibrosis pathology: the critical role of abnormal reduced glutathione (GSH) transport caused by CFTR mutation. *Free Radic. Biol. Med.* 30, 1440–1461. doi: 10.1016/S0891-5849(01)00530-5

Hughes, G. W., Ridley, C., Collins, R., Roseman, A., Ford, R., and Thornton, D. J. (2019). The MUC5B mucin polymer is dominated by repeating structural motifs and its topology is regulated by calcium and pH. *Sci. Rep.* 9, 17350. doi: 10.1038/s41598-019-53768-0

Hybiske, K., Fu, Z., Schwarzer, C., Tseng, J., Do, J., Huang, N., et al. (2007). Effects of cystic fibrosis transmembrane conductance regulator and ΔF508CFTR on inflammatory response, ER stress, and Ca^{2+} of airway epithelia. *Am. J. Physiol.-Lung Cell. Mol. Physiol.* 293, L1250–L1260. doi: 10.1152/ajplung.00231.2007

Illek, B., Yankaskas, J. R., and Machen, T. E. (1997). cAMP and genistein stimulate HCO3- conductance through CFTR in human airway epithelia. *Am. J. Physiol.-Lung Cell. Mol. Physiol.* 272, L752–L761. doi: 10.1152/ajplung.1997.272.4.L752

Immler, R., Simon, S.II, and Sperandio, M. (2018). Calcium signalling and related ion channels in neutrophil recruitment and function. *Eur. J. Clin. Invest.* 48, e12964. doi: 10.1111/eci.12964

Inglis, S. K., Corboz, M. R., Taylor, A. E., and Ballard, S. T. (1997). Effect of anion transport inhibition on mucus secretion by airway submucosal glands. *Am. J. Physiol.-Lung Cell. Mol. Physiol.* 272, L372–L377. doi: 10.1152/ajplung.1997.272.2.L372

Inglis, S. K., Corboz, M. R., and Ballard, S. T. (1998). Effect of anion secretion inhibitors on mucin content of airway submucosal gland ducts. *Am. J. Physiol.-Lung Cell. Mol. Physiol.* 274, L762–L766. doi: 10.1152/ajplung.1998.274.5.L762

Inglis, S. K., Collett, A., McAlroy, H. L., Wilson, S. M., and Olver, R. E. (1999). Effect of luminal nucleotides on Cl- secretion and Na+ absorption in distal bronchi. *Pflugers Arch.* 438, 621–627. doi: 10.1007/s004249900096

Ismailov, I.II, Awayda, M. S., Jovov, B., Berdiev, B. K., Fuller, C. M., Dedman, J. R., et al. (1996). Regulation of epithelial sodium channels by the cystic fibrosis transmembrane conductance regulator. *J. Biol. Chem.* 271, 4725–4732. doi: 10.1074/jbc.271.9.4725

Isobe, Y., Arita, M., Matsueda, S., Iwamoto, R., Fujihara, T., Nakanishi, H., et al. (2012). Identification and structure determination of novel anti-inflammatory mediator resolvin E3, 17,18-dihydroxyeicosapentaenoic acid. *J. Biol. Chem.* 287, 10525–10534. doi: 10.1074/jbc.M112.340612

Isopi, E., Mattoscio, D., Codagnone, M., Mari, V. C., Lamolinara, A., Patruno, S., et al. (2020). Resolvin D1 Reduces Lung Infection and Inflammation Activating Resolution in Cystic Fibrosis. *Front. Immunol.* 11, 581. doi: 10.3389/fimmu.2020.00581

Itani, O. A., Chen, J.-H., Karp, P. H., Ernst, S., Keshavjee, S., Parekh, K., et al. (2011). Human cystic fibrosis airway epithelia have reduced Cl- conductance but not increased Na+ conductance. *Proc. Natl. Acad. Sci. U. S. A.* 108, 10260–10265. doi: 10.1073/pnas.1106695108

Itokazu, Y., Pagano, R. E., Schroeder, A. S., O'Grady, S. M., Limper, A. H., and Marks, D. L. (2014). Reduced GM1 ganglioside in CFTR-deficient human airway cells results in decreased β_1 -integrin signaling and delayed wound repair. *Am. J. Physiol.-Cell Physiol.* 306, C819–C830. doi: 10.1152/ajpcell.00168.2013

Jarosz-Griffiths, H. H., Scambler, T., Wong, C. H., Lara-Reyna, S., Holbrook, J., Martinon, F., et al. (2020). Different CFTR modulator combinations downregulate inflammation differently in cystic fibrosis. *eLife* 9, e54556. doi: 10.7554/eLife.54556

Jeanson, L., Guerrera, I. C., Papon, J. F., Chhuon, C., Zadigue, P., Prulière-Escabasse, V., et al. (2014). Proteomic analysis of nasal epithelial cells from cystic fibrosis patients. *PLoS One* 9, e108671. doi: 10.1371/journal.pone.0108671

Jiajia, D., Mingke, Z., Zenglin, L., Wei, W., Tao, W., Lei, C., et al. (2014). Resolvin-D1 inhibits interleukin-8 and hydrogen peroxide production induced by cigarette smoke extract in 16HBE cells via attenuating NF-κB activation. *Chin. Med. J. (Engl.)* 127 (3), 511–517. doi: 10.3760/cma.j.issn.0366-6999.20131674

Jozsef, L., Zouki, C., Petasis, N. A., Serhan, C. N., and Filep, J. G. (2002). Lipoxin A4 and aspirin-triggered 15-epi-lipoxin A4 inhibit peroxynitrite formation, NF- B and AP-1 activation, and IL-8 gene expression in human leukocytes. *Proc. Natl. Acad. Sci.* 99, 13266–13271. doi: 10.1073/pnas.202296999

Jungas, T., Motta, I., Duffieux, F., Fanen, P., Stoven, V., and Ojcius, D. M. (2002). Glutathione Levels and BAX Activation during Apoptosis Due to Oxidative Stress in Cells Expressing Wild-type and Mutant Cystic Fibrosis Transmembrane Conductance Regulator. *J. Biol. Chem.* 277, 27912–27918. doi: 10.1074/jbc.M110288200

Kakazu, A., He, J., Kenchegowda, S., and Bazan, H. E. P. (2012). Lipoxin A4 inhibits platelet-activating factor inflammatory response and stimulates corneal wound healing of injuries that compromise the stroma. *Exp. Eye Res.* 103, 9–16. doi: 10.1016/j.exer.2012.07.008

Karp, C. L., Flick, L. M., Park, K. W., Softic, S., Greer, T. M., Keledjian, R., et al. (2004). Defective lipoxin-mediated anti-inflammatory activity in the cystic fibrosis airway. *Nat. Immunol.* 5, 388–392. doi: 10.1038/ni1056

Karra, L., Haworth, O., Priluck, R., Levy, B. D., and Levi-Schaffer, F. (2015). Lipoxin B_4; promotes the resolution of allergic inflammation in the upper and lower airways of mice. *Mucosal Immunol.* 8, 852–862. doi: 10.1038/mi.2014.116

Katz, S., Schöni, M. H., and Bridges, M. A. (1984). The calcium hypothesis of Cystic Fibrosis. *Cell Calcium* 5, 421–440. doi: 10.1016/0143-4160(84)90021-6

Keiser, N. W., Birket, S. E., Evans, I. A., Tyler, S. R., Crooke, A. K., Sun, X., et al. (2015). Defective innate immunity and hyperinflammation in newborn cystic fibrosis transmembrane conductance regulator-knockout ferret lungs. *Am. J. Respir. Cell Mol. Biol.* 52, 683–694. doi: 10.1165/rcmb.2014-0250OC

Kelly-Aubert, M., Trudel, S., Fritsch, J., Nguyen-Khoa, T., Baudouin-Legros, M., Moriceau, S., et al. (2011). GSH monoethyl ester rescues mitochondrial defects in cystic fibrosis models. *Hum. Mol. Genet.* 20, 2745–2759. doi: 10.1093/hmg/ddr173

Kenchegowda, S., Bazan, N. G., and Bazan, H. E. P. (2011). EGF Stimulates Lipoxin A4 Synthesis and Modulates Repair in Corneal Epithelial Cells through ERK and p38 Activation. *Investig. Opthalmol. Vis. Sci.* 52, 2240. doi: 10.1167/iovs.10-6199

Kerbiriou, M., Le Drévo, M.-A., Férec, C., and Trouvé, P. (2007). Coupling cystic fibrosis to endoplasmic reticulum stress: Differential role of Grp78 and ATF6. *Biochim. Biophys. Acta BBA - Mol. Basis Dis.* 1772, 1236–1249. doi: 10.1016/j.bbadis.2007.10.004

Kerem, B., Rommens, J. M., Buchanan, J. A., Markiewicz, D., Cox, T. K., Chakravarti, A., et al. (1989). Identification of the cystic fibrosis gene: genetic analysis. *Science* 245, 1073–1080. doi: 10.1126/science.2570460

Kerem, E., Corey, M., Kerem, B. S., Rommens, J., Markiewicz, D., Levison, H., et al. (1990). The relation between genotype and phenotype in cystic fibrosis–analysis of the most common mutation (delta F508). *N. Engl. J. Med.* 323, 1517–1522. doi: 10.1056/NEJM199011293232203

Kettle, A. J., Turner, R., Gangell, C. L., Harwood, D. T., Khalilova, I. S., Chapman, A. L., et al. (2014). Oxidation contributes to low glutathione in the airways of children with cystic fibrosis. *Eur. Respir. J.* 44, 122–129. doi: 10.1183/09031936.00170213

Khan, T. Z., Wagener, J. S., Bost, T., Martinez, J., Accurso, F. J., and Riches, D. W. (1995). Early pulmonary inflammation in infants with cystic fibrosis. *Am. J. Respir. Crit. Care Med.* 151, 1075–1082. doi: 10.1164/ajrccm/151.4.1075

Kim, D., Kim, J., Burghardt, B., Best, L., and Steward, M. C. (2014). Role of anion exchangers in Cl- and HCO3- secretion by the human airway epithelial cell line Calu-3. *Am. J. Physiol.-Cell Physiol.* 307, C208–C219. doi: 10.1152/ajpcell.00083.2014

Knorre, A., Wagner, M., Schaefer, H.-E., Colledge, W. H., and Pahl, H. L. (2002). deltaF508-CFTR Causes Constitutive NF-kB Activation through an ER-Overload Response in Cystic Fibrosis Lungs. *Biol. Chem.* 383, 271–282. doi: 10.1515/BC.2002.029

Knowles, M. R., and Boucher, R. C. (2002). Mucus clearance as a primary innate defense mechanism for mammalian airways. *J. Clin. Invest.* 109, 571–577. doi: 10.1172/JCI15217

König, J., Schreiber, R., Voelcker, T., Mall, M., and Kunzelmann, K. (2001). The cystic fibrosis transmembrane conductance regulator (CFTR) inhibits ENaC through an increase in the intracellular Cl– concentration. *EMBO Rep.* 2, 1047–1051. doi: 10.1093/embo-reports/kve232

Konstan, M. W., Walenga, R. W., Hilliard, K. A., and Hilliard, J. B. (1993). Leukotriene B4 markedly elevated in the epithelial lining fluid of patients with cystic fibrosis. *Am. Rev. Respir. Dis.* 148, 896–901. doi: 10.1164/ajrccm/148.4_Pt_1.896

Konstan, M. W., Morgan, W. J., Butler, S. M., Pasta, D. J., Craib, M. L., Silva, S. J., et al. (2007). Risk factors for rate of decline in forced expiratory volume in one second in children and adolescents with cystic fibrosis. *J. Pediatr.* 151134–139, 139.e1. doi: 10.1016/j.jpeds.2007.03.006

Kotas, M. E., and Medzhitov, R. (2015). Homeostasis, inflammation, and disease susceptibility. *Cell* 160, 816–827. doi: 10.1016/j.cell.2015.02.010

Krishnamoorthy, S., Recchiuti, A., Chiang, N., Yacoubian, S., Lee, C.-H., Yang, R., et al. (2010). Resolvin D1 binds human phagocytes with evidence for proresolving receptors. *Proc. Natl. Acad. Sci. U. S. A.* 107, 1660–1665. doi: 10.1073/pnas.0907342107

Krishnamoorthy, N., Burkett, P. R., Dalli, J., Abdulnour, R. E., Colas, R., Ramon, S., et al. (2015). Cutting edge: maresin-1 engages regulatory T cells to limit type 2 innate lymphoid cell activation and promote resolution of lung inflammation. *J. Immunol.* 194, 863–867. doi: 10.4049/jimmunol.1402534

Kunzelmann, K., Kathöfer, S., and Greger, R. (1995). Na+ and Cl- conductances in airway epithelial cells: increased Na+ conductance in cystic fibrosis. *Pflugers Arch.* 431, 1–9. doi: 10.1007/bf00374371

Kunzelmann, K., Schreiber, R., Nitschke, R., and Mall, M. (2000). Control of epithelial Na+ conductance by the cystic fibrosis transmembrane conductance regulator. *Pflugers Arch.* 440, 193–201. doi: 10.1007/s004240000255

Kunzelmann, K. (2003). ENaC is inhibited by an increase in the intracellular Cl(-) concentration mediated through activation of Cl(-) channels. *Pflugers Arch.* 445, 504–512. doi: 10.1007/s00424-002-0958-y

Kuo, P. T., Huang, N. N., and Bassett, D. R. (1962). The fatty acid composition of the serum chylomicrons and adipose tissue of children with cystic fibrosis of the pancreas. *J. Pediatr.* 60, 394–403. doi: 10.1016/s0022-3476(62)80065-1

Kushwah, R., Gagnon, S., and Sweezey, N. B. (2014). T cell unresponsiveness in a pediatric cystic fibrosis patient: a case report. *Allergy Asthma Clin. Immunol.* 10:2. doi: 10.1186/1710-1492-10-2

Lance, K. D., Chatterjee, A., Wu, B., Mottola, G., Nuhn, H., Lee, P. P., et al. (2017). Unidirectional and Sustained Delivery of the Pro-Resolving Lipid Mediator Resolvin D1 from a Biodegradable Thin Film Device. *J. Biomed. Mater. Res. A* 105, 31–41. doi: 10.1002/jbm.a.35861

Lands, L. C., and Stanojevic, S. (2013). Oral non-steroidal anti-inflammatory drug therapy for lung disease in cystic fibrosis. *Cochrane Database Syst. Rev.* 6: CD001505. doi: 10.1002/14651858.CD001505.pub3

Lara-Reyna, S., Scambler, T., Holbrook, J., Wong, C., Jarosz-Griffiths, H. H., Martinon, F., et al. (2019). Metabolic Reprograming of Cystic Fibrosis Macrophages via the IRE1α Arm of the Unfolded Protein Response Results in Exacerbated Inflammation. *Front. Immunol.* 10, 1789. doi: 10.3389/fimmu.2019.01789

Lazrak, A., Jurkuvenaite, A., Chen, L., Keeling, K. M., Collawn, J. F., Bedwell, D. M., et al. (2011). Enhancement of alveolar epithelial sodium channel activity with decreased cystic fibrosis transmembrane conductance regulator expression in mouse lung. *Am. J. Physiol. Lung Cell. Mol. Physiol.* 301, L557–L567. doi: 10.1152/ajplung.00094.2011

Lee, H. N., and Surh, Y. J. (2013). Resolvin D1-mediated NOX2 inactivation rescues macrophages undertaking efferocytosis from oxidative stress-induced apoptosis. *Biochem. Pharmacol.* 86, 759–769. doi: 10.1016/j.bcp.2013.07.002

Lee, T. H., Horton, C. E., Kyan-Aung, U., Haskard, D., Crea, A. E., and Spur, B. W. (1989). Lipoxin A4 and lipoxin B4 inhibit chemotactic responses of human neutrophils stimulated by leukotriene B4 and N-formyl-L-methionyl-L-leucyl-L-phenylalanine. *Clin. Sci. Lond. Engl. 1979* 77, 195–203. doi: 10.1042/cs0770195

Lee, T. H., Crea, A. E., Gant, V., Spur, B. W., Marron, B. E., Nicolaou, K. C., et al. (1990). Identification of lipoxin A4 and its relationship to the sulfidopeptide leukotrienes C4, D4, and E4 in the bronchoalveolar lavage fluids obtained from patients with selected pulmonary diseases. *Am. Rev. Respir. Dis.* 141, 1453–1458. doi: 10.1164/ajrccm/141.6.1453

Lee, H.-N., Kundu, J. K., Cha, Y.-N., and Surh, Y.-J. (2013). Resolvin D1 stimulates efferocytosis through p50/p50-mediated suppression of tumor necrosis factor-expression. *J. Cell Sci.* 126, 4037–4047. doi: 10.1242/jcs.131003

Levy, B. D., and Serhan, C. N. (2000). A novel polyisoprenyl phosphate signaling cascade in human neutrophils. *Ann. N. Acad. Sci.* 905, 69–80. doi: 10.1111/j.1749-6632.2000.tb06539.x

Levy, B. D., Fokin, V. V., Clark, J. M., Wakelam, M. J., Petasis, N. A., and Serhan, C. N. (1999). Polyisoprenyl phosphate (PIPP) signaling regulates phospholipase D activity: a "stop" signaling switch for aspirin-triggered lipoxin A4. *FASEB J.* 13, 903–911. doi: 10.1096/fasebj.13.8.903

Levy, B. D., Clish, C. B., Schmidt, B., Gronert, K., and Serhan, C. N. (2001). Lipid mediator class switching during acute inflammation: signals in resolution. *Nat. Immunol.* 2, 612–619. doi: 10.1038/89759

Levy, B. D., Bonnans, C., Silverman, E. S., Palmer, L. J., Marigowda, G., Israel, E., et al. (2005a). Diminished lipoxin biosynthesis in severe asthma. *Am. J. Respir. Crit. Care Med.* 172, 824–830. doi: 10.1164/rccm.200410-1413OC

Levy, B. D., Hickey, L., Morris, A. J., Larvie, M., Keledjian, R., Petasis, N. A., et al. (2005b). Novel polyisoprenyl phosphates block phospholipase D and human neutrophil activation in vitro and murine peritoneal inflammation in vivo. *Br. J. Pharmacol.* 146, 344–351. doi: 10.1038/sj.bjp.0706338

Levy, B. D., Kohli, P., Gotlinger, K., Haworth, O., Hong, S., Kazani, S., et al. (2007). Protectin D1 is generated in asthma and dampens airway inflammation and hyperresponsiveness. *J. Immunol.* 178, 496–502. doi: 10.4049/jimmunol.178.1.496

Ley, K., Laudanna, C., Cybulsky, M.II, and Nourshargh, S. (2007). Getting to the site of inflammation: the leukocyte adhesion cascade updated. *Nat. Rev. Immunol.* 7, 678–689. doi: 10.1038/nri2156

Li, D., Hodges, R. R., Jiao, J., Carozza, R. B., Shatos, M. A., Chiang, N., et al. (2013). Resolvin D1 and aspirin-triggered resolvin D1 regulate histamine-stimulated conjunctival goblet cell secretion. *Mucosal Immunol.* 6, 1119–1130. doi: 10.1038/mi.2013.7

Liao, Z., Dong, J., Wu, W., Yang, T., Wang, T., Guo, L., et al. (2012). Resolvin D1 attenuates inflammation in lipopolysaccharide-induced acute lung injury through a process involving the PPARγ/NF-κB pathway. *Respir. Res.* 13:110. doi: 10.1186/1465-9921-13-110

Lim, S. H., Legere, E.-A., Snider, J., and Stagljar, I. (2018). Recent Progress in CFTR Interactome Mapping and Its Importance for Cystic Fibrosis. *Front. Pharmacol.* 8, 997. doi: 10.3389/fphar.2017.00997

Lin, J. H., Walter, P., and Yen, T. S. B. (2008). Endoplasmic Reticulum Stress in Disease Pathogenesis. *Annu. Rev. Pathol. Mech. Dis.* 3, 399–425. doi: 10.1146/annurev.pathmechdis.3.121806.151434

Linsdell, P., and Hanrahan, J. W. (1998). Glutathione permeability of CFTR. *Am. J. Physiol.-Cell Physiol.* 275, C323–C326. doi: 10.1152/ajpcell.1998.275.1.C323

Linsdell, P. (2017). Architecture and functional properties of the CFTR channel pore. *Cell. Mol. Life Sci. CMLS* 74, 67–83. doi: 10.1007/s00018-016-2389-5

Lippestad, M., Hodges, R. R., Utheim, T. P., Serhan, C. N., and Dartt, D. A. (2017). Resolvin D1 Increases Mucin Secretion in Cultured Rat Conjunctival Goblet Cells via Multiple Signaling Pathways. *Investig. Opthalmol. Vis. Sci.* 58, 4530. doi: 10.1167/iovs.17-21914

Lippestad, M., Hodges, R. R., Utheim, T. P., Serhan, C. N., and Dartt, D. A. (2018). Signaling pathways activated by resolvin E1 to stimulate mucin secretion and increase intracellular Ca 2+ in cultured rat conjunctival goblet cells. *Exp. Eye Res.* 173, 64–72. doi: 10.1016/j.exer.2018.04.015

Liu, M., Chen, S., Shang, Y., and Yao, S. (2018). Aspirin-triggered lipoxin A4 attenuates lipopolysaccharide-induced acute lung injury by inhibiting activation of mitogen-activated protein kinases and NF-κB in mice. *Int. J. Clin. Exp. Pathol.* 11, 2570–2578.

Lloyd-Still, J. D., Powers, C. A., Hoffman, D. R., Boyd-Trull, K., Lester, L. A., Benisek, D. C., et al. (2006). Bioavailability and safety of a high dose of docosahexaenoic acid triacylglycerol of algal origin in cystic fibrosis patients: a randomized, controlled study. *Nutr. Burbank Los Angel. Cty. Calif* 22, 36–46. doi: 10.1016/j.nut.2005.05.006

Lopes-Pacheco, M. (2019). CFTR Modulators: The Changing Face of Cystic Fibrosis in the Era of Precision Medicine. *Front. Pharmacol.* 10, 1662. doi: 10.3389/fphar.2019.01662

MacNee, W. (2001). Oxidative stress and lung inflammation in airways disease. *Eur. J. Pharmacol.* 429, 195–207. doi: 10.1016/S0014-2999(01)01320-6

Maddox, J. F., Hachicha, M., Takano, T., Petasis, N. A., Fokin, V. V., and Serhan, C. N. (1997). Lipoxin A4 stable analogs are potent mimetics that stimulate human monocytes and THP-1 cells via a G-protein-linked lipoxin A4 receptor. *J. Biol. Chem.* 272, 6972–6978. doi: 10.1074/jbc.272.11.6972

Mall, M., Grubb, B. R., Harkema, J. R., O'Neal, W. K., and Boucher, R. C. (2004). Increased airway epithelial Na+ absorption produces cystic fibrosis-like lung disease in mice. *Nat. Med.* 10, 487–493. doi: 10.1038/nm1028

Marino, C. R., Matovcik, L. M., Gorelick, F. S., and Cohn, J. A. (1991). Localization of the cystic fibrosis transmembrane conductance regulator in pancreas. *J. Clin. Invest.* 88, 712–716. doi: 10.1172/JCI115358

Marson, F. A., de, L., Bertuzzo, C. S., Secolin, R., Ribeiro, A. F., and Ribeiro, J. D. (2013). Genetic interaction of GSH metabolic pathway genes in cystic fibrosis. *BMC Med. Genet.* 14, 60. doi: 10.1186/1471-2350-14-60

Marson, F. A., de, F. A., Bertuzzo, C. S., Ribeiro, A. F., and Ribeiro, J. D. (2014). Polymorphisms in the glutathione pathway modulate cystic fibrosis severity: a cross-sectional study. *BMC Med. Genet.* 15, 27. doi: 10.1186/1471-2350-15-27

Martínez, T. M., Llapur, C. J., Williams, T. H., Coates, C., Gunderman, R., Cohen, M. D., et al. (2005). High-resolution computed tomography imaging of airway disease in infants with cystic fibrosis. *Am. J. Respir. Crit. Care Med.* 172, 1133–1138. doi: 10.1164/rccm.200412-1665OC

Mas, E., Croft, K. D., Zahra, P., Barden, A., and Mori, T. A. (2012). Resolvins D1, D2, and other mediators of self-limited resolution of inflammation in human blood following n-3 fatty acid supplementation. *Clin. Chem.* 58, 1476–1484. doi: 10.1373/clinchem.2012.190199

Matte, A., Recchiuti, A., Federti, E., Koehl, B., Mintz, T., El Nemer, W., et al. (2019). Resolution of sickle cell disease–associated inflammation and tissue damage with 17R-resolvin D1. *Blood* 133, 252–265. doi: 10.1182/blood-2018-07-865378

Mattoscio, D., Evangelista, V., De Cristofaro, R., Recchiuti, A., Pandolfi, A., Di Silvestre, S., et al. (2010). Cystic fibrosis transmembrane conductance regulator (CFTR) expression in human platelets: impact on mediators and mechanisms of the inflammatory response. *FASEB J.* 24, 3970–3980. doi: 10.1096/fj.10-159921

Maurice, N. M., Bedi, B., Yuan, Z., Goldberg, J. B., Koval, M., Hart, C. M., et al. (2019). Pseudomonas aeruginosa Induced Host Epithelial Cell Mitochondrial Dysfunction. *Sci. Rep.* 9, 11929. doi: 10.1038/s41598-019-47457-1

McKiernan, P. J., and Greene, C. M. (2015). MicroRNA Dysregulation in Cystic Fibrosis. *Mediators Inflamm.* 2015:529642. doi: 10.1155/2015/529642

McShane, D., Davies, J. C., Davies, M. G., Bush, A., Geddes, D. M., and Alton, E. W. F. W. (2003). Airway surface pH in subjects with cystic fibrosis. *Eur. Respir. J.* 21, 37–42. doi: 10.1183/09031936.03.00027603

Mekus, F., Ballmann, M., Bronsveld, I., Bijman, J., Veeze, H., and Tümmler, B. (2000). Categories of deltaF508 homozygous cystic fibrosis twin and sibling pairs with distinct phenotypic characteristics. *Twin Res.* 3, 277–293. doi: 10.1375/136905200320565256

Miele, L., Cordella-Miele, E., Xing, M., Frizzell, R., and Mukherjee, A. B. (1997). Cystic fibrosis gene mutation (deltaF508) is associated with an intrinsic abnormality in Ca2+-induced arachidonic acid release by epithelial cells. *DNA Cell Biol.* 16, 749–759. doi: 10.1089/dna.1997.16.749

Mills, C. D., Kincaid, K., Alt, J. M., Heilman, M. J., and Hill, A. M. (2000). M-1/M-2 macrophages and the Th1/Th2 paradigm. *J. Immunol. Baltim. Md 1950* 164, 6166–6173. doi: 10.4049/jimmunol.164.12.6166

Mirakaj, V., Dalli, J., Granja, T., Rosenberger, P., and Serhan, C. N. (2014). Vagus nerve controls resolution and pro-resolving mediators of inflammation. *J. Exp. Med.* 211, 1037–1048. doi: 10.1084/jem.20132103

Mitchell, S., Thomas, G., Harvey, K., Cottell, D., Reville, K., Berlasconi, G., et al. (2002). Lipoxins, aspirin-triggered epi-lipoxins, lipoxin stable analogues, and the resolution of inflammation: stimulation of macrophage phagocytosis of apoptotic neutrophils in vivo. *J. Am. Soc. Nephrol.* 13, 2497–2507. doi: 10.1097/01.asn.0000032417.73640.72

Montgomery, S. T., Mall, M. A., Kicic, A., Stick, S. M., and AREST, C. F. (2017). Hypoxia and sterile inflammation in cystic fibrosis airways: mechanisms and potential therapies. *Eur. Respir. J.* 49 (1), 1600903. doi: 10.1183/13993003.00903-2016

Morris, T., Stables, M., Hobbs, A., de Souza, P., Colville-Nash, P., Warner, T., et al. (2009). Effects of low-dose aspirin on acute inflammatory responses in humans. *J. Immunol. Baltim. Md 1950* 183, 2089–2096. doi: 10.4049/jimmunol.0900477

Motwani, M. P., Bennett, F., Norris, P. C., Maini, A. A., George, M. J., Newson, J., et al. (2018a). Potent Anti-Inflammatory and Pro-Resolving Effects of Anabasum in a Human Model of Self-Resolving Acute Inflammation. *Clin. Pharmacol. Ther.* 104, 675–686. doi: 10.1002/cpt.980

Motwani, M. P., Colas, R. A., George, M. J., Flint, J. D., Dalli, J., Richard-Loendt, A., et al. (2018b). Pro-resolving mediators promote resolution in a human skin model of UV-killed Escherichia coli-driven acute inflammation. *JCI Insight* 3 (6), e94463. doi: 10.1172/jci.insight.94463

Muhlebach, M. S., and Noah, T. L. (2002). Endotoxin activity and inflammatory markers in the airways of young patients with cystic fibrosis. *Am. J. Respir. Crit. Care Med.* 165, 911–915. doi: 10.1164/ajrccm.165.7.2107114

Muhlebach, M. S., Stewart, P. W., Leigh, M. W., and Noah, T. L. (1999). Quantitation of inflammatory responses to bacteria in young cystic fibrosis and control patients. *Am. J. Respir. Crit. Care Med.* 160, 186–191. doi: 10.1164/ajrccm.160.1.9808096

Nathan, C., and Ding, A. (2010). Nonresolving inflammation. *Cell* 140, 871–882. doi: 10.1016/j.cell.2010.02.029

Nathan, C. (2002). Points of control in inflammation. *Nature* 420, 846–852. doi: 10.1038/nature01320

Nigam, S., Fiore, S., Luscinskas, F. W., and Serhan, C. N. (1990). Lipoxin A4 and lipoxin B4 stimulate the release but not the oxygenation of arachidonic acid in human neutrophils: dissociation between lipid remodeling and adhesion. *J. Cell Physiol.* 143, 512–523. doi: 10.1002/jcp.1041430316

Nixon, G. M., Armstrong, D. S., Carzino, R., Carlin, J. B., Olinsky, A., Robertson, C. F., et al. (2001). Clinical outcome after early Pseudomonas aeruginosa infection in cystic fibrosis. *J. Pediatr.* 138, 699–704. doi: 10.1067/mpd.2001.112897

Noah, T. L., Black, H. R., Cheng, P. W., Wood, R. E., and Leigh, M. W. (1997). Nasal and bronchoalveolar lavage fluid cytokines in early cystic fibrosis. *J. Infect. Dis.* 175, 638–647. doi: 10.1093/infdis/175.3.638

Norling, L. V., Headland, S. E., Dalli, J., Arnardottir, H. H., Haworth, O., Jones, H. R., et al. (2016). Proresolving and cartilage-protective actions of resolvin D1 in inflammatory arthritis. *JCI Insight* 1, e85922. doi: 10.1172/jci.insight.85922

Norris, P. C., Libreros, S., and Serhan, C. N. (2019). Resolution metabolomes activated by hypoxic environment. *Sci. Adv.* 5, eaax4895. doi: 10.1126/sciadv.aax4895

Odusanwo, O., Chinthamani, S., McCall, A., Duffey, M. E., and Baker, O. J. (2012). Resolvin D1 prevents TNF-α-mediated disruption of salivary epithelial formation. *Am. J. Physiol.-Cell Physiol.* 302, C1331–C1345. doi: 10.1152/ajpcell.00207.2011

Oh, S. F., Dona, M., Fredman, G., Krishnamoorthy, S., Irimia, D., and Serhan, C. N. (2012). Resolvin E2 formation and impact in inflammation-resolution. *J. Immunol. Baltim. Md 1950* 188, 4527–4534. doi: 10.4049/jimmunol.1103652

Oliver, C., and Watson, H. (2016). Omega-3 fatty acids for cystic fibrosis. *Cochrane Database Syst. Rev.* 2016 (1), CD002201. doi: 10.1002/14651858.CD002201.pub5

Olsen, M. V., Lyngstadaas, A. V., Bair, J. A., Hodges, R. R., Utheim, T. P., Serhan, C. N., et al. (2020). Maresin 1, a specialized proresolving mediator, stimulates intracellular [Ca2+] and secretion in conjunctival goblet cells. *J. Cell. Physiol.* 1–14. doi: 10.1002/jcp.29846

Olveira, C., Padilla, A., Dorado, A., Contreras, V., Garcia-Fuentes, E., Rubio-Martin, E., et al. (2017). Inflammation and Oxidation Biomarkers in Patients with Cystic Fibrosis: The Influence of Azithromycin. *Eurasian J. Med.* 49, 118–123. doi: 10.5152/eurasianjmed.2017.17010

Orr, S. K., Colas, R. A., Dalli, J., Chiang, N., and Serhan, C. N. (2015). Proresolving actions of a new resolvin D1 analog mimetic qualifies as an immunoresolvent. *Am. J. Physiol. Lung Cell Mol. Physiol.* 308, L904–L911. doi: 10.1152/ajplung.00370.2014

Ostedgaard, L. S., Moninger, T. O., McMenimen, J. D., Sawin, N. M., Parker, C. P., Thornell, I. M., et al. (2017). Gel-forming mucins form distinct morphologic structures in airways. *Proc. Natl. Acad. Sci. U. S. A.* 114, 6842–6847. doi: 10.1073/pnas.1703228114

Owens, J. M., Shroyer, K. R., and Kingdom, T. T. (2008). Expression of cyclooxygenase and lipoxygenase enzymes in sinonasal mucosa of patients with cystic fibrosis. *Arch. Otolaryngol. Head Neck Surg.* 134, 825–831. doi: 10.1001/archotol.134.8.825

Papayianni, A., Serhan, C. N., and Brady, H. R. (1996). Lipoxin A4 and B4 inhibit leukotriene-stimulated interactions of human neutrophils and endothelial cells. *J. Immunol.* 156, 2264–2272.

Park, H. S., Kim, S. R., and Lee, Y. C. (2009). Impact of oxidative stress on lung diseases. *Respirology* 14, 27–38. doi: 10.1111/j.1440-1843.2008.01447.x

Perez-Vilar, J., and Boucher, R. C. (2004). Reevaluating gel-forming mucins' roles in cystic fibrosis lung disease. *Free Radic. Biol. Med.* 37, 1564–1577. doi: 10.1016/j.freeradbiomed.2004.07.027

Perretti, M., and D'Acquisto, F. (2009). Annexin A1 and glucocorticoids as effectors of the resolution of inflammation. *Nat. Rev. Immunol.* 9, 62–70. doi: 10.1038/nri2470

Perretti, M., Chiang, N., La, M., Fierro, I. M., Marullo, S., Getting, S. J., et al. (2002a). Endogenous lipid- and peptide-derived anti-inflammatory pathways generated with glucocorticoid and aspirin treatment activate the lipoxin A4 receptor. *Nat. Med.* 8, 1296–1302. doi: 10.1038/nm786

Perretti, M., Chiang, N., La, M., Fierro, I. M., Marullo, S., Getting, S. J., et al. (2002b). Endogenous lipid- and peptide-derived anti-inflammatory pathways generated with glucocorticoid and aspirin treatment activate the lipoxin A4 receptor. *Nat. Med.* 8, 1296–1302. doi: 10.1038/nm786

Pezzulo, A. A., Tang, X. X., Hoegger, M. J., Abou Alaiwa, M. H., Ramachandran, S., Moninger, T. O., et al. (2012). Reduced airway surface pH impairs bacterial killing in the porcine cystic fibrosis lung. *Nature* 487, 109–113. doi: 10.1038/nature11130

Philippe, R., and Urbach, V. (2018). Specialized Pro-Resolving Lipid Mediators in Cystic Fibrosis. *Int. J. Mol. Sci.* 19 (10), 2865. doi: 10.3390/ijms19102865

Philippe, R., Antigny, F., Buscaglia, P., Norez, C., Becq, F., Frieden, M., et al. (2015). SERCA and PMCA pumps contribute to the deregulation of Ca2+ homeostasis in human CF epithelial cells. *Biochim. Biophys. Acta BBA - Mol. Cell Res.* 1853, 892–903. doi: 10.1016/j.bbamcr.2015.01.010

Pierdomenico, A. M., Recchiuti, A., Simiele, F., Codagnone, M., Mari, V. C., Davì, G., et al. (2015). MicroRNA-181b Regulates ALX/FPR2 Receptor Expression and Proresolution Signaling in Human Macrophages. *J. Biol. Chem.* 290, 3592–3600. doi: 10.1074/jbc.M114.592352

Pierdomenico, A. M., Patruno, S., Codagnone, M., Simiele, F., Mari, V. C., Plebani, R., et al. (2017). microRNA-181b is increased in cystic fibrosis cells and impairs lipoxin A4 receptor-dependent mechanisms of inflammation resolution and antimicrobial defense. *Sci. Rep.* 7, 13519. doi: 10.1038/s41598-017-14055-y

Pillarisetti, N., Williamson, E., Linnane, B., Skoric, B., Robertson, C. F., Robinson, P., et al. (2011). Infection, inflammation, and lung function decline in infants with cystic fibrosis. *Am. J. Respir. Crit. Care Med.* 184, 75–81. doi: 10.1164/rccm.201011-1892OC

Pinhal-Enfield, G., Ramanathan, M., Hasko, G., Vogel, S. N., Salzman, A. L., Boons, G.-J., et al. (2003). An Angiogenic Switch in Macrophages Involving Synergy between Toll-Like Receptors 2, 4, 7, and 9 and Adenosine A2A Receptors. *Am. J. Pathol.* 163, 711–721. doi: 10.1016/S0002-9440(10)63698-X

Pistorius, K., Souza, P. R., De Matteis, R., Austin-Williams, S., Primdahl, K. G., Vik, A., et al. (2018). PDn-3 DPA Pathway Regulates Human Monocyte Differentiation and Macrophage Function. *Cell Chem. Biol.* 25, 749–760.e9. doi: 10.1016/j.chembiol.2018.04.017

Planagumà, A., Kazani, S., Marigowda, G., Haworth, O., Mariani, T. J., Israel, E., et al. (2008). Airway lipoxin A4 generation and lipoxin A4 receptor expression are decreased in severe asthma. *Am. J. Respir. Crit. Care Med.* 178, 574–582. doi: 10.1164/rccm.200801-061OC

Pongnimitprasert, N., Hurtado, M., Lamari, F., El Benna, J., Dupuy, C., Fay, M., et al. (2012). Implication of NADPH Oxidases in the Early Inflammation Process Generated by Cystic Fibrosis Cells. *ISRN Inflamm.* 2012, 1–11. doi: 10.5402/2012/481432

Porto, P. D., Cifani, N., Guarnieri, S., Di Domenico, E. G., Mariggiò, M. A., Spadaro, F., et al. (2011). Dysfunctional CFTR Alters the Bactericidal Activity of Human Macrophages against Pseudomonas aeruginosa. *PLoS One* 6 (5), e19970. doi: 10.1371/journal.pone.0019970

Posso, S. V., Quesnot, N., Moraes, J. A., Brito-Gitirana, L., Kennedy-Feitosa, E., Barroso, M. V., et al. (2018). AT-RVD1 repairs mouse lung after cigarette smoke-induced emphysema via downregulation of oxidative stress by NRF2/KEAP1 pathway. *Int. Immunopharmacol.* 56, 330–338. doi: 10.1016/j.intimp.2018.01.045

Poulsen, J. H., Fischer, H., Illek, B., and Machen, T. E. (1994). Bicarbonate conductance and pH regulatory capability of cystic fibrosis transmembrane conductance regulator. *Proc. Natl. Acad. Sci.* 91, 5340–5344. doi: 10.1073/pnas.91.12.5340

Psychogios, N., Hau, D. D., Peng, J., Guo, A. C., Mandal, R., Bouatra, S., et al. (2011). The Human Serum Metabolome. *PLoS One* 6 (2), e16957. doi: 10.1371/journal.pone.0016957

Quinton, P. M. (2008). Cystic fibrosis: impaired bicarbonate secretion and mucoviscidosis. *Lancet* 372, 415–417. doi: 10.1016/S0140-6736(08)61162-9

Raetz, C. R. H., and Whitfield, C. (2002). Lipopolysaccharide Endotoxins. *Annu. Rev. Biochem.* 71, 635–700. doi: 10.1146/annurev.biochem.71.110601.135414

Ranganathan, S. C., Hall, G. L., Sly, P. D., Stick, S. M., Douglas, T. A.Australian Respiratory Early Surveillance Team for Cystic Fibrosis (AREST-CF) (2017). Early Lung Disease in Infants and Preschool Children with Cystic Fibrosis. What Have We Learned and What Should We Do about It? *Am. J. Respir. Crit. Care Med.* 195, 1567–1575. doi: 10.1164/rccm.201606-1107CI

Recchiuti, A., Krishnamoorthy, S., Fredman, G., Chiang, N., and Serhan, C. N. (2011). MicroRNAs in resolution of acute inflammation: identification of novel resolvin D1-miRNA circuits. *FASEB J.* 25, 544–560. doi: 10.1096/fj.10-169599

Recchiuti, A., Codagnone, M., Pierdomenico, A. M., Rossi, C., Mari, V. C., Cianci, E., et al. (2014). Immunoresolving actions of oral resolvin D1 include selective regulation of the transcription machinery in resolution-phase mouse macrophages. *FASEB J.* 28, 3090–3102. doi: 10.1096/fj.13-248393

Ribeiro, C. M. P., Zhang, G., Lubamba, B. A., and Tepper, M. A. (2017). Anabasum Reduces Excessive Inflammatory Responses in Cystic Fibrosis Patient-Derived Lung Macrophages. In: *PEDIATRIC PULMONOLOGY* (NJ USA: WILEY). Vol. 52, pp. S251–S251.

Ribeiro, C. M. P., Paradiso, A. M., Carew, M. A., Shears, S. B., and Boucher, R. C. (2005a). Cystic Fibrosis Airway Epithelial Ca2+i Signaling: The Mechanism For The Larger Agonist-Mediated Ca2+i Signals In Human Cystic Fibrosis Airway Epithelia. *J. Biol. Chem.* 280, 10202–10209. doi: 10.1074/jbc.M410617200

Ribeiro, C. M. P., Paradiso, A. M., Schwab, U., Perez-Vilar, J., Jones, L., O'Neal, W., et al. (2005b). Chronic Airway Infection/Inflammation Induces a Ca2+i-dependent Hyperinflammatory Response in Human Cystic Fibrosis Airway Epithelia. *J. Biol. Chem.* 280, 17798–17806. doi: 10.1074/jbc.M410618200

Ribeiro, C. M. P. (2006). The Role of Intracellular Calcium Signals in Inflammatory Responses of Polarised Cystic Fibrosis Human Airway Epithelia. *Drugs R. D.* 7, 17–31. doi: 10.2165/00126839-200607010-00002

Ringholz, F. C., Buchanan, P. J., Clarke, D. T., Millar, R. G., McDermott, M., Linnane, B., et al. (2014). Reduced 15-lipoxygenase 2 and lipoxin A4/leukotriene B4 ratio in children with cystic fibrosis. *Eur. Respir. J.* 44, 394–404. doi: 10.1183/09031936.00106013

Ringholz, F. C., Higgins, G., Hatton, A., Sassi, A., Moukachar, A., Fustero-Torre, C., et al. (2018). Resolvin D1 regulates epithelial ion transport and inflammation in cystic fibrosis airways. *J. Cyst. Fibros.* 17, 607–615. doi: 10.1016/j.jcf.2017.11.017

Riordan, J. R., Rommens, J. M., Kerem, B., Alon, N., Rozmahel, R., Grzelczak, Z., et al. (1989). Identification of the cystic fibrosis gene: cloning and characterization of complementary DNA. *Science* 245, 1066–1073. doi: 10.1126/science.2475911

Roca-Ferrer, J., Pujols, L., Gartner, S., Moreno, A., Pumarola, F., Mullol, J., et al. (2006). Upregulation of COX-1 and COX-2 in nasal polyps in cystic fibrosis. *Thorax* 61, 592–596. doi: 10.1136/thx.2004.039842

Rogerio, A. P., Haworth, O., Croze, R., Oh, S. F., Uddin, M., Carlo, T., et al. (2012). Resolvin D1 and aspirin-triggered resolvin D1 promote resolution of allergic airways responses. *J. Immunol.* 189, 1983–1991. doi: 10.4049/jimmunol.1101665

Romano, M., Maddox, J. F., and Serhan, C. N. (1996). Activation of human monocytes and the acute monocytic leukemia cell line (THP-1) by lipoxins involves unique signaling pathways for lipoxin A4 versus lipoxin B4: evidence for differential Ca2+ mobilization. *J. Immunol.* 157, 2149–2154.

Rommens, J. M., Iannuzzi, M. C., Kerem, B., Drumm, M. L., Melmer, G., Dean, M., et al. (1989). Identification of the cystic fibrosis gene: chromosome walking and jumping. *Science* 245, 1059–1065. doi: 10.1126/science.2772657

Rosen, B. H., Evans, T.II, Moll, S. R., Gray, J. S., Liang, B., Sun, X., et al. (2018). Infection Is Not Required for Mucoinflammatory Lung Disease in CFTR-Knockout Ferrets. *Am. J. Respir. Crit. Care Med.* 197, 1308–1318. doi: 10.1164/rccm.201708-1616OC

Rottner, M., Tual-Chalot, S., Mostefai, H. A., Andriantsitohaina, R., Freyssinet, J.-M., and Martínez, M. C. (2011). Increased Oxidative Stress Induces Apoptosis in Human Cystic Fibrosis Cells. *PLoS One* 6, e24880. doi: 10.1371/journal.pone.0024880

Roulet, M., Frascarolo, P., Rappaz, I., and Pilet, M. (1997). Essential fatty acid deficiency in well nourished young cystic fibrosis patients. *Eur. J. Pediatr.* 156, 952–956. doi: 10.1007/s004310050750

Roum, J. H., Buhl, R., McElvaney, N. G., Borok, Z., and Crystal, R. G. (1993). Systemic deficiency of glutathione in cystic fibrosis. *J. Appl. Physiol.* 75, 2419–2424. doi: 10.1152/jappl.1993.75.6.2419

Ruffin, M., Voland, M., Marie, S., Bonora, M., Blanchard, E., Blouquit-Laye, S., et al. (2013). Anoctamin 1 dysregulation alters bronchial epithelial repair in cystic fibrosis. *Biochim. Biophys. Acta BBA - Mol. Basis Dis.* 1832, 2340–2351. doi: 10.1016/j.bbadis.2013.09.012

Ruffin, M., Roussel, L., Maillé, É., Rousseau, S., and Brochiero, E. (2018). Vx-809/Vx-770 treatment reduces inflammatory response to Pseudomonas aeruginosa in primary differentiated cystic fibrosis bronchial epithelial cells. *Am. J. Physiol. Lung Cell. Mol. Physiol.* 314, L635–L641. doi: 10.1152/ajplung.00198.2017

Ruh, C., Banjade, R., Mandadi, S., Marr, C., Sumon, Z., and Crane, J. K. (2017). Immunomodulatory Effects of Antimicrobial Drugs. *Immunol. Invest.* 46, 847–863. doi: 10.1080/08820139.2017.1373900

Sala, A., Folco, G., and Murphy, R. C. (2010). Transcellular biosynthesis of eicosanoids. *Pharmacol. Rep. PR* 62, 503–510. doi: 10.1016/s1734-1140(10)70306-6

Samuelsson, B., Borgeat, P., Hammarström, S., and Murphy, R. C. (1980). Leukotrienes: a new group of biologically active compounds. *Adv. Prostaglandin Thromboxane Res.* 6, 1–18.

Samuelsson, B., Dahlén, S. E., Lindgren, J. A., Rouzer, C. A., and Serhan, C. N. (1987). Leukotrienes and lipoxins: structures, biosynthesis, and biological effects. *Science* 237, 1171–1176. doi: 10.1126/science.2820055

Sasaki, A., Fukuda, H., Shiida, N., Tanaka, N., Furugen, A., Ogura, J., et al. (2015). Determination of ω-6 and ω-3 PUFA metabolites in human urine samples using UPLC/MS/MS. *Anal. Bioanal. Chem.* 407, 1625–1639. doi: 10.1007/s00216-014-8412-5

Scannell, M., Flanagan, M. B., deStefani, A., Wynne, K. J., Cagney, G., Godson, C., et al. (2007). Annexin-1 and Peptide Derivatives Are Released by Apoptotic Cells and Stimulate Phagocytosis of Apoptotic Neutrophils by Macrophages. *J. Immunol.* 178, 4595–4605. doi: 10.4049/jimmunol.178.7.4595

Schett, G., and Neurath, M. F. (2018). Resolution of chronic inflammatory disease: universal and tissue-specific concepts. *Nat. Commun.* 9, 3261. doi: 10.1038/s41467-018-05800-6

Schiller, K. R., Maniak, P. J., and O'Grady, S. M. (2010). Cystic fibrosis transmembrane conductance regulator is involved in airway epithelial wound repair. *Am. J. Physiol.-Cell Physiol.* 299, C912–C921. doi: 10.1152/ajpcell.00215.2010

Schultz, A., Puvvadi, R., Borisov, S. M., Shaw, N. C., Klimant, I., Berry, L. J., et al. (2017). Airway surface liquid pH is not acidic in children with cystic fibrosis. *Nat. Commun.* 8, 1409. doi: 10.1038/s41467-017-00532-5

Schwab, J. M., Chiang, N., Arita, M., and Serhan, C. N. (2007). Resolvin E1 and protectin D1 activate inflammation-resolution programmes. *Nature* 447, 869–874. doi: 10.1038/nature05877

Schwarzer, C., Illek, B., Suh, J. H., Remington, S. J., Fischer, H., and Machen, T. E. (2007). Organelle redox of CF and CFTR-corrected airway epithelia. *Free Radic. Biol. Med.* 43, 300–316. doi: 10.1016/j.freeradbiomed.2007.04.015

Scudieri, P., Musante, I., Caci, E., Venturini, A., Morelli, P., Walter, C., et al. (2018). Increased expression of ATP12A proton pump in cystic fibrosis airways. *JCI Insight* 3, e123616. doi: 10.1172/jci.insight.123616

Serhan, C. N., and Levy, B. D. (2018). Resolvins in inflammation: emergence of the pro-resolving superfamily of mediators. *J. Clin. Invest.* 128, 2657–2669. doi: 10.1172/JCI97943

Serhan, C. N., Hamberg, M., and Samuelsson, B. (1984). Trihydroxytetraenes: a novel series of compounds formed from arachidonic acid in human leukocytes. *Biochem. Biophys. Res. Commun.* 118, 943–949. doi: 10.1016/0006-291x(84)91486-4

Serhan, C. N., Maddox, J. F., Petasis, N. A., Akritopoulou-Zanze, I., Papayianni, A., Brady, H. R., et al. (1995). Design of lipoxin A4 stable analogs that block transmigration and adhesion of human neutrophils. *Biochemistry* 34, 14609–14615. doi: 10.1021/bi00044a041

Serhan, C. N., Arita, M., Hong, S., and Gotlinger, K. (2004). Resolvins, docosatrienes, and neuroprotectins, novel omega-3-derived mediators, and their endogenous aspirin-triggered epimers. *Lipids* 39, 1125–1132. doi: 10.1007/s11745-004-1339-7

Serhan, C. N., Chiang, N., and Dalli, J. (2018). New pro-resolving n-3 mediators bridge resolution of infectious inflammation to tissue regeneration. *Mol. Aspects Med.* 64, 1–17. doi: 10.1016/j.mam.2017.08.002

Shanthikumar, S., Neeland, M. N., Saffery, R., and Ranganathan, S. (2019). Gene modifiers of cystic fibrosis lung disease: A systematic review. *Pediatr. Pulmonol.* 54, 1356–1366. doi: 10.1002/ppul.24366

Shei, R.-J., Peabody, J. E., and Rowe, S. M. (2018). Functional Anatomic Imaging of the Airway Surface. *Ann. Am. Thorac. Soc* 15, S177–S183. doi: 10.1513/AnnalsATS.201806-407AW

Simonin, J., Bille, E., Crambert, G., Noel, S., Dreano, E., Edwards, A., et al. (2019). Airway surface liquid acidification initiates host defense abnormalities in Cystic Fibrosis. *Sci. Rep.* 9, 6516. doi: 10.1038/s41598-019-42751-4

Six, D. A., and Dennis, E. A. (2000). The expanding superfamily of phospholipase A(2) enzymes: classification and characterization. *Biochim. Biophys. Acta* 1488, 1–19. doi: 10.1016/s1388-1981(00)00105-0

Song, Y., Salinas, D., Nielson, D. W., and Verkman, A. S. (2006). Hyperacidity of secreted fluid from submucosal glands in early cystic fibrosis. *Am. J. Physiol.-Cell Physiol.* 290, C741–C749. doi: 10.1152/ajpcell.00379.2005

Southern, K. W., and Barker, P. M. (2004). Azithromycin for cystic fibrosis. *Eur. Respir. J.* 24, 834–838. doi: 10.1183/09031936.04.00084304

Soyombo, O., Spur, B. W., and Lee, T. H. (1994). Effects of lipoxin A4 on chemotaxis and degranulation of human eosinophils stimulated by platelet-activating factor and N-formyl-L-methionyl-L-leucyl-L-phenylalanine. *Allergy* 49, 230–234. doi: 10.1111/j.1398-9995.1994.tb02654.x

Spite, M., Norling, L. V., Summers, L., Yang, R., Cooper, D., Petasis, N. A., et al. (2009). Resolvin D2 is a potent regulator of leukocytes and controls microbial sepsis. *Nature* 461, 1287–1291. doi: 10.1038/nature08541

Stanke, F., van Barneveld, A., Hedtfeld, S., Wölfl, S., Becker, T., and Tümmler, B. (2014). The CF-modifying gene EHF promotes p.Phe508del-CFTR residual function by altering protein glycosylation and trafficking in epithelial cells. *Eur. J. Hum. Genet.* 22, 660–666. doi: 10.1038/ejhg.2013.209

Stanton, B. A., Coutermarsh, B., Barnaby, R., and Hogan, D. (2015). Pseudomonas aeruginosa Reduces VX-809 Stimulated F508del-CFTR Chloride Secretion by Airway Epithelial Cells. *PLoS One* 10 (5), e0127742. doi: 10.1371/journal.pone.0127742

Starosta, V., Ratjen, F., Rietschel, E., Paul, K., and Griese, M. (2006). Anti-inflammatory cytokines in cystic fibrosis lung disease. *Eur. Respir. J.* 28, 581–587. doi: 10.1183/09031936.06.00071405

Stick, S. M., Brennan, S., Murray, C., Douglas, T., von Ungern-Sternberg, B. S., Garratt, L. W., et al. (2009). Bronchiectasis in infants and preschool children diagnosed with cystic fibrosis after newborn screening. *J. Pediatr.* 155, 623–628.e1. doi: 10.1016/j.jpeds.2009.05.005

Strandvik, B., Gronowitz, E., Enlund, F., Martinsson, T., and Wahlström, J. (2001). Essential fatty acid deficiency in relation to genotype in patients with cystic fibrosis. *J. Pediatr.* 139, 650–655. doi: 10.1067/mpd.2001.118890

Stutts, M. J., Canessa, C. M., Olsen, J. C., Hamrick, M., Cohn, J. A., Rossier, B. C., et al. (1995). CFTR as a cAMP-dependent regulator of sodium channels. *Science* 269, 847–850. doi: 10.1126/science.7543698

Sun, Y.-P., Oh, S. F., Uddin, J., Yang, R., Gotlinger, K., Campbell, E., et al. (2007). Resolvin D1 and its aspirin-triggered 17R epimer. Stereochemical assignments, anti-inflammatory properties, and enzymatic inactivation. *J. Biol. Chem.* 282, 9323–9334. doi: 10.1074/jbc.M609212200

Sun, X., Olivier, A. K., Liang, B., Yi, Y., Sui, H., Evans, T.II, et al. (2014). Lung Phenotype of Juvenile and Adult Cystic Fibrosis Transmembrane Conductance Regulator–Knockout Ferrets. *Am. J. Respir. Cell Mol. Biol.* 50, 502–512. doi: 10.1165/rcmb.2013-0261OC

Takamiya, R., Fukunaga, K., Arita, M., Miyata, J., Seki, H., Minematsu, N., et al. (2012). Resolvin E1 maintains macrophage function under cigarette smoke-induced oxidative stress. *FEBS Open Bio* 2, 328–333. doi: 10.1016/j.fob.2012.10.001

Taminelli, G. L., Sotomayor, V., Valdivieso, Á.G., Teiber, M. L., Marín, M. C., and Santa-Coloma, T. A. (2008). CISD1 codifies a mitochondrial protein upregulated by the CFTR channel. *Biochem. Biophys. Res. Commun.* 365, 856–862. doi: 10.1016/j.bbrc.2007.11.076

Tarique, A. A., Sly, P. D., Holt, P. G., Bosco, A., Ware, R. S., Logan, J., et al. (2017). CFTR-dependent defect in alternatively-activated macrophages in cystic fibrosis. *J. Cyst. Fibros.* 16, 475–482. doi: 10.1016/j.jcf.2017.03.011

Tarran, R., Grubb, B. R., Gatzy, J. T., Davis, C. W., and Boucher, R. C. (2001). The relative roles of passive surface forces and active ion transport in the modulation of airway surface liquid volume and composition. *J. Gen. Physiol.* 118, 223–236. doi: 10.1085/jgp.118.2.223

Tarran, R. (2004). Regulation of Airway Surface Liquid Volume and Mucus Transport by Active Ion Transport. *Proc. Am. Thorac. Soc.* 1, 42–46. doi: 10.1513/pats.2306014

Teopompi, E., Risé, P., Pisi, R., Buccellati, C., Aiello, M., Pisi, G., et al. (2019). Arachidonic Acid and Docosahexaenoic Acid Metabolites in the Airways of Adults With Cystic Fibrosis: Effect of Docosahexaenoic Acid Supplementation. *Front. Pharmacol.* 10, 938. doi: 10.3389/fphar.2019.00938

Thompson, G. N. (1989). Relationships between essential fatty acid levels, pulmonary function and fat absorption in pre-adolescent cystic fibrosis children with good clinical scores. *Eur. J. Pediatr.* 148, 327–329. doi: 10.1007/bf00444126

Tirouvanziam, R., de Bentzmann, S., Hubeau, C., Hinnrasky, J., Jacquot, J., Péault, B., et al. (2000). Inflammation and infection in naive human cystic fibrosis airway grafts. *Am. J. Respir. Cell Mol. Biol.* 23, 121–127. doi: 10.1165/ajrcmb.23.2.4214

Tjonahen, E., Oh, S. F., Siegelman, J., Elangovan, S., Percarpio, K. B., Hong, S., et al. (2006). Resolvin E2: identification and anti-inflammatory actions: pivotal role of human 5-lipoxygenase in resolvin E series biosynthesis. *Chem. Biol.* 13, 1193–1202. doi: 10.1016/j.chembiol.2006.09.011

Trinh, N. T. N., Privé, A., Maillé, E., Noël, J., and Brochiero, E. (2008). EGF and K+ channel activity control normal and cystic fibrosis bronchial epithelia repair. *Am. J. Physiol.-Lung Cell. Mol. Physiol.* 295, L866–L880. doi: 10.1152/ajplung.90224.2008

Trinh, N. T. N., Bardou, O., Privé, A., Maillé, E., Adam, D., Lingée, S., et al. (2012). Improvement of defective cystic fibrosis airway epithelial wound repair after CFTR rescue. *Eur. Respir. J.* 40, 1390–1400. doi: 10.1183/09031936.00221711

Tuggle, K. L., Birket, S. E., Cui, X., Hong, J., Warren, J., Reid, L., et al. (2014). Characterization of defects in ion transport and tissue development in cystic fibrosis transmembrane conductance regulator (CFTR)-knockout rats. *PLoS One* 9, e91253. doi: 10.1371/journal.pone.0091253

Tugores, A., Le, J., Sorokina, I., Snijders, A. J., Duyao, M., Reddy, P. S., et al. (2001). The epithelium-specific ETS protein EHF/ESE-3 is a context-dependent transcriptional repressor downstream of MAPK signaling cascades. *J. Biol. Chem.* 276, 20397–20406. doi: 10.1074/jbc.M010930200

Uluçkan, Ö., and Wagner, E. F. (2017). Chronic systemic inflammation originating from epithelial tissues. *FEBS J.* 284, 505–516. doi: 10.1111/febs.13904

Underwood, B. A., Denning, C. R., and Navab, M. (1972). Polyunsaturated fatty acids and tocopherol levels in patients with cystic fibrosis. *Ann. N. Y. Acad. Sci.* 203, 237–247. doi: 10.1111/j.1749-6632.1972.tb27879.x

Vachier, I., Bonnans, C., Chavis, C., Farce, M., Godard, P., Bousquet, J., et al. (2005). Severe asthma is associated with a loss of LX4, an endogenous anti-inflammatory compound. *J. Allergy Clin. Immunol.* 115, 55–60. doi: 10.1016/j.jaci.2004.09.038

Valdivieso, Á.G., Marcucci, F., Taminelli, G., Guerrico, A. G., Álvarez, S., Teiber, M. L., et al. (2007). The expression of the mitochondrial gene MT-ND4 is downregulated in cystic fibrosis. *Biochem. Biophys. Res. Commun.* 356, 805–809. doi: 10.1016/j.bbrc.2007.03.057

Valdivieso, A. G., Clauzure, M., Marín, M. C., Taminelli, G. L., Massip Copiz, M. M., Sánchez, F., et al. (2012). The Mitochondrial Complex I Activity Is Reduced in Cells with Impaired Cystic Fibrosis Transmembrane Conductance Regulator (CFTR) Function. *PLoS One* 7, e48059. doi: 10.1371/journal.pone.0048059

Van Dyke, T. E., Hasturk, H., Kantarci, A., Freire, M. O., Nguyen, D., Dalli, J., et al. (2015). Proresolving Nanomedicines Activate Bone Regeneration in Periodontitis. *J. Dent. Res.* 94, 148–156. doi: 10.1177/0022034514557331

Vass, G., and Horvath, I. (2008). Adenosine and Adenosine Receptors in the Pathomechanism and Treatment of Respiratory Diseases. *Curr. Med. Chem.* 15, 917–922. doi: 10.2174/092986708783955392

Velsor, L. W., Kariya, C., Kachadourian, R., and Day, B. J. (2006). Mitochondrial Oxidative Stress in the Lungs of Cystic Fibrosis Transmembrane Conductance Regulator Protein Mutant Mice. *Am. J. Respir. Cell Mol. Biol.* 35, 579–586. doi: 10.1165/rcmb.2005-0473OC

Verrière, V., Higgins, G., Al-Alawi, M., Costello, R. W., McNally, P., Chiron, R., et al. (2012). Lipoxin A4 Stimulates Calcium-Activated Chloride Currents and Increases Airway Surface Liquid Height in Normal and Cystic Fibrosis Airway Epithelia. *PLoS One* 7, e37746. doi: 10.1371/journal.pone.0037746

Viart, V., Bergougnoux, A., Bonini, J., Varilh, J., Chiron, R., Tabary, O., et al. (2015). Transcription factors and miRNAs that regulate fetal to adult CFTR expression change are new targets for cystic fibrosis. *Eur. Respir. J.* 45, 116–128. doi: 10.1183/09031936.00113214

Volkova, N., Moy, K., Evans, J., Campbell, D., Tian, S., Simard, C., et al. (2020). Disease progression in patients with cystic fibrosis treated with ivacaftor: Data from national US and UK registries. *J. Cyst. Fibros. Off. J. Eur. Cyst. Fibros. Soc* 19, 68–79. doi: 10.1016/j.jcf.2019.05.015

Von Ruecker, A. A., Bertele, R., and Karsten Harms, H. (1984). Calcium Metabolism and Cystic Fibrosis: Mitochondrial Abnormalities Suggest a Modification of the Mitochondrial Membrane. *Pediatr. Res.* 18, 594–599. doi: 10.1203/00006450-198407000-00005

Wallace, J. L., Ianaro, A., Flannigan, K. L., and Cirino, G. (2015). Gaseous mediators in resolution of inflammation. *Semin. Immunol.* 27, 227–233. doi: 10.1016/j.smim.2015.05.004

Wang, L., Ruixia, Y., Chengyue, Y., Qingping, W., Christelle, M., Wanli, X., et al. (2014). Effects of resolvin D1 on inflammatory responses and oxidative stress of lipopolysaccharide-induced acute lung injury in mice. *Chin. Med. J. (Engl.)* 127 (5), 803–809. doi: 10.3760/cma.j.issn.0366-6999.20131044

Wang, Q., Zheng, X., Cheng, Y., Zhang, Y.-L., Wen, H.-X., Tao, Z., et al. (2014). Resolvin D1 Stimulates Alveolar Fluid Clearance through Alveolar Epithelial Sodium Channel, Na,K-ATPase via ALX/cAMP/PI3K Pathway in Lipopolysaccharide-Induced Acute Lung Injury. *J. Immunol.* 192, 3765–3777. doi: 10.4049/jimmunol.1302421

Wang, H., Anthony, D., Yatmaz, S., Wijburg, O., Satzke, C., Levy, B., et al. (2017). Aspirin-triggered resolvin D1 reduces pneumococcal lung infection and inflammation in a viral and bacterial coinfection pneumonia model. *Clin. Sci. Lond. Engl. 1979* 131, 2347–2362. doi: 10.1042/CS20171006

Weber, A. J., Soong, G., Bryan, R., Saba, S., and Prince, A. (2001). Activation of NF-κB in airway epithelial cells is dependent on CFTR trafficking and Cl^- channel function. *Am. J. Physiol.-Lung Cell. Mol. Physiol.* 281, L71–L78. doi: 10.1152/ajplung.2001.281.1.L71

Weiss, G. A., Troxler, H., Klinke, G., Rogler, D., Braegger, C., and Hersberger, M. (2013). High levels of anti-inflammatory and pro-resolving lipid mediators lipoxins and resolvins and declining docosahexaenoic acid levels in human milk during the first month of lactation. *Lipids Health Dis.* 12, 89. doi: 10.1186/1476-511X-12-89

Wheelock, C. E., and Strandvik, B. (2020). Abnormal n-6 fatty acid metabolism in cystic fibrosis contributes to pulmonary symptoms. *Prostaglandins Leukot. Essent. Fatty Acids* 160, 102156. doi: 10.1016/j.plefa.2020.102156

Wood, L. G., Fitzgerald, D. A., Gibson, P. G., Cooper, D. M., and Garg, M. L. (2002). Increased plasma fatty acid concentrations after respiratory exacerbations are associated with elevated oxidative stress in cystic fibrosis patients. *Am. J. Clin. Nutr.* 75, 668–675. doi: 10.1093/ajcn/75.4.668

Wright, F. A., Strug, L. J., Doshi, V. K., Commander, C. W., Blackman, S. M., Sun, L., et al. (2011). Genome-wide association and linkage identify modifier loci of lung disease severity in cystic fibrosis at 11p13 and 20q13.2. *Nat. Genet.* 43, 539–546. doi: 10.1038/ng.838

Xu, K.-P., Li, Y., Ljubimov, A. V., and Yu, F.-S. X. (2009). High Glucose Suppresses Epidermal Growth Factor Receptor/Phosphatidylinositol 3-Kinase/Akt Signaling Pathway and Attenuates Corneal Epithelial Wound Healing. *Diabetes* 58, 1077–1085. doi: 10.2337/db08-0997

Yang, Y., Cheng, Y., Lian, Q.-Q., Yang, L., Qi, W., Wu, D.-R., et al. (2013). Contribution of CFTR to Alveolar Fluid Clearance by Lipoxin A_4 via PI3K/Akt Pathway in LPS-Induced Acute Lung Injury. *Mediators Inflamm.* 2013, 1–10. doi: 10.1155/2013/862628

Zhang, F., Yang, H., Pan, Z., Wang, Z., Wolosin, J. M., Gjorstrup, P., et al. (2010). Dependence of Resolvin-Induced Increases in Corneal Epithelial Cell Migration on EGF Receptor Transactivation. *Investig. Opthalmol. Vis. Sci.* 51, 5601. doi: 10.1167/iovs.09-4468

Zhang, J.-L., Zhuo, X.-J., Lin, J., Luo, L.-C., Ying, W.-Y., Xie, X., et al. (2017). Maresin1 stimulates alveolar fluid clearance through the alveolar epithelial sodium channel Na,K-ATPase via the ALX/PI3K/Nedd4-2 pathway. *Lab. Invest.* 97, 543–554. doi: 10.1038/labinvest.2016.150

Zhang, Z., Hu, X., Qi, X., Di, G., Zhang, Y., Wang, Q., et al. (2018). Resolvin D1 promotes corneal epithelial wound healing and restoration of mechanical sensation in diabetic mice. *Mol. Vis.* 24, 274.

Zheng, S., Wang, Q., D'Souza, V., Bartis, D., Dancer, R., Parekh, D., et al. (2018). ResolvinD1 stimulates epithelial wound repair and inhibits TGF-β-induced EMT whilst reducing fibroproliferation and collagen production. *Lab. Invest.* 98, 130–140. doi: 10.1038/labinvest.2017.114

Zurier, R. B., Sun, Y., George, K. L., Stebulis, J. A., Rossetti, R. G., Skulas, A., et al. (2009). Ajulemic acid, a synthetic cannabinoid, increases formation of the endogenous proresolving and anti-inflammatory eicosanoid, lipoxin A4. *FASEB J.* 23, 1503–1509. doi: 10.1096/fj.08-118323

2

Targeting the Heme Oxygenase 1/Carbon Monoxide Pathway to Resolve Lung Hyper-Inflammation and Restore a Regulated Immune Response in Cystic Fibrosis

*Caterina Di Pietro, Hasan H. Öz, Thomas S. Murray and Emanuela M. Bruscia**

Department of Pediatrics, Yale University School of Medicine, New Haven, CT, United States

Correspondence:
Emanuela M. Bruscia
emanuela.bruscia@yale.edu

In individuals with cystic fibrosis (CF), lung hyper-inflammation starts early in life and is perpetuated by mucus obstruction and persistent bacterial infections. The continuous tissue damage and scarring caused by non-resolving inflammation leads to bronchiectasis and, ultimately, respiratory failure. Macrophages (MΦs) are key regulators of immune response and host defense. We and others have shown that, in CF, MΦs are hyper-inflammatory and exhibit reduced bactericidal activity. Thus, MΦs contribute to the inability of CF lung tissues to control the inflammatory response or restore tissue homeostasis. The non-resolving hyper-inflammation in CF lungs is attributed to an impairment of several signaling pathways associated with resolution of the inflammatory response, including the heme oxygenase-1/carbon monoxide (HO-1/CO) pathway. HO-1 is an enzyme that degrades heme groups, leading to the production of potent antioxidant, anti-inflammatory, and bactericidal mediators, such as biliverdin, bilirubin, and CO. This pathway is fundamental to re-establishing cellular homeostasis in response to various insults, such as oxidative stress and infection. Monocytes/MΦs rely on abundant induction of the HO-1/CO pathway for a controlled immune response and for potent bactericidal activity. Here, we discuss studies showing that blunted HO-1 activation in CF-affected cells contributes to hyper-inflammation and defective host defense against bacteria. We dissect potential cellular mechanisms that may lead to decreased HO-1 induction in CF cells. We review literature suggesting that induction of HO-1 may be beneficial for the treatment of CF lung disease. Finally, we discuss recent studies highlighting how endogenous HO-1 can be induced by administration of controlled doses of CO to reduce lung hyper-inflammation, oxidative stress, bacterial infection, and dysfunctional ion transport, which are all hallmarks of CF lung disease.

Keywords: monocyte/macrophages, heme oxygenase-1 (HO-1), carbon monoxide (CO), CO-releasing molecules, lung inflammation, cystic fibrosis (CF)

INTRODUCTION

The hallmarks of cystic fibrosis (CF) lung disease are mucus obstruction, chronic hyper-inflammation, chronic infections, and excessive oxidative stress, which severely damage lung tissue over time and ultimately lead to lung failure. Several anti-inflammatory pathways are compromised in CF (Cantin et al., 2015), which further perpetuates lung inflammation. Despite the role of inflammation in CF lung disease, corticosteroids, or high-dose ibuprofen are the only approved long-term treatments for CF airway inflammation. Both treatments are often poorly tolerated (Mogayzel et al., 2013; Cantin et al., 2015). In addition, when treating CF lung disease, a fine balance must be maintained between dampening the pro-inflammatory response and preserving the host defense against microorganisms (Konstan et al., 2014). This situation calls for novel therapeutic targets, which allow a potent anti-inflammatory/antimicrobial host defense followed by restoration of lung tissue homeostasis.

One of the defective anti-inflammatory pathways in CF is the heme-oxygenase-1/carbon monoxide (HO-1/CO) signaling pathway. The stress response enzyme HO-1 catabolizes heme groups to CO and biliverdin, both strong anti-inflammatory and antioxidant agents. CO also has potent bactericidal properties, and acts in a positive feedback loop to increase HO-1 expression. Due to these combined anti-inflammatory and bactericidal properties, modulation of this pathway is an attractive target in CF.

Here, we will discuss: (1) how the shortcomings of CF lung immunity perpetuate inflammatory signaling and poor bacterial clearance; (2) the role of the HO-1/CO signaling pathway; and (3) the potential of CO-based therapy to reduce lung hyper-inflammation, counteract oxidative stress, and improve bacterial clearance, ultimately restoring lung homeostasis in CF lung disease.

CF LUNG DISEASE AND INFLAMMATION

Lung hyper-inflammation in CF patients starts early in life and is likely driven by accumulation of viscous mucus in the airways (Montgomery et al., 2017). Mucus airway obstruction and impaired mucociliarly clearance create a favorable environment for respiratory infections (Khan et al., 1995; Brennan et al., 2009; Sturges et al., 2010), which intensify the lung inflammatory response. In the early years, infections by *Haemophilus influenza* and *Staphylococcus aureus* (*S. aureus*) are predominant. Over time, the CF airways become susceptible to chronic infections by the opportunistic pathogen *Pseudomonas aeruginosa* (*P. aeruginosa*) (Khan et al., 1995; Brennan et al., 2009; Sturges et al., 2010; Elborn, 2016). In addition to the increased bacterial burden, the epithelial cells and immune cells display altered immune sensing *via* pathogen- or danger-associated molecular patterns (PAMPs or DAMPs), which lead to uncontrolled inflammatory responses. This leads to excessive infiltration of neutrophils, which are impaired in clearing the ongoing infection. Furthermore, CF-affected neutrophils have altered apoptosis (Tirouvanziam et al., 2008) and increased neutrophil extracellular trap formation (Gray et al., 2018), which is accompanied by high levels of neutrophil elastase in the airways of CF patients (Garratt et al., 2015; Kanik et al., 2020). This vicious cycle of persistent infections and uncontrolled pro-inflammatory responses also causes severe oxidative stress through the release of reactive oxygen species (ROS) from neutrophils and CF epithelia, and the irreversible damage of lung tissues (Bonfield et al., 1995; Chmiel and Davis, 2003; Davis, 2006; Cantin et al., 2015; Elborn, 2016; Turnbull et al., 2020). The oxidative stress is worsened by the impaired efflux of chloride, bicarbonate, and other solutes (e.g., glutathione) (Galli et al., 2012).

The failure to efficiently resolve the inflammatory response contributes to the development of chronic hyper-inflammation in CF (Cantin et al., 2015; Roesch et al., 2018; Recchiuti et al., 2019). Indeed, resolution of lung inflammation is an active, tightly coordinated process, whereby counterregulatory mechanisms are induced to clear inflammatory cells from sites of infection or injury in order to restore tissue homeostasis. Successful resolution includes arrest of neutrophil tissue infiltration, apoptosis of neutrophils and their subsequent removal [e.g., *via* efferocytosis (Yurdagul et al., 2017)], dampening of pro-inflammatory signals, clearance of pathogens and cell debris, and initiation of tissue repair processes (Headland and Norling, 2015).

Macrophages (MΦs) play a critical role in maintaining lung tissue homeostasis. During an inflammatory response, they acquire different pro- or anti-inflammatory properties and tissue-reparative phenotypes. Upon recognition of pathogens, they shift toward a pro-inflammatory phenotype, recruiting other immune cells and initiating inflammation. As the inflammation progresses, MΦs not only phagocytose pathogens, but also clear apoptotic cells and cell debris from the lungs. With other signals from surrounding cells or from the pathogen, this efferocytosis transforms MΦs into an anti-inflammatory phenotype, thus limiting inflammation and promoting the resolution/termination of inflammation (Doran et al., 2020). Furthermore, in the later phases of lung injury, MΦs tightly coordinate parenchymal repair processes, which are essential for reestablishing tissue homeostasis. Due to these key roles, it is not surprising that many chronic lung inflammatory diseases such asthma, chronic obstructive pulmonary disease (COPD), CF (Bruscia and Bonfield, 2016a; Bruscia and Bonfield, 2016b), and pulmonary fibrosis (Misharin et al., 2017; Reyfman et al., 2019), are associated with abnormal MΦ behavior.

Monocytes/MΦs from CF patients are dysregulated at many levels. *In vitro* and ex vivo studies from patients with CF and animal models of the disease suggest that both inherited factors (lack of functional CFTR) and acquired factors (CF lung environment) contribute to this dysfunction. As a result, monocytes/MΦs fail to properly handle inflammatory triggers (PAMPs, DAMPs, cytokines, growth factors), struggle to resolve inflammation, and fail to clear dead cells, kill bacteria, and adapt to the environment (reviewed in Bruscia et al. [Bruscia and Bonfield, 2016a; Bruscia and Bonfield, 2016b)].

The exact mechanisms for the exaggerated and dysfunctional inflammatory response observed in CF are not fully understood. However, it appears that the fine balance between the pro- and anti-inflammatory regulatory pathways is disrupted, with heightened pro-inflammatory stimuli and reduced counter-regulatory response, which would ordinarily promote resolution of inflammation.

Ibuprofen (Konstan et al., 1995), glucocorticosteroids (Ross et al., 2009), mucolytics (Paul et al., 2004), and antibiotics (Ratjen et al., 2012) are all treatments that have improved CF lung disease and are associated with a reduction in lung inflammation. However, there are concerns about using anti-inflammatory therapies in chronically infected CF patients. Indeed, blocking induction of inflammation may have immunosuppressive effects that compromise the host defense and thus worsen lung infections. This was observed in clinical studies assessing the effect of the LTB4-receptor antagonist BIIL 284, an inhibitor of neutrophil migration, in children and adults with CF. This study was terminated prematurely due to a significant increase in the frequency of pulmonary exacerbations (due to bacterial infections) in adult patients who received the treatment (Doring et al., 2014; Konstan et al., 2014).

The use of CFTR modulators, which correct mutant CFTR trafficking to the plasma membrane (correctors) and enhance its activity (potentiators), are now FDA-approved for most CF patients (Middleton et al., 2019). However, there are few long-term studies of their impact on immune response and monocyte/MΦs function. While Rowe et al. (2014) reported that the CFTR modulator VX-770 (Ivacaftor) did not reverse lung inflammation, other studies showed partial reduction of lung inflammation (Hisert et al., 2017). Ex vivo studies on monocytes and monocyte derived MΦs from patients with CF suggest that Ivacaftor modulates the inflammatory response (Hisert et al., 2017; Zhang et al., 2018; Jarosz-Griffiths et al., 2020) and improves bacterial killing (Hisert et al., 2017; Riquelme et al., 2017; Barnaby et al., 2018). The newly approved triple combination CFTR modulator therapy elexacaftor/tezacaftor/ivacaftor (Trikafta) (Middleton et al., 2019) has shown great promise for many CF patients. However, its effect on the abnormal inflammatory response in CF has not been fully elucidated, and it is not known whether it will help control lung hyper-inflammation over the longer life expectancy achieved. Moreover, these therapies are not applicable for all mutations and, therefore, for all patients with CF. Thus, novel therapeutic approaches are needed that, in combination with CFTR modulators, will rescue the abnormal anti-inflammatory regulatory mechanisms and facilitate the resolution of the inflammatory response, while maintaining a potent antimicrobial host defense. Below, we discuss the HO-1/CO pathway, which facilitates anti-inflammatory and antioxidant activities while strengthening the host's bactericidal functions. This pathway is thus an attractive therapeutic target for CF.

HO-1 FUNCTION AND REGULATION

Heme oxygenases (HO) are enzymes that facilitate the degradation of heme, a ubiquitous molecular complex consisting of iron and tetrapyrrole protoporphyrin IX. The heme from the hemoglobin in red blood cells and myoglobin in muscles is involved in the transport and storage of oxygen, respectively. However, many other proteins also use a heme group for fundamental cellular processes. If released from proteins, an excess of free heme is highly toxic because it promotes oxidative stress (Biswas et al., 2014; Wegiel et al., 2015). HO enzymes thus play a crucial role in cells (Gozzelino et al., 2010). HO activity is represented by two separate isoforms: an inducible isoform HO-1 and a constitutively expressed isoform HO-2. A suspected third isozyme, HO-3, turned out to be a pseudogene derived from processed HO-2 transcripts (Mccoubrey et al., 1997). HO-1 and HO-2 are the products of distinct genes, *hmox1* and *hmox2*, respectively. They differ in primary amino acid sequence, biochemical and biophysical properties (Cruse and Maines, 1988; Ryter and Choi, 2016). HO-1 is an integral membrane component of the smooth endoplasmic reticulum (Gottlieb et al., 2012), but it is also localized in plasma membrane caveolae (Kim et al., 2004), mitochondria (Converso et al., 2006), and nuclei (Biswas et al., 2014). HO-1 is undetectable under physiological conditions but is highly induced after exposure to a broad range of chemical and physical stimuli including heme, ultraviolet-A radiation, hydrogen peroxide, redox cycling compounds, heavy metals, hypoxia, hyperoxia, cytokines, hormones, growth factors, and microorganisms. HO-1 is mainly induced in hepatic, endothelial, myeloid, and respiratory epithelial cells. One exception is the spleen, where constantly high levels of HO-1 ensure an efficient recycling of iron from senescent erythrocytes (Ryter et al., 2006). Monocytes/MΦs rely on abundant induction of the HO-1 for a controlled immune response and for potent bactericidal activity. In liver endothelial and epithelial cells HO-1 plays a critical anti-oxidant and pro-survival function in response to cellular stressors (Ryter et al., 2006). In contrast to HO-1, HO-2 is constitutively expressed in most tissues, including brain, testis, endothelial, and smooth muscle cells (Zakhary et al., 1996), and is refractory to HO-1 inducers (Maines et al., 1986). The inducible nature of HO-1 makes it an attractive target for drug discovery.

HO-1 catalyzes the first and rate-limiting step in the oxidative catabolism of heme groups. With the use of cytochrome P-450, nicotinamide adenine dinucleotide phosphate (NADPH), and molecular oxygen, HO-1 catabolizes heme into equimolar amounts of carbon monoxide (CO), free iron (Fe^{2+}), and biliverdin IXa. The cytoprotective effects of HO-1 are enhanced by its catabolites. Biliverdin is rapidly metabolized to bilirubin (a highly antioxidant compound) by the biliverdin reductase. The free iron, which can stimulate free radical formation, is promptly sequestered by ferritin and recycled for heme synthesis. Degradation of heme is the only mammalian pathway known to produce CO. This gaseous molecule is toxic at higher concentrations because it binds hemoglobin and thus prevents the transport of oxygen. However, at physiological concentrations, CO has strong cytoprotective, anti-inflammatory, antioxidant, and bactericidal properties (**Figure 1**) (Motterlini and Otterbein, 2010; Ryter et al., 2018).

The essential cytoprotective role of HO-1 has been demonstrated by the phenotype of HO-1-null mice (HO-1 KO), which display increased embryonic lethality, anemia, and chronic inflammatory disorders. Cells isolated from HO-1 KO animals are also more susceptible to oxidative stress (Poss and Tonegawa, 1997a; Poss and Tonegawa, 1997b). HO-1 KO animals display increased mortality after lipopolysaccharide (LPS) administration, which supports the importance of HO-1 in mediating protection during bacterial infection (Wiesel et al., 2000). Importantly, the phenotypical alterations in the uniquely observed case of human HO-1 deficiency are similar to those in HO-1 KO mice, with severe hemolytic anemia, endothelial degradation, reduced serum bilirubin, renal and hepatic iron accumulation, and a pro-inflammatory phenotype (Yachie et al., 1999).

The expression of HO-1 is regulated primarily at the transcriptional level *via* regulatory element sites localized at the 5′-untranslated region of the *hmox1* gene promoter. These include binding sites for several prominent transcriptional factors (TFs), such as nuclear factor E2–related factor-2 (Nrf2) (Alam et al., 1999), activator protein-1 (AP-1) family (Alam and Den, 1992; Alam et al., 1999), nuclear factor-kappa B (NF-*k*B) (Lavrovsky et al., 1994), and hypoxia-inducible factor-1 alpha (HIF-1α) (Lee et al., 1997). For a comprehensive review of HO-1 regulation, please refer to (Alam and Cook, 2007; Waza et al., 2018; Medina et al., 2020). Many of the TFs and signaling pathways involved in modulating HO-1 expression are dysregulated in CF cells, resulting in decreased HO-1 induction (discussed in *HO-1 Dysregulation in CF*).

Nrf2 is a major transcriptional regulator of HO-1 (Chan and Kan, 1999). At steady state, Nrf2 localizes in the cytoplasm of the cells, where it is inactivated when associated with its cytosolic repressor Kelch-like ECH-associated protein-1 (Keap1). Keap1 actively promotes Nrf2's rapid degradation by the ubiquitin–proteasome pathway to ensure low Nrf2 levels in the cell. Exposure to electrophilic or oxidative stresses causes a conformational change in Keap1, with the subsequent dissociation of Nrf2. Nrf2 then translocates into the nucleus, where it forms a heterodimer with small masculoaponeurotic

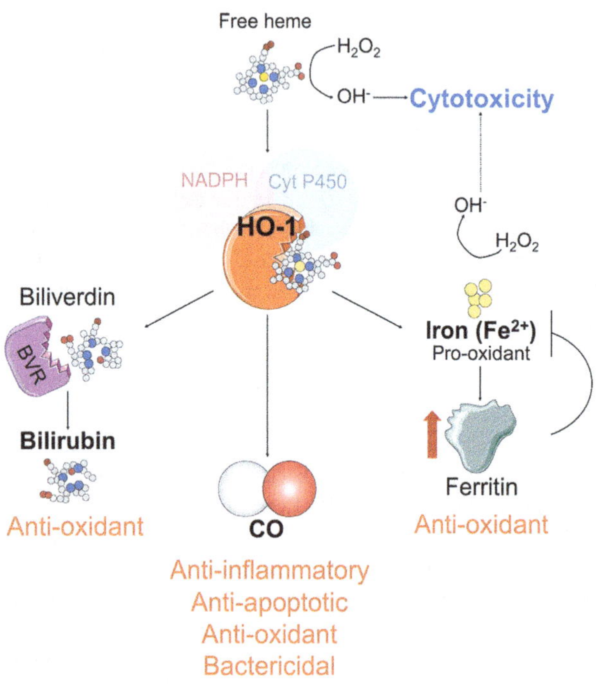

FIGURE 1 | HO-1 enzymatic activity. HO-1 enzymatic activity generates biliverdin and releases carbon monoxide (CO) and Fe^{2+}. Biliverdin is transformed into bilirubin by the biliverdin reductase (BVR). Fe^{2+} is sequestered by the iron storage protein ferritin.

fibrosarcoma (Maf) proteins and binds to the antioxidant response elements (ARE) in the promoter region of genes coding for antioxidant and detoxifying enzymes. These include HO-1, NAD(P)H quinone oxidoreductase 1 (NQO1), glutamate-cysteine ligase (GCL), and glutathione S transferases (GSTs), which all execute antioxidative functions in cells (Bryan et al., 2013). The Nrf2-mediated HO-1 expression is also finely regulated by TF BTB and CNC Homology 1 (Bach1), which also forms heterodimers with Maf and competes with Nrf2 for the binding sites in the *hmox1* promoter region, thus suppressing HO-1 expression (Dhakshinamoorthy et al., 2005). Thus, HO-1 induction is highly regulated and requires the release of Nrf2 from Keap1, the inactivation of its competitor Bach1, and the availability of Maf to initiate transcriptional signaling (Ogawa et al., 2001; Bryan et al., 2013) (**Figures 2A, B**).

Functional binding sites for AP-1 (Alam et al., 1999), HIF-1α (Lee et al., 1997), and NF-*k*B (Lee et al., 1997) have been identified within the promoter region of *hmox1* gene (details in **Figures 2C–E**). In response to hypoxia, HIF-1α is phosphorylated by the MAPK p38. This leads to its translocation to the nucleus, where it associates with HIF-1β, the transcriptional co-activator CREB-binding protein (CBP), and p300, thereby leading to transcription of HO-1 (Lee et al., 1997; Medina et al., 2020). Several studies have shown that NF-*k*B not only positively modulates HO-1 expression by directly binding to its promoter (Naidu et al., 2008; Rushworth et al., 2012), but it may also work as a negative regulator for HO-1 expression. Some of these conflicting data can be reconciled by the complex NF-κB crosstalk with Nrf2 in modulating HO-1 induction during specific cellular responses (Liu et al., 2008; Yu et al., 2011). For instance, NF-*k*B decreases the availability of CBP/p300 for Nrf2, thus preventing Nrf2 transcriptional activity (Liu et al., 2008). This is relevant for CF, where shifting the competitive binding of CBP/p300 in favor of Nrf2 (over NF-*k*B) leads to increased expression of antioxidant and anti-inflammatory genes and decreased cellular inflammation (Ziady et al., 2012). The molecular mechanisms underpinning the dynamic crosstalk between NF-κB and the Nrf2 are extensively reviewed in (Wardyn et al., 2015) and are still under investigation.

Post-transcriptional and post-translational modifications are also potential regulatory mechanisms for controlling HO-1 levels. A number of microRNAs (e.g., miR-24, miR-200c, miR-204, miR-211, miR-155, miR-378, miR-377, miR-217) directly regulate HO-1 levels by decreasing *hmox1* messenger RNA stability or translation. Other miRNAs indirectly modulate HO-1 by affecting the expression of upstream regulatory factors, such as Nrf2, Keap1, and Bach1 [Review in (Cheng et al., 2013)]. The GT-microsatellite polymorphism, located in the proximal human *hmox1* promoter region, also contributes to the regulation of HO-1 expression. These short GT repetitions increase HO-1 expression, which correlates with a reduced risk of developing rheumatoid arthritis, chronic pulmonary emphysema, and other diseases (Exner et al., 2004).

Activation of several signaling cascades mediates induction of HO-1, including the mitogen-activated protein kinase (MAPKs) superfamily (p38, ERK, and JNK), protein kinase C (PKC), and phosphatidylinositol 3-kinase (PI3K) (**Figures 2B–E**). Protein kinase C facilitates Nrf2 nuclear translocation by

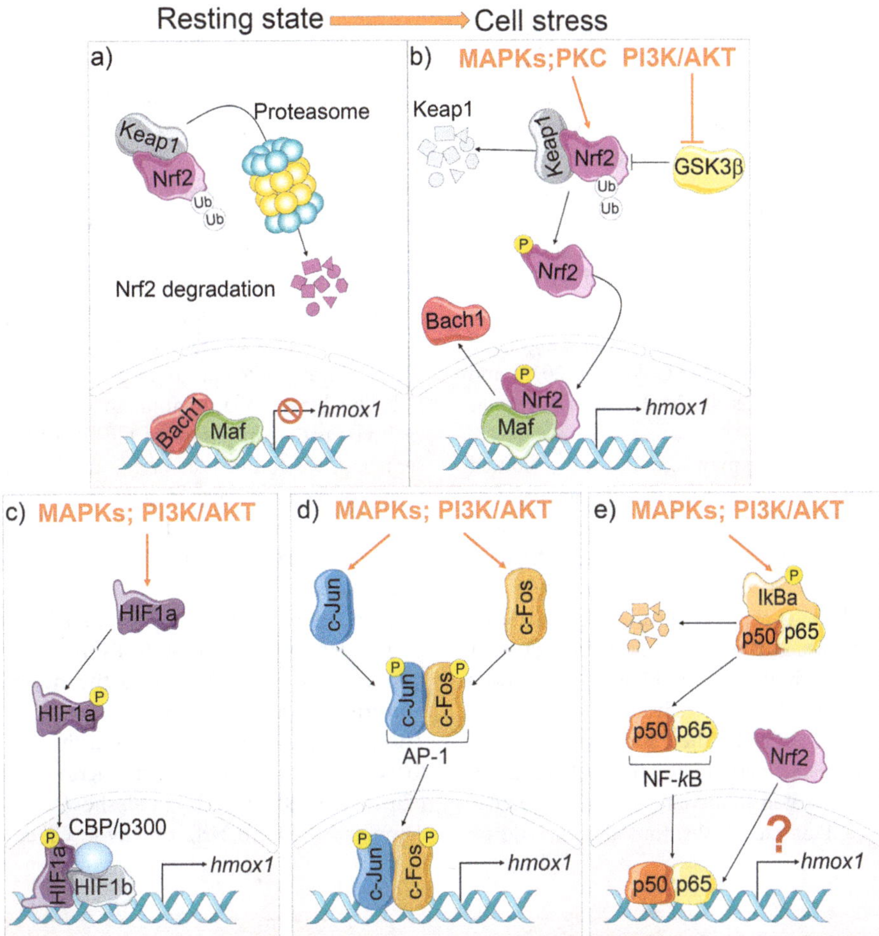

FIGURE 2 | *Hmox1* transcriptional regulation. **(A)** At steady state, Nrf2 is bound to Keap1 in the cytoplasm and targeted for proteasomal degradation. Bach-1 is bound to Maf at the promoter region of the *hmox1*, suppressing its transcription. **(B)** During cellular stress, *hmox1* expression is activated in several ways: mitogen-activated protein kinase (MAPKs) and protein kinase C (PKC) phosphorylate Nrf2. This stabilizes Nrf2, leading to its translocation into the nucleus. PI3K/AKT inhibits GSK3β. When activated, GSK3β facilitates the ubiquitination and proteasomal degradation of Nrf2. Once in the nucleus, Nrf2 displaces Bach-1 at the *hmox1* promoter leading to transcription. **(C)** HIF-1 is a heterodimer composed of HIF-1α and HIF-1β. HIF-1α phosphorylation leads to its translocation to the nucleus and association to HIF-1β and CBP/p300, thus inducing *hmox1* transcription. **(D)** Phosphorylation of *c-Fos* and *c-Jun* leads to their translocation to the nucleus and formation of the AP-1 complex, which induces *hmox1* expression; **(E)** NF-κB is sequestered in the cytosol under basal conditions by the inhibitor IκB. Phosphorylation results in the proteasomal degradation of IκB and the consequent release and nuclear translocation of NF-κB dimers (p50/p65) which targets *hmox1* activation. A complex crosstalk between NF-κB and Nrf2 can also inhibit *hmox1* transcription.

phosphorylation of Nrf2 at the Keap1 binding site freeing Nrf2 from Keap1 (Huang et al., 2002). MAPKs and PI3K/AKT can directly (*via* phosphorylation) or indirectly regulate transcription factors required for the HO-1 induction. The MAPKs and PI3K/AKT signaling cascades have been extensively investigated in the context of Nrf-2-dependent HO-1 activation. PI3K/AKT signaling can indirectly promote HO-1 transcription by inhibiting glycogen synthase kinase 3β (GSK3β)-mediated phosphorylation and subsequent ubiquitination and proteasomal degradation of Nrf2 (Bryan et al., 2013). Furthermore, PI3K/AKT signaling activation in response to oxidative stress results in actin polymerization and depolymerization, which promotes translocation of actin-bound Nrf2 into the nucleus (Kang et al., 2002).

HO-1 DYSREGULATION IN CF

In CF, *hmox1* has been reported to be a modifier gene, as a specific *hmox1* allele correlated with improved lung function in pediatric CF patients chronically infected with *P. aeruginosa* (Park et al., 2011). On top of genetic variants, studies comparing nasal epithelial cells and blood cells of CF patients with healthy donors have revealed altered epigenetic modifications of the *hmox1* gene (Magalhaes et al., 2017). An early study showed that the lungs of patients with CF have increased HO-1 expression compared to control lung resections from patients with cancer (Zhou et al., 2004). This is expected given the inflammatory environment of CF lungs. A better control would be tissues from patients with other lung inflammatory conditions. In the same study, the authors provided the first evidence for the beneficial effect of HO-1 in CF cells. Namely, overexpression of HO-1 in CF human bronchial epithelial (HBE) cell lines (IB3.1) led to potent cytoprotective properties against *P. aeruginosa* infections (Zhou et al., 2004). HO-1 expression in CF HBE cell lines (CFBE41o-) was decreased at baseline and its induction was hampered following stimulation by LPS or hypoxia compared with a HBE cell line control (Chillappagari et al., 2014; Chillappagari et al., 2020). This suggests that, while HO-1 can still be induced in the absence of CFTR, the amount produced may not be sufficient to provide beneficial effects. The lack of HO-1 correlates with an increased iron load (Chillappagari et al., 2014), that is also observed in lavages and lung tissues of CF patients (Stites et al., 1999; Ghio et al., 2013) and favors *P. aeruginosa* infections (Reid et al., 2002; Moreau-Marquis et al., 2008).

Several dysfunctional mechanisms may account for the blunted HO-1 induction in CF cells (**Figure 3**). Our group has demonstrated that HO-1 is inefficiently induced in human and murine CF MΦs in response to inflammatory or infectious triggers, which correlate with exaggerated inflammation and prolonged inflammatory signaling (Zhang et al., 2013; Zhang et al., 2015; Di Pietro et al., 2017). We have also shown that the defective induction of HO-1 is due to blunted activation of the PI3K/AKT pathway downstream of toll-like receptor 4 (TLR4) activation in MΦs from CF mouse models and patients with CF. Alteration of this pathway decreases HO-1 expression and perpetuates the inflammatory response. In addition to decreased induction, the HO-1 cellular distribution is altered in CF-affected MΦs, thus diminishing its beneficial effect. In response to LPS, HO-1 normally translocate to plasma membrane lipid rafts in a caveolin 1 (Cav1)- dependent manner, where it destabilizes the binding between TLR4 and its adapter protein myeloid differentiation factor 88 (MyD88) *via* CO production, thus ending inflammatory signaling (Wang X. et al., 2009). We found that HO-1 does not compartmentalize to the cell surface in CF MΦs, but rather accumulates intracellularly due to decreased Cav1 expression (Zhang et al., 2013). We linked the decreased levels of Cav1 expression to high levels of miR-199a-5p (which targets caveolin 1 3'-UTR) downstream of blunted PI3K/AKT signaling in CF MΦs (Zhang et al., 2015). Importantly, modulation of this pathway *via* overexpression of HO-1 or treatment with CO-releasing molecules (discussed in the next section) was sufficient to improve the signaling cascade, thus reducing hyper-inflammation in CF MΦs (Zhang et al., 2013). In investigating how loss of CFTR leads to blunted PI3K/AKT signaling, we found that ezrin, an F-actin binding protein that forms a macromolecular complex with CFTR at the plasma membrane (Guggino and Stanton, 2006), links CFTR, TLR4, PI3K/AKT signaling, and HO-1 expression in MΦs (Di Pietro et al., 2017).

Ziady et al. (Chen et al., 2008; Ziady et al., 2012) showed that CFTR deficiency in HBE cells reduces translocation of the transcription factor Nrf2 into the nuclear compartment, thus impairing the transcription of antioxidant genes, including HO-1. This group also found that the co-activator CBP favors the binding to NF-*k*B (over Nrf2), which increases inflammatory signaling (Chen et al., 2008). Kelley et al. showed that Rp-cAMPS, a cAMP competitor, rescued Nrf2 activity in CF epithelial cells by shifting

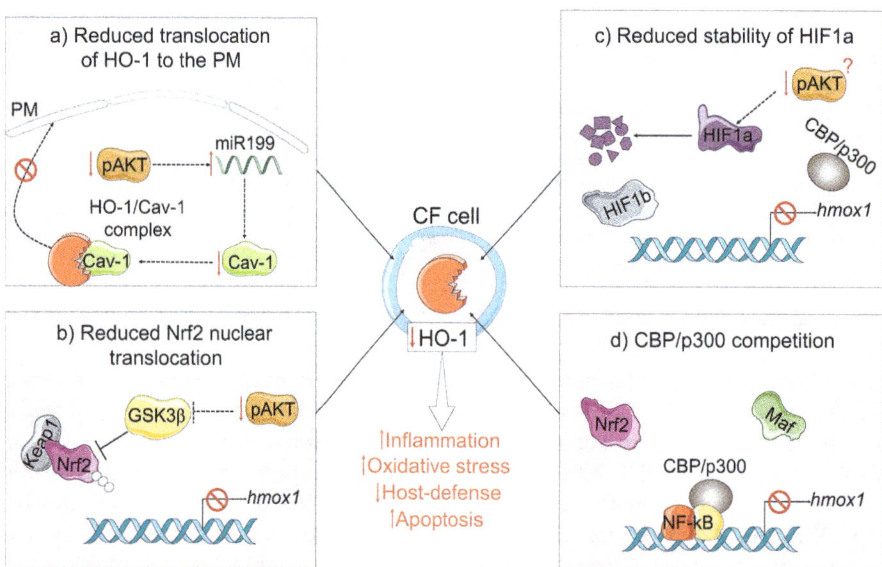

FIGURE 3 | Mechanisms of HO-1 dysregulation in cystic fibrosis (CF). In the absence of functional CFTR: **(A)** MΦs have a blunted PI3K/AKT signaling in response to TLR4 activation, which leads to accumulation of miR-199a-5p, which reduces Cav1 expression. Loss of Cav1 impairs translocation and compartmentalization of HO-1 at the plasma membrane (PM); **(B)** blunted PI3K/AKT signaling in CF cells results in elevated levels of active GSK3β, which leads to Nrf2 ubiquitination and proteasomal degradation and **(C)** affects the stability of HIF-1α. **(D)** NF-*k*B in CF cells competes for the Nrf2 co-activator CBP/p300, thus preventing Nrf2 transcriptional activity.

the CBP association in favor of Nrf2 (over NF-*k*B), thus decreasing inflammatory signaling and increasing antioxidant and anti-inflammatory activity (Ziady et al., 2012). In this study HO-1 expression was not tested, however, the rescued Nrf2 activity should result in increased HO-1 expression. Importantly, Ziady's group recently showed that the broadly used CFTR modulators VX-809 (Lumacaftor) and VX-661 (Tezacaftor) significantly increase Nrf2 activity after correction of CFTR expression in primary epithelial cells of CF patients with homozygous F508del mutations (Borcherding et al., 2019). VX-809 also stabilizes PTEN association with the mutant CFTR protein (upstream regulator of PI3K) (Riquelme et al., 2017) and increases cellular levels and phosphorylation of ezrin (Matos et al., 2019). This helps the mutant CFTR to form a stable macromolecular complex at the plasma membrane, thus improving function (Abbattiscianni et al., 2016). Plasma membrane stabilized mutant CFTR, restores the CFTR downstream signaling transduction events that reestablish the Nrf2-HO-1 axis in VX809-treated cells (Borcherding et al., 2019). In addition to Nrf2, stabilization of HIF-1α is downregulated in unstimulated and hypoxia-stimulated CFTR-deficient HBE cells, which decreases HO-1 expression (Legendre et al., 2011).

While CFTR modulators decreased the inflammatory response (Hisert et al., 2017; Zhang et al., 2018; Jarosz-Griffiths et al., 2020), and improved their bacterial clearance (Barnaby et al., 2018; Zhang et al., 2018) in monocyte/MΦs from patients with CF, these studies did not investigate a possible increase (and thus beneficial effect) of HO-1 levels. In CF patients, CFTR modulators initially decreased the bacterial burden in the lungs, but the bacteria re-emerged over time (Hisert et al., 2017). Thus, to preserve lung function in patients with CF in the long term, we propose that targeting the HO-1/CO pathway can complement existing treatments.

Several trials and studies have indirectly tested HO-1 induction in patients with CF. The first tested candidate was sulphoraphane, an antioxidant compound that induces Nrf2 signaling and improves bacterial clearance by alveolar MΦs (Harvey et al., 2011). The study found no adverse effects of increased dietary sulphoraphane intake. However, larger studies are needed to test sulphoraphane's efficacy in CF (NCT01315665). GSK Pharmaceuticals have developed a promising small molecule for therapeutically inducing HO-1 (Davies et al., 2016). This molecule activates Nrf2 by binding the Keap1-Nrf2 binding site, favoring their dissociation. It thus improves opsonic phagocytosis in MΦs isolated from COPD patients (Bewley et al., 2018), and may be beneficial for CF patients. As an alternative approach, exogenous delivery of low doses of CO, a potent inducer of HO-1, can be considered to improve CF lung disease. We have proven that exogenous CO delivery can overcome the defective plasma membrane localization of HO-1 in CF MΦs challenged with LPS (Zhang et al., 2013). However, certain epigenetic changes present at the *hmox1* gene in CF- affected cells (Magalhaes et al., 2017), may reduce the efficacy of such a therapeutic approach. In the following sections, we discuss the cellular effects of CO administration, and its relevance to CF.

CO ANTI-INFLAMMATORY AND ANTIOXIDANT FUNCTIONS, AND RELEVANCE TO CF

Similarly, to nitric oxide (NO) and hydrogen sulfide (H_2S), CO is a potent gaseous signaling molecule that can freely diffuse through membranes (Fagone et al., 2018). The biological activity of CO depends on its ability to bind with ferrous (Fe^{2+}) ions, thus controlling the activity of several heme-containing proteins (e.g., nitric oxide synthase (NOS), NADPH oxidase, cytochrome C oxidase, guanylate cyclase) (Wang et al., 2014; Ji et al., 2016; Motterlini and Foresti, 2017; Ryter et al., 2018). These proteins activate signaling pathways that are implicated in cell protection/survival against stress, in antioxidant responses, and in regulating inflammation. CO's downstream targets include p38, HIF-1α, PPARγ, glutathione, nitric oxide, and PI3K/AKT, many of which are altered in CF (Cantin et al., 2015). The current understanding of CO's biological function derives from studies in which cells and animal models were exposed to non-toxic doses of free CO, or were treated with small molecules able to release controlled amounts of CO, i.e., CO-releasing molecules (CO-RMs). CO-RMs were initially engineered by Motterlini and colleagues (Motterlini et al., 2002). They contain a transition metal (e.g., ruthenium, cobalt, iron) surrounded by carbonyl (CO) groups. Different CO-RMs have been developed to minimize toxicity, improve solubility, and increase control of CO release. Exogenous delivery of low doses of CO mimics the physiological/non-toxic effects elicited by the production of endogenous cellular CO (Motterlini and Otterbein, 2010; Wegiel et al., 2013; Wang et al., 2014; Ji et al., 2016; Motterlini and Foresti, 2017; Ryter et al., 2018).

Several *in vivo* studies, including ours in CF-affected mice (Zhang et al., 2013), support the notion that exogenous delivery of CO prevents hyper-inflammation and tissue damage in the context of sepsis, sterile inflammation, and hyperoxia (Motterlini and Otterbein, 2010). CO reduces the number of neutrophils in septic lungs by controlling transendothelial migration (Mizuguchi et al., 2009). Moreover, at low concentrations, CO attenuates the lung inflammatory response in mice challenged with LPS or live bacteria (Macgarvey et al., 2012; Wegiel et al., 2014b; Wilson et al., 2017; Kim et al., 2018). It differentially and selectively inhibits LPS-induced expression of pro-inflammatory cytokines (e.g., TNF-α, IL-6), while increasing levels of anti-inflammatory molecules (e.g., IL-10, IL-1 receptor antagonist (IL-1Ra, PPAR-γ) (Bilban et al., 2006; Haschemi et al., 2011; Piantadosi et al., 2011; Macgarvey et al., 2012; Uddin et al., 2015). This is relevant to CF because CF airway epithelial cells (Perez et al., 2007) and CF MΦs (Bruscia et al., 2009) both secrete more pro-inflammatory cytokines during inflammatory stimuli compared to non-CF cells. Moreover, CO can help reestablish the secretion levels of IL-10, which are lower in CF lungs (Bonfield et al., 1995), and of PPAR-γ, which are lower in CF epithelial cells and MΦs (Andersson et al., 2008; Harmon et al., 2010). Murine (Sawle et al., 2005) and human (Chhikara et al., 2009) MΦs are particularly responsive to CO treatment, which attenuates the inflammatory response to LPS (Sawle et al., 2005).

The anti-inflammatory effect of CO in response to LPS may be mediated by augmenting the caveolin 1(Cav-1)/TLR4 interaction at plasma membrane caveolae by a p38 MAPK-dependent mechanism (Otterbein et al., 2000; Sawle et al., 2005; Bilban et al., 2006; Chhikara et al., 2009; Tsoyi et al., 2009; Wang X. et al., 2009), which favors termination of pro-inflammatory signal transduction events. Importantly, CF MΦs have increased levels of plasma membrane TLR4 receptors (Bruscia et al., 2011) and decreased Cav1 expression in response to LPS (Zhang et al., 2013). We have shown that low levels of Cav1 prevent translocation of HO-1 to the plasma membrane of activated CF MΦs (Zhang et al., 2013), where it normally localizes (Wang X. et al., 2009). CO-RM treatment reversed this dysfunction in CF cells (Zhang et al., 2013).

CO's anti-inflammatory effects also rely on its ability to strongly induce expression of endogenous HO-1, thus increasing autonomous, cellular CO production. HO-1 expression is driven by several TFs and upstream signaling events (see *HO-1 Function and Regulation*, **Figure 2**). Exogenous CO administration can activate all the shown/mentioned TFs to induce HO-1 expression, with activation of preferential pathways depending on the experimental conditions, cell type, and cellular stressors (Piantadosi et al., 2008; Zhang et al., 2013) (**Figure 4**). Mechanistically, low doses of CO transiently increase mitochondrial ROS (mtROS) levels (Wang et al., 2007). This temporary increase in mtROS activates the MKK3/p38 MAPKs and PI3K/AKT signaling pathway, which ultimately strongly induces HO-1 expression (Otterbein et al., 2000; Otterbein et al., 2003).

More recently, it has been proposed that CO promotes resolution of inflammation by inducing expression of specialized pro-resolving lipid mediators (SPMs) derived from the metabolism of polyunsaturated fatty acids (Serhan et al., 2014). In a mouse model of peritonitis (Chiang et al., 2013) and a primate model of pneumonia (Dalli et al., 2015), CO induces expression of a key biosynthetic enzyme (12/15-LOX in mice, and 15-LOX-1 in humans), which induces the production of SPMs. In these models, CO increases levels of Resolvin (Rv)-D1, RvD2, and Lipoxin A4 (LXA4), and reduces levels of pro-inflammatory lipid mediators, such as thromboxane B2 (TXB2), leukotriene B4 (LTB4), and prostaglandin E2 (PGE2). This is relevant because CF patients have a reduced capacity to biosynthesize SPMs. Clinical studies have shown that the arachidonic-acid-derived LXA4 is reduced in the bronchoalveolar lavage fluid (BALF) of patients with CF (Karp et al., 2004; Chiron et al., 2008; Yang et al., 2012; Ringholz et al., 2014). The presence of the omega-3 fatty-acid-derived RvE1 in CF BALF correlates with better lung function compared to patients with undetectable RvE1 (Yang et al., 2012). Moreover, *P. aeruginosa* infection inhibits 15-epi-LXA4 production in HBE cells, thus promoting mucosal hyper-inflammation (Flitter et al., 2017; Recchiuti et al., 2019)

CO modulates several pathways in a way that may counteract the dysfunctions in the CF epithelium that lead to oxidative stress (Galli et al., 2012). These actions include inducing the aforementioned Nrf2-dependent and Nrf2-independent induction

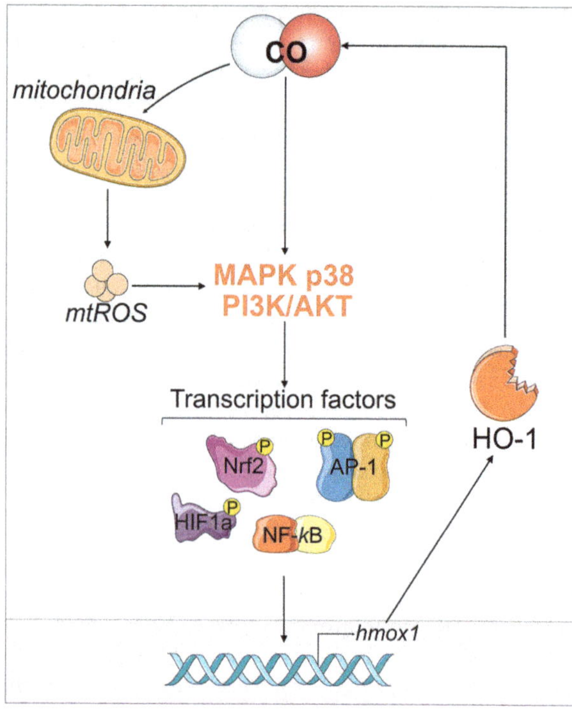

FIGURE 4 | CO-mediated induction of HO-1. Low dose CO can activate all the transcriptional factors (TFs) that drive the expression of HO-1, *via* either direct or indirect activation of MKK3/p38 MAPKs and PI3K/AKT signaling.

of HO-1, preventing ROS production downstream of NADPH oxidase activity, and rebalancing the defective glutathione homeostasis observed in CF cells (Gao et al., 1999; Velsor et al., 2001; Day et al., 2004; Galli et al., 2012; Yamamoto et al., 2014; De Bari et al., 2018).

CO STIMULATES CELLULAR HOST DEFENSE AGAINST INFECTIONS: IMPLICATIONS IN CF

Activating the HO-1/CO pathway or delivering exogenous CO has a promising additional clinical benefit. Namely, CO enhances MΦ bacterial killing capability and protects the lung epithelium from infection-associated damage (Chin and Otterbein, 2009). Several proposed mechanisms could explain how exposure to CO primes MΦs to better clear bacteria. For example, CO may stimulate bacterial uptake by redistribution of TLR4 at the plasma membrane (Otterbein et al., 2005). Moreover, the uptake of microorganisms such as *P. aeruginosa* by MΦs requires proper activation of the PI3K/AKT pathway (Araki et al., 2003; Bohdanowicz et al., 2010; Lovewell et al., 2014; Di Pietro et al., 2017; Demirdjian et al., 2018), which is stimulated by CO (Otterbein et al., 2000; Otterbein et al., 2003). TLR4 trafficking and its regulation at the plasma membrane of MΦs is altered in CF (Zhang et al., 2013). CF MΦs also show blunted induction of the PI3K/AKT signaling pathway in response to LPS or *P. aeruginosa* (Zhang et al., 2015; Di Pietro et al., 2017).

Wegiel et al. (2014a) have shown that modulation of the HO-1/CO pathway or exogenous delivery of CO increases the efficiency of MΦs in killing bacteria such as *Escherichia coli* and *Enterococcus faecalis*. The mechanism relies on CO promoting ATP production from bacteria, which, in turn, activates the Nacht, LRR, and PYD domains-containing protein 3 (NALP3) inflammasome system *via* binding of the purinergic receptor P2X7 (Wegiel et al., 2014a). An additional *in vivo* study has shown that CO-driven inflammasome activation facilitates bacterial clearance in a mouse model of polymicrobial infection caused by cecal ligation and puncture (Lancel et al., 2009). This may help macrophages kill *P. aeruginosa* clinical strains that are adapted to the altered CF environment (Riquelme et al., 2019). However, the effect of CO on inflammasome activation may depend on the type of stimuli, since Nakahira et al. have demonstrated that CO negatively regulates NLRP3 inflammasome activation in MΦs challenged with LPS but not with live bacteria (Jung et al., 2015).

Autophagy is another cellular mechanism that is fundamental to efficient bacterial clearance by immune cells. CO stimulates autophagy by inducing the expression and activation of the microtubule-associated protein 1A/1B light chain 3 (LC3) (Lee et al., 2011). Autophagy is impaired in CF HBE (Luciani et al., 2010) and MΦs of CF patients (Abdulrahman et al., 2011). This contributes to the hyper-inflammation (Luciani et al., 2010) and poor bacterial killing of organisms such as *Burkholderia cepacia* (Abdulrahman et al., 2011) and *P. aeruginosa* (Ferrari et al., 2017). CO also increases acidification of the phagolysosome (Onyiah et al., 2013). Although controversial (Haggie and Verkman, 2007), this may be an additional dysregulated mechanism in CF MΦs that contributes to the failure to efficiently kill bacteria (Di et al., 2006).

Mitochondrial metabolic reprogramming is a key response by MΦs to efficiently fight pathogens during infection (Mills and O'Neill, 2016). CO affects mitochondrial function by binding to the cytochrome-c oxidase. At high doses, CO damages mitochondria. However, at physiological/non-toxic levels, CO has positive effects on mitochondrial metabolism. CO shifts the cellular energetic metabolism from glycolysis to oxidative phosphorylation and the pentose phosphate pathway, increasing oxygen consumption and ATP production. This may be a key mechanism in CO's modulation of the MΦ response to infections. CO also induces mitochondrial and lysosomal biogenesis by activating the guanylate cyclase and the PI3K/AKT pathway, and upregulating transcription factors such as Nrf1, Transcription Factor A, mitochondrial (TFAM), Nrf2, Transcription Factor EB (TFEB), and PGC-1α (Zuckerbraun et al., 2007; Piantadosi et al., 2011; Queiroga et al., 2012; Wegiel et al., 2013; Motterlini and Foresti, 2017; Kim et al., 2018). These data suggest that cellular CO primes MΦs to better respond to cellular stressors. Although CO treatment has been associated with increased bacterial killing (Chin and Otterbein, 2009), caution is required when considering CO as a treatment for infection. This is because CO can inhibit the activity of NADPH oxidase 2 (NOX2) proteins. However, in other experimental settings, the beneficial effect of CO requires the presence of functional NOX2 (Nakahira et al., 2006; Lin et al., 2019). Thus, the inhibitory effect of CO on NADPH oxidases may depend on the CO dose used, cellular status (steady state or in response to stress), and type of stressor. This must be carefully evaluated when considering CO as a potential CF therapy because MΦs from CF patients may have an intrinsically lower capacity to activate NOX2 in response to bacterial infections (Assani et al., 2017).

A few *in vivo* studies suggest that administration of CO or CO-RMs protects against mortality after infectious challenge. Systemic delivery of CO-RMs reduced the mortality from 80% to 0% compared with controls in neutropenic mice infected with *P. aeruginosa*. This correlated with reduced bacterial recovery from the spleen due to either direct CO-mediated killing or enhanced bacterial clearance by the host immune system (Desmard et al., 2009). The authors demonstrate that mitochondrial function was protected in the CO-RM-treated mice and the pro-inflammatory response of sepsis was blunted (Lancel et al., 2009). Similarly, in a mouse peritonitis sepsis model, lower dose of CO-RM (10 mg/kg) resulted in an 80% survival rate. Additionally, upregulation of the HO-1/CO pathway, or delivery of inhaled CO, improved survival of mice in an *S. aureus* sepsis model. In this model, the mechanism of action relies on mitochondrial energetic metabolism reprogramming and biogenesis, increasing host cell survival, and countering the exuberant pro-inflammatory response in an AKT1-Nrf2 dependent manner (Macgarvey et al., 2012).

Finally, and particularly relevant in the context of CF lung disease, increased cellular levels of CO protect the bronchial epithelium from damage associated with *P. aeruginosa* infection. Secreted virulence factors from *P. aeruginosa* (e.g., *P. aeruginosa* quinolone signaling compound, PQS) decrease levels of HO-1 and Nrf2 expression in lung epithelial cells and primary HBE cells. This increases oxidative stress in epithelial cells, contributing to the pathogenicity of *P. aeruginosa* (Abdalla et al., 2017). In another study by Roussel et al., the *P. aeruginosa* biofilm-derived quorum sensing molecule N-(3-oxododecanoyl)-l-homoserine lactone (3OC12-HSL) decreased the activation of the Nrf2-HO-1 axis in HBE cells, increasing cellular ROS production (Roussel and Rousseau, 2017). Importantly, we and others have shown that stimulating the HO-1 pathway (with genetic manipulation (Zhou et al., 2004) or exposure to CO-RMs (Murray et al., 2012)) is sufficient to improve HBE cell survival following acute *P. aeruginosa* infection (Zhou et al., 2004) or exposure to *P. aeruginosa* biofilms (Murray et al., 2012). Improved CO cellular survival in response to infections may be mediated by stabilization of HIF-1α (Chin et al., 2007) and activation of the PI3K/AKT-driven induction of Bcl-2-mediated protection to apoptotic stimuli (Otterbein et al., 2003; Martin et al., 2004; Zhang et al., 2015; Shi et al., 2019).

THE DIRECT EFFECTS OF CO ON BACTERIA AND RELEVANCE TO CF

Along with the previously discussed stimulation of the host cells, CO treatment has an additional potential clinical benefit in its direct bactericidal activity. Multiple studies have documented that CO and CO-RM treatment results in killing of a variety of pathogenic bacteria including *P. aeruginosa*, *E. coli*, *Salmonella enterica*, *S. aureus*, and *Helicobacter pylori* (Nobre et al., 2007; Murray et al., 2012; Bang et al., 2014; Rana et al., 2014; Flanagan et al., 2018). This has generally been true regardless of the carrier molecule used to deliver the CO, which accumulates inside bacterial cells before they release CO (Nobre et al., 2016). CO's killing efficiency and mechanism of action against microorganisms likely differs based on the CO dose, microorganism, and the metabolic status of the microorganism (Chin and Otterbein, 2009; Chung et al., 2009; Tavares et al., 2012; Wilson et al., 2012). There are many explanations for how CO-RMs induce bacterial cell death (for a comprehensive review, see (Wilson et al., 2012)). One mechanism is that bacterial CO exposure generates reactive oxidative species (ROS) and subsequent DNA damage (Nobre et al., 2009). Another demonstrated mechanism is that CO directly targets respiration by binding to terminal cytochrome oxidases (Desmard et al., 2009; Tavares et al., 2013).

P. aeruginosa demonstrates the promises and limitations of CO and CO-RMs as antimicrobial therapies. We and others have shown that CO-RMs are effective at killing or aiding in the killing of *P. aeruginosa* clinical strains recovered from CF patients and grown in liquid culture or in biofilms (Murray et al., 2012; Flanagan et al., 2018). However, these studies also show that certain *P. aeruginosa* clinical isolates are less susceptible to CO (Murray et al., 2012; Flanagan et al., 2018). Moreover, the bacterial growth conditions influence CO's effectiveness. CO does not effectively kill the common *P. aeruginosa* strain PAO1 in rich media, but it is highly effective in glucose-based media (Murray et al., 2012). CO-RMs also kill *P. aeruginosa* in anaerobic conditions (Desmard et al., 2009), similar to those found in the CF lung.

Riquelme & Prince recently pointed out that the metabolic environment is important for CF infections (Riquelme et al., 2019). The CF lung has high levels of succinate, and thus preferentially selects for *P. aeruginosa*, which efficiently metabolize succinate (Riquelme et al., 2017). This metabolic adaptation drives a transcriptional reprogramming of the bacteria, leading to expression of genes for extracellular molecules that favor bacterial biofilm formation. Interestingly, one study of a novel photo-activated CO-RM demonstrated CO-RM-dependent killing of *E. coli* when succinate was supplied as the sole carbon source (Nagel et al., 2014). Riquelme & Prince also provide evidence that *P. aeruginosa* clinical strains adapt to the altered CF environment and change the host immune response to induce recruitment of immune cells (monocytes and neutrophils) to the lungs, while retaining the ability to activate mitochondrial ROS. However, the recruited immune cells display immune dysfunction when challenged with CF-adapted *P. aeruginosa*, including failure to stabilize HIF-1α and to secrete IL-1β. Thus, CF-adapted bacterial isolates can evade clearance by MΦs (Riquelme et al., 2019). As discussed above (Wegiel et al., 2014a), by stabilizing HIF-1α and restoring IL-1β secretion, CO treatment may enhance the ability of host immune cells to better sense and eradicate *P. aeruginosa* isolates that are metabolically adapted to the CF lung environment.

CO AS A MODULATOR OF ION CHANNEL ACTIVITY: RELEVANCE TO CF

CO is also emerging as a modulator of ion channel activity. CO regulates the function of the Ca^{2+}-activated K (BK_{Ca}), voltage-activated K+ (Kv), and Ca^{2+} channel (L-type) families, ligand-gated P2X receptors, tandem P domain K+ channels (TREK1), and the epithelial Na+ channel (ENaC). The mechanism/s by which CO modulates their activity is unclear. However, activation of the BK_{Ca} channel seems to be directly mediated by CO binding to a metal-based center in BK_{Ca} channels (Brazier et al., 2009; Telezhkin et al., 2011). Generation of cGMP by soluble guanylyl cyclase activation (Murad, 2006) and generation of mtROS (Wilkinson and Kemp, 2011; Peers et al., 2015) are two indirect mechanisms that have been proposed to mediate CO-dependent modulation of ion channel activity.

Relevance to CF

Loss of CFTR function leads to reduced expression of the inducible nitric oxide synthase, a target of CO, in CF murine and human airway epithelial cells (Kelley et al., 1997a; Kelley and Drumm, 1998; Elmer et al., 1999; Steagall et al., 2000). This reduces NO production, thus decreasing cGMP levels in CF cells and dysregulating transepithelial sodium and chloride transport (Elmer et al., 1999). Importantly, cGMPs activate CFTR in a PKA-independent manner (Kelley et al., 1997b), and promote trafficking of CFTR to the plasma membrane of the intestinal epithelium (Ahsan et al., 2017). Stimulating this pathway may also correct/potentiate mutant CFTR and thus ameliorate the intestinal fluid deficit in the CF intestine (Arora et al., 2017). Thus, by increasing cGMP cellular levels (Foresti and Motterlini, 1999), CO may help stimulate wild-type and mutant CFTR ion transport. A thought-provoking study by Wang suggests that CO may activate CFTR-dependent Cl^- and HCO_3^- currents across the apical membrane of the rat distal colon. This study reported that the CFTR protein has a high-affinity ferric ion (Fe^{3+}) binding site at the interface between the regulatory domain and intracellular loop 3. The binding of Fe^{3+} to CFTR prevents channel opening, and CO leads to release of the inhibitive Fe^{3+} ions, thus activating CFTR (Wang, 2017).

In addition to potentially regulating the CFTR function, CO also modulates the function of ion channels involved in CF lung disease, i.e., the large conductance calcium-activated potassium channels (BK_{Ca}) and the epithelial Na+ channels (ENaC). The BK_{Ca} channels are expressed on the apical membrane of airways. Apical secretion of K^+ provides a driving force for Cl^- flow, which maintains the airway surface liquid (ASL) volume. Its depletion leads to mucociliary dysfunction (Manzanares et al., 2011; Manzanares et al., 2015; Kim et al., 2020). Importantly, Salathe's group recently reported that CF HBE cells have reduced BK_{Ca} channel activity due to increased lung inflammation, and that restoring BK_{Ca} channel activity reduces CF and inflammation-associated mucociliary dysfunction (Kim et al., 2020). Thus, CO's ability to activate BK_{Ca} may reduce inflammation and help re-balance ion secretions in CF.

CO also inhibits the sodium channel ENaC, an established pharmacological target for CF lung disease (Mall, 2009). The ENaC channel absorbs Na^+ from the apical side, thus reducing the ASL volume. CO inhibits ENaC in rat cultured alveolar type II cells and human airway epithelial cell line, and it prevents alveolar fluid reabsorption in perfused rabbit lungs (Althaus et al., 2009). Thus, CO can potentially block the hyperabsorption of sodium through the ENaC channel, which may restore ASL volumes (Mall et al., 2004). However, a different study has reported that CO has the opposite effect on ENaC in a mouse kidney cortical collecting duct cell line (Wang S. et al., 2009). These data are not easy to reconcile, but they may reflect tissue-specific differences in ENaC subunit composition, the CO doses, and experimental conditions. More studies are needed to clarify CO's effect on ENaC in CF epithelium.

In summary, CO targets the signaling cascade associated with NO production and cGMP levels. It also directly targets the activity of ion channels such as BK_{Ca} (and potentially CFTR). It may thus help rebalance ion transport across the CF epithelium and restore physiological ASL levels.

EXOGENOUS DELIVERY OF CO AND CLINICAL APPLICATIONS

Based on encouraging studies in preclinical models, the pharmacological use of CO has been tested in humans. In this rapidly evolving field, the current approaches to delivering controlled levels of CO in humans are: (a) inhalation and (b) a hemoglobin based-CO carrier.

CO Inhalation

At high concentrations (10,000 ppm), inhalation of CO is toxic. However, at controlled low concentrations (10–200 ppm), exogenous CO delivery is safe in humans [NCT00531856 (Mayr et al., 2005) (Bathoorn et al., 2007)] and is beneficial against numerous diseases and pathological conditions featuring hyper-inflammation, tissue damage, pulmonary arterial hypertension, and ischemic conditions (Motterlini and Otterbein, 2010; Ji et al., 2016; Ryter and Choi, 2016; Ryter et al., 2018). Inhalation of 100–125 ppm CO by patients with stable chronic obstructive pulmonary disease (COPD) is safe, reduces sputum eosinophil levels and improves responsiveness to methacholine [NCT00122694 (Bathoorn et al., 2007)]. Results from a multicenter, double-blinded, clinical trial of inhaled CO in patients with idiopathic pulmonary fibrosis show that CO inhalation (100-200 ppm) was not associated with adverse events, but also did not result in significant changes in the study end points. These end points included differences in matrix metalloproteinase-7 serum concentration and pulmonary function test measures [NCT01214187 (Rosas et al., 2018)]. However, treatment with CO lead to a change in the expression profile of peripheral blood mononuclear cells dominated by oxidative phosphorylation-related genes (Casanova et al., 2019). Clinical implications for such transcriptional changes are not clear. Following successful preclinical studies in primates (Dalli et al., 2015; Fredenburgh et al., 2015), CO inhalation was tested in an initial safety study with patients with sepsis induced by acute respiratory distress syndrome (ARDS). Subjects were administered inhaled CO (100 ppm or 200 ppm) or placebo for 90 min for up to

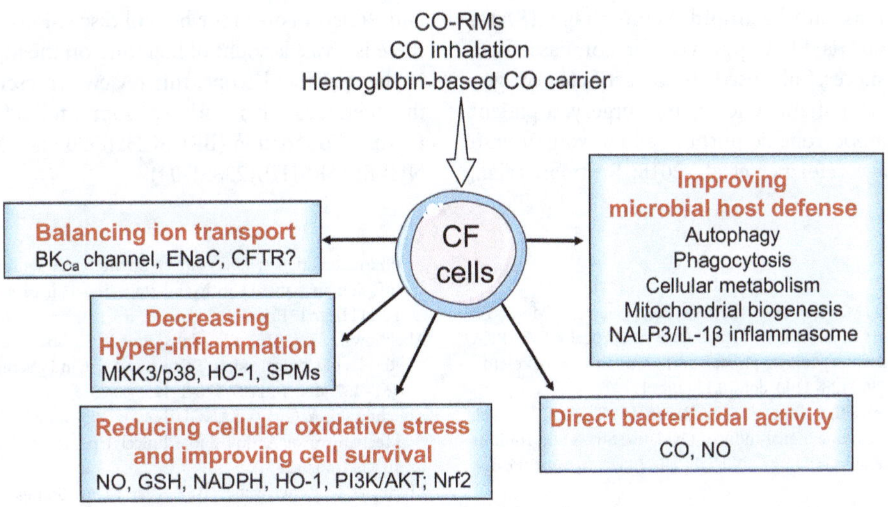

FIGURE 5 | CO beneficial effects in cystic fibrosis (CF). CO may have several beneficial effects in CF. In addition to transcriptional induction of HO-1, CO helps to rebalance ion transport in bronchial epithelial cells by modulating the activity of BK_{Ca} channels, ENaC, and, possibly, CFTR. It has direct bactericidal activity and also primes the macrophages. It thus improves the host defense mechanisms by modulating autophagy, phagocytosis, the inflammasome, and immunometabolic responses. CO reduces cellular oxidative stress and improves cell survival by activating/inducing NO, GSH, NADPH, HO-1, PI3K/AKT, and Nrf2. CO also decreases hyper-inflammation by increasing levels of anti-inflammatory mediators, HO-1 and SPMs.

5 consecutive days. The treatment was well-tolerated and appeared to be safe (Fredenburgh et al., 2018). A multi-center Phase II clinical trial of inhaled CO for the treatment of ARDS involving 5 US-based medical centers is currently ongoing (NCT03799874).

Hemoglobin-Based CO Carrier

Prolong Pharmaceuticals has developed PP-007 (formerly known as *Sanguinate*), a polyethylene-glycol-modified (PEGylated) form of bovine hemoglobin loaded with CO. CO is released within 2 h of infusion and exchanged for oxygen, which is then delivered to areas of low oxygen tension (Abuchowski, 2017). This dual mode of action targets inflammation (CO) and hypoxia (O_2), two complications in the CF lung. PP-007 is also PEGylated, which ensures stability and prolongs retention of the molecules in the circulation. PP-007 is being studied for several clinical situations to treat hypoxia and/or inflammation, including sickle cell disease (SCD), reperfusion injury, and cerebral hemorrhage (Misra et al., 2014; Abuchowski, 2016; Abuchowski, 2017; Dhar et al., 2017; Misra et al., 2017; Abu Jawdeh et al., 2018). PP-007 is safe in a phase I clinical trials in both healthy controls and patients with SCD. After a single intravenous dose (80, 120, or 160 mg/kg) in a randomized phase I single-blinded placebo-controlled study, the only observed adverse effect was a transient trend toward increased blood pressure, likely due to temporary intravascular volume expansion, which resolved within 24 h. In addition, a dose-dependent decrease in serum haptoglobin was observed, which binds to PP-007, forming a complex that is cleared from the circulation. Importantly, no Hb was detected in the urine, and no signs of nephrotoxicity were found (Abuchowski, 2016; Abuchowski, 2017). A second Phase I study in SCD patients also showed the transient increase in blood pressure, as well as an asymptomatic increase in troponin. Currently, PP-007 is being tested in several Phase II clinical trials in SCD (NCT02672540; NCT02600390). PP-007 is also well-tolerated in patients with other diseases, such as subarachnoid hemorrhage (SAH) (NCT02323685). PP-007 is FDA-approved for compassionate care, and has been successfully used as an artificial oxygen transfusion agent in two patients undergoing surgery, a patient with thrombotic thrombocytopenic purpura and a woman with postpartum hemorrhage (Holzner et al., 2018; Brotman et al., 2019). Patients were eventually stabilized, and no adverse events were reported (Sam et al., 2017; Thenuwara et al., 2017). Given PP-007's cytoprotective effects and its use in ischemia-reperfusion injury in renal transplant patients (clinicaltrials.gov, ID: NCT02490202; Phase II/III), PP-007 may be able to prevent/reduce ischemia-reperfusion injury in CF patients after lung transplant (Porteous et al., 2015). The anti-inflammatory effects of PP-007 in preclinical mouse models of CF lung disease are currently being tested by our laboratory.

CONCLUDING REMARKS

Modulating the HO-1/CO pathway, e.g., *via* CO administration, can attenuate hyper-inflammation, counteract oxidative stress, improve bacterial clearance by strengthening the host defense mechanisms or by direct killing, and rehydrate the airways (**Figure 5**). We therefore propose that the HO-1/CO pathway may be targeted as an adjuvant therapy to minimize lung disease in CF.

AUTHOR CONTRIBUTIONS

CP, HÖ, TM, and EB wrote the manuscript. CP designed the figures. EB initiated and overseen the work. All authors contributed to the article and approved the submitted version.

ACKNOWLEDGMENTS

We thank the Yale CF Research Center and Dr. Marie Egan for the continuous support, and Drs. Diane Krause, Roberto Motterlini, and Roberta Foresti for helpful discussions. We acknowledge that there is a vast amount of literature on the topic. Due to limitations in the space and scope, this review represents only a selection of this literature. This work was supported by The American Cystic Fibrosis Foundation (BRUSCHI18G0 and OZ18F0), and by NIH/NHLBI (5R01HL123851-04).

REFERENCES

Abbattiscianni, A. C., Favia, M., Mancini, M. T., Cardone, R. A., Guerra, L., Monterisi, S., et al. (2016). Correctors of mutant CFTR enhance subcortical cAMP-PKA signaling through modulating ezrin phosphorylation and cytoskeleton organization. *J. Cell Sci.* 129, 1128–1140. doi: 10.1242/jcs.177907

Abdalla, M. Y., Hoke, T., Seravalli, J., Switzer, B. L., Bavitz, M., Fliege, J. D., et al. (2017). Pseudomonas Quinolone Signal Induces Oxidative Stress and Inhibits Heme Oxygenase-1 Expression in Lung Epithelial Cells. *Infect. Immun.* 85. doi: 10.1128/IAI.00176-17

Abdulrahman, B. A., Khweek, A. A., Akhter, A., Caution, K., Kotrange, S., Abdelaziz, D. H., et al. (2011). Autophagy stimulation by rapamycin suppresses lung inflammation and infection by Burkholderia cenocepacia in a model of cystic fibrosis. *Autophagy* 7, 1359–1370. doi: 10.4161/auto.7.11.17660

Abu Jawdeh, B. G., Woodle, E. S., Leino, A. D., Brailey, P., Tremblay, S., Dorst, T., et al. (2018). A phase Ib, open-label, single arm study to assess the safety, pharmacokinetics, and impact on humoral sensitization of SANGUINATE infusion in patients with end-stage renal disease. *Clin. Transplant.* 32. doi: 10.1111/ctr.13155

Abuchowski, A. (2016). PEGylated Bovine Carboxyhemoglobin (SANGUINATE): Results of Clinical Safety Testing and Use in Patients. *Adv. Exp. Med. Biol.* 876, 461–467. doi: 10.1007/978-1-4939-3023-4_58

Abuchowski, A. (2017). SANGUINATE (PEGylated Carboxyhemoglobin Bovine): Mechanism of Action and Clinical Update. *Artif. Organs* 41, 346–350. doi: 10.1111/aor.12934

Ahsan, M. K., Tchernychev, B., Kessler, M. M., Solinga, R. M., Arthur, D., Linde, C. I., et al (2017). Linaclotide activates guanylate cyclase-C/cGMP/protein kinase-II-dependent trafficking of CFTR in the intestine. *Physiol. Rep.* 5. doi: 10.14814/phy2.13299

Alam, J., and Cook, J. L. (2007). How many transcription factors does it take to turn on the heme oxygenase-1 gene? *Am. J. Respir. Cell Mol. Biol.* 36, 166–174. doi: 10.1165/rcmb.2006-0340TR

Alam, J., and Den, Z.(1992). Distal AP-1 binding sites mediate basal level enhancement and TPA induction of the mouse heme oxygenase-1 gene. *J. Biol. Chem.* 267, 21894–21900.

Alam, J., Stewart, D., Touchard, C., Boinapally, S., Choi, A. M., and Cook, J. L. (1999). Nrf2, a Cap'n'Collar transcription factor, regulates induction of the heme oxygenase-1 gene. *J. Biol. Chem.* 274, 26071–26078. doi: 10.1074/jbc.274.37.26071

Althaus, M., Fronius, M., Buchackert, Y., Vadasz, I., Clauss, W. G., Seeger, W., et al. (2009). Carbon monoxide rapidly impairs alveolar fluid clearance by inhibiting epithelial sodium channels. *Am. J. Respir. Cell Mol. Biol.* 41, 639–650. doi: 10.1165/rcmb.2008-0458OC

Andersson, C., Zaman, M. M., Jones, A. B., and Freedman, S. D. (2008). Alterations in immune response and PPAR/LXR regulation in cystic fibrosis macrophages. *J. Cyst. Fibros* 7, 68–78. doi: 10.1016/j.jcf.2007.05.004

Araki, N., Hatae, T., Furukawa, A., and Swanson, J. A. (2003). Phosphoinositide-3-kinase-independent contractile activities associated with Fcgamma-receptor-mediated phagocytosis and macropinocytosis in macrophages. *J. Cell Sci.* 116, 247–257. doi: 10.1242/jcs.00235

Arora, K., Huang, Y., Mun, K., Yarlagadda, S., Sundaram, N., Kessler, M. M., et al. (2017). Guanylate cyclase 2C agonism corrects CFTR mutants. *JCI Insight* 2. doi: 10.1172/jci.insight.93686

Assani, K., Shrestha, C. L., Robledo-Avila, F., Rajaram, M. V., Partida-Sanchez, S., Schlesinger, L. S., et al. (2017). Human Cystic Fibrosis Macrophages Have Defective Calcium-Dependent Protein Kinase C Activation of the NADPH Oxidase, an Effect Augmented by Burkholderia cenocepacia. *J. Immunol.* 198, 1985–1994. doi: 10.4049/jimmunol.1502609

Bang, C. S., Kruse, R., Demirel, I., Onnberg, A., Soderquist, B., and Persson, K. (2014). Multiresistant uropathogenic extended-spectrum beta-lactamase (ESBL)-producing Escherichia coli are susceptible to the carbon monoxide releasing molecule-2 (CORM-2). *Microb. Pathog.* 66, 29–35. doi: 10.1016/j.micpath.2013.12.003

Barnaby, R., Koeppen, K., Nymon, A., Hampton, T. H., Berwin, B., Ashare, A., et al. (2018). Lumacaftor (VX-809) restores the ability of CF macrophages to phagocytose and kill Pseudomonas aeruginosa. *Am. J. Physiol. Lung Cell Mol. Physiol.* 314, L432–L438. doi: 10.1152/ajplung.00461.2017

Bathoorn, E., Slebos, D. J., Postma, D. S., Koeter, G. H., Van Oosterhout, A. J., Van Der Toorn, M., et al. (2007). Anti-inflammatory effects of inhaled carbon monoxide in patients with COPD: a pilot study. *Eur. Respir. J.* 30, 1131–1137. doi: 10.1183/09031936.00163206

Bewley, M. A., Budd, R. C., Ryan, E., Cole, J., Collini, P., Marshall, J., et al. (2018). Opsonic Phagocytosis in Chronic Obstructive Pulmonary Disease Is Enhanced by Nrf2 Agonists. *Am. J. Respir. Crit. Care Med.* 198, 739–750. doi: 10.1164/rccm.201705-0903OC

Bilban, M., Bach, F. H., Otterbein, S. L., Ifedigbo, E., D'avila, J. C., Esterbauer, H., et al. (2006). Carbon monoxide orchestrates a protective response through PPARgamma. *Immunity* 24, 601–610. doi: 10.1016/j.immuni.2006.03.012

Biswas, C., Shah, N., Muthu, M., La, P., Fernando, A. P., Sengupta, S., et al. (2014). Nuclear heme oxygenase-1 (HO-1) modulates subcellular distribution and activation of Nrf2, impacting metabolic and anti-oxidant defenses. *J. Biol. Chem.* 289, 26882–26894. doi: 10.1074/jbc.M114.567685

Bohdanowicz, M., Cosio, G., Backer, J. M., and Grinstein, S. (2010). Class I and class III phosphoinositide 3-kinases are required for actin polymerization that propels phagosomes. *J. Cell Biol.* 191, 999–1012. doi: 10.1083/jcb.201004005

Bonfield, T. L., Panuska, J. R., Konstan, M. W., Hilliard, K. A., Hilliard, J. B., Ghnaim, H., et al. (1995). Inflammatory cytokines in cystic fibrosis lungs. *Am. J. Respir. Crit. Care Med.* 152, 2111–2118. doi: 10.1164/ajrccm.152.6.8520783

Borcherding, D. C., Siefert, M. E., Lin, S., Brewington, J., Sadek, H., Clancy, J. P., et al. (2019). Clinically-approved CFTR modulators rescue Nrf2 dysfunction in cystic fibrosis airway epithelia. *J. Clin. Invest.* 129, 3448–3463. doi: 10.1172/JCI96273

Brazier, S. P., Telezhkin, V., Mears, R., Muller, C. T., Riccardi, D., and Kemp, P. J. (2009). Cysteine residues in the C-terminal tail of the human BK(Ca)alpha subunit are important for channel sensitivity to carbon monoxide. *Adv. Exp. Med. Biol.* 648, 49–56. doi: 10.1007/978-90-481-2259-2_5

Brennan, S., Sly, P. D., Gangell, C. L., Sturges, N., Winfield, K., Wikstrom, M., et al. (2009). Alveolar macrophages and CC chemokines are increased in children with cystic fibrosis. *Eur. Respir. J.* 34, 655–661. doi: 10.1183/09031936.00178508

Brotman, I., Kocher, M., and Mchugh, S. (2019). Bovine Hemoglobin-Based Oxygen Carrier Treatment in a Severely Anemic Jehovah's Witness Patient After Cystoprostatectomy and Nephrectomy: A Case Report. *A. A. Pract.* 12, 243–245. doi: 10.1213/XAA.0000000000000901

Bruscia, E. M., and Bonfield, T. L. (2016a). Cystic Fibrosis Lung Immunity: The Role of the Macrophage. *J. Innate Immun.* 8, 550–563. doi: 10.1159/000446825

Bruscia, E. M., and Bonfield, T. L. (2016b). Innate and Adaptive Immunity in Cystic Fibrosis. *Clin. Chest Med.* 37, 17–29. doi: 10.1016/j.ccm.2015.11.010

Bruscia, E. M., Zhang, P. X., Ferreira, E., Caputo, C., Emerson, J. W., Tuck, D., et al. (2009). Macrophages directly contribute to the exaggerated inflammatory response in cystic fibrosis transmembrane conductance regulator-/- mice. *Am. J. Respir. Cell Mol. Biol.* 40, 295–304. doi: 10.1165/rcmb.2008-0170OC

Bruscia, E. M., Zhang, P. X., Satoh, A., Caputo, C., Medzhitov, R., Shenoy, A., et al. (2011). Abnormal trafficking and degradation of TLR4 underlie the elevated inflammatory response in cystic fibrosis. *J. Immunol.* 186, 6990–6998. doi: 10.4049/jimmunol.1100396

Bryan, H. K., Olayanju, A., Goldring, C. E., and Park, B. K. (2013). The Nrf2 cell defence pathway: Keap1-dependent and -independent mechanisms of regulation. *Biochem. Pharmacol.* 85, 705–717. doi: 10.1016/j.bcp.2012.11.016

Cantin, A. M., Hartl, D., Konstan, M. W., and Chmiel, J. F. (2015). Inflammation in cystic fibrosis lung disease: Pathogenesis and therapy. *J. Cyst. Fibros* 14, 419–430. doi: 10.1016/j.jcf.2015.03.003

Casanova, N., Zhou, T., Gonzalez-Garay, M. L., Rosas, I. O., Goldberg, H. J., Ryter, S. W., et al. (2019). Low Dose Carbon Monoxide Exposure in Idiopathic Pulmonary Fibrosis Produces a CO Signature Comprised of Oxidative Phosphorylation Genes. *Sci. Rep.* 9, 14802. doi: 10.1038/s41598-019-50585-3

Chan, K., and Kan, Y. W. (1999). Nrf2 is essential for protection against acute pulmonary injury in mice. *Proc. Natl. Acad. Sci. U.S.A.* 96, 12731–12736. doi: 10.1073/pnas.96.22.12731

Chen, J., Kinter, M., Shank, S., Cotton, C., Kelley, T. J., and Ziady, A. G. (2008). Dysfunction of Nrf-2 in CF epithelia leads to excess intracellular H2O2 and inflammatory cytokine production. *PloS One* 3, e3367. doi: 10.1371/journal.pone.0003367

Cheng, X., Ku, C. H., and Siow, R. C. (2013). Regulation of the Nrf2 antioxidant pathway by microRNAs: New players in micromanaging redox homeostasis. *Free Radic. Biol. Med.* 64, 4–11. doi: 10.1016/j.freeradbiomed.2013.07.025

Chhikara, M., Wang, S., Kern, S. J., Ferreyra, G. A., Barb, J. J., Munson, P. J., et al. (2009). Carbon monoxide blocks lipopolysaccharide-induced gene expression by interfering with proximal TLR4 to NF-kappaB signal transduction in human monocytes. *PloS One* 4, e8139. doi: 10.1371/journal.pone.0008139

Chiang, N., Shinohara, M., Dalli, J., Mirakaj, V., Kibi, M., Choi, A. M., et al. (2013). Inhaled carbon monoxide accelerates resolution of inflammation via unique proresolving mediator-heme oxygenase-1 circuits. *J. Immunol.* 190, 6378–6388. doi: 10.4049/jimmunol.1202969

Chillappagari, S., Venkatesan, S., Garapati, V., Mahavadi, P., Munder, A., Seubert, A., et al. (2014). Impaired TLR4 and HIF expression in cystic fibrosis bronchial epithelial cells downregulates hemeoxygenase-1 and alters iron homeostasis in vitro. *Am. J. Physiol. Lung Cell Mol. Physiol.* 307, L791–L799. doi: 10.1152/ajplung.00167.2014

Chillappagari, S., Garapati, V., Mahavadi, P., Naehrlich, L., Schmeck, B. T., Schmitz, M. L., et al. (2020). Defective BACH1/HO-1 regulatory circuits in cystic fibrosis bronchial epithelial cells. *J. Cyst. Fibros.* doi: 10.1016/j.jcf.2020.05.006

Chin, B. Y., and Otterbein, L. E. (2009). Carbon monoxide is a poison... to microbes! CO as a bactericidal molecule. *Curr. Opin. Pharmacol.* 9, 490–500. doi: 10.1016/j.coph.2009.06.025

Chin, B. Y., Jiang, G., Wegiel, B., Wang, H. J., Macdonald, T., Zhang, X. C., et al. (2007). Hypoxia-inducible factor 1alpha stabilization by carbon monoxide results in cytoprotective preconditioning. *Proc. Natl. Acad. Sci. U.S.A.* 104, 5109–5114. doi: 10.1073/pnas.0609611104

Chiron, R., Grumbach, Y. Y., Quynh, N. V., Verriere, V., and Urbach, V. (2008). Lipoxin A(4) and interleukin-8 levels in cystic fibrosis sputum after antibiotherapy. *J. Cyst. Fibros* 7, 463–468. doi: 10.1016/j.jcf.2008.04.002

Chmiel, J. F., and Davis, P. B. (2003). State of the art: why do the lungs of patients with cystic fibrosis become infected and why can't they clear the infection? *Respir. Res.* 4, 8. doi: 10.1186/1465-9921-4-8

Chung, S. W., Hall, S. R., and Perrella, M. A. (2009). Role of haem oxygenase-1 in microbial host defence. *Cell Microbiol.* 11, 199–207. doi: 10.1111/j.1462-5822.2008.01261.x

Converso, D. P., Taille, C., Carreras, M. C., Jaitovich, A., Poderoso, J. J., and Boczkowski, J. (2006). HO-1 is located in liver mitochondria and modulates mitochondrial heme content and metabolism. *FASEB J.* 20, 1236–1238. doi: 10.1096/fj.05-4204fje

Cruse, I., and Maines, M. D. (1988). Evidence suggesting that the two forms of heme oxygenase are products of different genes. *J. Biol. Chem.* 263, 3348–3353.

Dalli, J., Kraft, B. D., Colas, R. A., Shinohara, M., Fredenburgh, L. E., Hess, D. R., et al. (2015). The Regulation of Proresolving Lipid Mediator Profiles in Baboon Pneumonia by Inhaled Carbon Monoxide. *Am. J. Respir. Cell Mol. Biol.* 53, 314–325. doi: 10.1165/rcmb.2014-0299OC

Davies, T. G., Wixted, W. E., Coyle, J. E., Griffiths-Jones, C., Hearn, K., Mcmenamin, R., et al. (2016). Monoacidic Inhibitors of the Kelch-like ECH-Associated Protein 1: Nuclear Factor Erythroid 2-Related Factor 2 (KEAP1:NRF2) Protein-Protein Interaction with High Cell Potency Identified by Fragment-Based Discovery. *J. Med. Chem.* 59, 3991–4006. doi: 10.1021/acs.jmedchem.6b00228

Davis, P. B. (2006). Cystic fibrosis since 1938. *Am. J. Respir. Crit. Care Med.* 173, 475–482. doi: 10.1164/rccm.200505-840OE

Day, B. J., Van Heeckeren, A. M., Min, E., and Velsor, L. W. (2004). Role for cystic fibrosis transmembrane conductance regulator protein in a glutathione response to bronchopulmonary pseudomonas infection. *Infect. Immun.* 72, 2045–2051. doi: 10.1128/IAI.72.4.2045-2051.2004

De Bari, L., Favia, M., Bobba, A., Lassandro, R., Guerra, L., and Atlante, A. (2018). Aberrant GSH reductase and NOX activities concur with defective CFTR to pro-oxidative imbalance in cystic fibrosis airways. *J. Bioenerg. Biomembr.* 50, 117–129. doi: 10.1007/s10863-018-9748-x

Demirdjian, S., Hopkins, D., Sanchez, H., Libre, M., Gerber, S. A., and Berwin, B. (2018). Phosphatidylinositol-(3,4,5)-Trisphosphate Induces Phagocytosis of Nonmotile Pseudomonas aeruginosa. *Infect. Immun.* 86. doi: 10.1128/IAI.00215-18

Desmard, M., Davidge, K. S., Bouvet, O., Morin, D., Roux, D., Foresti, R., et al. (2009). A carbon monoxide-releasing molecule (CORM-3) exerts bactericidal activity against Pseudomonas aeruginosa and improves survival in an animal model of bacteraemia. *FASEB J.* 23, 1023–1031. doi: 10.1096/fj.08-122804

Dhakshinamoorthy, S., Jain, A. K., Bloom, D. A., and Jaiswal, A. K. (2005). Bach1 competes with Nrf2 leading to negative regulation of the antioxidant response element (ARE)-mediated NAD(P)H:quinone oxidoreductase 1 gene expression and induction in response to antioxidants. *J. Biol. Chem.* 280, 16891–16900. doi: 10.1074/jbc.M500166200

Dhar, R., Misra, H., and Diringer, M. N. (2017). SANGUINATE (PEGylated Carboxyhemoglobin Bovine) Improves Cerebral Blood Flow to Vulnerable Brain Regions at Risk of Delayed Cerebral Ischemia After Subarachnoid Hemorrhage. *Neurocrit. Care* 27, 341–349. doi: 10.1007/s12028-017-0418-3

Di, A., Brown, M. E., Deriy, L. V., Li, C., Szeto, F. L., Chen, Y., et al. (2006). CFTR regulates phagosome acidification in macrophages and alters bactericidal activity. *Nat. Cell Biol.* 8, 933–944. doi: 10.1038/ncb1456

Di Pietro, C., Zhang, P. X., O'rourke, T. K., Murray, T. S., Wang, L., Britto, C. J., et al. (2017). Ezrin links CFTR to TLR4 signaling to orchestrate anti-bacterial immune response in macrophages. *Sci. Rep.* 7, 10882. doi: 10.1038/s41598-017-11012-7

Doran, A. C., Yurdagul, A.Jr., and Tabas, I. (2020). Efferocytosis in health and disease. *Nat. Rev. Immunol.* 20, 254–267. doi: 10.1038/s41577-019-0240-6

Doring, G., Bragonzi, A., Paroni, M., Akturk, F. F., Cigana, C., Schmidt, A., et al. (2014). BIIL 284 reduces neutrophil numbers but increases P. aeruginosa bacteremia and inflammation in mouse lungs. *J. Cyst. Fibros* 13, 156–163. doi: 10.1016/j.jcf.2013.10.007

Elborn, J. S. (2016). Cystic fibrosis. *Lancet* 388, 2519–2531. doi: 10.1016/S0140-6736(16)00576-6

Elmer, H. L., Brady, K. G., Drumm, M. L., and Kelley, T. J. (1999). Nitric oxide-mediated regulation of transepithelial sodium and chloride transport in murine nasal epithelium. *Am. J. Physiol.* 276, L466–L473. doi: 10.1152/ajplung.1999.276.3.L466

Exner, M., Minar, E., Wagner, O., and Schillinger, M. (2004). The role of heme oxygenase-1 promoter polymorphisms in human disease. *Free Radic. Biol. Med.* 37, 1097–1104. doi: 10.1016/j.freeradbiomed.2004.07.008

Fagone, P., Mazzon, E., Bramanti, P., Bendtzen, K., and Nicoletti, F. (2018). Gasotransmitters and the immune system: Mode of action and novel therapeutic targets. *Eur. J. Pharmacol.* 834, 92–102. doi: 10.1016/j.ejphar.2018.07.026

Ferrari, E., Monzani, R., Villella, V. R., Esposito, S., Saluzzo, F., Rossin, F., et al. (2017). Cysteamine re-establishes the clearance of Pseudomonas aeruginosa by macrophages bearing the cystic fibrosis-relevant F508del-CFTR mutation. *Cell Death Dis.* 8, e2544. doi: 10.1038/cddis.2016.476

Flanagan, L., Steen, R. R., Saxby, K., Klatter, M., Aucott, B. J., Winstanley, C., et al. (2018). The Antimicrobial Activity of a Carbon Monoxide Releasing Molecule (EBOR-CORM-1) Is Shaped by Intraspecific Variation within Pseudomonas aeruginosa Populations. *Front. Microbiol.* 9, 195. doi: 10.3389/fmicb.2018.00195

Flitter, B. A., Hvorecny, K. L., Ono, E., Eddens, T., Yang, J., Kwak, D. H., et al. (2017). Pseudomonas aeruginosa sabotages the generation of host proresolving lipid mediators. *Proc. Natl. Acad. Sci. U.S.A.* 114, 136–141. doi: 10.1073/pnas.1610242114

Foresti, R., and Motterlini, R. (1999). The heme oxygenase pathway and its interaction with nitric oxide in the control of cellular homeostasis. *Free Radic. Res.* 31, 459–475. doi: 10.1080/10715769900301031

Fredenburgh, L. E., Kraft, B. D., Hess, D. R., Harris, R. S., Wolf, M. A., Suliman, H. B., et al. (2015). Effects of inhaled CO administration on acute lung injury in baboons with pneumococcal pneumonia. *Am. J. Physiol. Lung Cell Mol. Physiol.* 309, L834–L846. doi: 10.1152/ajplung.00240.2015

Fredenburgh, L. E., Perrella, M. A., Barragan-Bradford, D., Hess, D. R., Peters, E., Welty-Wolf, K. E., et al. (2018). A phase I trial of low-dose inhaled carbon monoxide in sepsis-induced ARDS. *JCI Insight* 3. doi: 10.1172/jci.insight.124039

Galli, F., Battistoni, A., Gambari, R., Pompella, A., Bragonzi, A., Pilolli, F., et al. (2012). Oxidative stress and antioxidant therapy in cystic fibrosis. *Biochim. Biophys. Acta* 1822, 690–713. doi: 10.1016/j.bbadis.2011.12.012

Gao, L., Kim, K. J., Yankaskas, J. R., and Forman, H. J. (1999). Abnormal glutathione transport in cystic fibrosis airway epithelia. *Am. J. Physiol.* 277, L113–L118. doi: 10.1152/ajplung.1999.277.1.L113

Garratt, L. W., Sutanto, E. N., Ling, K. M., Looi, K., Iosifidis, T., Martinovich, K. M., et al. (2015). Matrix metalloproteinase activation by free neutrophil elastase contributes to bronchiectasis progression in early cystic fibrosis. *Eur. Respir. J.* 46, 384–394. doi: 10.1183/09031936.00212114

Ghio, A. J., Roggli, V. L., Soukup, J. M., Richards, J. H., Randell, S. H., and Muhlebach, M. S. (2013). Iron accumulates in the lavage and explanted lungs of cystic fibrosis patients. *J. Cyst. Fibros* 12, 390–398. doi: 10.1016/j.jcf.2012.10.010

Gottlieb, Y., Truman, M., Cohen, L. A., Leichtmann-Bardoogo, Y., and Meyron-Holtz, E. G. (2012). Endoplasmic reticulum anchored heme-oxygenase 1 faces the cytosol. *Haematologica* 97, 1489–1493. doi: 10.3324/haematol.2012.063651

Gozzelino, R., Jeney, V., and Soares, M. P. (2010). Mechanisms of cell protection by heme oxygenase-1. *Annu. Rev. Pharmacol. Toxicol.* 50, 323–354. doi: 10.1146/annurev.pharmtox.010909.105600

Gray, R. D., Hardisty, G., Regan, K. H., Smith, M., Robb, C. T., Duffin, R., et al. (2018). Delayed neutrophil apoptosis enhances NET formation in cystic fibrosis. *Thorax* 73, 134–144. doi: 10.1136/thoraxjnl-2017-210134

Guggino, W. B., and Stanton, B. A. (2006). New insights into cystic fibrosis: molecular switches that regulate CFTR. *Nat. Rev. Mol. Cell Biol.* 7, 426–436. doi: 10.1038/nrm1949

Haggie, P. M., and Verkman, A. S. (2007). Cystic fibrosis transmembrane conductance regulator-independent phagosomal acidification in macrophages. *J. Biol. Chem.* 282, 31422–31428. doi: 10.1074/jbc.M705296200

Harmon, G. S., Dumlao, D. S., Ng, D. T., Barrett, K. E., Dennis, E. A., Dong, H., et al. (2010). Pharmacological correction of a defect in PPAR-gamma signaling ameliorates disease severity in Cftr-deficient mice. *Nat. Med.* 16, 313–318. doi: 10.1038/nm.2101

Harvey, C. J., Thimmulappa, R. K., Sethi, S., Kong, X., Yarmus, L., Brown, R. H., et al. (2011). Targeting Nrf2 signaling improves bacterial clearance by alveolar macrophages in patients with COPD and in a mouse model. *Sci. Transl. Med.* 3, 78ra32. doi: 10.1126/scitranslmed.3002042

Haschemi, A., Chin, B. Y., Jeitler, M., Esterbauer, H., Wagner, O., Bilban, M., et al. (2011). Carbon monoxide induced PPARgamma SUMOylation and UCP2 block inflammatory gene expression in macrophages. *PloS One* 6, e26376. doi: 10.1371/journal.pone.0026376

Headland, S. E., and Norling, L. V. (2015). The resolution of inflammation: Principles and challenges. *Semin. Immunol.* 27, 149–160. doi: 10.1016/j.smim.2015.03.014

Hisert, K. B., Heltshe, S. L., Pope, C., Jorth, P., Wu, X., Edwards, R. M., et al. (2017). Restoring Cystic Fibrosis Transmembrane Conductance Regulator Function Reduces Airway Bacteria and Inflammation in People with Cystic Fibrosis and Chronic Lung Infections. *Am. J. Respir. Crit. Care Med.* 195, 1617–1628. doi: 10.1164/rccm.201609-1954OC

Holzner, M. L., Demaria, S., Haydel, B., Smith, N., Flaherty, D., and Florman, S. (2018). Pegylated Bovine Carboxyhemoglobin (SANGUINATE) in a Jehovah's Witness Undergoing Liver Transplant: A Case Report. *Transplant. Proc.* 50, 4012–4014. doi: 10.1016/j.transproceed.2018.09.006

Huang, H. C., Nguyen, T., and Pickett, C. B. (2002). Phosphorylation of Nrf2 at Ser-40 by protein kinase C regulates antioxidant response element-mediated transcription. *J. Biol. Chem.* 277, 42769–42774. doi: 10.1074/jbc.M206911200

Jarosz-Griffiths, H. H., Scambler, T., Wong, C. H., Lara-Reyna, S., Holbrook, J., Martinon, F., et al. (2020). Different CFTR modulator combinations downregulate inflammation differently in cystic fibrosis. *Elife* 9. doi: 10.7554/eLife.54556

Ji, X., Damera, K., Zheng, Y., Yu, B., Otterbein, L. E., and Wang, B. (2016). Toward Carbon Monoxide-Based Therapeutics: Critical Drug Delivery and Developability Issues. *J. Pharm. Sci.* 105, 406–416. doi: 10.1016/j.xphs.2015.10.018

Jung, S. S., Moon, J. S., Xu, J. F., Ifedigbo, E., Ryter, S. W., Choi, A. M., et al. (2015). Carbon monoxide negatively regulates NLRP3 inflammasome activation in macrophages. *Am. J. Physiol. Lung Cell Mol. Physiol.* 308, L1058–L1067. doi: 10.1152/ajplung.00400.2014

Kang, K. W., Lee, S. J., Park, J. W., and Kim, S. G. (2002). Phosphatidylinositol 3-kinase regulates nuclear translocation of NF-E2-related factor 2 through actin rearrangement in response to oxidative stress. *Mol. Pharmacol.* 62, 1001–1010. doi: 10.1124/mol.62.5.1001

Kanik, E. T., Yilmaz, O., Ozdogru, E., Alper, H., Ulman, C., Kanik, A., et al. (2020). Relevance between clinical status and exhaled molecules related to neutrophilic inflammation in pediatric cystic fibrosis. *J. Breath Res.* doi: 10.1088/1752-7163/ab670d

Karp, C. L., Flick, L. M., Park, K. W., Softic, S., Greer, T. M., Keledjian, R., et al. (2004). Defective lipoxin-mediated anti-inflammatory activity in the cystic fibrosis airway. *Nat. Immunol.* 5, 388–392. doi: 10.1038/ni1056

Kelley, T. J., and Drumm, M. L. (1998). Inducible nitric oxide synthase expression is reduced in cystic fibrosis murine and human airway epithelial cells. *J. Clin. Invest.* 102, 1200–1207. doi: 10.1172/JCI2357

Kelley, T. J., Al-Nakkash, L., and Drumm, M. L. (1997a). C-type natriuretic peptide increases chloride permeability in normal and cystic fibrosis airway cells. *Am. J. Respir. Cell Mol. Biol.* 16, 464–470. doi: 10.1165/ajrcmb.16.4.9115758

Kelley, T. J., Cotton, C. U., and Drumm, M. L. (1997b). In vivo activation of CFTR-dependent chloride transport in murine airway epithelium by CNP. *Am. J. Physiol.* 273, L1065–L1072. doi: 10.1152/ajplung.1997.273.5.L1065

Khan, T. Z., Wagener, J. S., Bost, T., Martinez, J., Accurso, F. J., and Riches, D. W. (1995). Early pulmonary inflammation in infants with cystic fibrosis. *Am. J. Respir. Crit. Care Med.* 151, 1075–1082. doi: 10.1164/ajrccm.151.4.7697234

Kim, H. P., Wang, X., Galbiati, F., Ryter, S. W., and Choi, A. M. (2004). Caveolae compartmentalization of heme oxygenase-1 in endothelial cells. *FASEB J.* 18, 1080–1089. doi: 10.1096/fj.03-1391com

Kim, H. J., Joe, Y., Rah, S. Y., Kim, S. K., Park, S. U., Park, J., et al. (2018). Carbon monoxide-induced TFEB nuclear translocation enhances mitophagy/mitochondrial biogenesis in hepatocytes and ameliorates inflammatory liver injury. *Cell Death Dis.* 9, 1060. doi: 10.1038/s41419-018-1112-x

Kim, M. D., Baumlin, N., Yoshida, M., Polineni, D., Salathe, S. F., David, J. K., et al. (2020). Losartan Rescues Inflammation-related Mucociliary Dysfunction in Relevant Models of Cystic Fibrosis. *Am. J. Respir. Crit. Care Med.* 201, 313–324. doi: 10.1164/rccm.201905-0990OC

Konstan, M. W., Byard, P. J., Hoppel, C. L., and Davis, P. B. (1995). Effect of high-dose ibuprofen in patients with cystic fibrosis. *N. Engl. J. Med.* 332, 848–854. doi: 10.1056/NEJM199503303321303

Konstan, M. W., Doring, G., Heltshe, S. L., Lands, L. C., Hilliard, K. A., Koker, P., et al. (2014). A randomized double blind, placebo controlled phase 2 trial of BIIL 284 BS (an LTB4 receptor antagonist) for the treatment of lung disease in children and adults with cystic fibrosis. *J. Cyst. Fibros* 13, 148–155. doi: 10.1016/j.jcf.2013.12.009

Lancel, S., Hassoun, S. M., Favory, R., Decoster, B., Motterlini, R., and Neviere, R. (2009). Carbon monoxide rescues mice from lethal sepsis by supporting mitochondrial energetic metabolism and activating mitochondrial biogenesis. *J. Pharmacol. Exp. Ther.* 329, 641–648. doi: 10.1124/jpet.108.148049

Lavrovsky, Y., Schwartzman, M. L., Levere, R. D., Kappas, A., and Abraham, N. G. (1994). Identification of binding sites for transcription factors NF-kappa B and AP-2 in the promoter region of the human heme oxygenase 1 gene. *Proc. Natl. Acad. Sci. U.S.A.* 91, 5987–5991. doi: 10.1073/pnas.91.13.5987

Lee, P. J., Jiang, B. H., Chin, B. Y., Iyer, N. V., Alam, J., Semenza, G. L., et al. (1997). Hypoxia-inducible factor-1 mediates transcriptional activation of the heme oxygenase-1 gene in response to hypoxia. *J. Biol. Chem.* 272, 5375–5381. doi: 10.1074/jbc.272.9.5375

Lee, S. J., Ryter, S. W., Xu, J. F., Nakahira, K., Kim, H. P., Choi, A. M., et al. (2011). Carbon monoxide activates autophagy via mitochondrial reactive oxygen species formation. *Am. J. Respir. Cell Mol. Biol.* 45, 867–873. doi: 10.1165/rcmb.2010-0352OC

Legendre, C., Mooij, M. J., Adams, C., and O'gara, F. (2011). Impaired expression of hypoxia-inducible factor-1alpha in cystic fibrosis airway epithelial cells - a role for HIF-1 in the pathophysiology of CF? *J. Cyst. Fibros* 10, 286–290. doi: 10.1016/j.jcf.2011.02.005

Lin, C. C., Hsiao, L. D., Cho, R. L., and Yang, C. M. (2019). CO-Releasing Molecule-2 Induces Nrf2/ARE-Dependent Heme Oxygenase-1 Expression Suppressing TNF-alpha-Induced Pulmonary Inflammation. *J. Clin. Med.* 8. doi: 10.3390/jcm8040436

Liu, G. H., Qu, J., and Shen, X. (2008). NF-kappaB/p65 antagonizes Nrf2-ARE pathway by depriving CBP from Nrf2 and facilitating recruitment of HDAC3 to MafK. *Biochim. Biophys. Acta* 1783, 713–727. doi: 10.1016/j.bbamcr.2008.01.002

Lovewell, R. R., Hayes, S. M., O'toole, G. A., and Berwin, B. (2014). Pseudomonas aeruginosa flagellar motility activates the phagocyte PI3K/Akt pathway to induce phagocytic engulfment. *Am. J. Physiol. Lung Cell Mol. Physiol.* 306, L698–L707. doi: 10.1152/ajplung.00319.2013

Luciani, A., Villella, V. R., Esposito, S., Brunetti-Pierri, N., Medina, D., Settembre, C., et al. (2010). Defective CFTR induces aggresome formation and lung inflammation in cystic fibrosis through ROS-mediated autophagy inhibition. *Nat. Cell Biol.* 12, 863–875. doi: 10.1038/ncb2090

Macgarvey, N. C., Suliman, H. B., Bartz, R. R., Fu, P., Withers, C. M., Welty-Wolf, K. E., et al. (2012). Activation of mitochondrial biogenesis by heme oxygenase-1-mediated NF-E2-related factor-2 induction rescues mice from lethal Staphylococcus aureus sepsis. *Am. J. Respir. Crit. Care Med.* 185, 851–861. doi: 10.1164/rccm.201106-1152OC

Magalhaes, M., Rivals, I., Claustres, M., Varilh, J., Thomasset, M., Bergougnoux, A., et al. (2017). DNA methylation at modifier genes of lung disease severity is altered in cystic fibrosis. *Clin. Epigenet.* 9, 19. doi: 10.1186/s13148-016-0300-8

Maines, M. D., Trakshel, G. M., and Kutty, R. K. (1986). Characterization of two constitutive forms of rat liver microsomal heme oxygenase. Only one molecular species of the enzyme is inducible. *J. Biol. Chem.* 261, 411–419.

Mall, M., Grubb, B. R., Harkema, J. R., O'neal, W. K., and Boucher, R. C. (2004). Increased airway epithelial Na+ absorption produces cystic fibrosis-like lung disease in mice. *Nat. Med.* 10, 487–493. doi: 10.1038/nm1028

Mall, M. A. (2009). Role of the amiloride-sensitive epithelial Na+ channel in the pathogenesis and as a therapeutic target for cystic fibrosis lung disease. *Exp. Physiol.* 94, 171–174. doi: 10.1113/expphysiol.2008.042994

Manzanares, D., Gonzalez, C., Ivonnet, P., Chen, R. S., Valencia-Gattas, M., Conner, G. E., et al. (2011). Functional apical large conductance, Ca2+-activated, and voltage-dependent K+ channels are required for maintenance of airway surface liquid volume. *J. Biol. Chem.* 286, 19830–19839. doi: 10.1074/jbc.M110.185074

Manzanares, D., Krick, S., Baumlin, N., Dennis, J. S., Tyrrell, J., Tarran, R., et al. (2015). Airway Surface Dehydration by Transforming Growth Factor beta (TGF-beta) in Cystic Fibrosis Is Due to Decreased Function of a Voltage-dependent Potassium Channel and Can Be Rescued by the Drug Pirfenidone. *J. Biol. Chem.* 290, 25710–25716. doi: 10.1074/jbc.M115.670885

Martin, D., Rojo, A. I., Salinas, M., Diaz, R., Gallardo, G., Alam, J., et al. (2004). Regulation of heme oxygenase-1 expression through the phosphatidylinositol 3-kinase/Akt pathway and the Nrf2 transcription factor in response to the antioxidant phytochemical carnosol. *J. Biol. Chem.* 279, 8919–8929. doi: 10.1074/jbc.M309660200

Matos, A. M., Pinto, F. R., Barros, P., Amaral, M. D., Pepperkok, R., and Matos, P. (2019). Inhibition of calpain 1 restores plasma membrane stability to pharmacologically rescued Phe508del-CFTR variant. *J. Biol. Chem.* 294, 13396–13410. doi: 10.1074/jbc.RA119.008738

Mayr, F. B., Spiel, A., Leitner, J., Marsik, C., Germann, P., Ullrich, R., et al. (2005). Effects of carbon monoxide inhalation during experimental endotoxemia in humans. *Am. J. Respir. Crit. Care Med.* 171, 354–360. doi: 10.1164/rccm.200404-446OC

Mccoubrey, W. K.Jr., Huang, T. J., and Maines, M. D. (1997). Isolation and characterization of a cDNA from the rat brain that encodes hemoprotein heme oxygenase-3. *Eur. J. Biochem.* 247, 725–732. doi: 10.1111/j.1432-1033.1997.00725.x

Medina, M. V., Sapochnik, D., Garcia Sola, M., and Coso, O. (2020). Regulation of the Expression of Heme Oxygenase-1: Signal Transduction, Gene Promoter Activation, and Beyond. *Antioxid. Redox Signal* 32, 1033–1044. doi: 10.1089/ars.2019.7991

Middleton, P. G., Mall, M. A., Drevinek, P., Lands, L. C., Mckone, E. F., Polineni, D., et al. (2019). Elexacaftor-Tezacaftor-Ivacaftor for Cystic Fibrosis with a Single Phe508del Allele. *N. Engl. J. Med.* 381, 1809–1819. doi: 10.1056/NEJMoa1908639

Mills, E. L., and O'Neill, L. A. (2016). Reprogramming mitochondrial metabolism in macrophages as an anti-inflammatory signal. *Eur. J. Immunol.* 46, 13–21. doi: 10.1002/eji.201445427

Misharin, A. V., Morales-Nebreda, L., Reyfman, P. A., Cuda, C. M., Walter, J. M., Mcquattie-Pimentel, A. C., et al. (2017). Monocyte-derived alveolar macrophages drive lung fibrosis and persist in the lung over the life span. *J. Exp. Med.* 214, 2387–2404. doi: 10.1084/jem.20162152

Misra, H., Lickliter, J., Kazo, F., and Abuchowski, A. (2014). PEGylated carboxyhemoglobin bovine (SANGUINATE): results of a phase I clinical trial. *Artif. Organs* 38, 702–707. doi: 10.1111/aor.12341

Misra, H., Bainbridge, J., Berryman, J., Abuchowski, A., Galvez, K. M., Uribe, L. F., et al. (2017). A Phase Ib open label, randomized, safety study of SANGUINATE in patients with sickle cell anemia. *Rev. Bras. Hematol. Hemoter.* 39, 20–27. doi: 10.1016/j.bjhh.2016.08.004

Mizuguchi, S., Stephen, J., Bihari, R., Markovic, N., Suehiro, S., Capretta, A., et al. (2009). CORM-3-derived CO modulates polymorphonuclear leukocyte migration across the vascular endothelium by reducing levels of cell surface-bound elastase. *Am. J. Physiol. Heart Circ. Physiol.* 297, H920–H929. doi: 10.1152/ajpheart.00305.2009

Mogayzel, P. J.Jr., Naureckas, E. T., Robinson, K. A., Mueller, G., Hadjiliadis, D., Hoag, J. B., et al. (2013). Cystic fibrosis pulmonary guidelines. Chronic medications for maintenance of lung health. *Am. J. Respir. Crit. Care Med.* 187, 680–689. doi: 10.1164/rccm.201207-1160OE

Montgomery, S. T., Mall, M. A., Kicic, A., Stick, S. M., and Arest, C. F. (2017). Hypoxia and sterile inflammation in cystic fibrosis airways: mechanisms and potential therapies. *Eur. Respir. J.* 49. doi: 10.1183/13993003.00903-2016

Moreau-Marquis, S., Bomberger, J. M., Anderson, G. G., Swiatecka-Urban, A., Ye, S., O'toole, G. A., et al. (2008). The DeltaF508-CFTR mutation results in increased biofilm formation by Pseudomonas aeruginosa by increasing iron availability. *Am. J. Physiol. Lung Cell Mol. Physiol.* 295, L25–L37. doi: 10.1152/ajplung.00391.2007

Motterlini, R., and Foresti, R. (2017). Biological signaling by carbon monoxide and carbon monoxide-releasing molecules. *Am. J. Physiol. Cell Physiol.* 312, C302–C313. doi: 10.1152/ajpcell.00360.2016

Motterlini, R., and Otterbein, L. E. (2010). The therapeutic potential of carbon monoxide. *Nat. Rev. Drug Discovery* 9, 728–743. doi: 10.1038/nrd3228

Motterlini, R., Clark, J. E., Foresti, R., Sarathchandra, P., Mann, B. E., and Green, C. J. (2002). Carbon monoxide-releasing molecules: characterization of biochemical and vascular activities. *Circ. Res.* 90, E17–E24. doi: 10.1161/hh0202.104530

Murad, F. (2006). Shattuck Lecture. Nitric oxide and cyclic GMP in cell signaling and drug development. *N. Engl. J. Med.* 355, 2003–2011. doi: 10.1056/NEJMsa063904

Murray, T. S., Okegbe, C., Gao, Y., Kazmierczak, B. I., Motterlini, R., Dietrich, L. E., et al. (2012). The carbon monoxide releasing molecule CORM-2 attenuates Pseudomonas aeruginosa biofilm formation. *PloS One* 7, e35499. doi: 10.1371/journal.pone.0035499

Nagel, C., Mclean, S., Poole, R. K., Braunschweig, H., Kramer, T., and Schatzschneider, U. (2014). Introducing [Mn(CO)3(tpa-kappa(3)N)](+) as a novel photoactivatable CO-releasing molecule with well-defined iCORM intermediates - synthesis, spectroscopy, and antibacterial activity. *Dalton. Trans.* 43, 9986–9997. doi: 10.1039/c3dt51848e

Naidu, S., Wijayanti, N., Santoso, S., Kietzmann, T., and Immenschuh, S. (2008). An atypical NF-kappa B-regulated pathway mediates phorbol ester-dependent heme oxygenase-1 gene activation in monocytes. *J. Immunol.* 181, 4113–4123. doi: 10.4049/jimmunol.181.6.4113

Nakahira, K., Kim, H. P., Geng, X. H., Nakao, A., Wang, X., Murase, N., et al. (2006). Carbon monoxide differentially inhibits TLR signaling pathways by regulating ROS-induced trafficking of TLRs to lipid rafts. *J. Exp. Med.* 203, 2377–2389. doi: 10.1084/jem.20060845

Nobre, L. S., Seixas, J. D., Romao, C. C., and Saraiva, L. M. (2007). Antimicrobial action of carbon monoxide-releasing compounds. *Antimicrob. Agents Chemother.* 51, 4303–4307. doi: 10.1128/AAC.00802-07

Nobre, L. S., Al-Shahrour, F., Dopazo, J., and Saraiva, L. M. (2009). Exploring the antimicrobial action of a carbon monoxide-releasing compound through whole-genome transcription profiling of Escherichia coli. *Microbiology* 155, 813–824. doi: 10.1099/mic.0.023911-0

Nobre, L. S., Jeremias, H., Romao, C. C., and Saraiva, L. M. (2016). Examining the antimicrobial activity and toxicity to animal cells of different types of CO-releasing molecules. *Dalton. Trans.* 45, 1455–1466. doi: 10.1039/C5DT02238J

Ogawa, K., Sun, J., Taketani, S., Nakajima, O., Nishitani, C., Sassa, S., et al. (2001). Heme mediates derepression of Maf recognition element through direct binding to transcription repressor Bach1. *EMBO J.* 20, 2835–2843. doi: 10.1093/emboj/20.11.2835

Onyiah, J. C., Sheikh, S. Z., Maharshak, N., Steinbach, E. C., Russo, S. M., Kobayashi, T., et al. (2013). Carbon monoxide and heme oxygenase-1 prevent intestinal inflammation in mice by promoting bacterial clearance. *Gastroenterology* 144, 789–798. doi: 10.1053/j.gastro.2012.12.025

Otterbein, L. E., Bach, F. H., Alam, J., Soares, M., Tao Lu, H., Wysk, M., et al. (2000). Carbon monoxide has anti-inflammatory effects involving the mitogen-activated protein kinase pathway. *Nat. Med.* 6, 422–428. doi: 10.1038/74680

Otterbein, L. E., Otterbein, S. L., Ifedigbo, E., Liu, F., Morse, D. E., Fearns, C., et al. (2003). MKK3 mitogen-activated protein kinase pathway mediates carbon monoxide-induced protection against oxidant-induced lung injury. *Am. J. Pathol.* 163, 2555–2563. doi: 10.1016/S0002-9440(10)63610-3

Otterbein, L. E., May, A., and Chin, B. Y. (2005). Carbon monoxide increases macrophage bacterial clearance through Toll-like receptor (TLR)4 expression. *Cell Mol. Biol. (Noisy-le-grand)* 51, 433–440.

Park, J. E., Yung, R., Stefanowicz, D., Shumansky, K., Akhabir, L., Durie, P. R., et al. (2011). Cystic fibrosis modifier genes related to Pseudomonas aeruginosa infection. *Genes Immun.* 12, 370–377. doi: 10.1038/gene.2011.5

Paul, K., Rietschel, E., Ballmann, M., Griese, M., Worlitzsch, D., Shute, J., et al. (2004). Effect of treatment with dornase alpha on airway inflammation in patients with cystic fibrosis. *Am. J. Respir. Crit. Care Med.* 169, 719–725. doi: 10.1164/rccm.200307-959OC

Peers, C., Boyle, J. P., Scragg, J. L., Dallas, M. L., Al-Owais, M. M., Hettiarachichi, N. T., et al. (2015). Diverse mechanisms underlying the regulation of ion channels by carbon monoxide. *Br. J. Pharmacol.* 172, 1546–1556. doi: 10.1111/bph.12760

Perez, A., Issler, A. C., Cotton, C. U., Kelley, T. J., Verkman, A. S., and Davis, P. B. (2007). CFTR inhibition mimics the cystic fibrosis inflammatory profile. *Am. J. Physiol. Lung Cell Mol. Physiol.* 292, L383–L395. doi: 10.1152/ajplung.00403.2005

Piantadosi, C. A., Carraway, M. S., Babiker, A., and Suliman, H. B. (2008). Heme oxygenase-1 regulates cardiac mitochondrial biogenesis via Nrf2-mediated transcriptional control of nuclear respiratory factor-1. *Circ. Res.* 103, 1232–1240. doi: 10.1161/01.RES.0000338597.71702.ad

Piantadosi, C. A., Withers, C. M., Bartz, R. R., Macgarvey, N. C., Fu, P., Sweeney, T. E., et al. (2011). Heme oxygenase-1 couples activation of mitochondrial biogenesis to anti-inflammatory cytokine expression. *J. Biol. Chem.* 286, 16374–16385. doi: 10.1074/jbc.M110.207738

Porteous, M. K., Diamond, J. M., and Christie, J. D. (2015). Primary graft dysfunction: lessons learned about the first 72 h after lung transplantation. *Curr. Opin. Organ Transplant.* 20, 506–514. doi: 10.1097/MOT.0000000000000232

Poss, K. D., and Tonegawa, S. (1997a). Heme oxygenase 1 is required for mammalian iron reutilization. *Proc. Natl. Acad. Sci. U.S.A.* 94, 10919–10924. doi: 10.1073/pnas.94.20.10919

Poss, K. D., and Tonegawa, S. (1997b). Reduced stress defense in heme oxygenase 1-deficient cells. *Proc. Natl. Acad. Sci. U.S.A.* 94, 10925–10930. doi: 10.1073/pnas.94.20.10925

Queiroga, C. S., Almeida, A. S., and Vieira, H. L. (2012). Carbon monoxide targeting mitochondria. *Biochem. Res. Int.* 2012, 749845. doi: 10.1155/2012/749845

Rana, N., Mclean, S., Mann, B. E., and Poole, R. K. (2014). Interaction of the carbon monoxide-releasing molecule Ru(CO)3Cl(glycinate) (CORM-3) with Salmonella enterica serovar Typhimurium: in situ measurements of carbon monoxide binding by integrating cavity dual-beam spectrophotometry. *Microbiology* 160, 2771–2779. doi: 10.1099/mic.0.081042-0

Ratjen, F., Saiman, L., Mayer-Hamblett, N., Lands, L. C., Kloster, M., Thompson, V., et al. (2012). Effect of azithromycin on systemic markers of inflammation in patients with cystic fibrosis uninfected with Pseudomonas aeruginosa. *Chest* 142, 1259–1266. doi: 10.1378/chest.12-0628

Recchiuti, A., Mattoscio, D., and Isopi, E. (2019). Roles, Actions, and Therapeutic Potential of Specialized Pro-resolving Lipid Mediators for the Treatment of Inflammation in Cystic Fibrosis. *Front. Pharmacol.* 10, 252. doi: 10.3389/fphar.2019.00252

Reid, D. W., Withers, N. J., Francis, L., Wilson, J. W., and Kotsimbos, T. C. (2002). Iron deficiency in cystic fibrosis: relationship to lung disease severity and chronic Pseudomonas aeruginosa infection. *Chest* 121, 48–54. doi: 10.1378/chest.121.1.48

Reyfman, P. A., Walter, J. M., Joshi, N., Anekalla, K. R., Mcquattie-Pimentel, A. C., Chiu, S., et al. (2019). Single-Cell Transcriptomic Analysis of Human Lung Provides Insights into the Pathobiology of Pulmonary Fibrosis. *Am. J. Respir. Crit. Care Med.* 199, 1517–1536. doi: 10.1164/rccm.201712-2410OC

Ringholz, F. C., Buchanan, P. J., Clarke, D. T., Millar, R. G., Mcdermott, M., Linnane, B., et al. (2014). Reduced 15-lipoxygenase 2 and lipoxin A4/ leukotriene B4 ratio in children with cystic fibrosis. *Eur. Respir. J.* 44, 394–404. doi: 10.1183/09031936.00106013

Riquelme, S. A., Hopkins, B. D., Wolfe, A. L., Dimango, E., Kitur, K., Parsons, R., et al. (2017). Cystic Fibrosis Transmembrane Conductance Regulator Attaches Tumor Suppressor PTEN to the Membrane and Promotes Anti Pseudomonas aeruginosa Immunity. *Immunity* 47, 1169–1181 e1167. doi: 10.1016/j.immuni.2017.11.010

Riquelme, S. A., Lozano, C., Moustafa, A. M., Liimatta, K., Tomlinson, K. L., Britto, C., et al. (2019). CFTR-PTEN-dependent mitochondrial metabolic dysfunction promotes Pseudomonas aeruginosa airway infection. *Sci. Transl. Med.* 11. doi: 10.1126/scitranslmed.aav4634

Roesch, E. A., Nichols, D. P., and Chmiel, J. F. (2018). Inflammation in cystic fibrosis: An update. *Pediatr. Pulmonol.* 53, S30–S50. doi: 10.1002/ppul.24129

Rosas, I. O., Goldberg, H. J., Collard, H. R., El-Chemaly, S., Flaherty, K., Hunninghake, G. M., et al. (2018). A Phase II Clinical Trial of Low-Dose Inhaled Carbon Monoxide in Idiopathic Pulmonary Fibrosis. *Chest* 153, 94–104. doi: 10.1016/j.chest.2017.09.052

Ross, K. R., Chmiel, J. F., and Konstan, M. W. (2009). The role of inhaled corticosteroids in the management of cystic fibrosis. *Paediatr. Drugs* 11, 101–113. doi: 10.2165/00148581-200911020-00002

Roussel, L., and Rousseau, S. (2017). Exposure of airway epithelial cells to Pseudomonas aeruginosa biofilm-derived quorum sensing molecules decrease the activity of the anti-oxidant response element bound by NRF2. *Biochem. Biophys. Res. Commun.* 483, 829–833. doi: 10.1016/j.bbrc.2017.01.009

Rowe, S. M., Heltshe, S. L., Gonska, T., Donaldson, S. H., Borowitz, D., Gelfond, D., et al. (2014). Clinical mechanism of the cystic fibrosis transmembrane conductance regulator potentiator ivacaftor in G551D-mediated cystic fibrosis. *Am. J. Respir. Crit. Care Med.* 190, 175–184. doi: 10.1164/rccm.201404-0703OC

Rushworth, S. A., Zaitseva, L., Murray, M. Y., Shah, N. M., Bowles, K. M., and Macewan, D. J. (2012). The high Nrf2 expression in human acute myeloid leukemia is driven by NF-kappaB and underlies its chemo-resistance. *Blood* 120, 5188–5198. doi: 10.1182/blood-2012-04-422121

Ryter, S. W., and Choi, A. M. (2016). Targeting heme oxygenase-1 and carbon monoxide for therapeutic modulation of inflammation. *Transl. Res.* 167, 7–34. doi: 10.1016/j.trsl.2015.06.011

Ryter, S. W., Alam, J., and Choi, A. M. (2006). Heme oxygenase-1/carbon monoxide: from basic science to therapeutic applications. *Physiol. Rev.* 86, 583–650. doi: 10.1152/physrev.00011.2005

Ryter, S. W., Ma, K. C., and Choi, A. M. K. (2018). Carbon monoxide in lung cell physiology and disease. *Am. J. Physiol. Cell Physiol.* 314, C211–C227. doi: 10.1152/ajpcell.00022.2017

Sam, C., Desai, P., Laber, D., Patel, A., Visweshwar, N., and Jaglal, M. (2017). Pegylated bovine carboxyhaemoglobin utilisation in a thrombotic thrombocytopenic purpura patient. *Transfus. Med.* 27, 300–302. doi: 10.1111/tme.12407

Sawle, P., Foresti, R., Mann, B. E., Johnson, T. R., Green, C. J., and Motterlini, R. (2005). Carbon monoxide-releasing molecules (CO-RMs) attenuate the inflammatory response elicited by lipopolysaccharide in RAW264.7 murine macrophages. *Br. J. Pharmacol.* 145, 800–810. doi: 10.1038/sj.bjp.0706241

Serhan, C. N., Chiang, N., Dalli, J., and Levy, B. D. (2014). Lipid mediators in the resolution of inflammation. *Cold Spring Harb. Perspect. Biol.* 7, a016311. doi: 10.1101/cshperspect.a016311

Shi, J., Yu, J., Zhang, Y., Wu, L., Dong, S., Wu, L., et al. (2019). PI3K/Akt pathway-mediated HO-1 induction regulates mitochondrial quality control and attenuates endotoxin-induced acute lung injury. *Lab. Invest.* 99, 1795–1809. doi: 10.1038/s41374-019-0286-x

Steagall, W. K., Elmer, H. L., Brady, K. G., and Kelley, T. J. (2000). Cystic fibrosis transmembrane conductance regulator-dependent regulation of epithelial inducible nitric oxide synthase expression. *Am. J. Respir. Cell Mol. Biol.* 22, 45–50. doi: 10.1165/ajrcmb.22.1.3789

Stites, S. W., Plautz, M. W., Bailey, K., O'brien-Ladner, A. R., and Wesselius, L. J. (1999). Increased concentrations of iron and isoferritins in the lower respiratory tract of patients with stable cystic fibrosis. *Am. J. Respir. Crit. Care Med.* 160, 796–801. doi: 10.1164/ajrccm.160.3.9811018

Sturges, N. C., Wikstrom, M. E., Winfield, K. R., Gard, S. E., Brennan, S., Sly, P. D., et al. (2010). Monocytes from children with clinically stable cystic fibrosis show enhanced expression of Toll-like receptor 4. *Pediatr. Pulmonol.* 45, 883–889. doi: 10.1002/ppul.21230

Tavares, A. F., Nobre, L. S., and Saraiva, L. M. (2012). A role for reactive oxygen species in the antibacterial properties of carbon monoxide-releasing molecules. *FEMS Microbiol. Lett.* 336, 1–10. doi: 10.1111/j.1574-6968.2012.02633.x

Tavares, A. F., Parente, M. R., Justino, M. C., Oleastro, M., Nobre, L. S., and Saraiva, L. M. (2013). The bactericidal activity of carbon monoxide-releasing molecules against Helicobacter pylori. *PloS One* 8, e83157. doi: 10.1371/journal.pone.0083157

Telezhkin, V., Brazier, S. P., Mears, R., Muller, C. T., Riccardi, D., and Kemp, P. J. (2011). Cysteine residue 911 in C-terminal tail of human BK(Ca)alpha channel subunit is crucial for its activation by carbon monoxide. *Pflugers Arch.* 461, 665–675. doi: 10.1007/s00424-011-0924-7

Thenuwara, K., Thomas, J., Ibsen, M., Ituk, U., Choi, K., Nickel, E., et al. (2017). Use of hyperbaric oxygen therapy and PEGylated carboxyhemoglobin bovine in a Jehovah's Witness with life-threatening anemia following postpartum hemorrhage. *Int. J. Obstet. Anesth.* 29, 73–80. doi: 10.1016/j.ijoa.2016.10.006

Tirouvanziam, R., Gernez, Y., Conrad, C. K., Moss, R. B., Schrijver, I., Dunn, C. E., et al. (2008). Profound functional and signaling changes in viable inflammatory neutrophils homing to cystic fibrosis airways. *Proc. Natl. Acad. Sci. U.S.A.* 105, 4335–4339. doi: 10.1073/pnas.0712386105

Tsoyi, K., Ha, Y. M., Kim, Y. M., Lee, Y. S., Kim, H. J., Kim, H. J., et al. (2009). Activation of PPAR-gamma by carbon monoxide from CORM-2 leads to the inhibition of iNOS but not COX-2 expression in LPS-stimulated macrophages. *Inflammation* 32, 364–371. doi: 10.1007/s10753-009-9144-0

Turnbull, A. R., Pyle, C. J., Patel, D. F., Jackson, P. L., Hilliard, T. N., Regamey, N., et al. (2020). Abnormal pro-gly-pro pathway and airway neutrophilia in pediatric cystic fibrosis. *J. Cyst. Fibros* 19, 40–48. doi: 10.1016/j.jcf.2019.05.017

Uddin, M. J., Li, C. S., Joe, Y., Chen, Y., Zhang, Q., Ryter, S. W., et al. (2015). Carbon Monoxide Inhibits Tenascin-C Mediated Inflammation via IL-10 Expression in a Septic Mouse Model. *Mediators Inflammation* 2015, 613249. doi: 10.1155/2015/613249

Velsor, L. W., Van Heeckeren, A., and Day, B. J. (2001). Antioxidant imbalance in the lungs of cystic fibrosis transmembrane conductance regulator protein mutant mice. *Am. J. Physiol. Lung Cell Mol. Physiol.* 281, L31–L38. doi: 10.1152/ajplung.2001.281.1.L31

Wang, X., Wang, Y., Kim, H. P., Nakahira, K., Ryter, S. W., and Choi, A. M. (2007). Carbon monoxide protects against hyperoxia-induced endothelial cell apoptosis by inhibiting reactive oxygen species formation. *J. Biol. Chem.* 282, 1718–1726. doi: 10.1074/jbc.M607610200

Wang, S., Publicover, S., and Gu, Y. (2009). An oxygen-sensitive mechanism in regulation of epithelial sodium channel. *Proc. Natl. Acad. Sci. U.S.A.* 106, 2957–2962. doi: 10.1073/pnas.0809100106

Wang, X. M., Kim, H. P., Nakahira, K., Ryter, S. W., and Choi, A. M. (2009). The heme oxygenase-1/carbon monoxide pathway suppresses TLR4 signaling by regulating the interaction of TLR4 with caveolin-1. *J. Immunol.* 182, 3809–3818. doi: 10.4049/jimmunol.0712437

Wang, D., Viennois, E., Ji, K., Damera, K., Draganov, A., Zheng, Y., et al. (2014). A click-and-release approach to CO prodrugs. *Chem. Commun. (Camb)* 50, 15890–15893. doi: 10.1039/C4CC07748B

Wang, G. (2017). Mechanistic insight into the heme-independent interplay between iron and carbon monoxide in CFTR and Slo1 BKCa channels. *Metallomics* 9, 634–645. doi: 10.1039/C7MT00065K

Wardyn, J. D., Ponsford, A. H., and Sanderson, C. M. (2015). Dissecting molecular cross-talk between Nrf2 and NF-kappaB response pathways. *Biochem. Soc. Trans.* 43, 621–626. doi: 10.1042/BST20150014

Waza, A. A., Hamid, Z., Ali, S., Bhat, S. A., and Bhat, M. A. (2018). A review on heme oxygenase-1 induction: is it a necessary evil. *Inflammation Res.* 67, 579–588. doi: 10.1007/s00011-018-1151-x

Wegiel, B., Hanto, D. W., and Otterbein, L. E. (2013). The social network of carbon monoxide in medicine. *Trends Mol. Med.* 19, 3–11. doi: 10.1016/ j.molmed.2012.10.001

Wegiel, B., Larsen, R., Gallo, D., Chin, B. Y., Harris, C., Mannam, P., et al. (2014a). Macrophages sense and kill bacteria through carbon monoxide-dependent inflammasome activation. *J. Clin. Invest.* 124, 4926–4940. doi: 10.1172/JCI72853

Wegiel, B., Nemeth, Z., Correa-Costa, M., Bulmer, A. C., and Otterbein, L. E. (2014b). Heme oxygenase-1: a metabolic nike. *Antioxid. Redox Signal* 20, 1709–1722. doi: 10.1089/ars.2013.5667

Wegiel, B., Hauser, C. J., and Otterbein, L. E. (2015). Heme as a danger molecule in pathogen recognition. *Free Radic. Biol. Med.* 89, 651–661. doi: 10.1016/j.freeradbiomed.2015.08.020

Wiesel, P., Patel, A. P., Difonzo, N., Marria, P. B., Sim, C. U., Pellacani, A., et al. (2000). Endotoxin-induced mortality is related to increased oxidative stress and end-organ dysfunction, not refractory hypotension, in heme oxygenase-1-deficient mice. *Circulation* 102, 3015–3022. doi: 10.1161/01.CIR.102.24.3015

Wilkinson, W. J., and Kemp, P. J. (2011). Carbon monoxide: an emerging regulator of ion channels. *J. Physiol.* 589, 3055–3062. doi: 10.1113/jphysiol.2011.206706

Wilson, J. L., Jesse, H. E., Poole, R. K., and Davidge, K. S. (2012). Antibacterial effects of carbon monoxide. *Curr. Pharm. Biotechnol.* 13, 760–768. doi: 10.2174/138920112800399329

Wilson, J. L., Bouillaud, F., Almeida, A. S., Vieira, H. L., Ouidja, M. O., Dubois-Rande, J. L., et al. (2017). Carbon monoxide reverses the metabolic adaptation of microglia cells to an inflammatory stimulus. *Free Radic. Biol. Med.* 104, 311–323. doi: 10.1016/j.freeradbiomed.2017.01.022

Yachie, A., Niida, Y., Wada, T., Igarashi, N., Kaneda, H., Toma, T., et al. (1999). Oxidative stress causes enhanced endothelial cell injury in human heme oxygenase-1 deficiency. *J. Clin. Invest.* 103, 129–135. doi: 10.1172/JCI4165

Yamamoto, T., Takano, N., Ishiwata, K., Ohmura, M., Nagahata, Y., Matsuura, T., et al. (2014). Reduced methylation of PFKFB3 in cancer cells shunts glucose towards the pentose phosphate pathway. *Nat. Commun.* 5, 3480. doi: 10.1038/ncomms4480

Yang, J., Eiserich, J. P., Cross, C. E., Morrissey, B. M., and Hammock, B. D. (2012). Metabolomic profiling of regulatory lipid mediators in sputum from adult cystic fibrosis patients. *Free Radic. Biol. Med.* 53, 160–171. doi: 10.1016/j.freeradbiomed.2012.05.001

Yu, M., Li, H., Liu, Q., Liu, F., Tang, L., Li, C., et al. (2011). Nuclear factor p65 interacts with Keap1 to repress the Nrf2-ARE pathway. *Cell Signal* 23, 883–892. doi: 10.1016/j.cellsig.2011.01.014

Yurdagul, A.Jr., Doran, A. C., Cai, B., Fredman, G., and Tabas, I. A. (2017). Mechanisms and Consequences of Defective Efferocytosis in Atherosclerosis. *Front. Cardiovasc. Med.* 4, 86. doi: 10.3389/fcvm.2017.00086

Zakhary, R., Gaine, S. P., Dinerman, J. L., Ruat, M., Flavahan, N. A., and Snyder, S. H. (1996). Heme oxygenase 2: endothelial and neuronal localization and role in endothelium-dependent relaxation. *Proc. Natl. Acad. Sci. U.S.A.* 93, 795–798. doi: 10.1073/pnas.93.2.795

Zhang, P. X., Murray, T. S., Villella, V. R., Ferrari, E., Esposito, S., D'souza, A., et al. (2013). Reduced caveolin-1 promotes hyperinflammation due to abnormal heme oxygenase-1 localization in lipopolysaccharide-challenged macrophages with dysfunctional cystic fibrosis transmembrane conductance regulator. *J. Immunol.* 190, 5196–5206. doi: 10.4049/jimmunol.1201607

Zhang, P. X., Cheng, J., Zou, S., D'souza, A. D., Koff, J. L., Lu, J., et al. (2015). Pharmacological modulation of the AKT/microRNA-199a-5p/CAV1 pathway ameliorates cystic fibrosis lung hyper-inflammation. *Nat. Commun.* 6, 6221. doi: 10.1038/ncomms7221

Zhang, S., Shrestha, C. L., and Kopp, B. T. (2018). Cystic fibrosis transmembrane conductance regulator (CFTR) modulators have differential effects on cystic fibrosis macrophage function. *Sci. Rep.* 8, 17066. doi: 10.1038/s41598-018-35151-7

Zhou, H., Lu, F., Latham, C., Zander, D. S., and Visner, G. A. (2004). Heme oxygenase-1 expression in human lungs with cystic fibrosis and cytoprotective effects against Pseudomonas aeruginosa in vitro. *Am. J. Respir. Crit. Care Med.* 170, 633–640. doi: 10.1164/rccm.200311-1607OC

Ziady, A. G., Sokolow, A., Shank, S., Corey, D., Myers, R., Plafker, S., et al. (2012). Interaction with CREB binding protein modulates the activities of Nrf2 and NF-kappaB in cystic fibrosis airway epithelial cells. *Am. J. Physiol. Lung Cell Mol. Physiol.* 302, L1221–L1231. doi: 10.1152/ajplung.00156.2011

Zuckerbraun, B. S., Chin, B. Y., Bilban, M., D'avila, J. C., Rao, J., Billiar, T. R., et al. (2007). Carbon monoxide signals via inhibition of cytochrome c oxidase and generation of mitochondrial reactive oxygen species. *FASEB J.* 21, 1099–1106. doi: 10.1096/fj.06-6644com

3

Nasal Delivery of Hesperidin/Chitosan Nanoparticles Suppresses Cytokine Storm Syndrome in a Mouse Model of Acute Lung Injury

Hua Jin[1†*], *Zuguo Zhao*[1†], *Qian Lan*[1], *Haotong Zhou*[1], *Zesen Mai*[1], *Yuan Wang*[1], *Xiaowen Ding*[1], *Wenting Zhang*[1], *Jiang Pi*[2], *Colin E. Evans*[3] *and Xinguang Liu*[1*]

[1]*College of Pharmacy, Guangdong Provincial Key Laboratory of Medical Molecular Diagnostics, Guangdong Medical University, Dongguan, China,* [2]*Department of Microbiology and Immunology, University of Illinois at Chicago, Chicago, IL, United States,* [3]*Feinberg School of Medicine, Northwestern University, Chicago, IL, United States*

***Correspondence:**
Hua Jin
jinhua0413@gdmu.edu.cn
Xinguang Liu
xgliu@gdmu.edu.cn

[†]*These authors have contributed equally to this work*

The cytokine storm or cytokine storm syndrome (CSS) is associated with high mortality in patients with acute lung injury (ALI) and acute respiratory distress syndrome (ARDS), for example following sepsis or infectious diseases including COVID-19. However, there are no effective treatments for CSS-associated ALI or ALI/ARDS. Thus, there remains an urgent need to develop effective drugs and therapeutic strategies against CSS and ALI/ARDS. Nasal and inhaled drug delivery methods represent a promising strategy in the treatment of inflammatory lung disease as a result of their ability to improve drug delivery to lungs. Improving the nasal mucosa absorption of poorly water-soluble drugs with poor mucosa bioavailability to a therapeutically effective level is another promising strategy in the fight against ALI/ARDS. Here, chitosan nanoparticles loaded with hesperidin (HPD/NPs) were developed for nasal delivery of the anti-inflammatory HPD compound to inflammatory lungs. *In vitro* and *in vivo*, HPD/NPs exhibited enhanced cellular uptake in the inflammatory microenvironment compared with free HPD. In a mouse model of inflammatory lung disease, the HPD/NPs markedly inhibited lung injury as evidenced by reduced inflammatory cytokine levels and suppressed vascular permeability compared with free HPD. Collectively, our study demonstrates that nasal delivery of HPD/NPs suppresses CSS and ALI/ARDS in a murine model of inflammatory lung disease, and that nanoparticle-based treatment strategies with anti-inflammatory effects could be used to reduce CSS and ALI in patients with inflammatory lung injury.

Keywords: cytokine storm syndrome, hesperidin, chitosan nanoparticle, lung inflammation, nasal drug delivery

INTRODUCTION

Inflammatory lung injury, including sepsis-induced acute lung injury (ALI) and acute respiratory distress syndrome (ARDS), is associated with increased expression of pro-inflammatory cytokines. This so-called cytokine storm syndrome (CSS) is characterized by excessive amounts of pro-inflammatory cytokines, such as the interleukins (IL), interferons (IFN), and tumor necrosis factors (TNF) (Gupta et al., 2020). CSS is associated with clinical deterioration and high mortality in patients with viral infections, such as COVID-19 (Mehta et al., 2020), SARS (Channappanavar and Perlman, 2017) and influenza. At present, there are no efficient drugs or strategies to treat CSS and CSS-associated ALI/ARDS in severe COVID-19 cases.

Although corticosteroids have been used to inhibit CSS in COVID-19 patients, such drugs are limited by their side effects (Russell et al., 2020). Furthermore, several antiinflammatory agents have been shown to reduce ALI and inflammation in experimental studies, but have failed in clinical trials of ALI/ARDS patients (Matthay et al., 2017). Alternative anti-inflammatory methods targeting CSS are under development, such as interleukin-6 antibodies, and have been used to combat COVID-19 (Zhang et al., 2020). Long-term use of antibody treatments, however, could cause chronic immunosuppression. Thus, the development of novel therapies to effectively control and target ALI and CSS is an urgent requirement in the fight against sepsis-induced ALI/ARDS, COVID-19, or other infectious inflammatory lung diseases. One potential limitation of anti-inflammatory agents is the off-target delivery to, and short-term retention of, the agents in lungs. In this work, a nasal nanoparticle (NP)-based drug delivery system was designed to deliver an inflammatory agent (Hesperidin, HPD) to inflammatory lungs with the view to reducing CSS and ALI/ARDS. HPD is an active flavonoid aglycone (Hemanth Kumar et al., 2017) found in citrus fruits, which has shown no side effects or toxicity in experimental animal studies (Li et al., 2019). Along with its anti-inflammatory properties, HPD exhibits analgesic, anti-carcinogenic, anti-viral (Ciftci et al., 2015), and anticoagulant activities (Roohbakhsh et al., 2015).

Many investigators are aiming to improve the development of drug-loaded NPs and the delivery of drugs to infectious sites via cell- or tissue-specific targeting techniques (Wang et al., 2018). Nasal drug delivery systems can be employed to reduce elimination by the liver, kidneys, and gastrointestinal tract (Sukumar et al., 2019), compared with oral, intraperitoneal, or intravenous delivery routes. However, nasal administration of HPD is limited *in vivo* because of its poor aqueous solubility and bioavailability. To address this drawback, PLGA or chitosan nanoparticle (NP) delivery systems have been developed to improve the aqueous solubility, safety, and efficacy of pharmacological agents (Jin et al., 2017). Chitosan (CS)-based NPs, for example, can significantly improve mucosal drug delivery, as a result of the electrostatic attraction between positively charged CS chains and negatively charged sialic acid of nasal mucosa (Gholizadeh et al., 2019).

In this work, we synthesized an HPD-loaded PLGA-CS NP delivery system (HPD/NPs) to target HPD to inflammatory lungs via the nasal delivery route, and assessed the capacity of these HPD/NPs to suppress CSS and ALI in a mouse model of endotoxic lung injury.

METHODS AND MATERIALS

Preparation and Characterization of Hesperidin-Loaded PLGA-Chitosan NPs (HPD/NPs)

HPD-NPs were synthesized by emulsification and evaporation methods. Briefly, 20 mg HPD and 80 mg PLGA-PEG (1:1 lactide: glycolide, Sigma, USA) were dissolved in 5 ml of dichloromethane and homogenized for 40 seconds to form the oil phase emulsification. The oil phase emulsification was combined with 20 ml PVA (1% w/w, Sigma, USA) containing of 0.2% of chitosan and homogenized for another 40 s to form the second water phase emulsification. This water phase emulsification was added to 100 ml water and stirred for 6 h to achieve organic reagent evaporation and nanoparticle hardening. Finally, HPD/NPs were harvested by centrifugation at 12,000 rpm for 20 min and washed 3 times with ultrapure water then lyophilized for 48 h for storage at 4 °C.

Characterization of NPs

Size distribution and zeta potential were estimated by dynamic laser scattering using a Zetasizer Nano ZS (Malvern Instruments, UK). NPs were visualized by scanning electron microscopy (Philips Co, Holland). For measuring HPD loading capacity in HPD/NPs, 10 mg lyophilized NPs were dissolved in 1 ml of dichloromethane, and then, the amount of HPD in the solution was determined by high-pressure liquid chromatography (HPLC). HPLC detection was performed using a C18 column (5 µm, 250 mm × 4.6 mm), whereas the mobile phase, consisting of methanol and 0.1% acetic acid (88:12) (v/v), was maintained at a flow rate of 1.0 ml/min. The ultraviolet detector wavelength was 285 nm, and the injection volume was 20 µl.

Evaluation of HPD Release *in vitro*

HPD release from NPs was evaluated *in vitro* using the dialysis method as previously described (Jin et al., 2017). Briefly, dialysis bags with a molecular weight cut-off of 10,000 Da containing 10 mg of compounds were immersed in a water bath containing 20 ml of PBS (pH 7.4) at 37 °C. At indicated times, 1 ml of receiving buffer was withdrawn and replaced with 1 ml of PBS. HPD release from dialysis bag into the water bath was determined by ultraviolet spectrophotometry (Agilent 8,453, Agilent Technologies, USA) at 285 nm.

Cell Culture

Mouse macrophage RAW264.7 cells and human umbilical vein endothelial cells (HUVECs, Lonza) were cultured in DMEM (Gibco) with 10% fetal bovine serum (Gibco) containing 100 µg/ml streptomycin and 100 IU/ml penicillin. Cells were sub-cultured twice/week and incubated in a humidified incubator (Thermo) at 5% CO2 and 37 °C.

Cell Viability Assay

RAW264.7 cells or HUVECs were cultured in 96-well plates for 24 h, then exposed to 10 µg/ml HPD or HPD/NPs or vehicle (0.02% DMSO) for 3 h, followed by activation with 1 µg/ml of LPS for 24 h. Cell viability was assessed using the Cell Counting Kit assay (Beyotime Institute of Biotechnology, Nanjing, China) according to the manufacturer's instructions. All experiments were performed three times.

Endothelial Permeability Assay

The endothelial permeability assay was performed as described (Monfoulet et al., 2017) with the following modifications. In brief,

HUVECs were seeded onto Corning Transwell filters for 24 h in medium with 0.2% FBS then exposed to 10 μg/ml HPD or HPD/NPs or vehicle (0.02% DMSO) for 3 h, followed by activation with 1 μg/ml of LPS for 24 h. Permeability of the endothelium was evaluated by assessing the passage of FITC-dextran (40 kDa) through endothelial monolayer. One hundred microliters of FITC-dextran were added to the upper chamber and allowed to equilibrate for 1 h, after which FITC fluorescence (excitation 488 nm; emission 525 nm) in the lower chamber was measured using a microplate reader. Three independent experiments were performed.

Immunofluorescence Staining

F-actin expression was evaluated by staining with phalloidin FITC. In brief, HUVECs were cultured on coverslips, then fixed with 4% paraformaldehyde for 30 min and incubated with 1 mM phalloidin-FITC for 60 min in the dark at room temperature, and then washed twice with PBS. Cytoskeleton organization was imaged with a laser scanning confocal microscope (LCM 880, Carl Zeiss, Germany). Fluorescence was measured by flow cytometer at excitation wavelength 488 nm, emission wavelength 530 nm to quantitatively elucidate the alterations of cytoskeleton proteins.

HUVECs cultured on coverslips were fixed with 4% paraformaldehyde and stained with primary anti VE-cadherin (1:1,000; Sigma-Aldrich) and fluorescence-conjugated secondary antibodies (1:500; Sigma-Aldrich). Nuclei were counterstained with DAPI (DAPI Fluoromount-GTM, thermofisher). Cells were imaged with LCM 880.

In vivo Studies

Mice

C57BL/6 mice were used throughout at 12–14 weeks of age. The experimental protocols were conducted according to National Institutes of Health guidelines on the use of laboratory animals. The animal care and study protocols were approved by the Institutional Animal Care and Use Committee of Guangdong Medical University (GDY2002094).

Mouse Model of Acute Lung Injury

Lipopolysaccharide (LPS, *E. coli* 055:B5, Santa Cruz), a component of the cell wall of Gram-negative bacterium, was dissolved in PBS. To induce sepsis, LPS was administered intraperitoneally to mice at 3.5 mg/kg body weight in 100 μL PBS. HPD or HPD/NPs was nasally administrated at 3 h-post LPS challenge, and the animals were sacrificed to collect samples at 24 h post-LPS challenge.

Histology

Lung tissues were fixed and processed for H&E staining. Briefly, lung tissues were fixed by 5 min instillation of 10% PBS-buffered formalin through trachea catheterization at a transpulmonary pressure of 15 cm H_2O, and then overnight at 4°C with agitation. After paraffin processing, the tissues were cut into 5 μm sections and stained with H&E for histological analysis.

Assessment of Lung Vascular Permeability

The Evans blue-conjugated albumin (EBA) extravasation assay was used to assess pulmonary vascular permeability (Huang et al., 2016). Briefly, EBA (20 mg/kg) was injected retro-orbitally at 45 min before sacrifice and lung collection following perfusion free of blood with PBS. The extravasated EBA in lung homogenates was expressed as μg of EBA per g of lung.

Total protein levels in bronchiolar alveolar lavage fluid (BALF) were measured via bicinchoninacid-assay (BCA) according to the manufacturer's instructions (Pierce BCA Protein Assay, Thermo Scientific, USA).

Immunohistochemistry

The Lung sections were incubated overnight at 4 °C in a humidified chamber with anti-caspase 1 (Proteintech: 22915-1-AP) or anti- IL-1β antibodies (Abcam: ab9722) diluted 1:500 in PBS containing 1% BSA. Primary antibodies were incubated at 4 °C overnight followed by secondary antibodies for 1 h at 37 °C. Proteins were visualized using the DAB chromogen kit (ZSGB-BIO, Beijing, China). Finally, the lung sections were counter-stained with hematoxylin.

Statistical Analysis

Results are expressed as mean ± SD. Statistical significance was determined by 1-way ANOVA with a Games-Howell post hoc analysis for multiple-group comparisons. Two-group comparisons were analyzed by the 2-tailed unpaired Student *t*-test.

RESULTS

Preparation and Characterization of HPD/NPs

To improve the water solubility and bioavailability of HPD, biodegradable polymer PLGA was employed to encapsulate HPD to form soluble NP carriers, and chitosan was employed to modulate the surface zeta potential of the NPs to positive (Bruinsmann et al., 2019). After formulation of the HPD/NPs, the particle size, zetapotential, morphology, entrapment efficiency, and HPD release were determined by dynamic laser light scattering (DLS), scanning electronic microscopy (SEM) and HPLC, respectively. The size distribution of HPD/NPs was approximately 200 nm (**Figures 1A,B**). The surface charge (zeta potential) was +22 mV (**Figure 1C**). The loading rate of HPD into the NPs was 8.1%, and encapsulation rate was 81.02%. The HPD/NP diameter did not change significantly for up to 4 weeks at 37 °C (**Figure 1D**). The release of HPD from the HPD/NPs occurred steadily in the first 12 h, with ~75% and ~90% of the HPD being released by 12 and 24 h, respectively (**Figure 1E**). Notably, free NPs had a similar appearance and diameter to HPD/NPs (**Supplementary Figure S1A**).

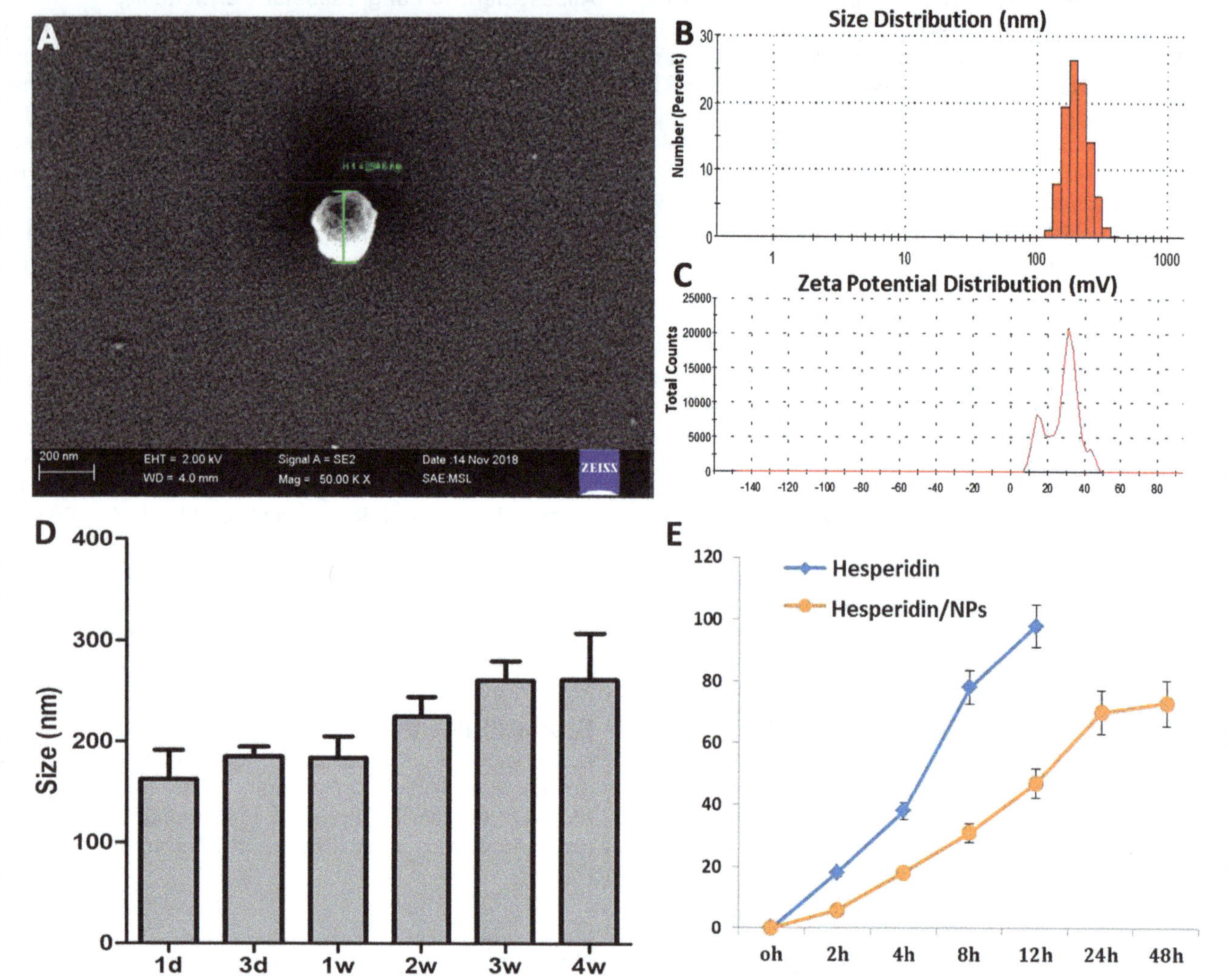

FIGURE 1 | Characterization of HPD/NPs. **(A)** Scanning electron microscopy (SEM) image of an HPD/NP in suspension. **(B)** Mean size and **(C)** zeta potentials of HPD/NPs. **(D)** HPD/NP size over time (n = 4/group). **(E)** *In vitro* release of HPD from HPD/NPs in PBS (0.01 M, PH = 7.4, n = 4/group).

In vitro Anti-Cytokine Storm Syndrome Activity of HPD and HPD/NPs

Figure 2A showed that 10 or 50 μg/ml of HPD or HPD/NPs did not induce toxic effects on RAW264.7 cells, while 100 μg/ml of HPD or HPD/NPs caused decreases in cell viability. Therefore, 10 μg/ml concentrations of HPD or HPD/NPs were selected as the dose in the following *in vitro* and *in vivo* experiments. Next, RAW264.7 cells were treated with LPS (1 μg/ml) for 24 h. **Figure 2B** showed that the decreases in cell viability resulting from LPS exposure could be restored by pre-treatment with 10 μg/ml of HPD/NPs, demonstrating that HPD/NPs can protect against LPS-induced cell death *in vitro*. **Figures 2C,D** indicate that 10 μg/ml of HPD/NPs can significantly suppress the level of inflammation cytokines (NO and IL-6) in LPS-treated RAW264.7 cells. Notably, 2% DMSO aggravated the inflammatory profile of the RAW264.7 cells, which implied that the DMSO-free delivery of water-soluble HPD/NPs could decrease the side effects of DMSO-based drug delivery. We also found that free NPs did not alter LPS-induced cell viability vs. vehicle-treated cells (**Supplementary Figure S1B**).

HPD/NPs Preserved Endothelial Permeability *in vitro*

To delineate the effects of HPD and HPD/NPs on regulating endothelial barrier function, we employed a Transwell system to quantify changes in the integrity of endothelial junctions activated by LPS. HUVECs were plated at >90% confluence on Transwell filters to form cell-to-cell contacts and intact monolayers before treatment with compounds and/or LPS. Upon addition of PBS, HPD or HPD/NPs for 2 h, followed by activation with LPS for 24 h, the PBS-treated group exhibited significantly increased permeability compared with the LPS-free basal group, indicative of decreased endothelial barrier function.

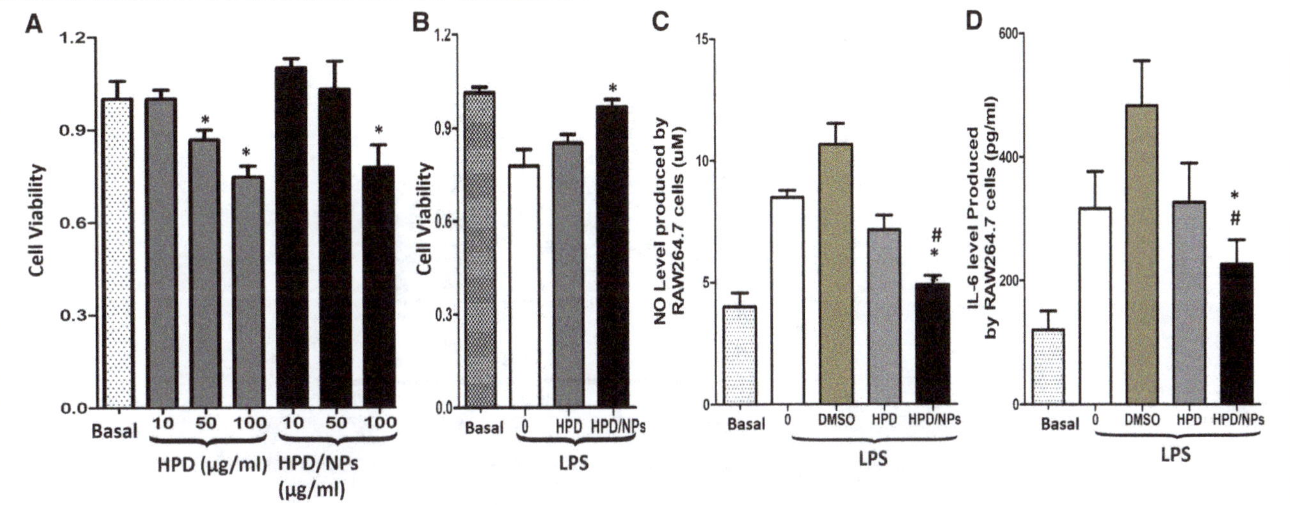

FIGURE 2 | Impact of HPD and HPD/NPs on LPS-induced inflammatory response *in vitro*. **(A)**. Viability of RAW264.7 macrophages exposed to different doses of HPD or HPD/NPs for 24 h. **(B)** Viability of RAW264.7 macrophages exposed to 10 mg/ml HPD or HPD/NPs or vehicle (0.02% DMSO) for 3 h, followed by stimulation with 1 µg/ml of LPS for 24 h. **(C)** NO and **(D)** IL-6 production by RAW264.7 macrophages exposed to 10 mg/ml HPD or HPD/NPs or vehicle (0.02% DMSO) for 3 h, followed by stimulation with 1 µg/ml of LPS for 24 h **(A)** $N = 4$/group, *$p < 0.05$ vs. basal group or 10 µg/ml group. **(B–D)**. $N = 4$/group, *$p < 0.05$ vs. vehicle control; #$p < 0.05$ vs. HPD group.

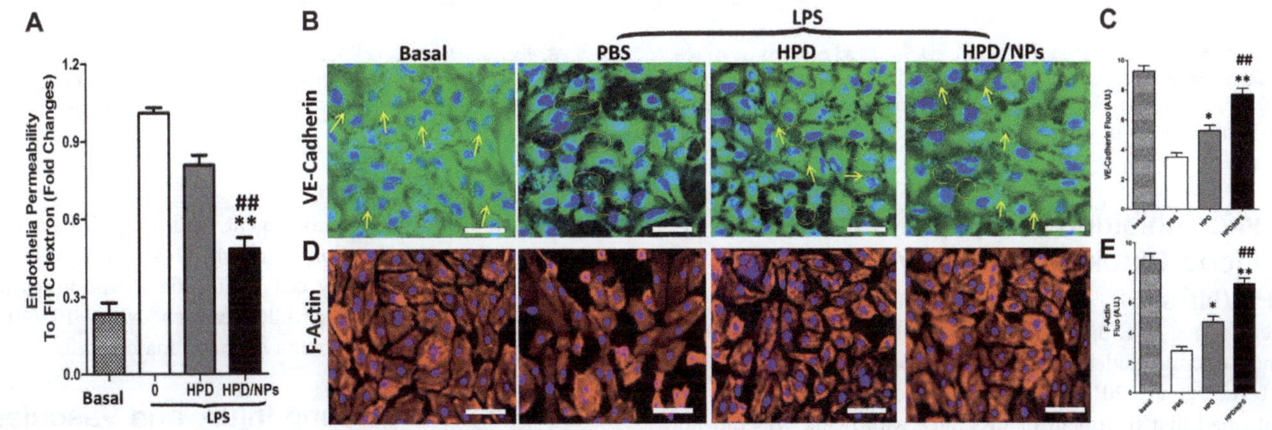

FIGURE 3 | Impact of HPD and HPD/NPs on LPS-induced endothelial integrity *in vitro*. **(A)** Permeability of the HUVEC monolayer to FITC-dextran (40 kDa) after 3 h exposure to PBS or HPD or HPD/NPs (10 µg/ml) followed by 24 h LPS exposure. Data expressed as a percentage of PBS + LPS treatment group ($n = 4$/group, **$p < 0.001$ vs. vehicle control group; ##$p < 0.001$ vs. HPD group). **(B)** Representative images and **(C)** quantification of immunostaining for VE-cadherin (green) in HUVEC monolayers Arrows indicate VE-cadherin-positive cell junctions; circles indicate weak or absent VE-cadherin signal at cell junction. **(D)** Representative images and **(E)** quantification of F-actin (red) immunostaining of HUVECs after 3 h exposure to PBS or HPD or HPD/NPs followed by 24 h LPS (3.5 mg/kg). Nuclei were counterstained with DAPI (blue). Scale bar, 50 µm *$p < 0.05$ and **$p < 0.01$ vs. PBS group; ##$p < 0.01$ vs. HPD group. A.U., arbitrary units.

Figure 3A shows that stimulation of HUVECs by LPS resulted in an approximately 5-fold increase in endothelial permeability compared to the basal group. This increase in permeability was inhibited by 25% and 58% following pre-incubation with 10 µg/ml of HPD and HPD/NPs, respectively. Interestingly, there was no significant change in endothelial permeability in the cells treated with 10 µg/ml HPD/NPs compared with the basal group, indicative of restored endothelial barrier function. To assess the morphological properties of the HUVEC monolayers, VE-cadherin and F-actin expression was observed by immunofluorescence microscopy. **Figure 3B,E** shows that LPS induced EC shrinkage and decreased expression of VE-cadherin and F-actin. Excitingly, 10 µg/ml of HPD/NPs could restore normal EC shape and reverse the reduced expression of VE-cadherin and F-actin. Treatment with 10 µg/ml of free HPD, however, failed to decrease the LPS-induced increases in HUVEC permeability or restore VE-cadherin and F-actin expression. These studies showed that HPD/NPs can be used to alleviate LPS-induced increases in endothelial permeability and morphology disruption.

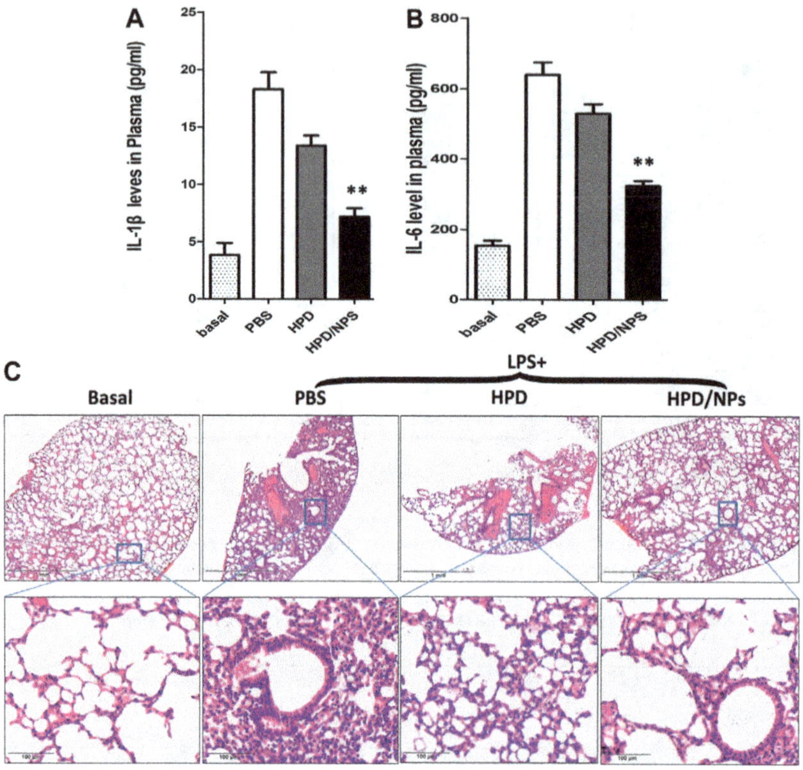

FIGURE 4 | Impact of HPD and HPD/NPs on LPS-induced inflammation in mice. At 3 h postLPS, PBS (vehicle), HPD, or HPD/NPs were nasally administered to mice. Lung tissues were collected at 24 h post-LPS challenge. **(A)** Expression levels of IL-1β and **(B)** IL-6 in mouse plasma at 24 h post-LPS challenge ($n = 4$/group; $^{**}p < 0.001$ vs. PBS vehicle and vs. HPD). **(C)** Representative micrographs of H&E stained lung tissue cross-sections at 24 h post-LPS challenge. Scale bar, 1 mm (upper row) or 100 μm (lower row).

In vivo Inhibition of Lipopolysaccharide-Induced Cytokine Storm by HPD/NPs

The effects of HPD or HPD/NPs were further examined *in vivo* in a mouse sepsis model. LPS injection is commonly used to induce ALI (Lei et al., 2018) and CSS (Du et al., 2018). First, we confirmed that treatment of LPS mice with blank NPs did not alter the level of lung injury vs. LPS mice, as shown by absence of change in BALF protein concentration (**Supplementary Figure S1C**). **Figures 4A,B** demonstrates that IL-1β and IL-6 levels in peripheral blood promptly ascended at 24 h after intraperitoneal injection of LPS.

Treatment with 10 mg/kg of HPD/NPs efficiently depressed the LPS-induced increases in these inflammatory factors over this short period of time. Moreover, pro-inflammation cytokines such as TNF-α and IL-17 play crucial roles in lung inflammation, so we also determined the levels of such cytokines in BALF. As shown in **Supplementary Figure S2A, B**, treatment with HPD/NPs inhibited the LPS-induced increases in these inflammatory cytokines. In addition to pro-inflammatory cytokines, the LPS-induced expression of NO (**Supplementary Figure S2C**) was also decreased by HPD/NPs treatment. Treatment with blank NPs, however, had no discernable effects on inflammatory cytokine levels or NO production in LPS-treated mice, which implied that HPD acts as the anti-inflammatory agent, while the chitosan NPs act as passive drug carriers. Consistent with these findings, H&E staining showed inflammatory cell infiltration in the lungs of LPS-treated mice (**Figure 4C**), while treatment with HPD/NPs effectively alleviated the infiltration of inflammatory cells.

HPD/NPs Reduce Lung Injury and Vascular Permeability

We next investigated the impact of the HPD/NPs on LPS-induced lung injury. We determined alterations in vascular permeability by assessing pulmonary transvascular flux of Evans blue dye-conjugated albumin (EBA) (Huang et al., 2016), bronchiolar-alveolar lavage (BAL) protein and wet/dry ratio of lungs. **Figure 5A** demonstrates the experimental scheme of the EBA assay. **Figure 5B** shows representative images of lungs extracted from EBA-injected-mice. As expected, LPS treatment resulted in increases in EBA flux, BAL protein, and wet/dry ratio at 24 h post-LPS compared to basal controls (**Figures 5C–E**). In mice receiving HPD at 3 h post-LPS, there were no discernable improvements in wet/dry ratio or BAL protein at 24 h post-LPS compared to PBS treatment. Mice receiving HPD/NPs, however, showed decreased levels of LPS-induced vascular permeability (EBA flux and BAL protein), and edema (wet/dry ratio). These data demonstrated that nasally administered HPD/

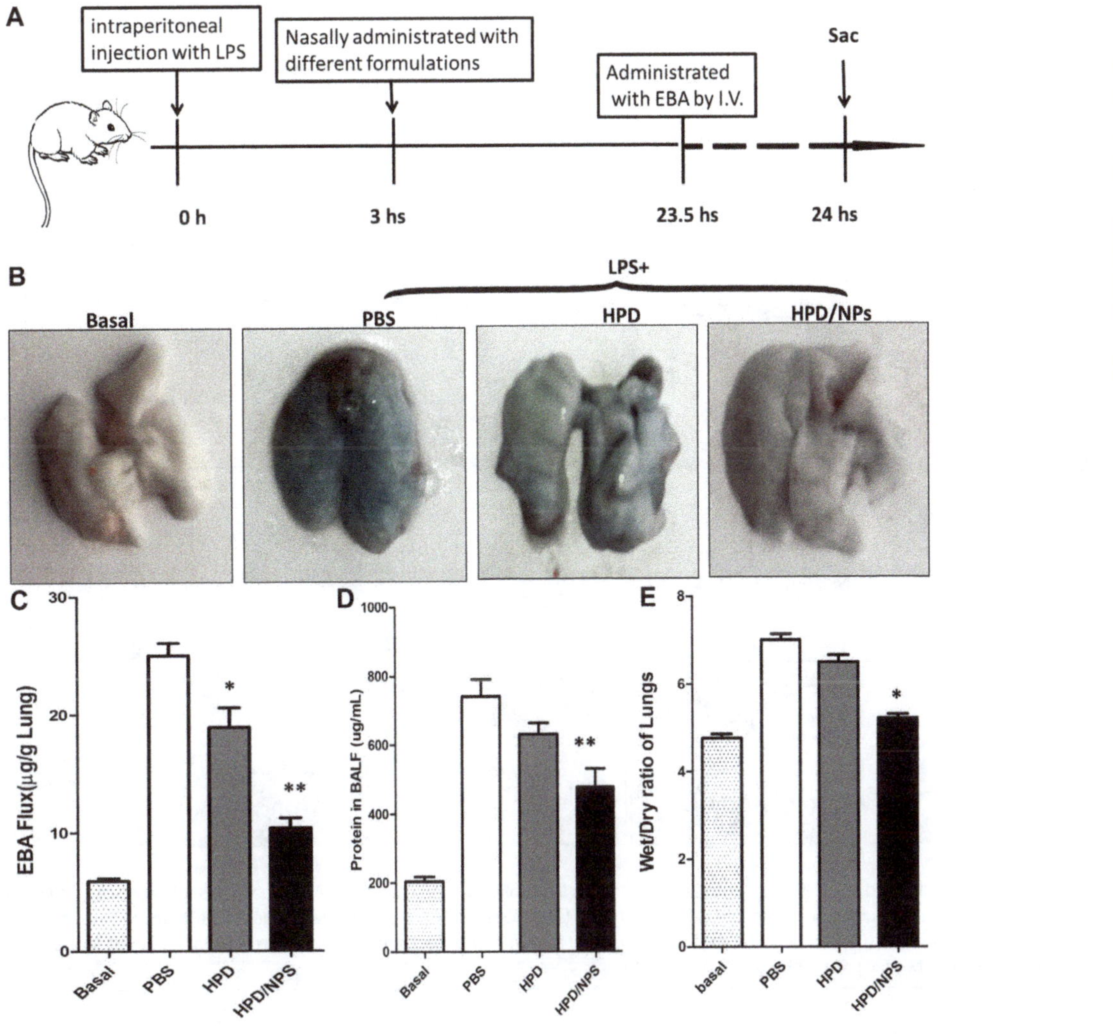

FIGURE 5 | Impact of HPD and HPD/NPs on LPS-induced ALI in mice. At 3 h post-LPS, PBS (vehicle), HPD, or HPD/NPs were nasally administered to mice. Lung tissues were collected at 24 h post-LPS challenge. **(A)** EBA assay schematic. **(B)** Representative images of murine lung tissues after EBA-injection. **(C)** EBA flux, **(D)** BAL protein, and **(E)** wet/dry weight ratio. **(C–E)** N = 5; **p* < 0.05 and ***p* < 0.001 vs. PBS group.

NPs result in targeted delivery of HPD to the inflammatory lungs and inhibition of lung injury.

HPD/NPs Suppress Pyroptosis in Septic Mouse Lungs

To investigate whether cell pyroptosis (Bergsbaken et al., 2009) was involved in the pathogenesis of ALI in LPS-treated mice and to explore the possible inhibition of LPS-induced pyroptosis by HPD/NPs, immunohistochemical staining was performed to detect the expression levels of IL-1β and caspase 1 in the lung of septic mice (**Figure 6**). The septic lung tissues in the PBS-treated group showed significantly increased expressions of IL-1β and caspase 1 compared with mice in the basal group. Excitingly, the expression of IL-1β and caspase 1 decreased significantly following treatment of LPS mice with HPD/NPs. The inhibitory effect of HPD on pyroptosis was once more less than that of HPD/NPs, again suggesting that these modified NPs can be used to improve drug delivery and treatment efficacy in inflammatory lung.

DISCUSSION

ALI following sepsis or infection with SARS-CoV, MERS-CoV, or SARS-CoV-2, represent major healthcare and financial problems worldwide (Su et al., 2016). Despite the threats to human survival and well-being, there are still no effective therapeutic drugs against ALI/ARDS. Additionally, human studies have shown that patients with severe COVID-19 also demonstrate CSS (He et al., 2020). Thus, the develop of novel drugs or treatment strategies against ALI/ARDS and/or CSS is of upmost importance. Wu et al. (Wu et al., 2020) employed computational methods to identify therapeutic targets for

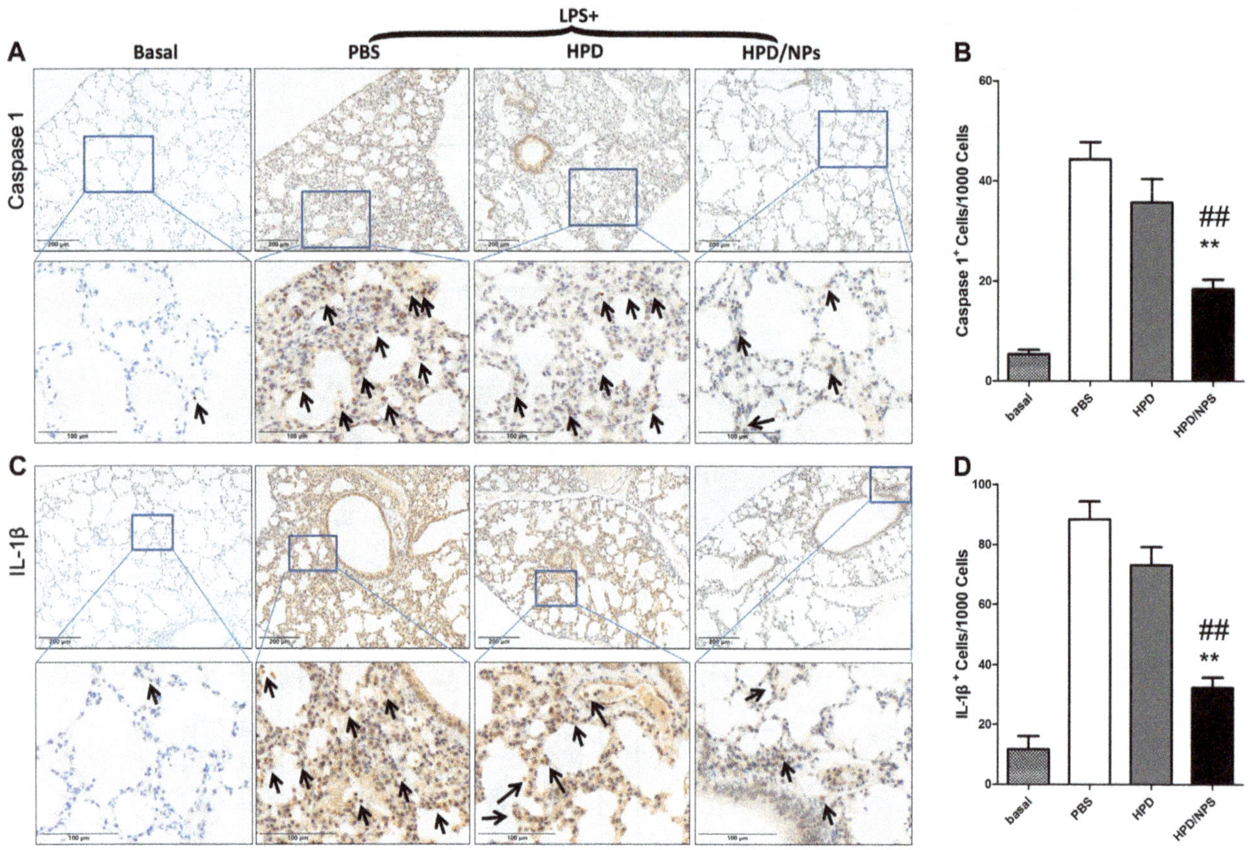

FIGURE 6 | Impact of HPD and HPD/NPs on markers of pyroptosis in lungs of LPS-challenged mice. At 3 h post-LPS, PBS (vehicle), HPD, or HPD/NPs were nasally administered to mice. Lung tissues were collected at 24 h post-LPS challenge. **(A)** Representative images and **(B)** quantification of lung tissue cross-sections immune-stained for caspase 1. **(C)** Representative images and **(D)** quantification of lung tissue cross-sections immune-stained for IL-1β. Arrows indicate brown/positive staining. *N* = 4/group; $^{**}p < 0.01$ vs. PBS, $^{\#\#}p < 0.01$ vs. HPD.

COVID-19 and discovered that HPD could be used as a potential anti- COVID-19 drug. Although this anti-inflammatory and anti-viral agent (Lin et al., 2005) can be easily extracted from *Isatis indigotica* roots and phenolic Chinese herbs, and was extensively used for the prevention of SARS in China, the poor water solubility and bioavailability of HPD limit its efficiency, especially when delivery intranasally.

Herein, we designed a HPD/NP delivery system to target inflammatory lung tissue and reduce CSS. To improve the adsorption rate of the HPD/NPs by nasal mucosa, chitosan was added to the surface of the PLGA NPs (Garg et al., 2019). The zeta potential of the HPD/NPs was +22 mV, suggestive of good adsorption of HPD/NPs into nasal mucosa. However, the impact of different types of NP on nasal mucosal absorption per se should be assessed in future studies.

In vitro, we identified 10 μg/ml as a dose of HPD/NPs that does not induce cytotoxicity in RAW264.7 cells, while 50 μg/ml or 100 μg/ml of both HPD and HPD/NPs did decrease cell viability. Thus, the dose of 10 μg/ml was selected to be assessed in the *in vitro* and *in vivo* experiments. While both HPD and HPD/NPs could significantly inhibit the production of inflammatory cytokines (NO and IL-6) *in vitro*, this inhibition was greater when cells were treated with HPD/NPs compared with HPD alone. *In vivo*, 10 mg/kg of HPD/NPs but not free HPD significantly suppressed CSS. These studies suggest that the anti-inflammatory impact of HPD is enhanced by delivery in chitosan NPs. This delivery system also alleviated the need for DMSO as a solubility agent *in vivo*, which could damage nasal mucosa when administrated nasally. Furthermore, excessive amounts of NO can promote cytokine and matrix metalloproteinase production, mitochondrial dysfunction, and cell apoptosis, which aggravates inflammation and tissue injury (Wu et al., 2018). The HPD/NPs significantly inhibited NO release in LPS-challenged mice, implying that nasal delivery of HPD/NPs can enhance the anti-CSS effects of HPD through reductions in multiple different cytokines and signaling molecules.

To determine the impact of HPD/NPs on CSS-associated ALI, we next investigated the effects of HPD/NPs on endothelial barrier function, which plays a vital role in lung inflammation and ALI We showed that the damaged integrity of endothelial monolayers following LPS treatment could be restored by HPD/NP treatment *in vitro*. Consistent with these findings, we also showed that nasal HPD/NPs significantly attenuated LPS-induced increases in ALI in mice, as shown by reductions in vascular permeability, CSS, infiltration of leukocytes, and presence of protein-rich liquid in pulmonary alveoli. Importantly, we showed that the NPs alone did not alter inflammatory cytokine levels or NO production in LPS-treated mice, suggesting that HPD/NPs but not the NPs alone were active pharmacological agents against CSS-associated ALI. Pyroptosis is involved in the development of inflammatory lung diseases such as ALI/ARDS, and we demonstrated that the HPD/NPs inhibited pulmonary cell pyroptosis markers in LPS-treated mice. These findings together support the possibility that HPD/NPs reduce CSS-associated ALI through decreases in cytokine release, vascular permeability, and cell pyroptosis, and have potential for the development of novel treatment strategies for sepsis and CSS in infectious diseases.

It is worth mentioning that the HPD dose that had protective effects on CSS-induced lung injury in our study is 5-fold lower than HPD dose in free form used to reduce smoke-induced lung inflammation in a previous study (Yu et al., 2019). Previous experimental studies have shown that treatment efficacy can be improved through delivery strategies that target inflammatory tissues (Zhang et al., 2019) (Gao et al., 2019). In this work, the anti-inflammatory effects of HPD on macrophages and lungs of LPS challenged mice was improved by using the nasal NP-based drug delivery system. In summary, our data provide strong evidence that nasal NP-delivery of HPD protects against CSS-associated ALI and that the nasal NP delivery system could be used to enhance the efficacy of anti-inflammatory agents in the treatment of CSS and ALI/ARDS.

ETHICS STATEMENT

The animal study was reviewed and approved by Guangdong Medical University.

AUTHOR CONTRIBUTIONS

HJ, ZZ, and XL proposed and supervised the project. HJ, QL, ZM, HZ, YW, XD, WZ, and JP performed the experiments. HJ wrote the paper. CE revised and polished the manuscript. XL provided the funding in this study. All authors have given approval to the final version of the manuscript.

FUNDING

This work was supported by National Natural Science Foundation of China (No. 81971329, 81671399), Special Funds for the Cultivation of Guangdong College Students'Scientific, Technological Innovation (Climbing Program Special Funds, No. pdjh2019b0224), PhD early development program of Guangdong medical University (B2019012) and "Group-type" Special Supporting Project for Educational Talents in Universities (4SG19057G). CE received an American Heart Association Career Development Award (19CDA34500000).

REFERENCES

Bergsbaken, T., Fink, S. L., and Cookson, B. T. (2009). Pyroptosis: host cell death and inflammation. *Nat. Rev. Microbiol.*, 7 (2), 99–109. doi:10.1038/nrmicro2070

Bruinsmann, F. A., Pigana, S., Aguirre, T., Dadalt Souto, G., Garrastazu Pereira, G., Bianchera, A., et al. (2019). Chitosan-coated nanoparticles: effect of chitosan molecular weight on nasal transmucosal delivery. *Pharmaceutics* 11 (2), 86. doi:10.3390/pharmaceutics11020086

Channappanavar, R., and Perlman, S. (2017). Pathogenic human coronavirus infections: causes and consequences of cytokine storm and immunopathology. *Semin. Immunopathol.*, 39 (5), 529–539. doi:10.1007/s00281-017-0629-x

Ciftci, O., Ozcan, C., Kamisli, O., Cetin, A., Basak, N., and Aytac, B. (2015). Hesperidin, a citrus flavonoid, has the ameliorative effects against experimental autoimmune encephalomyelitis (EAE) in a C57BL/J6 mouse model. *Neurochem. Res.*, 40 (6), 1111–1120. doi:10.1007/s11064-015-1571-8

Du, Z. A., Sun, M. N., and Hu, Z. S. (2018). Saikosaponin a ameliorates LPS-induced acute lung injury in mice. *Inflammation*, 41 (1), 193–198. doi:10.1007/s10753-017-0677-3

Gao, W., Wang, Y., Xiong, Y., Sun, L., Wang, L., Wang, K., et al. (2019). Size-dependent anti-inflammatory activity of a peptide-gold nanoparticle hybrid *in vitro* and in a mouse model of acute lung injury. *Acta Biomater.* 85, 203–217. doi:10.1016/j.actbio.2018.12.046

Garg, U., Chauhan, S., Nagaich, U., and Jain, N. (2019). Current advances in chitosan nanoparticles based drug delivery and targeting. *Adv. Pharmaceut. Bull.* 9 (2), 195–204. doi:10.15171/apb.2019.023

Gholizadeh, H., Messerotti, E., Pozzoli, M., Cheng, S., Traini, D., Young, P., et al. (2019). Application of a thermosensitive in situ gel of ChitosanBased nasal spray loaded with tranexamic acid for localised treatment of nasal wounds. *AAPS PharmSciTech*, 20 (7), 299. doi:10.1208/s12249-019-1517-6

Gupta, K. K., Khan, M. A., and Singh, S. K. (2020). Constitutive inflammatory cytokine storm: a major threat to human Health. *J. Interferon Cytokine Res.* 40 (1), 19–23. doi:10.1089/jir.2019.00851

He, J., Tao, H., Yan, Y., Huang, S. Y., and Xiao, Y. (2020). Molecular mechanism of evolution and human infection with SARS-CoV-2. *Viruses* 12 (4), 428. doi:10.3390/v12040428

Hemanth Kumar, B., Dinesh Kumar, B., and Diwan, P. V. (2017). Hesperidin, a citrus flavonoid, protects against l-methionine-induced hyperhomocysteinemia by abrogation of oxidative stress, endothelial dysfunction and neurotoxicity in Wistar rats. *Pharm. Biol.*, 55 (1), 146–155. doi:10.1080/13880209.2016.1231695

Huang, X., Dai, Z., Cai, L., Sun, K., Cho, J., Albertine, K. H., et al. (2016). Endothelial p110γPI3K mediates endothelial regeneration and vascular repair after inflammatory vascular injury. *Circulation*, 133 (11), 1093–1103. doi:10.1161/CIRCULATIONAHA.115.020918

Jin, H., Pi, J., Zhao, Y., Jiang, J., Li, T., Zeng, X., et al. (2017). EGFR-targeting PLGA-PEG nanoparticles as a curcumin delivery system for breast cancer therapy. *Nanoscale*, 9 (42), 16365–16374. doi:10.1039/c7nr06898k

Lei, J., Wei, Y., Song, P., Li, Y., Zhang, T., Feng, Q., Xu, G., et al. (2018). Cordycepin inhibits LPS-induced acute lung injury by inhibiting inflammation and oxidative stress. *Eur. J. Pharmacol.*, 818, 110–114. doi:10.1016/j.ejphar.2017.10.029

Li, Y., Kandhare, A. D., Mukherjee, A. A., and Bodhankar, S. L. (2019). Acute and sub-chronic oral toxicity studies of hesperidin isolated from orange peel extract in Sprague Dawley rats. *Regul. Toxicol. Pharmacol.*, 105, 77–85. doi:10.1016/j.yrtph.2019.04.001

Lin, C. W., Tsai, F. J., Tsai, C. H., Lai, C. C., Wan, L., Ho, T. Y., et al. (2005). Anti-SARS coronavirus 3C-like protease effects of Isatis indigotica root and plant-derived phenolic compounds. *Antivir. Res.*, 68 (1), 36–42. doi:10.1016/j.antiviral.2005.07.002

Matthay, M. A., McAuley, D. F., and Ware, L. B. (2017). Clinical trials in acute respiratory distress syndrome: challenges and opportunities. *Lancet Respir. Med.* 5 (6), 524–534. doi:10.1016/S2213-2600(17)30188-1

Mehta, P., McAuley, D. F., Brown, M., Sanchez, E., Tattersall, R. S., and Manson, J. J., and HLH Across Speciality Collaboration, UK (2020). COVID-19: consider cytokine storm syndromes and immunosuppression. *Lancet* 395 (10229), 1033–1034. doi:10.1016/S0140

Monfoulet, L. E., Mercier, S., Bayle, D., Tamaian, R., Barber-Chamoux, N., Morand, C., et al. (2017). Curcumin modulates endothelial permeability and monocyte transendothelial migration by affecting endothelial cell dynamics. *Free Radic. Biol. Med.* 112, 109–120. doi:10.1016/j.freeradbiomed.2017.07.019

Roohbakhsh, A., Parhiz, H., Soltani, F., Rezaee, R., and Iranshahi, M. (2015). Molecular mechanisms behind the biological effects of hesperidin and hesperetin for the prevention of cancer and cardiovascular diseases. *Life Sci.* 124, 64–74. doi:10.1016/j.lfs.2014.12.030

Russell, C. D., Millar, J. E., and Baillie, J. K. (2020). Clinical evidence does not support corticosteroid treatment for 2019-nCoV lung injury. *Lancet* 395 (10223), 473–475. doi:10.1016/S0140-6736(20)30317-2

Su, S., Wong, G., Shi, W., Liu, J., Lai, A., Zhou, J., et al. (2016). Epidemiology, genetic recombination, and pathogenesis of coronaviruses. *Trends Microbiol.*, 24 (6), 490–502. doi:10.1016/j.tim.2016.03.003

Sukumar, U. K., Bose, R. J. C., Malhotra, M., Babikir, H. A., Afjei, R., Robinson, E., et al. (2019). Intranasal delivery of targeted polyfunctional gold-iron oxide nanoparticles loaded with therapeutic microRNAs for combined theranostic multimodality imaging and presensitization of glioblastoma to temozolomide. *Biomaterials*, 218, 119342. doi:10.1016/j.biomaterials.2019.119342

Wang, Y., Li, L., Zhao, W., Dou, Y., An, H., Tao, H., et al. (2018). Targeted therapy of atherosclerosis by a broad-spectrum reactive oxygen species scavenging nanoparticle with intrinsic anti-inflammatory activity. *ACS Nano*, 12 (9), 8943–8960. doi:10.1021/acsnano.8b02037

Wu, C., Liu, Y., Yang, Y., Zhang, P., Zhong, W., Wang, Y., et al. (2020). Analysis of therapeutic targets for SARS-CoV-2 and discovery of potential drugs by computational methods. *Acta Pharm. Sin. B* 10 (5), 766–788. doi:10.1016/j.apsb.2020.02.008

Wu, Y. X., He, H. Q., Nie, Y. J., Ding, Y. H., Sun, L., and Qian, F. (2018). Protostemonine effectively attenuates lipopolysaccharide-induced acute lung injury in mice. *Acta Pharmacol. Sin.* 39 (1), 85–96. doi:10.1038/aps.2017.131

Yu, X. H., Wang, Y. F., Dai, F. Y., Zhao, J. H., and Li, P. (2019). The protective effects of Berberine and Hesperidin on inflammatory factor-stimulating cardiac fibroblasts. *Eur. Rev. Med. Pharmacol. Sci.* 23 (12), 5468–5476. doi:10.26355/eurrev_201906_18216

Zhang, C., Wu, Z., Li, J. W., Zhao, H., and Wang, G. Q. (2020). Cytokine release syndrome in severe COVID-19: interleukin-6 receptor antagonist tocilizumab may be the key to reduce mortality. *Int. J. Antimicrob. Agents*, 55 (5), 105954. doi:10.1016/j.ijantimicag.2020.105954

Zhang, C. Y., Lin, W., Gao, J., Shi, X., Davaritouchaee, M., Nielsen, A. E., et al. (2019). pH-responsive nanoparticles targeted to lungs for improved therapy of acute lung inflammation/injury. *ACS Appl. Mater. Interfaces* 11 (18), 16380–16390. doi:10.1021/acsami.9b04051

4

Cystic Fibrosis Lung Disease in the Aging Population

*Lisa Künzi[1,2], Molly Easter[1], Meghan June Hirsch[1] and Stefanie Krick[1,3,4]**

[1]Division of Pulmonary, Allergy and Critical Care Medicine, University of Alabama at Birmingham, Birmingham, AL, United States, [2]Epidemiology, Biostatistics and Prevention Institute, Department of Public and Global Health, University of Zürich, Zürich, Switzerland, [3]Gregory Fleming Cystic Fibrosis Research Center, University of Alabama at Birmingham, Birmingham, AL, United States, [4]Comprehensive Center for Healthy Aging, University of Alabama at Birmingham, Birmingham, AL, United States

***Correspondence:**
Stefanie Krick
skrick@uabmc.edu

The demographics of the population with cystic fibrosis (CF) is continuously changing, with nowadays adults outnumbering children and a median predicted survival of over 40 years. This leads to the challenge of treating an aging CF population, while previous research has largely focused on pediatric and adolescent patients. Chronic inflammation is not only a hallmark of CF lung disease, but also of the aging process. However, very little is known about the effects of an accelerated aging pathology in CF lungs. Several chronic lung disease pathologies show signs of chronic inflammation with accelerated aging, also termed "inflammaging"; the most notable being chronic obstructive pulmonary disease (COPD) and idiopathic pulmonary fibrosis (IPF). In these disease entities, accelerated aging has been implicated in the pathogenesis via interference with tissue repair mechanisms, alterations of the immune system leading to impaired defense against pulmonary infections and induction of a chronic pro-inflammatory state. In addition, CF lungs have been shown to exhibit increased expression of senescence markers. Sustained airway inflammation also leads to the degradation and increased turnover of cystic fibrosis transmembrane regulator (CFTR). This further reduces CFTR function and may prevent the novel CFTR modulator therapies from developing their full efficacy. Therefore, novel therapies targeting aging processes in CF lungs could be promising. This review summarizes the current research on CF in an aging population focusing on accelerated aging in the context of chronic airway inflammation and therapy implications.

Keywords: cystic fibrosis, aging, inflammaging, oxidative stress, mitochondrial dysfunction, senescence

INTRODUCTION

30 years ago, mutations in the cystic fibrosis transmembrane regulator (CFTR) gene were characterized as single gene defect leading to the pathology of cystic fibrosis (CF) (Kerem et al., 1989; Tsui, 1995). Since then, our understanding of the pathological processes has largely improved with CFTR targeted modulator therapies in clinical use (Wainwright et al., 2015; Rowe et al., 2017; Taylor-Cousar et al., 2017; Davies et al., 2018; Keating et al., 2018). Nevertheless, progressive lung disease is still the major cause for morbidity and mortality in individuals born with CF (Elborn, 2016). Functional failure of CFTR results in impaired ciliary function, mucus obstruction, bacterial

---

Abbreviations: BAL, bronchoalveolar lavage; BK, large-conductance Ca2+- and voltage-dependent K+; ECM, extracellular matrix; FEV1, forced expiratory volume in 1s; FVC, forced ventilator capacity; GSH, reduced glutathione; HBE, human bronchial epithelial; IGF-1, Insulin-like growth factor 1; MAPK, mitogen-activated protein kinase; NE, neutrophil elastase; oh8dG, urinary 8-hydroxydeoxyguanosine; PBMCs, peripheral blood mononuclear cells; PMN, polymorphnuclear leukocyte; ROS, reactive oxygen species; TG2, tissue trans-glutaminase 2; TIMP-1 tissue inhibitor of metalloprotease-1; wt, wild-type.

colonization and chronic inflammation (Matsui et al., 1998; Mall et al., 2004; Boucher, 2007). This sets the stage for smoldering chronic infections interrupted by episodic exacerbations due to newly acquired pathogens leading to progressive loss of lung function (Nichols et al., 2008; Elborn, 2016). Elevated levels of pro-inflammatory mediators, reactive oxygen species (ROS), and proteases, which further propagate airway inflammation, can accelerate cellular senescence (Bezzerri et al., 2019).

Major improvements in supportive therapies and the development of CFTR targeted therapies increased life expectancy in CF patients to a median survival of 40 years or more in industrialized nations (Dodge et al., 2007; MacKenzie et al., 2014). Hence, CF is no longer considered primarily a pediatric disease. This entails new challenges, including treatment of CF in an aging population with CF dependent and independent comorbidities. Diabetes, osteopenia and osteoporosis, renal, and vestibulocholear complications from aminoglycoside toxicity, cardiovascular disease, and worsening lung disease are medical issues often emerging in the aging CF population (Hodson et al., 2008; Simmonds et al., 2009). Chronic local and systemic inflammation is a key pathogenic mechanisms suspected of promoting these comorbidities (Nichols et al., 2008; Bezzerri et al., 2019). Aging impairs lung function through several mechanisms, a central being chronic, low-grade inflammation termed "inflammaging" (Franceschi and Campisi, 2014). Accelerated aging has been implicated in several chronic inflammatory lung disease pathologies. As chronic inflammation is a hallmark of CF airway disease, the question arises whether this chronic inflammation may also cause premature aging in CF lung tissue; and if so whether novel therapies targeting "inflammaging" and aging pathomechanisms in CF lungs might prove to be beneficial.

HALLMARKS OF AGING IN CF LUNG DISEASE

Physiological aging is associated with considerable changes in lung structure and cell function, giving rise to reduced lung function, pulmonary remodeling, diminished regenerative capacity, and enhanced susceptibility to lung injury, and disease (Cho and Stout-Delgado, 2020). Considering the increased life expectancy of CF patients, the question whether chronic inflammation contributes to accelerated aging becomes more and more relevant. Interestingly, healthy aging lungs show a proinflammatory state with increased neutrophils and IL-8 (Meyer et al., 1998), bearing some similarity with chronic CF lung inflammation. In the following paragraphs we aim to provide an overview on the hallmarks of aging and their potential implications for CF lung disease. Central findings on accelerated aging in CF are also summarized in **Figure 1**.

Genomic Instability

Non-transplanted CF patients have a higher risk for lymphoid leukemia, testicular cancer and digestive tract cancers than the general population (Maisonneuve et al., 2013). Similarly, cancer risk in CF lung transplant recipients is more increased than in non-CF recipients, particularly for colorectal cancer, esophageal cancer, and non-Hodgkin lymphoma (Fink et al., 2017). Defects in CFTR themselves have been linked to cancers (Scott et al., 2020). The striking overlap of organ systems with elevated cancer risk and those that are primarily affected by CF-associated mucus hypersecretion, i.e., the respiratory, digestive, and reproductive systems, strongly implicates chronic inflammation as a potential causative factor. In CF airway inflammation, large numbers of activated neutrophils release reactive oxygen species (ROS) and proteases, such as neutrophil elastase, thereby inducing additional ROS production in lung cells (Brown and Kelly, 1994; Aoshiba et al., 2001). In addition, reduced antioxidant defense with systemic glutathione deficiency, reduced vitamin E plasma levels, and increased mitochondrial oxidative stress has been reported in CF patients (Roum et al., 1985; Brown et al., 1995; Starosta et al., 2006; Velsor et al., 2006). Not surprisingly, CF lungs are exposed to significantly higher oxidative stress levels (Starosta et al., 2006). As marker of oxidant-induced DNA damage, urinary 8-hydroxydeoxyguanosine (8-OHdG) was found to be significantly elevated in children with CF (Brown and Kelly, 1994). Further, airway epithelia from CF patients show increased expression of two DNA damage markers (phospho-Histone H2A.X (γH2A.X) and phospho-checkpoint 2 kinase (phospho-Chk2)) (Fischer et al., 2013). However, it would be too simplistic to attribute the increased cancer risk solely to oxidative stress. CFTR has been proposed a tumor suppressor protein and CFTR deficiency is implicated in airway and intestinal cancer progression and poor prognosis (Than et al., 2016; Li et al., 2015; Tu et al., 2016). In summary, aging-associated DNA repair deficiency in combination with increased oxidative damage can lead to accumulating genome damage and thus to genomic instability (Moskalev et al., 2013).

Telomere Attrition

The proliferative capacity of cells is limited by the gradual loss of their protective telomeric DNA with each division ultimately leading to cellular senescence (Blackburn et al., 2006). Chronic inflammation can not only increase cell turnover, it has also been shown to lead to telomere dysfunction and accelerated aging (Jurk et al., 2014; Gorenjak et al., 2020). Telomeres are highly sensitive to oxidative damage as it is ineffectively repaired causing accelerated telomere loss (Gorenjak et al., 2020; Hewitt et al., 2012). This raises the question whether oxidative stress associated with chronic airway inflammation can cause accelerated telomere shortening in CF patients.

In CF, decreased telomere length in peripheral blood leukocytes has been reported to be associated with disease severity (Lammertyn et al., 2017). However, telomere length was not reduced in explant lungs from CF patients, and no correlation between telomere length and disease severity at the sampling location was found (Everaerts et al., 2018). Similarly, telomere length in CF airway epithelial cells was not significantly different from control donor lungs; only a small subgroup of CF subjects had shorter telomeres (Fischer et al., 2013). Based on the limited scientific data available, we cannot conclude whether telomere attrition is a common feature in CF lungs. Further research is needed to determine its contribution to CF airway disease pathogenesis.

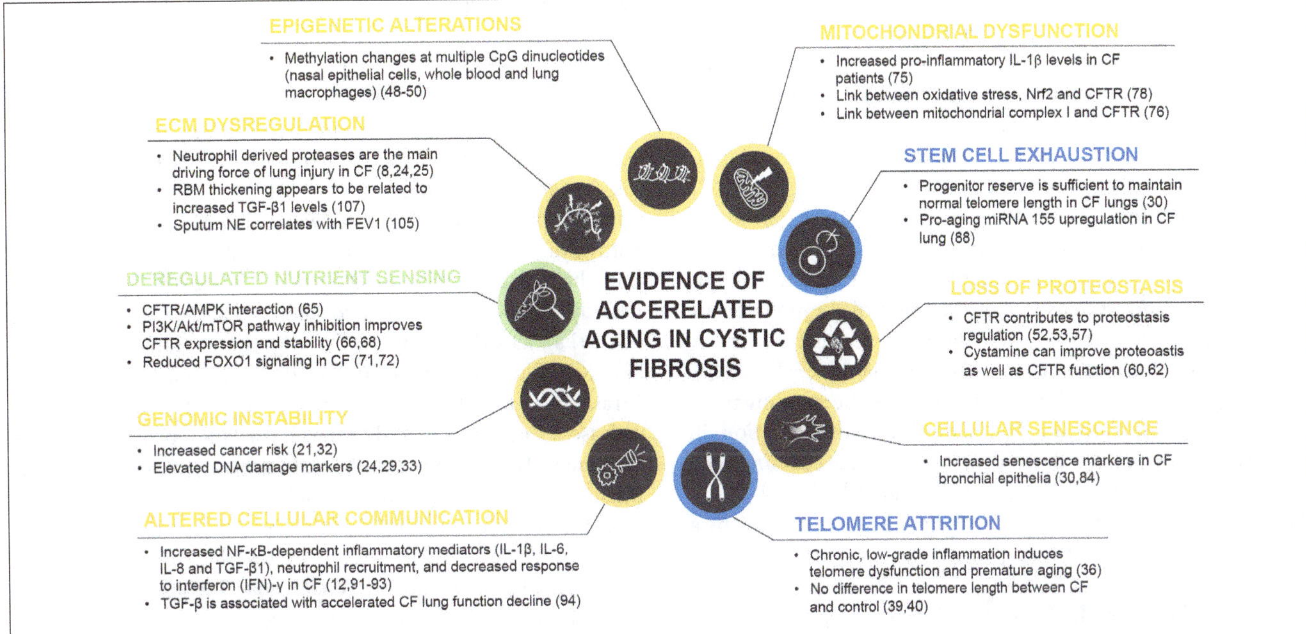

FIGURE 1 | Current state of evidence on accelerated aging processes in CF. Research findings on the role of each of the ten hallmarks of aging in CF disease are summarized and color coded based on their level of evidence with blue = no evidence for involvement in CF pathology, green = weak evidence, yellow = strong evidence.

Epigenetic Alterations

Epigenetic alterations are stable, heritable changes to the chemical DNA structure by alterations in its methylation pattern, post-translational histone modifications, and chromatin remodeling. They regulate gene expression without modifying the DNA sequence (Gonzalo, 1985; Berger et al., 2009). Specific changes in the histone modification pattern such as increased H4K20 and H3K4 trimethylation, and decreased H3K9 methylation as well as H3K27 trimethylation constitute markers of age-associated epigenetic alterations (Gonzalo, 1985; López-Otín et al., 2013). DNA methylation has been shown to play an important role in aging and disease. Global DNA methylation changes over the lifespan and methylation of specific CpG (cytosine guanine) sites correlate with age (Jones et al., 2015; Ashapkin et al., 2017; Levine et al., 2018). Alterations in DNA methylation patterns are associated with cancer, several genetic diseases and inflammatory lung conditions including CF (Robertson, 2005; Scott and De Sario, 2020). In CF, methylation changes were found at multiple CpG dinucleotides in nasal epithelial cells, whole blood and lung macrophages. Interestingly, these epigenetic alterations were preferentially located at genes important for the respective tissue, such as for cell adhesion, immune response or inflammation, and correlated with lung function (Scott and De Sario, 2020; Magalhães et al., 2018; Chen et al., 2018). Though the specific research is yet in its infancy, CFTR has been shown to be epigenetically regulated too which may open up novel therapeutic strategies to restore CFTR dysfunction in CF pathology (Sirinupong and Yang, 2015).

Loss of Proteostasis

Molecular chaperones and the proteolytic machinery assure continuous proteome renewal protecting cells from accumulation of misfolded or damaged proteins (López-Otín et al., 2013). Loss of adequate proteostasis occurs during the aging process and has been shown to be altered in CF epithelia. There is increasing evidence that CFTR function can regulate the proteostasis network (Villella et al., 2013; Esposito et al., 2016). CFTR carrying the ΔF508 mutation as well as other less frequent mutations does not mature into the fully glycosylated protein. Instead, the misfolded protein is mostly retained at the endoplasmic reticulum, where it is sequestered for degradation (Cheng et al., 1990; Van Goor et al., 2011). ΔF508 overexpression causes ER stress and activates the unfolded protein response *in vitro* leading to decreased wild type CFTR mRNA levels (Bartoszewski et al., 2008). This implicates defective CFTR leads to suppressed CFTR expression. The severity of the clinical disease spectrum varies considerably even within patients carrying the same mutation. Variations in the proteostasis network are suspected to be modifying factors contributing to those differences (Balch et al., 2011). A promising new therapeutic strategy aims at improving protein trafficking by the proteostasis network (Strub and McCray Jr, 2020). The proteostasis regulator cystamine promotes ΔF508-CFTR trafficking to the apical cell membrane and thereby allows it to respond to CFTR potentiators (Luciani et al., 2012). Cystamine combined with epigallocatechin gallate restored CFTR function, reduced lung inflammation and restored autophagy in a phase-2 trial, particularly in patients carrying the ΔF508 mutation (Tosco et al., 2016).

CFTR is not only subjected to degradation by the proteostasis network, it is a key player in its own regulation. Inhibition of CFTR function leads to CFTR protein ubiquitination and drastically reduced stability in the plasma membrane of bronchial epithelial cells (Esposito et al., 2016), with cystamine correcting this deranged proteostasis (Villella et al.,

2013). In addition, siRNA depleting CFTR interferes with endosomal trafficking of cell surface proteins demonstrated for transferrin receptor, epidermal growth factor receptor, and CFTR itself (Villella et al., 2013). Hence, insufficient CFTR function derails the proteostasis network in a feed-forward loop fostering its own degradation. Dysfunctional autophagy also appears to contribute to the exaggerated CF lung inflammation. Improving autophagosome clearance attenuates the hyperinflammatory response (Mayer et al., 2013). Oxidative stress from defective CFTR function inhibits ubiquitination and proteasome degradation of the pro-fibrotic tissue trans-glutaminase 2, thereby driving chronic inflammation (Esposito et al., 2016; Luciani et al., 2009). Autophagy restoration by cystamine has been shown to suppress trans-glutaminase 2 and diminish inflammation in CF mice and in patient derived nasal epithelial cells *in vitro*. In summary, loss of proteostasis as an aging hallmark in CF disease has been established by current evidence and might be a valuable target for future therapies.

Deregulated Nutrient Sensing

Aging is regulated by nutrient-sensing pathways including insulin/insulin-like growth factor (IGF-1), mTOR, AMP kinase, sirtuins, and FOXO transcription factors (Vellai, 2009; Kenyon, 2010). Pro-inflammatory signals are closely integrated in stress and nutrient signaling (Jurk et al., 2014). Hence, both inflammaging and chronic inflammatory conditions such as CF lung disease have the potential to interfere with nutrient sensing signaling pathways. An *in vitro* study identified the α1 (catalytic) subunit of AMP-activated protein kinase (AMPK) as a dominant and novel protein interacting with CFTR demonstrating a potential link between transepithelial transport and cell metabolic state (Hallows et al., 2000).

Oxidative stress as seen in CF airway inflammation leads to increased pro-growth signaling by the mTOR pathway (Chen et al., 2011). So far, only little is known about deregulated nutrient sensing in CF lung disease. CFTR has been found to interact with mTOR signaling pathway components, which can be affected by CFTR mutations such that ΔF508 CFTR exhibits a specific interactome different from wild type CFTR (Pankow et al., 2015; Reilly et al., 2017). mTOR activity in CF bronchial epithelial cells is upregulated, and PI3K/Akt/mTOR pathway inhibition improves CFTR expression and stability (Reilly et al., 2017). FOXO transcription factors down stream of insulin/IGF-1 signaling (IIS) regulate cellular processes involved in stress resistance, metabolism as well as cell cycle arrest, and are central to IIS attenuation-mediated lifespan expansion (Martins et al., 2016). FOXO1 and 3 have been shown to regulate innate immune mechanisms in respiratory epithelia in response to bacterial infections (Seiler et al., 2013). In a human CF bronchial epithelial cell line, reduced FOXO1 was found related to loss of CFTR function (Smerieri et al., 2014). Interestingly, four miRNAs that are predicted FOXO1 regulators were differently expressed in CF patient sera (Montanini et al., 2016). However, the implications of altered FOXO transcription factor signaling in terms of accelerated aging in CF patients remains unclear and calls for further investigation.

Mitochondrial Dysfunction

Age-associated mitochondrial dysfunction is most commonly caused by increased ROS ultimately leading to cell senescence (Chapman et al., 2019). Excessive oxidant levels from dysfunctional mitochondria can trigger inflammatory cytokine release inducing chronic inflammation and progression of airway diseases such as CF (Prakash et al., 2017). In addition, as cells age, DNA damage occurs and activates DNA damage response pathways. These chronically stimulated pathways cause mitochondrial stress leading to increased release of mitochondrial damage-associated molecular patterns (DAMPs). DAMPs along with ROS production, and/or ATP and K^+ efflux contribute to NLRP3 inflammasome activation (Prakash et al., 2017; dos Santos et al., 2012). This leads to caspase-1 activation and release of the proinflammatory cytokines IL-1β and IL-18, initiating a cycle of chronic inflammation, disease progression, and further accumulative damage to mitochondria resulting in accelerated aging (dos Santos et al., 2012). Recent research is showing that mitochondrial dysfunction could be involved in disease progression in CF. Cells with impaired CFTR function exhibit reduced mitochondrial complex I activity (Valdivieso et al., 2012). And increased IL-1β levels are very common among CF patients, which has been linked to inflammation triggered by underlying chronic *Pseudomonas aeruginosa* infections (Rimessi et al., 2015). As discussed, elevated IL-1β is not only a sign of inflammation, but also a hallmark of mitochondrial dysfunction. These two intrinsically connected hallmarks of aging both contribute to disease progression in CF. Furthermore, it will be of benefit to assess whether the triple CFTR modulator therapy affects these pathogenetic mechanisms favorably. A recent study has shown that CFTR modulation can restore Nrf2 phosphorylation, a major regulator of oxidative balance and inflammatory signaling (Borcherding et al., 2019).

Cellular Senescence

Accumulation of senescent cells is seen in normal aging and chronic pulmonary disease (Jeyapalan et al., 2007; Meiners et al., 2015). Senescence is triggered by a range of insults such as oxidative stress, DNA damage, telomere shortening, and inflammation, and is associated with a characteristic secretory profile termed senescence-associated secretory phenotype (SASP) (Naylor et al., 2013; Jurk et al., 2014). This includes release of proinflammatory mediators, growth factors, and matrix-remodeling proteases that may perpetuate inflammatory processes resulting in further accumulation of senescent cells (Naylor et al., 2013; Parikh et al., 2019). In CF, the liquid lung lining layer contains high amounts of neutrophil elastase that has been shown to trigger cell cycle arrest through elevated $p27^{Kip1}$ expression resulting in G1 arrest in normal human bronchial epithelial cells *in vitro* (Nakamura et al., 1992; Fischer et al., 2007). Cell cycle arrest may lead to cellular senescence (Fischer et al., 2013; Naylor et al., 2013). Indeed, a study by Fischer and colleagues confirmed airway epithelia from CF lungs have increased expression of the senescence markers $p16^{INK4a}$, γH2A.X, and phospho-Chk2 (Fischer et al., 2013). Their study showed that neutrophil elastase increases p16 expression resulting in inhibition of cyclin-dependent kinase 4 activity *in vitro* (Fischer et al., 2007). This suggests cellular senescence due to excessive neutrophil elastase release in CF lungs may contribute to accelerated aging. A recent review concluded there was consistent data supporting that cellular senescence may also be involved in CF lung disease, but the exact mechanisms leading from loss of CFTR function to cellular senescence and the precise role in CF lung disease remain unknown (Bezzerri et al., 2019).

Stem Cell Exhaustion

Lung tissue has a low steady-state cell turnover with the ability to increase proliferation of stem/progenitor cells in response to injury (Hogan et al., 2014). Aging is associated with a progressive decline of stem/progenitor cells that maintain homeostatic and regenerative capacity (Oh et al., 2014). Chronic inflammation is considered a main factor accelerating the deterioration of stem cell function with transforming growth factor (TGF)-β and ROS accumulation as important pathological factors (Oh et al., 2014). miRNA-155 is upregulated in aging and has been suggested to contribute to inflammation-associated stem cell dysfunction (Teramura and Onodera, 2018). High expression of this specific miRNA has been found in CF lung epithelial cells and circulating neutrophils (Bhattacharyya et al., 2011). Further, chronic airway inflammation in combination with recurrent exacerbations causes recurrent tissue damage thereby increasing the need for stem cell proliferation. This may exceed the supply the stem cell niche is capable of providing resulting in its depletion in CF lungs (Mora and Rojas, 2013). To this point, there are no reports on the exact role of stem cell exhaustion in CF lung disease. One study observed no telomere shortening in CF airway epithelial cells leading to the conclusion that the epithelial stem/progenitor reserve is sufficient to maintain normal telomere length despite enhanced cell turnover (Fischer et al., 2013). But this does not exclude an involvement of stem cell exhaustion in accelerated aging in CF lungs, and further studies are needed to draw definite conclusions.

Altered Cellular Communication

In addition to chronic lung inflammation, CFTR deficiency has been reported to causes abnormalities in diverse signaling pathways. Functional CFTR has been reported to downregulate NF-κB activity and CF associated hyper-inflammation may represent a consequence of insufficient inhibition of NF-κB signaling (Hunter et al., 2010). Chronic, progressive low-grade inflammation promoted by NF-κB can cause premature aging (Jurk et al., 2014). CF airway inflammation is associated with excessive production of NF-κB-dependent inflammatory mediators such as interleukin-1β (IL-1β), IL-6, IL-8, and TGF-β1, neutrophil recruitment, and decreased response to interferon (IFN)-γ as well as further abnormalities in various signaling pathways (Nichols et al., 2008; Harris et al., 2009; Peterson-Carmichael et al., 2009; Lara-Reyna et al., 2020). The profibrotic cytokine TGF-β is considered a pro-aging factor and is associated with accelerated lung function decline in CF patients (Arkwright et al., 2000). Several reports show that TGF-β causes CFTR dysfunction (Manzanares et al., 2015; Snodgrass et al., 2013; Sun et al., 2014). Chronic bacterial infections stimulate persistent IL-8 release from airway epithelia (McCuaig and Martin, 2013). Attracted neutrophils further potentiate airway inflammation by releasing high concentrations of inflammatory mediators such as TNFα and IL-8, oxidants, and proteases (Petit-Bertron et al., 2008). Neutrophil elastase promotes CFTR degradation and dysfunction by calpains (Le Gars et al., 2013). Recent drug developments have focused on restoring CFTR function; these therapies significantly improve lung function and reduce exacerbations in CF patients (Wainwright et al., 2015; Rowe et al., 2017; Davies et al., 2018; Keating et al., 2018). However, sustained airway inflammation leads to degradation and increased turnover of CFTR, hindering the targeted therapies from developing their full potential by inducing a state of accelerated aging at the tissue level (Rowe et al., 2014). Oxidative stress from ROS associated with neutrophilic airway inflammation can lead to accumulation of modified or damaged biomolecules impairing their function. Oxidatively damaged cellular structures can act as DAMPs that are recognized by receptors of the innate immune system, i.e., Toll-like-receptors (TLRs) and the NLRP3 inflammasome (Meiners et al., 2015). Hence, oxidative stress can further enhance cytokine production in the ongoing inflammation and maintain the proinflammatory state in inflammaging (Franceschi and Campisi, 2014; Meiners et al., 2015).

Extracellular Matrix Dysregulation

ECM remodeling in lung diseases is not only a consequence of tissue injury, it also contributes to disease progression by impaired repair mechanisms (Parker et al., 2014). The neutrophilic inflammation in CF is accompanied by protease/antiprotease imbalance with increased neutrophil elastase and matrix metalloprotease-9 and reduced tissue inhibitor of metalloprotease-1 (Gaggar et al., 2007). While proteolytic enzymes are beneficial for tissue repair, excessive release due to chronic inflammation may overwhelm anti-protease activity causing airway remodeling and obstruction (Gaggar et al., 2011). Neutrophil derived proteases are the main driving force of lung injury in CF (Elborn, 2016) and sputum neutrophil elastase correlates with FEV_1 in children with CF (Sagel et al., 2002). Furthermore, neutrophil elastase and proteolytic collagen and elastin breakdown products play a pathogenic role in fibrotic lung remodeling (Chua and Laurent, 2006). Ultrastructural evidence for ECM degradation includes lysis of elastic and collagen fibers, loss of arborescent elastic network distribution and alterations in the reticular basement membrane structure (RBM) (Durieu et al., 1998; Hilliard et al., 2007; Regamey et al., 2011). In CF, RBM thickening appears to be related to increased TGF-β1 levels (Hilliard et al., 2007). The elastic network reduction combined with increased collagen deposition in bronchial walls of CF patients resembles fibrotic ECM changes in aging lungs (Hilliard et al., 2007). Together, these data suggest that ECM dysregulation plays an important role in accelerated lung aging in CF.

THERAPEUTIC IMPLICATIONS

Current Effective CF Therapies Targeting Chronic Inflammation

Various drugs targeting inflammation have been studied in CF since 1990, but only few are recommended for clinical use. Due to the length of this review, only significant ones will be discussed here.

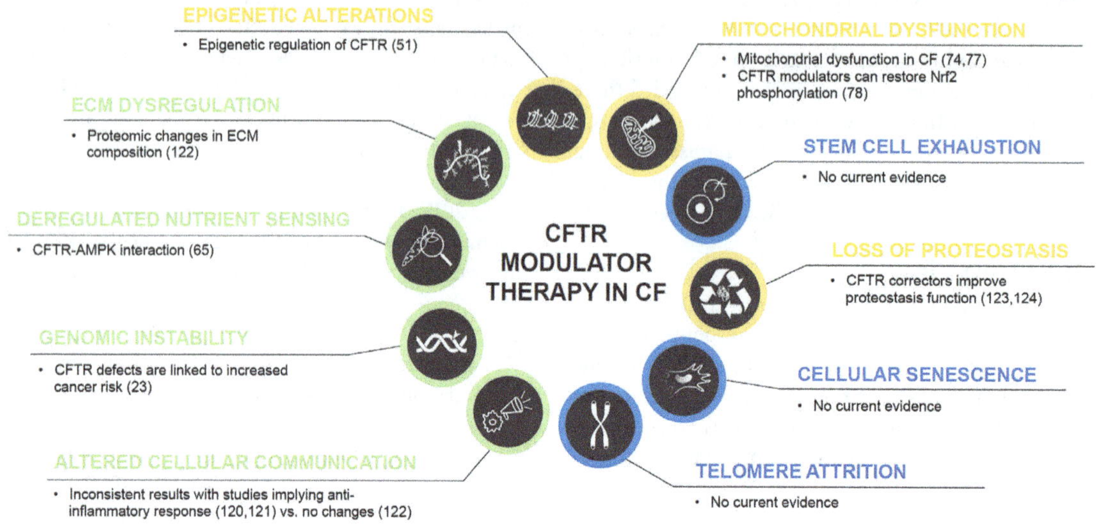

FIGURE 2 | CFTR modulator therapy in CF and potential effects on the hallmarks of aging. Color code for current level of evidence with blue = no evidence for involvement in CF pathology, green = weak evidence, yellow = strong evidence.

Corticosteroids were one of the first anti-inflammatory drugs studied as a chronic therapy attenuating CF airway inflammation (Auerbach et al., 1985; Eigen et al., 1995). Although beneficial effects on lung function were shown, overall adverse effects outweighed the benefits and long-term use of systemic corticosteroids to slow lung function decline is currently not recommended (Flume et al., 2007). Several studies investigated the effects of inhaled corticosteroids (ICS) on lung function decline, but their anti-inflammatory effect was never confirmed (Ren et al., 2008; De Boeck et al., 2011). The CF Foundation therefore is advising against the use of long-term ICS in patients with CF older than 6 years without coexistent asthma or allergic bronchopulmonary aspergillosis (Flume et al., 2007).

Nonsteroidal anti-inflammatory drugs (NSAIDs) have been studied as therapeutic options for CF due to similar properties as corticosteroids, but fewer adverse effects. Ibuprofen has specific activity against neutrophils and twice-daily high-dose ibuprofen use was linked to a slower lung function decline, a decreased exacerbation frequency and less weight loss in the pediatric CF population (Konstan et al., 1995; Konstan et al., 2003; Konstan et al., 2007; Lands et al., 2007). Nevertheless, ibuprofen is not widely used, but the CF Foundation expert panel recommends its use for CF patients with mild lung disease (Flume et al., 2007).

CFTR modulator therapy has demonstrated its efficacy and beneficial effect on restoration of CFTR function for approximately 90% CF genotypes (Wainwright et al., 2015; Rowe et al., 2017; Davies et al., 2018; Keating et al., 2018; Middleton et al., 2019). Interestingly, CFTR dysfunction has been linked to contribute to chronic inflammation as well as other hallmarks of aging, and two recent studies have demonstrated an anti-inflammatory effect of CFTR modulators (Jarosz-Griffiths et al., 2020; Hisert et al., 2017). A recent observational study though did not show any significant alterations in sputum inflammatory markers, but changes in ECM using whole proteome analysis (Kopp et al., 2020). Therefore, the validation of potential anti-inflammatory effects of CFTR correctors needs further investigation. CFTR correctors also have been shown to act as proteostasis regulators (Lopes-Pacheco et al., 2015; Lopes-Pacheco et al., 2016) and there is evidence that CFTR modulators can regulate mitochondrial dysfunction. **Figure 2** summarizes current evidence of CFTR modulators and their link to aging hallmarks.

Potential Novel CF Therapies

Modulation of ion channels other than CFTR has been evaluated as potential therapies. Most recently, potentiation of TMEM16A using ETX001 significantly increased the Ca^{2+}-activated Cl^- channel activity and anion secretion both *in vitro* and *in vivo* ovine models leading to improved mucociliary clearance without impacting calcium signaling (Danahay et al., 2020). Whether ETX001 also affects airway inflammation will be of great interest.

Anti-inflammatory cytokines and antibodies targeting cytokines may be valuable novel CF therapies. IL-10 has been demonstrated to terminate the inflammatory response and is deficient in CF patients (Bonfield et al., 1999). And its administration is anti-inflammatory in Pseudomonas infected mice (Chmiel et al., 1999; Soltys et al., 2002). Treatment with the anti-inflammatory cytokine IFN-γ was tested in a multicenter clinical trial but did not show any beneficial effect on pulmonary function or inflammatory sputum markers (Moss et al., 2005). This is in line with the above-mentioned reduced response of CF airways to IFN-γ. As an alternative to the treatment with anti-inflammatory cytokines, various blocking antibodies targeting pro-inflammatory cytokines have been assessed. Anti-IL-17 antibodies have been shown to decrease neutrophil recruitment in murine airways when exposed to lipopolysaccharide (Ferretti et al., 2003). Anti-IL-17 has been tested clinically in rheumatoid arthritis and psoriasis (Ly et al., 2019; Taams, 2020) and might be a potential novel therapeutic strategy for CF-associated airway inflammation. Anti-ICAM-1 and -IL-8 have been assessed preclinically, but never reached the clinical stage. Because of high concentrations of LTB_4 in CF airways (Konstan et al., 1993) BIIL 284 BS (amelubant), a specific LTB_4 receptor antagonist, has been tested in CF. Due to serious pulmonary adverse events, the clinical trial was terminated early (Konstan MW et al., 2005).

Fatty acid modulation may proof beneficial as alterations in fatty acid concentrations contributing to airway inflammation have been demonstrated in CF such as increases in arachidonic acid and decreases in docosahexaenoic acid (DHA) (Freedman et al., 1999; Horati et al., 2020). Cumulative data from *in vitro* studies and some small, non-placebo controlled trials using oral DHA supplementation imply this may be beneficial for pulmonary function preservation (Beharry et al., 2007; Van Biervliet et al., 2008; Aldámiz-Echevarría et al., 2009). To validate these results, larger placebo-controlled trials will be needed. Furthermore, Myriocin, an inhibitor of sphingolipid synthesis, induced changes in a transcriptional program of cell metabolism *in vitro* in CF airway epithelial cells. Therefore, the authors speculated that sphingolipid *de novo* synthesis could attenuate chronic inflammation, optimize energy supply, and anti-oxidant responses, implying a novel future therapeutic strategy for CF (Mingione et al., 2020)

Inhibiton of NF-κB activation has been demonstrated by both ibuprofen at high doses and IL-10. Furthermore, NF-κB signaling can be attenuated by glitazones through peroxisome proliferator activating receptor (PPAR) elevation (Zingarelli et al., 2003; Ruan et al., 2003) and there seems to be a deficiency of PPAR in CF (Perez et al., 2008). Both tiglitazone and troglitazone can activate PPAR in the CF epithelium and attenuate the inflammatory response to *P. aeruginosa* (Perez et al., 2008). One clinical trial using glitazones has not shown a beneficial effect towards inflammation, but this trial was very small and did not assess lung function outcomes (Konstan MW et al., 2009). Long term use of Azithromycin has not only been shown to improve functional outcomes, but some of the underlying mechanisms can be attributed to STAT and NF-κB inhibition (Haydar et al., 2019; Nichols et al., 2020). In summary, targeting NF-κB signaling in CF disease seems to be an attractive future therapeutic direction.

Inhibition of the NLRP3 Inflammasome has also been discussed as a potential anti-inflammatory strategy (Scambler et al., 2019). A recent report utilized MCC950 as a specific NLRP3 inhibitor *in vivo* in CF animal models, which resulted in significantly reduced airway inflammation and improved *Pseudomonas* clearance (McElvaney et al., 2019).

Statins exhibit anti-inflammatory effects through various mechanisms including inhibition of neutrophil migration, RhoGTPase/increase in nitric oxide (NO)/IL-8 production and other proinflammatory cytokines as well as increase of PPAR transcription (Dunzendorfer et al., 1997; Kraynack et al., 2002; Zelvyte et al., 2002). Agents that can increase NO, such as arginine, have been studied, since it has been shown that there is increased arginase activity in blood and sputum of CF patients. This leads to degradation of L-arginine, which is a substrate for NO production (Grasemann et al., 2005a). A small pilot study assessed oral supplementation with L-arginine in CF patients, which led to increased exhaled NO (Grasemann et al., 2005b). In order to show efficacy, large prospective clinical trials are needed.

The antioxidant N-Acetyl cysteine (NAC) is frequently used as a mucolytic, but has spiked recent interest as antioxidant due to its ability to increase glutathione levels and inhibit H_2O_2-induced damage. Supplementation of oral NAC was linked to significantly increased blood glutathione levels and decreased neutrophils, IL-8, and elastase activity in sputum of CF patients (Tirouvanziam et al., 2006) A randomized double-blind placebo-controlled trial including 70 CF patients for 24 weeks showed stability or a slight increase in spirometric lung function in NAC treated participants compared to the control group (Conrad et al., 2015). A second open-label randomized controlled trial demonstrated a non-significant improvement in lung function in adults with CF and chronic Pseudomonas infection (Skov et al., 2015). P3001, a mucolytic agent was also assessed and directly compared with NAC in a more recent study using both *in vitro* and *in vivo* CF models. Results indicated that P3001 acted faster and was more effective than NAC and DNAse, but investigators did not study its anti-oxidant or anti-inflammatory properties (Ehre et al., 2019). Since glutathione is transported by CFTR (Linsdell and Hanrahan, 1998), CFTR defects could potentially decrease levels of this antioxidant in the airway epithelium increasing susceptibility to oxidative stress. Indeed, decreased glutathione levels have been observed in CF mouse models and patients (Roum et al., 1985; Velsor et al., 2001). A small pilot study using twice daily treatment of aerosolized glutathione in CF patients led to a reduction in superoxide production, but no changes in oxidative stress markers in bronchoalveolar lavage fluid (Bishop et al., 2005; Hartl et al., 2005). A more recent Cochrane meta-analysis summarized antioxidant therapy approaches in CF and concluded that there does not seem to be a beneficial effect of antioxidant micronutrients on clinical outcomes; but oral supplementation with glutathione showed some benefit to lung function, nutritional status, and decrease in oxidative stress (Ciofu et al., 2019). Nevertheless, due to concurrent treatments including intensive antibiotic therapies, there is not sufficient evidence yet justifying their use in the CF population without larger trials and longer follow up.

Therapeutic use of protease inhibitors has been investigated in CF since 1990. Several groups demonstrated that α_1-antitrypsin delivered as an aerosol formulary decreases inflammatory markers and neutrophils (McElvaney et al., 1991; Griese et al., 2007). rSLPI and EPI-hNE4 are two neutrophil elastase inhibitors, which have shown beneficial effects in CF, but large cohort trials are still lacking (McElvaney et al., 1993; Grimbert et al., 2003).

Other potential anti-inflammatories are also being investigated. SB-656933, a CXCR2 antagonist, has shown a trend toward attenuating airway inflammation (Moss et al., 2013). Low-dose cyclosporin A was characterized as a potential steroid sparing agent in a small case series (Bhal et al., 2001). Furthermore, methotrexate was studied as a potential anti-inflammatory agent in cystic fibrosis,

TABLE 1 | Summary of *in vitro*, animal and human studies pointing towards an involvement of accelerated aging in CF disease.

***In vitro* studies**

Hallmark of aging	Cell culture model	Main findings	Ref
Genomic instability	Human fetal lung fibroblast cell line IMR-90, primary human bronchial epithelial cells, and lymphocytes isolated from human blood	ROS and proteases from activated neutrophils increase ROS in mitochondria and cytoplasm, which is associated with oxidative cell injury and death	(Aoshiba et al., 2001)
	Human CF lung epithelial cell line IB3-1 (compound heterozygot for ΔF508 and 128W2X) and isogenic stably wild-type (wt) CFTR transfected C38 cells	Decreased mitochondrial reduced glutathione (GSH) and increased ROS in CFTR deficient human lung epithelial cells	(Velsor et al., 2006)
	CFTR overexpression and knockdown in A549 cell line	Inhibition of CFTR activity promotes epithelial-mesenchymal transition through the uPA/uPAR pathway	(Li et al., 2015)
Loss of proteostasis	COS-7 cell line	Mutated CFTR such as ΔF508 remains in the endoplasmatic reticulum (ER) and is sequester for degradation	(Cheng et al., 1990)
	Calu-3 (wt and stably ΔF508-CFTR transfected) and CFPAC-1 (endogenous ΔF508-CFTR) cell line	ΔF508-CFTR overexpression causes ER stress and activates the unfolded protein response leading to decreased wt CFTR mRNA and protein maturation	(Bartoszewski et al., 2008)
	Normal and CFTR mutated CFBE41° bronchial epithelial cells, primary human bronchial/tracheal epithelial cells and HeLa cells	Functional CFTR controls its own surface expression in a positive feed-forward loop through its effects on the proteostasis network. siRNA depleting CFTR interferes with endosomal trafficking of cell surface proteins. Proteostasis regulator cystamine corrects the deranged proteostasis	(Villella et al., 2013)
	FRT cell line, HEK-293 cells, and primary human bronchial epithelial (HBE) cells	CFTR corrector VX-809 improves F508del-CFTR processing in the ER, leading to plasma residence time and susceptibility to proteolysis similar to normal CFTR.	(Van Goor et al., 2011)
	Human normal and CF bronchial epithelial cell lines (CFBE41o-, IB3-1, 16HBE14o-), ex-vivo cultures of nasal polyp mucosal biopsies and brushed nasal epithelial cells from ΔF508 homozygous patients and matched controls	Proteostasis regulators cystamine and EUK-134 (superoxide dismutase/catalase-mimetic) improve ΔF508-CFTR trafficking and stability at the epithelial cell surface by overexpressing BECN1 and depleting SQSTM1. This facilitates its response to CFTR potentiators and suppresses inflammation	(Luciani et al., 2012)
	IB3-1 and isogenic stably rescued C38 cells and peripheral blood mononuclear cells (PBMCs) from pediatric CF patients and healthy controls	Dysfunctional autophagy appears to contribute to the exaggerated CF lung inflammation. Improving autophagosome clearance attenuates the hyperinflammatory response	(Mayer et al., 2013)
	IB3-1 and isogenic stably rescued C38, 16HBE and A549 cell line, *ex vivo* cultures of nasal polyp mucosal biopsies from CF patients and controls	Defective CFTR function generates oxidative stress that leads to PIASy mediated tissue trans-glutaminase 2 (TG2) SUMOylation inhibiting its ubiquitination and proteasome degradation. TG2 inhibition increases NF-κB inhibitor Ikκα	(Luciani et al., 2009)
Deregulated nutrient sensing	CHO (wt and stably expressing CFTR), T84 and Calu-3 cell line, and Xenopus oocytes	AMPK and CFTR are endogenously expressed in the same tissue types and have been found to interact with each other leading to CFTR phosphorylation and altered CFTR Cl^- conductance. This may represent a link between transepithelial transport and cell metabolic state	(Hallows et al., 2000)
	CF human bronchial epithelial cell line CFBE41o- (ΔF508 mutation) and isogenic HBE41o- cells (wt CFTR)	ΔF508-CFTR interactome differs highly from its wt counterpart including differences in the mTOR, JAK/STAT and several other pathways, showing the catastrophic effects from one misfolded protein on protein-protein interactions	(Pankow et al., 2015)
	CFBE41o- and HBE41o- cells	Inhibition of the PI3K/Akt/mTOR pathway leads to improved CFTR stability, while select inhibitors of this pathway leads to restored autophagy and reduced ΔF508-CFTR aggregates	Reilly et al. (2017)
	CFBE41o- and 16HBE14o- cells	Reduced level of transcription factor FOXO1 and β2 arrestin, along with increased ERK1/2 in CF cells. FOXO1 reduction is linked to loss of CFTR function and increased after insulin-like growth factor 1 (IGF-1) administration. Reduced FOXO1 may explain insulin insensitivity in CF, with IGF-1 constituting a potential treatment of CF-related diabetes	(Smerieri et al., 2014)
	CFBE41o-, 16HBE14o-, and IB3-1 cells	Altered transcriptional profile of miRNAs in CF cells, four of which are potential FOXO1 regulators. These four miRNAs are also differentially expressed in CF patients, and dependent on genotype and glucose tolerance state. This may explain some of the variability in metabolism among CF patients	(Montanini et al., 2016)
Mitochondrial dysfunction	IB3-1 cell line	*Pseudomonas eruginosa* induced inflammation shows importance of mitochondria in the pro-inflammatory condition in CF including their role in Ca^{2+} signaling along with NLRP3 recruitment and activation	Rimessi et al. (2015)

(Continued on following page)

TABLE 1 | *(Continued)* Summary of *in vitro*, animal and human studies pointing towards an involvement of accelerated aging in CF disease.

***In vitro* studies**

Hallmark of aging	Cell culture model	Main findings	Ref
	CF and non-CF HBE cells	ΔF508-CFTR correctors recover diminished function of the major redox balance and inflammatory signaling regulator Nrf2, inducing its nuclear translocation and transcription of target genes. Nrf2 rescue is dependent on CFTR function	(Borcherding et al., 2019)
Cellular senescence	Normal HBE cells	Neutrophil elastase (NE) triggers cell cycle arrest through elevated p27Kip1 expression resulting in G1 arrest in normal HBE cells	(Fischer et al., 2007)
	Normal HBE cells	NE increases p16 expression and decreases CDK4 activity in HBE cells, which may explain how NE treatment triggers cell cycle arrest	(Fischer et al., 2013)
Stem cell exhaustion	HBE cells	No general telomere shortening in CF HBE cells leading to the conclusion that progenitor reserve is sufficient to maintain normal telomere length despite enhanced cell turnover	(Fischer et al., 2013)
	IB3-1 and control CFTR repaired IB3-S9 cells	CF lung epithelial cells hyperexpress miRNA-155, also upregulated in aging. This activates PI3K/Akt signaling through reduced SHIP1. Resulting activation of downstream MAPKs stabilizes IL-8 mRNA and thus increases IL-8 expression promoting inflammation	(Bhattacharyya et al., 2011)
Altered cellular communication	NCI-H441 and 16HBE14o- cells	Functional CFTR downregulates NF-κB activity. CF associated hyper-inflammation may represent a consequence of insufficient inhibition of NF-κB signaling	Hunter et al. (2010)
	HBE cells	TGF-β_1 decreases expression of the γ-subunit LRRC26 of the apically located large-conductance Ca^{2+}- and voltage-dependent K^+ (BK) channels. Thereby, TGF-β_1 reduces BK activity, airway surface liquid volume and ciliary beat frequency	Manzanares et al. (2015)
	Normal and homozygous Δ508-CFTR HBE cells	TGF-β_1, which is frequently elevated in CF patients, reduces CFTR mRNA and protein level in non-CF HBE cells. TGF-β_1 also impairs functional rescue of Δ508-CFTR suggesting it may interfere with therapies aiming at correcting the processing defect of Δ508-CFTR.	Snodgrass et al. (2013)
	T84 cell line and HBE cells	TGF-β reduces calcium activated chloride conductance (CaCC) and CFTR-dependent chloride currents. It reduces expression and activity of TMEM16A and CFTR, and reverses Δ508-CFTR correction by VX-809. Inhibition of Smad3 and p38 MAPK partially reverses TMEM16A and CFTR downregulation	Sun et al. (2014)
	NCI-H292 cell line infected with wt or Δ508-CFTR	NE promotes degradation of wt and Δ508-CFTR through activation of intracellular calpain protease causing loss of channel function	Le Gars et al. (2013)

***In vivo* animal studies**

Hallmark of aging	Animal model	Main findings	Ref
Genomic instability	Congenic CFTR KO strains (S489X and FABP) and C57B6 control mice	Decreased mitochondrial GSH in lungs of CFTR-knockout mice, and increased mitochondrial DNA oxidation and oxidative stress	Velsor et al. (2006)
	Athymic balb/c mice injected with CFTR knockdown or control A-549 cells	CFTR status affects cell invasion and migration. No difference in primary tumor growth between control and CFTR-knockdown A549-injected mice, but increased lung metastasis and increased tumor burden by CFTR-knockdown cells	Li et al. (2015)
Telomere attrition	Nfkb1$^{-/-}$ mice (C57B1/6 background) and fibroblast cultures from ear clippings, p55$^{\Delta ns/\Delta ns}$ mice, and late-generation (F3-F4) terc$^{-/-}$ mice bred from B6/Cg-TERC^{tm1Rdp}/J	Chronic, low-grade inflammation induces telomere dysfunction, senescence, impaired tissue regeneration and premature aging. Conversely, telomere dysfunction leads to a pro-inflammatory state. Anti-inflammatory or antioxidant treatment blocks accumulation of telomere-dysfunctional senescent cells in nfkb1$^{-/-}$ tissues	Jurk et al. (2014)
Loss of proteostasis	Cftr$^{F508del/F508del}$ mice (129/FVB outbred background) and wt littermates	Autophagy restoration by cystamine treatment, BECN1 overexpression and SQSTM1 depletion all considerably increase ΔF508-CFTR at the epithelial surface and decrease lung inflammation	Luciani et al. (2012)

(Continued on following page)

TABLE 1 | *(Continued)* Summary of *in vitro*, animal and human studies pointing towards an involvement of accelerated aging in CF disease.

***In vivo* animal studies**

Hallmark of aging	Animal model	Main findings	Ref
	$Cftr^{F508del/F508del}$, $cftr^{-/-}$ and $Cftr^{F508/-}$ mice, $Cftr^{F508/+}$ and $Cftr^{F508del/F508del}$ mice in *Becn1* haploinsufficient background ($Becn1^{+/-}$)	Cystamine plus epigallocatechin gallate restore CFTR function and reduce lung inflammation in $Cftr^{F508del/F508del}$ and $Cftr^{F508/-}$ mice. ΔF508-CFTR rescue is linked to autophagy restoration, i.e., no rescue in $Becn1^{+/-}$ background	Tosco et al. (2016)
	$Cftr^{F508del/F508del}$ mice (129/FVB outbred background) and wt littermates	TG2 inhibition by cystamine restores PPARγ levels and nuclear localization, and reduces TNFα in lungs of CF mice	Luciani et al. (2009)
Deregulated nutrient sensing	Young adult CF mice homozygous for F508del-CFTR and wt litter mates	Reduced FOXO1 in muscle, but not in liver and adipose tissue of CF mice. Insulin-like growth factor 1 (IGF-1) increases FOXO1 in CF muscle tissue similar to the wt level, and increases it in adipose tissue of both mouse models	Smerieri et al. (2014)
Mitochondrial dysfunction	CF mouse models ($Cftr^{tm1kth}$, $Cftr^{tm2Mrc}$, and $Cftr^{tm1Unc}$ in C57BL/6J background)	Reduced Nrf2-CFTR colocalization in CF mouse models with concomitantly reduced expression of Nrf2 target geneses HMOX1, NQO1, and GCLC.	Borcherding et al. (2019)
Cellular senescence	$Nfkb1^{-/-}$ mice (C57B1/6 background) and fibroblast cultures from ear clipping, $p55^{\Delta ns/\Delta ns}$ mice, and late-generation (F3-F4) $terc^{-/-}$ mice bred from B6/Cg-$TERC^{tm1Rdp}$/J	Chronic, low-grade inflammation induces telomere dysfunction, senescence, impaired tissue regeneration and premature aging. Anti-inflammatory or antioxidant treatment blocks accumulation of telomere-dysfunctional senescent cells in $nfkb1^{-/-}$ tissues	Jurk et al. (2014)
Altered cellular communication	$Nfkb1^{-/-}$ mice (C57B1/6 background) and fibroblast cultures from ear clippings, $p55^{\Delta ns/\Delta ns}$ mice, and late-generation (F3-F4) $terc^{-/-}$ mice bred from B6/Cg-$TERC^{tm1Rdp}$/J	Chronic, progressive low-grade inflammation promoted by NF-κB can cause premature aging	Jurk et al. (2014)
	C57/B16 and $NE^{-/-}$ mice	NE promotes CFTR degradation through activation of intracellular calpain protease causing loss of channel function	Le Gars et al. (2013)

Human studies

Hallmark of aging	Study design	Main findings	Ref
Genomic instability	20 years follow up of CF patients receiving care in United States CF care center programs comparing their cancer incidence with that of the general population	Increased risk for lymphoid leukemia, testicular cancer and digestive tract (esophago-gastric junction, biliary tract, small bowel and colon) cancers in non-transplanted patients compared to the general population. Particularly high risk for digestive tract (mostly bowel) cancers in transplanted patients	Maisonneuve et al. (2013)
	Cancer incidence in CF and non-CF lung transplant recipients compared to the general population based on the United States transplant and 16 cancer registries	Overall cancer risk in CF lung transplant recipients is more increased than in non-CF recipients, particularly for colorectal cancer, esophageal cancer and non-Hodgkin lymphoma	Fink et al. (2017)
	CFTR expression in non-small cell lung cancer (NSCLC) and normal lung samples	Downregulated CFTR expression in NSCLC samples; correlation of low CFTR expression with advanced stage, lymph node metastasis and poor prognosis	Li et al. (2015)
	Urinary 8-hydroxydeoxyguano-sine (oh^8dG, marker of free radical-induced DNA damage) from CF patients and age matched healthy controls and correlation with clinical status	Significantly higher urinary oh^8dG in CF group, but no correlation with markers of lung function (FEV_1, FVC) or clinical status assessed by Taussig-Schwachman score in CF patients; highly significant, positive correlation between urinary oh^8dG and plasma vitamin E	Brown et al. (1995)
	Bronchoalveloar lavage (BAL) of CF and nonsmoking control subjects	Glutathione deficiency with significant reduction in GSH in CF BAL fluid. Simultaneously marked deficiency of plasma GSH.	Roum et al. (1985)
	BAL of children with CF and normal control subjects	Highest oxidative stress level assessed by protein carbonyls in patients with FEV1 < 80% of predicted or highly elevated neutrophils	Starosta et al. (2006)
Telomere attrition	Telomere length of DNA extracted from airway epithelial cells of CF patients and controls	No significant difference in telomere length between CF and control airway epithelial cells, apart for a small subgroup of CF subjects showing shorter telomeres	Fischer et al. (2013)
	Telomere length of DNA extracted from peripheral blood leukocyte of CF patients	Decreased telomere length associated with severe disease characterized by lower FEV_1, ΔF508 homozygosity and CF asthma	Lammertyn et al. (2017)
	Telomere length of DNA extracted from tissue cores of healthy and diseased human lungs from (re-)transplantation or autopsy	Decreasing telomere length with age in normal, but not in CF lungs. No reduction in telomere length in CF explant lungs compared to normal lungs and no correlation between telomere length and disease severity	Everaerts et al. (2018)

(Continued on following page)

TABLE 1 | *(Continued)* Summary of *in vitro*, animal and human studies pointing towards an involvement of accelerated aging in CF disease.

Human studies

Hallmark of aging	Study design	Main findings	Ref
Epigenetic alterations	DNA methylation profiling in nasal epithelial cells and whole blood from CF and control subjects	Substantial DNA methylation differences between CF and control samples, and different methylation levels between mild and severe CF disease. DNA methylation changes in genes responsible for epithelial integrity, inflammatory and immune response, and over-represented in enhancers active in lung tissue	Magalhães et al. (2018)
	DNA methylation profiling in BAL cells, i.e., primarily lung macrophages, from CF and normal subjects	Multiple differentially methylated CpG sites in CF BAL cells, mostly hypo-methylated and located in non-promoter CpG island as well as putative enhancer regions and DNase hypersensitive regions. Altered DNA methylation significantly associated with CF disease status and may be a driving factor in CF innate immune dysfunction	Chen et al. (2018)
Loss of proteostasis	Single-center, open-label phase-2 clinical trial with CF patients orally treated with cysteamine and epigallocatechin	Beneficial effects of proteostasis regulators in patients with rescuable CFTR with decreased sweat chloride, increased CFTR expression and function, restored autophagy, decreased sputum CXCL8 and TNF-α and tendency for improved respiratory function	Tosco et al. (2016)
Cellular senescence	Immunohistochemistry for senescence markers on tissue sections of lungs from CF patients and normal controls	Significantly increased expression of senescence/DNA damage markers ($p16^{INK4a}$, γH2A.X and phospho-Chk2) in CF airways	Fischer et al. (2013)
Stem cell exhaustion	Bronchial epithelial cells from lung brush biopsies and blood neutrophils from CF patients homozygous for ΔF508 mutation and normal controls	miRNA-155, upregulated in aging and suspected to contribute to inflammation-associated stem cell dysfunction (Teramura and Onodera, 2018), is highly expressed in CF lung epithelial cells and blood neutrophils, where it reduces SHIP1 levels promoting PI3K/Akt activation that drives IL-8 expression	Bhattacharyya et al. (2011)
Altered cellular communication	TGF-β_1 gene polymorphism in CF patients homozygous for ΔF508	Patients with high levels of the profibrotic, pro-aging cytokine TGF-β_1 show accelerated lung function decline	Arkwright et al. (2000)
	TGF-β_1 level in BAL fluid of pediatric CF patients and non-CF controls, and assessment of clinical disease indicators	Elevated TGF-β_1 in CF patients is associated with neutrophilic inflammation, diminished lung function and recent hospitalization. No association of TGF-β_1 with presence or quantity of bacterial pathogens	Harris et al. (2009)
	Estimation of lung volumes and forced expiratory flows in children before clinically indicated BAL	TGF-β_1 and matrix metalloprotease (MMP)-2, both previously linked to airway remodeling, are associated with diminished flows as well as hyperinflation and air trapping	Peterson-Carmichael et al. (2009)
ECM dysregulation	Matrix metalloprotease (MMP) profile in lower airway secretions of CF in- and outpatients and normal controls	Increased active MMP-9 and NE, and decreased tissue inhibitor of metalloprotease-1 (TIMP-1) in CF. NE can activate pro-MMP-9 and degrade TIMP-1, hence not surprisingly a strong correlations between NE and MMP-9 activity in CF inpatient samples	Gaggar et al. (2007)
	BAL and endobronchial biopsies in children with CF and controls without lower airway symptoms	Increased elastin, glycosaminoglycan and collagen in BAL fluid from children with CF indicating matrix breakdown that positively correlates with age, neutrophil count and protease concentration. Increased reticular basement membrane thickness in CF group correlates with TGF-β_1 level in BAL fluid	Hilliard et al. (2007)

but studies were inconclusive with one showing beneficial effects on lung function and total serum immunoglobulin levels, whereas another study showed less tolerance and increased exacerbations (Ballmann et al., 2003; Oermann and Wheeler C, 2007).

Micro RNAs as a potential anti-inflammatory approach have recently become a focus of interest. mi-RNAs have been implicated in various diseases including cystic fibrosis (Bardin et al., 2019; Bartoszewska et al., 2017). Vencken et al. suggested the use of nebulized lipid-polymer hybrid nanoparticles for the delivery of a therapeutic anti-inflammatory microRNA, miR-17, to reduce IL-8 secretion, which was successfully tested *in vitro* (Vencken et al., 2019) In addition, targeting miRNAs to restore CFTR activity has also been suggested as a novel therapeutic strategy (De Santi et al., 2020). Please see **Table 1** for a summary of the evidence for accelerated aging in CF shown in in vitro and in vivo studies.

CONCLUSION AND FURTHER DIRECTIONS

Increasing evidence suggests that accelerated aging processes are involved in CF lung pathology. Based on the current state of research summarized in the paragraphs above, it appears sufficiently established that accelerated aging in CF patients is not only a consequence of chronic lung inflammation, but aging-associated processes are also driving disease progression. Of the ten hallmarks of aging, according to recent literature all but stem cell depletion and telomere attrition appear to be involved to varying degrees in CF lung disease (cp. **Figure 1**). For some hallmarks there is already considerable data on the specific mechanisms of their pathologic involvement, as in the case of altered proteostasis and intercellular communication. Others, such as mitochondrial dysfunction, deregulated nutrient sensing and cellular senescence, have been indicated to play a role in CF lung pathology and accelerated aging, but further research is needed to elucidate underlying pathomechanisms. And although each of the ten hallmarks was discussed individually, they should be considered as interdependent processes that influence each other.

Growing evidence on the role of accelerated aging processes in CF lung disease and progress in deciphering involved mechanisms also provide new therapeutic targets for future treatment strategy complementing established therapies as summarized in *Therapeutic Implications*. Some therapies targeting the ten hallmarks of aging are already in clinical use, and further can be expected to follow which may aid further reducing mortality and improving quality of life in CF patients.

AUTHOR CONTRIBUTIONS

LK, ME, MH, and SK contributed to the writing of the manuscript. LK designed the figures and helped to draft the manuscript. LK, ME, and MH contributed to the literature search. SK critically revised the manuscript. All authors read and approved the manuscript for publication.

ACKNOWLEDGMENTS

The authors would like to thank Eva Maria Künzi for her assistance in creating the illustrations.

REFERENCES

Aldámiz-Echevarría, L., Prieto, J. A., Andrade, F., Elorz, J., Sojo, A., Lage, S., et al. (2009). Persistence of essential fatty acid deficiency in cystic fibrosis despite nutritional therapy. *Pediatr. Res.* 66 (5), 585–589. doi:10.1203/pdr.0b013e3181b4e8d3

Aoshiba, K., Yasuda, K., Yasui, S., Tamaoki, J., and Nagai, A. (2001). Serine proteases increase oxidative stress in lung cells. *Am. J. Physiology-Lung Cell Mol. Physiol.* 281 (3), L556–L564. doi:10.1152/ajplung.2001.281.3.l556

Arkwright, P. D., Laurie, S., Super, M., Pravica, V., Schwarz, M. J., Webb, A. K., et al. (2000). TGF-beta 1 genotype and accelerated decline in lung function of patients with cystic fibrosis. *Thorax* 55 (6), 459–462. doi:10.1136/thorax.55.6.459

Ashapkin, V. V., Kutueva, L. I., and Vanyushin, B. F. (2017). Aging as an epigenetic phenomenon. *Curr. Genomics* 18 (5), 385–407. doi:10.2174/1389202918666170412112130

Auerbach, H., Kirkpatrick, J., Williams, M., and Colten, H. (1985). Alternate-day prednisone reduces morbidity and improves pulmonary function in cystic fibrosis. *The Lancet* 326 (8457), 686–688. doi:10.1016/s0140-6736(85)92929-0

Balch, W. E., Roth, D. M., and Hutt, D. M. (2011). Emergent properties of proteostasis in managing cystic fibrosis. *Cold Spring Harb Perspect. Biol.* 3 (2). doi:10.1101/cshperspect.a004499

Ballmann, M., Junge, S., and von der Hardt, H. (2003). Low-dose methotrexate for advanced pulmonary disease in patients with cystic fibrosis. *Respir. Med.* 97 (5), 498–500. doi:10.1053/rmed.2002.1471

Bardin, P., Foussignière, T., Rousselet, N., Rebeyrol, C., Porter, J. C., Corvol, H., et al. (2019). miR-636: a newly-identified actor for the regulation of pulmonary inflammation in cystic fibrosis. *Front. Immunol.* 10, 2643. doi:10.3389/fimmu.2019.02643

Bartoszewska, S., Kamysz, W., Jakiela, B., Sanak, M., Króliczewski, J., Bebok, Z., et al. (2017). miR-200b downregulates CFTR during hypoxia in human lung epithelial cells. *Cell Mol Biol Lett* 22, 23. doi:10.1186/s11658-017-0054-0

Bartoszewski, R., Rab, A., Jurkuvenaite, A., Mazur, M., Wakefield, J., Collawn, J. F., et al. (2008). Activation of the unfolded protein response by ΔF508 CFTR. *Am. J. Respir. Cel Mol Biol* 39 (4), 448–457. doi:10.1165/rcmb.2008-0065oc

Beharry, S., Ackerley, C., Corey, M., Kent, G., Heng, Y.-M., Christensen, H., et al. (2007). Long-term docosahexaenoic acid therapy in a congenic murine model of cystic fibrosis. *Am. J. Physiology-Gastrointestinal Liver Physiol.* 292 (3), G839–G848. doi:10.1152/ajpgi.00582.2005

Berger, S. L., Kouzarides, T., Shiekhattar, R., and Shilatifard, A. (2009). An operational definition of epigenetics. *Genes Development* 23 (7), 781–783. doi:10.1101/gad.1787609

Bezzerri, V., Piacenza, F., Caporelli, N., Malavolta, M., Provinciali, M., and Cipolli, M. (2019). Is cellular senescence involved in cystic fibrosis? *Respir. Res.* 20 (1), 32. doi:10.1186/s12931-019-0993-2

Bhal, G. K., Maguire, S. A., and Bowler, I. M. (2001). Use of cyclosporin A as a steroid sparing agent in cystic fibrosis. *Arch. Dis. Child.* 84 (1), 89. doi:10.1136/adc.84.1.89

Bhattacharyya, S., Balakathiresan, N. S., Dalgard, C., Gutti, U., Armistead, D., Jozwik, C., et al. (2011). Elevated miR-155 promotes inflammation in cystic fibrosis by driving hyperexpression of interleukin-8. *J. Biol. Chem.* 286 (13), 11604–11615. doi:10.1074/jbc.m110.198390

Bishop, C., Hudson, V. M., Hilton, S. C., and Wilde, C. (2005). A pilot study of the effect of inhaled buffered reduced glutathione on the clinical status of patients with cystic fibrosis. *Chest* 127 (1), 308–317. doi:10.1378/chest.127.1.308

Blackburn, E. H., Greider, C. W., and Szostak, J. W. (2006). Telomeres and telomerase: the path from maize, Tetrahymena and yeast to human cancer and aging. *Nat. Med.* 12 (10), 1133–1138. doi:10.1038/nm1006-1133

Bonfield, T. L., Konstan, M. W., and Berger, M. (1999). Altered respiratory epithelial cell cytokine production in cystic fibrosis☆☆☆★. *J. Allergy Clin. Immunol.* 104 (1), 72–78. doi:10.1016/s0091-6749(99)70116-8

Borcherding, D. C., Siefert, M. E., Lin, S., Brewington, J., Sadek, H., Clancy, J. P., et al. (2019). Clinically approved CFTR modulators rescue Nrf2 dysfunction in cystic fibrosis airway epithelia. *J. Clin. Invest.* 129 (8), 3448–3463. doi:10.1172/jci96273

Boucher, R. C. (2007). Cystic fibrosis: a disease of vulnerability to airway surface dehydration. *Trends Mol. Med.* 13 (6), 231–240. doi:10.1016/j.molmed.2007.05.001

Brown, R. K., and Kelly, F. J. (1994). Evidence for increased oxidative damage in patients with cystic fibrosis. *Pediatr. Res.* 36 (4), 487–492. doi:10.1203/00006450-199410000-00013

Brown, R. K., McBurney, A., Lunec, J., and Kelly, F. J. (1995). Oxidative damage to DNA in patients with cystic fibrosis. *Free Radic. Biol. Med.* 18 (4), 801–806. doi:10.1016/0891-5849(94)00172-g

Chapman, J., Fielder, E., and Passos, J. F. (2019). Mitochondrial dysfunction and cell senescence: deciphering a complex relationship. *FEBS Lett.* 593 (13), 1566–1579. doi:10.1002/1873-3468.13498

Chen, T., Shen, L., Yu, J., Wan, H., Guo, A., Chen, J., et al. (2011). Rapamycin and other longevity-promoting compounds enhance the generation of mouse induced pluripotent stem cells. *Aging Cell* 10 (5), 908–911. doi:10.1111/j.1474-9726.2011.00722.x

Chen, Y., Armstrong, D. A., Salas, L. A., Hazlett, H. F., Nymon, A. B., Dessaint, J. A., et al. (2018). Genome-wide DNA methylation profiling shows a distinct epigenetic signature associated with lung macrophages in cystic fibrosis. *Clin. Epigenetics* 10 (1), 152. doi:10.1186/s13148-018-0580-2

Cheng, S. H., Gregory, R. J., Marshall, J., Paul, S., Souza, D. W., White, G. A., et al. (1990). Defective intracellular transport and processing of CFTR is the molecular basis of most cystic fibrosis. *Cell* 63 (4), 827–834. doi:10.1016/0092-8674(90)90148-8

Chmiel, J. F., Konstan, M. W., Knesebeck, J. E., Hilliard, J. B., Bonfield, T. L., Dawson, D. V., et al. (1999). IL-10 attenuates excessive inflammation in ChronicPseudomonasInfection in mice. *Am. J. Respir. Crit. Care Med.* 160 (6), 2040–2047. doi:10.1164/ajrccm.160.6.9901043

Cho, S. J., and Stout-Delgado, H. W. (2020). Aging and lung disease. *Annu. Rev. Physiol.* 82, 433–459. doi:10.1146/annurev-physiol-021119-034610

Chua, F., and Laurent, G. J. (2006). Neutrophil elastase: mediator of extracellular matrix destruction and accumulation. *Proc. Am. Thorac. Soc.* 3 (5), 424–427. doi:10.1513/pats.200603-078aw

Ciofu, O., Lykkesfeldt, J., and Lykkesfeldt, J. (2019). Antioxidant supplementation for lung disease in cystic fibrosis. *Cochrane Database Syst. Rev.* 10, CD007020. doi:10.1002/14651858.CD007020.pub3

Conrad, C., Lymp, J., Thompson, V., Dunn, C., Davies, Z., Chatfield, B., et al. (2015). Long-term treatment with oral N-acetylcysteine: affects lung function but not sputum inflammation in cystic fibrosis subjects. A phase II randomized placebo-controlled trial. *J. Cystic Fibrosis* 14 (2), 219–227. doi:10.1016/j.jcf.2014.08.008

Danahay, H. L., Lilley, S., Fox, R., Charlton, H., Sabater, J., Button, B., et al. (2020). TMEM16A potentiation: a novel therapeutic approach for the treatment of cystic fibrosis. *Am. J. Respir. Crit. Care Med.* 201 (8), 946–954. doi:10.1164/rccm.201908-1641oc

Davies, J. C., Moskowitz, S. M., Brown, C., Horsley, A., Mall, M. A., McKone, E. F., et al. (2018). VX-659-Tezacaftor-Ivacaftor in Patients with Cystic Fibrosis and One or Two Phe508del Alleles. *N. Engl. J. Med.* 379 (17), 1599–1611. doi:10.1056/nejmoa1807119

De Boeck, K., Vermeulen, F., Wanyama, S., and Thomas, M. (2011). Inhaled corticosteroids and lower lung function decline in young children with cystic fibrosis. *Eur. Respir. J.* 37 (5), 1091–1095. doi:10.1183/09031936.00077210

De Santi, C., Fernández Fernández, E., Gaul, R., Vencken, S., Glasgow, A., Oglesby, I. K., et al. (2020). Precise targeting of miRNA sites restores CFTR activity in CF bronchial epithelial cells. *Mol. Ther.* 28 (4), 1190–1199. doi:10.1016/j.ymthe.2020.02.001

Dodge, J. A., Lewis, P. A., Stanton, M., and Wilsher, J. (2007). Cystic fibrosis mortality and survival in the UK: 1947-2003. *Eur. Respir. J.* 29 (3), 522–526. doi:10.1183/09031936.00099506

dos Santos, G., Kutuzov, M. A., and Ridge, K. M. (2012). The inflammasome in lung diseases. *Am. J. Physiology-Lung Cell Mol. Physiol.* 303 (8), L627–L633. doi:10.1152/ajplung.00225.2012

Dunzendorfer, S., Rothbucher, D., Schratzberger, P., Reinisch, N., Kähler, C. M., and Wiedermann, C. J. (1997). Mevalonate-dependent inhibition of transendothelial migration and chemotaxis of human peripheral blood neutrophils by pravastatin. *Circ. Res.* 81 (6), 963–969. doi:10.1161/01.res.81.6.963

Durieu, I., Peyrol, S., Gindre, D., Bellon, G., Durand, D. V., and Pacheco, Y. (1998). Subepithelial fibrosis and degradation of the bronchial extracellular matrix in cystic fibrosis. *Am. J. Respir. Crit. Care Med.* 158 (2), 580–588. doi:10.1164/ajrccm.158.2.9707126

Ehre, C., Rushton, Z. L., Wang, B., Hothem, L. N., Morrison, C. B., Fontana, N. C., et al. (2019). An improved inhaled mucolytic to treat airway muco-obstructive diseases. *Am. J. Respir. Crit. Care Med.* 199 (2), 171–180. doi:10.1164/rccm.201802-0245oc

Eigen, H., Rosenstein, B. J., FitzSimmons, S., and Schidlow, D. V. (1995). A multicenter study of alternate-day prednisone therapy in patients with cystic fibrosis. *J. Pediatr.* 126 (4), 515–523. doi:10.1016/s0022-3476(95)70343-8

Elborn, J. S. (2016). Cystic fibrosis. *The Lancet* 388 (10059), 2519–2531. doi:10.1016/s0140-6736(16)00576-6

Esposito, S., Tosco, A., Villella, V. R., Raia, V., Kroemer, G., and Maiuri, L. (2016). Manipulating proteostasis to repair the F508del-CFTR defect in cystic fibrosis. *Mol. Cel Pediatr* 3 (1), 13. doi:10.1186/s40348-016-0040-z

Everaerts, S., Lammertyn, E., Martens, D. S., Sadeleer, L. D., Maes, K., Goldschmeding, R., et al. (2018). The aging lung: tissue telomere shortening in health and disease. *Respir. Res.* 19 (1), 95. doi:10.1186/s12931-018-0794-z

Ferretti, S., Bonneau, O., Dubois, G. R., Jones, C. E., and Trifilieff, A. (2003). IL-17, produced by lymphocytes and neutrophils, is necessary for lipopolysaccharide-induced airway neutrophilia: IL-15 as a possible trigger. *J. Immunol.* 170 (4), 2106–2112. doi:10.4049/jimmunol.170.4.2106

Fink, A. K., Yanik, E. L., Marshall, B. C., Wilschanski, M., Lynch, C. F., Austin, A. A., et al. (2017). Cancer risk among lung transplant recipients with cystic fibrosis. *J. Cystic Fibrosis* 16 (1), 91–97. doi:10.1016/j.jcf.2016.07.011

Fischer, B. M., Wong, J. K., Degan, S., Kummarapurugu, A. B., Zheng, S., Haridass, P., et al. (2013). Increased expression of senescence markers in cystic fibrosis airways. *Am. J. Physiology-Lung Cell Mol. Physiol.* 304 (6), L394–L400. doi:10.1152/ajplung.00091.2012

Fischer, B. M., Zheng, S., Fan, R., and Voynow, J. A. (2007). Neutrophil elastase inhibition of cell cycle progression in airway epithelial cells *in vitro* is mediated by p27kip1. *Am. J. Physiology-Lung Cell Mol. Physiol.* 293 (3), L762–L768. doi:10.1152/ajplung.00067.2007

Flume, P. A., O'Sullivan, B. P., Robinson, K. A., Goss, C. H., Mogayzel, P. J., Willey-Courand, D. B., et al. (2007). Cystic fibrosis pulmonary guidelines. *Am. J. Respir. Crit. Care Med.* 176 (10), 957–969. doi:10.1164/rccm.200705-664oc

Franceschi, C., and Campisi, J. (2014). Chronic inflammation (inflammaging) and its potential contribution to age-associated diseases. *Journals Gerontol. Ser. A: Biol. Sci. Med. Sci.* 69 (Suppl. 1), S4–S9. doi:10.1093/gerona/glu057

Freedman, S. D., Katz, M. H., Parker, E. M., Laposata, M., Urman, M. Y., and Alvarez, J. G. (1999). A membrane lipid imbalance plays a role in the phenotypic expression of cystic fibrosis in cftr-/- mice. *Proc. Natl. Acad. Sci.* 96 (24), 13995–14000. doi:10.1073/pnas.96.24.13995

Gaggar, A., Hector, A., Bratcher, P. E., Mall, M. A., Griese, M., and Hartl, D. (2011). The role of matrix metalloproteinases in cystic fibrosis lung disease. *Eur. Respir. J.* 38 (3), 721–727. doi:10.1183/09031936.00173210

Gaggar, A., Li, Y., Weathington, N., Winkler, M., Kong, M., Jackson, P., et al. (2007). Matrix metalloprotease-9 dysregulation in lower airway secretions of cystic fibrosis patients. *Am. J. Physiology-Lung Cell Mol. Physiol.* 293 (1), L96–L104. doi:10.1152/ajplung.00492.2006

Gonzalo, S. (1985). Epigenetic alterations in aging. *J. Appl. Physiol.* 109 (2), 586–597. doi:10.1152/japplphysiol.00238.2010

Gorenjak, V., Petrelis, A. M., Stathopoulou, M. G., and Visvikis-Siest, S. (2020). Telomere length determinants in childhood. *Clin. Chem. Lab. Med.* 58 (2), 162–177. doi:10.1515/cclm-2019-0235

Grasemann, H., Grasemann, C., Kurtz, F., Tietze-Schillings, G., Vester, U., and Ratjen, F. (2005a). Oral L-arginine supplementation in cystic fibrosis patients: a placebo-controlled study. *Eur. Respir. J.* 25 (1), 62–68. doi:10.1183/09031936.04.00086104

Grasemann, H., Schwiertz, R., Matthiesen, S., Racké, K., and Ratjen, F. (2005b). Increased arginase activity in cystic fibrosis airways. *Am. J. Respir. Crit. Care Med.* 172 (12), 1523–1528. doi:10.1164/rccm.200502-253oc

Griese, M., Latzin, P., Kappler, M., Weckerle, K., Heinzlmaier, T., Bernhardt, T., et al. (2007). alpha1-Antitrypsin inhalation reduces airway inflammation in cystic fibrosis patients. *Eur. Respir. J.* 29 (2), 240–250. doi:10.1183/09031936.00047306

Grimbert, D., Vecellio, L., Delépine, P., Attucci, S., Boissinot, E., Poncin, A., et al. (2003). Characteristics of EPI-hNE4 aerosol: a new elastase inhibitor for treatment of cystic fibrosis. *J. Aerosol Med.* 16 (2), 121–129. doi:10.1089/089426803321919889

Hallows, K. R., Raghuram, V., Kemp, B. E., Witters, L. A., and Foskett, J. K. (2000). Inhibition of cystic fibrosis transmembrane conductance regulator by novel interaction with the metabolic sensor AMP-activated protein kinase. *J. Clin. Invest.* 105 (12), 1711–1721. doi:10.1172/jci9622

Harris, W. T., Muhlebach, M. S., Oster, R. A., Knowles, M. R., and Noah, T. L. (2009). Transforming growth factor-β1 in bronchoalveolar lavage fluid from children with cystic fibrosis. *Pediatr. Pulmonol.* 44 (11), 1057–1064. doi:10.1002/ppul.21079

Hartl, D., Starosta, V., Maier, K., Beck-Speier, I., Rebhan, C., Becker, B. F., et al. (2005). Inhaled glutathione decreases PGE2 and increases lymphocytes in cystic fibrosis lungs. *Free Radic. Biol. Med.* 39 (4), 463–472. doi:10.1016/j.freeradbiomed.2005.03.032

Haydar, D., Cory, T. J., Birket, S. E., Murphy, B. S., Pennypacker, K. R., Sinai, A. P., et al. (2019). Azithromycin polarizes macrophages to an M2 phenotype via inhibition of the STAT1 and NF-κB signaling pathways. *J.I.* 203 (4), 1021–1030. doi:10.4049/jimmunol.1801228

Hewitt, G., Jurk, D., Marques, F. D. M., Correia-Melo, C., Hardy, T., Gackowska, A., et al. (2012). Telomeres are favoured targets of a persistent DNA damage response in ageing and stress-induced senescence. *Nat. Commun.* 3, 708. doi:10.1038/ncomms1708

Hilliard, T. N., Regamey, N., Shute, J. K., Nicholson, A. G., Alton, E. W. F. W., Bush, A., et al. (2007). Airway remodelling in children with cystic fibrosis. *Thorax* 62 (12), 1074–1080. doi:10.1136/thx.2006.074641

Hisert, K. B., Heltshe, S. L., Pope, C., Jorth, P., Wu, X., Edwards, R. M., et al. (2017). Restoring cystic fibrosis transmembrane conductance regulator function reduces airway bacteria and inflammation in people with cystic fibrosis and chronic lung infections. *Am. J. Respir. Crit. Care Med.* 195 (12), 1617–1628. doi:10.1164/rccm.201609-1954oc

Hodson, M. E., Simmonds, N. J., Warwick, W. J., Tullis, E., Castellani, C., Assael, B., et al. (2008). An international/multicentre report on patients with cystic fibrosis (CF) over the age of 40 years. *J. Cystic Fibrosis* 7 (6), 537–542. doi:10.1016/j.jcf.2008.06.003

Hogan, B. L. M., Barkauskas, C. E., Chapman, H. A., Epstein, J. A., Jain, R., Hsia, C. C. W., et al. (2014). Repair and regeneration of the respiratory system: complexity, plasticity, and mechanisms of lung stem cell function. *Cell Stem Cell* 15 (2), 123–138. doi:10.1016/j.stem.2014.07.012

Horati, H., Janssens, H. M., Margaroli, C., Veltman, M., Stolarczyk, M., Kilgore, M. B., et al. (2020). Airway profile of bioactive lipids predicts early progression of lung disease in cystic fibrosis. *J. Cystic Fibrosis* 19 (6), 902–909. doi:10.1016/j.jcf.2020.01.010

Hunter, M. J., Treharne, K. J., Winter, AK, Cassidy, D. M., and Land, S. (2010). Expression of wild-type CFTR suppresses NF-kappaB-driven inflammatory signalling. *PLoS One* 5 (7), e11598. doi:10.1371/journal.pone.0011598

Jarosz-Griffiths, H. H., Scambler, T., Wong, C. H., Lara-Reyna, S., Holbrook, J., Martinon, F., et al. (2020). Different CFTR modulator combinations downregulate inflammation differently in cystic fibrosis. *Elife* 9. doi:10.7554/elife.54556

Jeyapalan, J. C., Ferreira, M., Sedivy, J. M., and Herbig, U. (2007). Accumulation of senescent cells in mitotic tissue of aging primates. *Mech. Ageing Development* 128 (1), 36–44. doi:10.1016/j.mad.2006.11.008

Jones, M. J., Goodman, S. J., and Kobor, M. S. (2015). DNA methylation and healthy human aging. *Aging Cell* 14 (6), 924–932. doi:10.1111/acel.12349

Jurk, D., Wilson, C., Passos, J. F., Oakley, F., Correia-Melo, C., Greaves, L., et al. (2014). Chronic inflammation induces telomere dysfunction and accelerates ageing in mice. *Nat. Commun.* 2, 4172. doi:10.1038/ncomms5172

Keating, D., Marigowda, G., Burr, L., Daines, C., Mall, M. A., McKone, E. F., et al. (2018). VX-445-Tezacaftor-Ivacaftor in Patients with Cystic Fibrosis and One or Two Phe508del Alleles. *N. Engl. J. Med.* 379 (17), 1612–1620. doi:10.1056/nejmoa1807120

Kenyon, C. J. (2010). The genetics of ageing. *Nature* 464 (7288), 504–512. doi:10.1038/nature08980

Kerem, B., Rommens, J., Buchanan, J., Markiewicz, D., Cox, T., Chakravarti, A., et al. (1989). Identification of the cystic fibrosis gene: genetic analysis. *Science* 245 (4922), 1073–1080. doi:10.1126/science.2570460

Konstan Mw, D. G., Lands, L. C., Hilliard, K. A., Koker, P., Bhattacharya, S., Staab, A., et al. (2005). Results of a phase II clinical trial of BIIL 284 BS (a LTB4 receptor antagonist) for the treatment of CF lung disease. *Pediatr. Pulmonol* 40, 125–127.

Konstan, M. W., Krenicky, J. E., Hilliard, K. A., and Hilliard, J. B. (2009). A pilot study evaluating the effect of pioglitazone, simvastatin and ibuprofen on neutrophil migration *in vivo* in healthy subjects. *Pediatr. Pulmonol* 44, 289–290.

Konstan, M. W., Byard, P. J., Hoppel, C. L., and Davis, P. B. (1995). Effect of high-dose ibuprofen in patients with cystic fibrosis. *N. Engl. J. Med.* 332 (13), 848–854. doi:10.1056/nejm199503303321303

Konstan, M. W., Krenicky, J. E., Finney, M. R., Kirchner, H. L., Hilliard, K. A., Hilliard, J. B., et al. (2003). Effect of ibuprofen on neutrophil migration *in vivo* in cystic fibrosis and healthy subjects. *J. Pharmacol. Exp. Ther.* 306 (3), 1086–1091. doi:10.1124/jpet.103.052449

Konstan, M. W., Schluchter, M. D., Xue, W., and Davis, P. B. (2007). Clinical use of ibuprofen is associated with slower FEV1Decline in children with cystic fibrosis. *Am. J. Respir. Crit. Care Med.* 176 (11), 1084–1089. doi:10.1164/rccm.200702-181oc

Konstan, M. W., Walenga, R. W., Hilliard, K. A., and Hilliard, J. B. (1993). Leukotriene B4Markedly elevated in the epithelial lining fluid of patients with cystic fibrosis. *Am. Rev. Respir. Dis.* 148 (4 Pt 1), 896–901. doi:10.1164/ajrccm/148.4_pt_1.896

Kopp, B. T., Fitch, J., Jaramillo, L., Shrestha, C. L., Robledo-Avila, F., Zhang, S., et al. (2020). Whole-blood transcriptomic responses to lumacaftor/ivacaftor therapy in cystic fibrosis. *J. Cystic Fibrosis* 19 (2), 245–254. doi:10.1016/j.jcf.2019.08.021

Kraynack, N. C., Corey, D. A., Elmer, H. L., and Kelley, T. J. (2002). Mechanisms of NOS2 regulation by Rho GTPase signaling in airway epithelial cells. *Am. J. Physiology-Lung Cell Mol. Physiol.* 283 (3), L604–L611. doi:10.1152/ajplung.00459.2001

Lammertyn, E. M. D., Colpaert, K., Goeminne, P., Proesmans, M., Vanaudenaerde, B., Nawrot, T., et al. (2017). The association between leukocyte telomere length, telomere attrition and disease severity in cystic fibrosis patients. *Eur. Respir. J.*, OA4402.

Lands, L. C., Milner, R., Cantin, A. M., Manson, D., and Corey, M. (2007). High-dose ibuprofen in cystic fibrosis: Canadian safety and effectiveness trial. *J. Pediatr.* 151 (3), 249–254. doi:10.1016/j.jpeds.2007.04.009

Lara-Reyna, S., Holbrook, J., Jarosz-Griffiths, H. H., Peckham, D., and McDermott, M. F. (2020). Dysregulated signalling pathways in innate immune cells with cystic fibrosis mutations. *Cell. Mol. Life Sci.* 77 (22), 4485–4503. doi:10.1007/s00018-020-03540-9

Le Gars, M., Descamps, D., Roussel, D., Saussereau, E., Guillot, L., Ruffin, M., et al. (2013). Neutrophil elastase degrades cystic fibrosis transmembrane conductance regulator via calpains and disables channel FunctionIn VitroandIn vivo. *Am. J. Respir. Crit. Care Med.* 187 (2), 170–179. doi:10.1164/rccm.201205-0875oc

Levine, M. E., Lu, A. T., Quach, A., Chen, B. H., Assimes, T. L., Bandinelli, S., et al. (2018). An epigenetic biomarker of aging for lifespan and healthspan. *Aging* 10 (4), 573–591. doi:10.18632/aging.101414

Li, J., Zhang, J. T., Jiang, X., Shi, X., Shen, J., Feng, F., et al. (2015). The cystic fibrosis transmembrane conductance regulator as a biomarker in non-small cell lung cancer. *Int. J. Oncol.* 46 (5), 2107–2115. doi:10.3892/ijo.2015.2921

Linsdell, P., and Hanrahan, J. W. (1998). Glutathione permeability of CFTR. *Am. J. Physiology-Cell Physiol.* 275 (1), C323–C326. doi:10.1152/ajpcell.1998.275.1.c323

Lopes-Pacheco, M., Boinot, C., Sabirzhanova, I., Morales, M. M., Guggino, W. B., and Cebotaru, L. (2015). Combination of correctors rescue df508-CFTR by reducing its association with Hsp40 and Hsp27. *J. Biol. Chem.* 290 (42), 25636–25645. doi:10.1074/jbc.m115.671925

Lopes-Pacheco, M., Sabirzhanova, I., Rapino, D., Morales, M. M., Guggino, W. B., and Cebotaru, L. (2016). Correctors rescue CFTR mutations in nucleotide-binding domain 1 (NBD1) by modulating proteostasis. *Chembiochem* 17 (6), 493–505. doi:10.1002/cbic.201500620

López-Otín, C., Blasco, M. A., Partridge, L., Serrano, M., and Kroemer, G. (2013). The hallmarks of aging. *Cell* 153 (6), 1194–1217. doi:10.1016/j.cell.2013.05.039

Luciani, A., Villella, V. R., Esposito, S., Gavina, M., Russo, I., Silano, M., et al. (2012). Targeting autophagy as a novel strategy for facilitating the therapeutic action of potentiators on ΔF508 cystic fibrosis transmembrane conductance regulator. *Autophagy* 8 (11), 1657–1672. doi:10.4161/auto.21483

Luciani, A., Villella, V. R., Vasaturo, A., Giardino, I., Raia, V., Pettoello-Mantovani, M., et al. (2009). SUMOylation of tissue transglutaminase as link between oxidative stress and inflammation. *J. Immunol.* 183 (4), 2775–2784. doi:10.4049/jimmunol.0900993

Ly, K., Smith, M. P., Thibodeaux, Q., Reddy, V., Liao, W., and Bhutani, T. (2019). Anti IL-17 in psoriasis. *Expert Rev. Clin. Immunol.* 15 (11), 1185–1194. doi:10.1080/1744666x.2020.1679625

MacKenzie, T., Gifford, A. H., Sabadosa, K. A., Quinton, H. B., Knapp, E. A., Goss, C. H., et al. (2014). Longevity of patients with cystic fibrosis in 2000 to 2010 and beyond: survival analysis of the Cystic Fibrosis Foundation patient registry. *Ann. Intern. Med.* 161 (4), 233–241. doi:10.7326/m13-0636

Magalhães, M., Tost, J., Pineau, F., Rivals, I., Busato, F., Alary, N., et al. (2018). Dynamic changes of DNA methylation and lung disease in cystic fibrosis: lessons from a monogenic disease. *Epigenomics* 10 (8), 1131–1145. doi:10.2217/epi-2018-0005

Maisonneuve, P., Marshall, B. C., Knapp, E. A., and Lowenfels, A. B. (2013). Cancer risk in cystic fibrosis: a 20-year nationwide study from the United States. *J. Natl. Cancer Inst.* 105 (2), 122–129. doi:10.1093/jnci/djs481

Mall, M., Grubb, B. R., Harkema, J. R., O'Neal, W. K., and Boucher, R. C. (2004). Increased airway epithelial Na+ absorption produces cystic fibrosis-like lung disease in mice. *Nat. Med.* 10 (5), 487–493. doi:10.1038/nm1028

Manzanares, D., Krick, S., Baumlin, N., Dennis, J. S., Tyrrell, J., Tarran, R., et al. (2015). Airway surface dehydration by transforming growth factor β (TGF-β) in cystic fibrosis is due to decreased function of a voltage-dependent potassium channel and can Be rescued by the drug pirfenidone. *J. Biol. Chem.* 290 (42), 25710–25716. doi:10.1074/jbc.m115.670885

Martins, R., Lithgow, G. J., and Link, W. (2016). Long live FOXO : unraveling the role of FOXO proteins in aging and longevity. *Aging Cell* 15 (2), 196–207. doi:10.1111/acel.12427

Matsui, H., Grubb, B. R., Tarran, R., Randell, S. H., Gatzy, J. T., Davis, C. W., et al. (1998). Evidence for periciliary liquid layer depletion, not abnormal ion composition, in the pathogenesis of cystic fibrosis airways disease. *Cell* 95 (7), 1005–1015. doi:10.1016/s0092-8674(00)81724-9

Mayer, M. L., Blohmke, C. J., Falsafi, R., Fjell, C. D., Madera, L., Turvey, S. E., et al. (2013). Rescue of dysfunctional autophagy attenuates hyperinflammatory responses from cystic fibrosis cells. *J.I.* 190 (3), 1227–1238. doi:10.4049/jimmunol.1201404

McCuaig, S., and Martin, J. G. (2013). How the airway smooth muscle in cystic fibrosis reacts in proinflammatory conditions: implications for airway hyper-responsiveness and asthma in cystic fibrosis. *Lancet Respir. Med.* 1 (2), 137–147. doi:10.1016/s2213-2600(12)70058-9

McElvaney, N. G., Doujaiji, B., Moan, M. J., Burnham, M. R., Wu, M. C., and Crystal, R. G. (1993). Pharmacokinetics of recombinant secretory leukoprotease inhibitor aerosolized to normals and individuals with cystic fibrosis. *Am. Rev. Respir. Dis.* 148 (4 Pt 1), 1056–1060. doi:10.1164/ajrccm/148.4_pt_1.1056

McElvaney, N. G., Hubbard, R. C., Birrer, P., Crystal, R. G., Chernick, M. S., Frank, M. M., et al. (1991). Aerosol α1 -antitrypsin treatment for cystic fibrosis. *The Lancet* 337 (8738), 392–394. doi:10.1016/0140-6736(91)91167-s

McElvaney, O. J., Zaslona, Z., Becker-Flegler, K., Palsson-McDermott, E. M., Boland, F., Gunaratnam, C., et al. (2019). Specific inhibition of the NLRP3 inflammasome as an antiinflammatory strategy in cystic fibrosis. *Am. J. Respir. Crit. Care Med.* 200 (11), 1381–1391. doi:10.1164/rccm.201905-1013oc

Meiners, S., Eickelberg, O., and Königshoff, M. (2015). Hallmarks of the ageing lung. *Eur. Respir. J.* 45 (3), 807–827. doi:10.1183/09031936.00186914

Meyer, K. C., Rosenthal, N. S., Soergel, P., and Peterson, K. (1998). Neutrophils and low-grade inflammation in the seemingly normal aging human lung. *Mech. Ageing Development* 104 (2), 169–181. doi:10.1016/s0047-6374(98)00065-7

Middleton, P. G., Mall, M. A., Dřevínek, P., Lands, L. C., McKone, E. F., Polineni, D., et al. (2019). Elexacaftor-Tezacaftor-Ivacaftor for Cystic Fibrosis with a Single Phe508del Allele. *N. Engl. J. Med.* 381 (19), 1809–1819. doi:10.1056/nejmoa1908639

Mingione, A., Dei Cas, M., Bonezzi, F., Caretti, A., Piccoli, M., Anastasia, L., et al. (2020). Inhibition of sphingolipid synthesis as a phenotype-modifying therapy in cystic fibrosis. *Cell Physiol Biochem* 54 (1), 110–125. doi:10.33594/000000208

Montanini, L., Smerieri, A., Gullì, M., Cirillo, F., Pisi, G., Sartori, C., et al. (2016). miR-146a, miR-155, miR-370, and miR-708 are CFTR-dependent, predicted FOXO1 regulators and change at onset of CFRDs. *J. Clin. Endocrinol. Metab.* 101 (12), 4955–4963. doi:10.1210/jc.2016-2431

Mora, A. L., and Rojas, M. (2013). Adult stem cells for chronic lung diseases. *Respirology* 18 (7), 1041–1046. doi:10.1111/resp.12112

Moskalev, A. A., Shaposhnikov, M. V., Plyusnina, E. N., Zhavoronkov, A., Budovsky, A., Yanai, H., et al. (2013). The role of DNA damage and repair in aging through the prism of Koch-like criteria. *Ageing Res. Rev.* 12 (2), 661–684. doi:10.1016/j.arr.2012.02.001

Moss, R. B., Mayer-Hamblett, N., Wagener, J., Daines, C., Hale, K., Ahrens, R., et al. (2005). Randomized, double-blind, placebo-controlled, dose-escalating study of aerosolized interferon gamma-1b in patients with mild to moderate cystic fibrosis lung disease. *Pediatr. Pulmonol.* 39 (3), 209–218. doi:10.1002/ppul.20152

Moss, R. B., Mistry, S. J., Konstan, M. W., Pilewski, J. M., Kerem, E., Tal-Singer, R., et al. (2013). Safety and early treatment effects of the CXCR2 antagonist SB-656933 in patients with cystic fibrosis. *J. Cystic Fibrosis* 12 (3), 241–248. doi:10.1016/j.jcf.2012.08.016

Nakamura, H., Yoshimura, K., McElvaney, N. G., and Crystal, R. G. (1992). Neutrophil elastase in respiratory epithelial lining fluid of individuals with cystic fibrosis induces interleukin-8 gene expression in a human bronchial epithelial cell line. *J. Clin. Invest.* 89 (5), 1478–1484. doi:10.1172/jci115738

Naylor, R. M., Baker, D. J., and van Deursen, J. M. (2013). Senescent cells: a novel therapeutic target for aging and age-related diseases. *Clin. Pharmacol. Ther.* 93 (1), 105–116. doi:10.1038/clpt.2012.193

Nichols, D., Chmiel, J., and Berger, M. (2008). Chronic inflammation in the cystic fibrosis lung: alterations in inter- and intracellular signaling. *Clinic Rev. Allerg Immunol.* 34 (2), 146–162. doi:10.1007/s12016-007-8039-9

Nichols, D. P., Odem-Davis, K., Cogen, J. D., Goss, C. H., Ren, C. L., Skalland, M., et al. (2020). Pulmonary outcomes associated with long-term Azithromycin therapy in cystic fibrosis. *Am. J. Respir. Crit. Care Med.* 201 (4), 430–437. doi:10.1164/rccm.201906-1206oc

Oermann, C. M. K. M., and Wheeler C, Cumming. S. (2007). A pilot study evaluating the potential use of low-dose methotrexate as an anti-inflammatory therapy for cystic fibrosis lung disease. *Pediatr. Pulmonol* 42, 292–293.

Oh, J., Lee, Y. D., and Wagers, A. J. (2014). Stem cell aging: mechanisms, regulators and therapeutic opportunities. *Nat. Med.* 20 (8), 870–880. doi:10.1038/nm.3651

Pankow, S., Bamberger, C., Calzolari, D., Martínez-Bartolomé, S., Lavallée-Adam, M., Balch, W. E., et al. (2015). ΔF508 CFTR interactome remodelling promotes rescue of cystic fibrosis. *Nature* 528 (7583), 510–516. doi:10.1038/nature15729

Parikh, P., Wicher, S., Khandalavala, K., Pabelick, C. M., Britt, R. D., and Prakash, Y. S. (2019). Cellular senescence in the lung across the age spectrum. *Am. J. Physiology-Lung Cell Mol. Physiol.* 316 (5), L826–L842. doi:10.1152/ajplung.00424.2018

Parker, M. W., Rossi, D., Peterson, M., Smith, K., Sikström, K., White, E. S., et al. (2014). Fibrotic extracellular matrix activates a profibrotic positive feedback loop. *J. Clin. Invest.* 124 (4), 1622–1635. doi:10.1172/jci71386

Perez, A., van Heeckeren, A. M., Nichols, D., Gupta, S., Eastman, J. F., and Davis, P. B. (2008). Peroxisome proliferator-activated receptor-γ in cystic fibrosis lung epithelium. *Am. J. Physiology-Lung Cell Mol. Physiol.* 295 (2), L303–L313. doi:10.1152/ajplung.90276.2008

Peterson-Carmichael, S. L., Harris, W. T., Goel, R., Noah, T. L., Johnson, R., Leigh, M. W., et al. (2009). Association of lower airway inflammation with physiologic findings in young children with cystic fibrosis. *Pediatr. Pulmonol.* 44 (5), 503–511. doi:10.1002/ppul.21044

Petit-Bertron, A.-F., Tabary, O., Corvol, H., Jacquot, J., Clément, A., Cavaillon, J.-M., et al. (2008). Circulating and airway neutrophils in cystic fibrosis display different TLR expression and responsiveness to interleukin-10. *Cytokine* 41 (1), 54–60. doi:10.1016/j.cyto.2007.10.012

Prakash, Y. S., Pabelick, C. M., and Sieck, G. C. (2017). Mitochondrial dysfunction in airway disease. *Chest* 152 (3), 618–626. doi:10.1016/j.chest.2017.03.020

Regamey, N., Jeffery, P. K., Alton, E. W. F. W., Bush, A., and Davies, J. C. (2011). Airway remodelling and its relationship to inflammation in cystic fibrosis. *Thorax* 66 (7), 624–629. doi:10.1136/thx.2009.134106

Reilly, R., Mroz, M. S., Dempsey, E., Wynne, K., Keely, S. J., McKone, E. F., et al. (2017). Targeting the PI3K/Akt/mTOR signalling pathway in Cystic Fibrosis. *Sci. Rep.* 7 (1), 7642. doi:10.1038/s41598-017-06588z

Ren, C. L., Pasta, D. J., Rasouliyan, L., Wagener, J. S., Konstan, M. W., and Morgan, W. J. (2008). Relationship between inhaled corticosteroid therapy and rate of lung function decline in children with cystic fibrosis. *J. Pediatr.* 153 (6), 746–751. doi:10.1016/j.jpeds.2008.07.010

Rimessi, A., Bezzerri, V., Patergnani, S., Marchi, S., Cabrini, G., and Pinton, P. (2015). Mitochondrial Ca2+-dependent NLRP3 activation exacerbates the Pseudomonas aeruginosa-driven inflammatory response in cystic fibrosis. *Nat. Commun.* 6, 6201. doi:10.1038/ncomms7201

Robertson, K. D. (2005). DNA methylation and human disease. *Nat. Rev. Genet.* 6 (8), 597–610. doi:10.1038/nrg1655

Roum, J. H., Buhl, R., McElvaney, N. G., Borok, Z., and Crystal, R. G. (1985). Systemic deficiency of glutathione in cystic fibrosis. *J. Appl. Physiol.* 75 (6), 2419–2424. doi:10.1152/jappl.1993.75.6.24191993

Rowe, S. M., Daines, C., Ringshausen, F. C., Kerem, E., Wilson, J., Tullis, E., et al. (2017). Tezacaftor-Ivacaftor in residual-function heterozygotes with cystic fibrosis. *N. Engl. J. Med.* 377 (21), 2024–2035. doi:10.1056/nejmoa1709847

Rowe, S. M., Heltshe, S. L., Gonska, T., Donaldson, S. H., Borowitz, D., Gelfond, D., et al. (2014). Clinical mechanism of the cystic fibrosis transmembrane conductance regulator potentiator ivacaftor in G551D-mediated cystic fibrosis. *Am. J. Respir. Crit. Care Med.* 190 (2), 175–184. doi:10.1164/rccm.201404-0703oc

Ruan, X. Z., Moorhead, J. F., Fernando, R., Wheeler, D. C., Powis, S. H., and Varghese, Z. (2003). PPAR agonists protect mesangial cells from interleukin 1 -induced intracellular lipid accumulation by activating the ABCA1 cholesterol efflux pathway. *J. Am. Soc. Nephrol.* 14 (3), 593–600. doi:10.1097/01.asn.0000050414.52908.da

Sagel, S. D., Sontag, M. K., Wagener, J. S., Kapsner, R. K., Osberg, I., and Accurso, F. J. (2002). Induced sputum inflammatory measures correlate with lung function in children with cystic fibrosis. *J. Pediatr.* 141 (6), 811–817. doi:10.1067/mpd.2002.129847

Scambler, T., Jarosz-Griffiths, H. H., Lara-Reyna, S., Pathak, S., Wong, C., Holbrook, J., et al. (2019). ENaC-mediated sodium influx exacerbates NLRP3-dependent inflammation in cystic fibrosis. *Elife* 8. doi:10.7554/elife.49248

Scott, M., and De Sario, A. (2020). DNA methylation changes in cystic fibrosis: cause or consequence? *Clin. Genet.* 98 (1), 3–9. doi:10.1111/cge.13731

Scott, P., Anderson, K., Singhania, M., and Cormier, R. (2020). Cystic fibrosis, CFTR, and colorectal cancer. *Int. J. Mol. Sci.* 21 (8). doi:10.3390/ijms21082891

Seiler, F., Hellberg, J., Lepper, P. M., Kamyschnikow, A., Herr, C., Bischoff, M., et al. (2013). FOXO transcription factors regulate innate immune mechanisms in respiratory epithelial cells. *J.I.* 190 (4), 1603–1613. doi:10.4049/jimmunol.1200596

Simmonds, N. J., Cullinan, P., and Hodson, M. E. (2009). Growing old with cystic fibrosis - the characteristics of long-term survivors of cystic fibrosis. *Respir. Med.* 103 (4), 629–635. doi:10.1016/j.rmed.2008.10.011

Sirinupong, N., and Yang, Z. (2015). Epigenetics in cystic fibrosis: epigenetic targeting of a genetic disease. *Cdt* 16 (9), 976–987. doi:10.2174/1389450116666150416114514

Skov, M., Pressler, T., Lykkesfeldt, J., Poulsen, H. E., Jensen, P. Ø., Johansen, H. K., et al. (2015). The effect of short-term, high-dose oral N-acetylcysteine treatment on oxidative stress markers in cystic fibrosis patients with chronic *P. aeruginosa* infection - a pilot study. *J. Cystic Fibrosis* 14 (2), 211–218. doi:10.1016/j.jcf.2014.09.015

Smerieri, A., Montanini, L., Maiuri, L., Bernasconi, S., and Street, M. (2014). FOXO1 content is reduced in cystic fibrosis and increases with IGF-I treatment. *Ijms* 15 (10), 18000–18022. doi:10.3390/ijms151018000

Snodgrass, S. M., Cihil, K. M., Cornuet, P. K., Myerburg, M. M., and Swiatecka-Urban, A. (2013). Tgf-beta1 inhibits Cftr biogenesis and prevents functional rescue of DeltaF508-Cftr in primary differentiated human bronchial epithelial cells. *PLoS One* 8 (5), e63167. doi:10.1371/journal.pone.0063167

Soltys, J., Bonfield, T., Chmiel, J., and Berger, M. (2002). Functional IL-10 deficiency in the lung of cystic fibrosis (cftr−/−) and IL-10 knockout mice causes increased expression and function of B7 costimulatory molecules on alveolar macrophages. *J. Immunol.* 168 (4), 1903–1910. doi:10.4049/jimmunol.168.4.1903

Starosta, V., Rietschel, E., Paul, K., Baumann, U., and Griese, M. (2006). Oxidative changes of bronchoalveolar proteins in cystic fibrosis. *Chest* 129 (2), 431–437. doi:10.1378/chest.129.2.431

Strub, M. D., and McCray, P. B., Jr. (2020). Transcriptomic and proteostasis networks of CFTR and the development of small molecule modulators for the treatment of cystic fibrosis lung disease. *Genes (Basel)* 11 (5). doi:10.3390/genes11050546

Sun, H., Harris, W. T., Kortyka, S., Kotha, K., Ostmann, A. J., Rezayat, A., et al. (2014). Tgf-beta downregulation of distinct chloride channels in cystic fibrosis-affected epithelia. *PLoS One* 9 (9), e106842. doi:10.1371/journal.pone.0106842

Taams, L. S. (2020). Interleukin-17 in rheumatoid arthritis: trials and tribulations. *J. Exp. Med.* 217 (3). doi:10.1084/jem.20192048

Taylor-Cousar, J. L., Munck, A., McKone, E. F., van der Ent, C. K., Moeller, A., Simard, C., et al. (2017). Tezacaftor-Ivacaftor in Patients with Cystic Fibrosis Homozygous for Phe508del. *N. Engl. J. Med.* 377 (21), 2013–2023. doi:10.1056/nejmoa1709846

Teramura, T., and Onodera, Y. (2018). Stem cell depletion by inflammation-associated miR-155. *Aging* 10 (1), 17–18. doi:10.18632/aging.101374

Than, B. L., Linnekamp, J. F., Starr, T. K., Largaespada, D. A., Rod, A., Zhang, Y., et al. (2016). CFTR is a tumor suppressor gene in murine and human intestinal cancer. *Oncogene* 35 (32), 4179–4187. doi:10.1038/onc.2015.483

Tirouvanziam, R., Conrad, C. K., Bottiglieri, T., Herzenberg, L. A., Moss, R. B., and Herzenberg, L. A. (2006). High-dose oral N-acetylcysteine, a glutathione prodrug, modulates inflammation in cystic fibrosis. *Proc. Natl. Acad. Sci.* 103 (12), 4628–4633. doi:10.1073/pnas.0511304103

Tosco, A., De Gregorio, F., Esposito, S., De Stefano, D., Sana, I., Ferrari, E., et al. (2016). A novel treatment of cystic fibrosis acting on-target: cysteamine plus epigallocatechin gallate for the autophagy-dependent rescue of class II-mutated CFTR. *Cell Death Differ* 23 (8), 1380–1393. doi:10.1038/cdd.2016.22

Tsui, L.-C. (1995). The cystic fibrosis transmembrane conductance regulator gene. *Am. J. Respir. Crit. Care Med.* 151 (3 Pt 2), S47–S53. doi:10.1164/ajrccm/151.3_pt_2.s47

Tu, Z., Chen, Q., Zhang, J. T., Jiang, X., Xia, Y., and Chan, H. C. (2016). CFTR is a potential marker for nasopharyngeal carcinoma prognosis and metastasis. *Oncotarget* 7 (47), 76955–76965. doi:10.18632/oncotarget.12762

Valdivieso, A. G., Clauzure, M., Marín, M. C., Taminelli, G. L., Massip Copiz, M. M., Sánchez, F., et al. (2012). The mitochondrial complex I activity is reduced in cells with impaired cystic fibrosis transmembrane conductance regulator (CFTR) function. *PLoS One* 7 (11), e48059. doi:10.1371/journal.pone.0048059

Van Biervliet, S., Devos, M., Delhaye, T., Van Biervliet, J. P., Robberecht, E., and Christophe, A. (2008). Oral DHA supplementation in ΔF508 homozygous cystic fibrosis patients. *Prostaglandins, Leukot. Essent. Fatty Acids* 78 (2), 109–115. doi:10.1016/j.plefa.2007.12.005

Van Goor, F., Hadida, S., Grootenhuis, P. D. J., Burton, B., Stack, J. H., Straley, K. S., et al. (2011). Correction of the F508del-CFTR protein processing defect *in vitro* by the investigational drug VX-809. *Proc. Natl. Acad. Sci.* 108 (46), 18843–18848. doi:10.1073/pnas.1105787108

Vellai, T. (2009). Autophagy genes and ageing. *Cel Death Differ* 16 (1), 94–102. doi:10.1038/cdd.2008.126

Velsor, L. W., Kariya, C., Kachadourian, R., and Day, B. J. (2006). Mitochondrial oxidative stress in the lungs of cystic fibrosis transmembrane conductance regulator protein mutant mice. *Am. J. Respir. Cel Mol Biol* 35 (5), 579–586. doi:10.1165/rcmb.2005-0473oc

Velsor, L. W., van Heeckeren, A., and Day, B. J. (2001). Antioxidant imbalance in the lungs of cystic fibrosis transmembrane conductance regulator protein mutant mice. *Am. J. Physiology-Lung Cell Mol. Physiol.* 281 (1), L31–L38. doi:10.1152/ajplung.2001.281.1.l31

Vencken, S., Foged, C., Ramsey, J. M., Sweeney, L., Cryan, S. A., MacLoughlin, R. J., et al. (2019). Nebulised lipid-polymer hybrid nanoparticles for the delivery of a therapeutic anti-inflammatory microRNA to bronchial epithelial cells. *ERJ Open Res.* 5 (2). doi:10.1183/23120541.00161-2018

Villella, V. R., Esposito, S., Bruscia, E. M., Vicinanza, M., Cenci, S., Guido, S., et al. (2013). Disease-relevant proteostasis regulation of cystic fibrosis transmembrane conductance regulator. *Cel Death Differ* 20 (8), 1101–1115. doi:10.1038/cdd.2013.46

Wainwright, C. E., Elborn, J. S., Ramsey, B. W., Marigowda, G., Huang, X., Cipolli, M., et al. (2015). Lumacaftor-Ivacaftor in Patients with Cystic Fibrosis Homozygous for Phe508del CFTR. *N. Engl. J. Med.* 373 (3), 220–231. doi:10.1056/nejmoa1409547

Zelvyte, I., Dominaitiene, R., Crisby, M., and Janciauskiene, S. (2002). Modulation of inflammatory mediators and pparγand nfκb expression by pravastatin in response to lipoproteins in human monocytes *in vitro*. *Pharmacol. Res.* 45 (2), 147–154. doi:10.1006/phrs.2001.0922

Zingarelli, B., Sheehan, M., Hake, P. W., O'Connor, M., Denenberg, A., and Cook, J. A. (2003). Peroxisome proliferator activator receptor-γ ligands, 15-deoxy-d12,14-prostaglandin J2 and ciglitazone, reduce systemic inflammation in polymicrobial sepsis by modulation of signal transduction pathways. *J. Immunol.* 171 (12), 6827–6837. doi:10.4049/jimmunol.171.12.6827

5

The Resolution Approach to Cystic Fibrosis Inflammation

Antonio Recchiuti, Sara Patruno, Roberto Plebani and Mario Romano**

Laboratory of Molecular Medicine, Center on Advanced Studies and Technology (CAST), Department of Medical, Oral e Biotechnological Sciences, "G. d'Annunzio" University of Chieti-Pescara, Chieti, Italy

***Correspondence:**
Antonio Recchiuti
a.recchiuti@unich.it
Mario Romano
mromano@unich.it

Despite the high expectations associated with the recent introduction of CFTR modulators, airway inflammation still remains a relevant clinical issue in cystic fibrosis (CF). The classical anti-inflammatory drugs have shown very limited efficacy, when not being harmful, raising the question of whether alternative approaches should be undertaken. Thus, a better knowledge of the mechanisms underlying the aberrant inflammation observed in CF is pivotal to develop more efficacious pharmacology. In this respect, the observation that endogenous proresolving pathways are defective in CF and that proresolving mediators, physiologically generated during an acute inflammatory reaction, do not completely suppress inflammation, but promote resolution, tissue healing and microbial clearance, without compromising immune host defense mechanisms, opens interesting therapeutic scenarios for CF. In this mini-review, we present the current knowledge and perspectives of proresolving pharmacology in CF, focusing on the specialized proresolving lipid mediators and selected peptides.

Keywords: inflammation resolution, specialized proresolving lipid mediators, ALX/FPR2 receptor, melanocortin system, melanocortin receptor (MCR), CFTR modulator therapy

INTRODUCTION

Pulmonary inflammation and infection, leading to lung failure, represent the main cause of morbidity and mortality in individuals with cystic fibrosis (CF) (Cantin et al., 2015). Accumulating evidence indicates that loss-of-function of the Cystic Fibrosis Transmembrane Conductance Regulator (CFTR) is per se associated with a proinflammatory phenotype, even in the absence of infection (Khan et al., 1995). This is consistent with the observation that CFTR dysfunction primarily affects cells of the immune response including platelets, leukocytes and vascular endothelial cells (Painter et al., 2006; Mattoscio et al., 2010; Del Porto et al., 2011; Sorio et al., 2011; Plebani et al., 2017; Totani et al., 2017), making the pathogenesis of inflammation in CF quite complex. This may represent one of the reasons why the current anti-inflammatory pharmacology is of limited benefit to patients with CF.

With the advent of CFTR modulators, the CF therapeutic landscape has considerably changed. New highly effective modulator therapy combining one potentiator (ivacaftor) with two correctors (elexacaftor and tezacaftor) was recently tested in subjects carrying the F508del/F508del mutation, which causes the premature degradation of CFTR. Results from two randomized short-term trials are encouraging (Heijerman et al., 2019; Middleton et al., 2019), although the long-term impact of this treatment remains to be determined. Main question is whether modulators can significantly reduce the bacterial burden and ameliorate chronic inflammation. A partial answer to this question may be provided by a subsequent study of the GOAL trial, showing a downward trend in the relative abundance of *P. aeruginosa* and *S. aureus* in the airways of study participants treated with ivacaftor, but no changes in interleukin (IL)-6, -8, -1β, and free elastase in sputum (Rowe et al., 2014; Heltshe et al., 2015). Moreover, bacterial load in sputum of subjects treated with ivacaftor was reported to decline during the 1st year of treatment but started to increase afterwards (Hisert et al., 2017), suggesting that inflammation will eventually revamp as infection rebounds. Thus, it is still unclear whether CFTR modulators may downtone the inflammatory response sufficiently to prevent or slowdown the progression of lung deterioration. Consequently, therapies targeting inflammation continue to represent an important component of CF treatment.

Until recently, much of the research on CF airway phlogosis has been focused on the activation phase of the inflammatory response and has looked like a "boulevard of broken dreams" (Cantin et al., 2015). High dose ibuprofen is to date the only treatment of some efficacy to control CF inflammation and its short- and long-term beneficial effects have been confirmed by several studies (Konstan et al., 1995; Konstan et al., 2003; Konstan et al., 2018). However, ibuprofen can carry relevant side effects that limit its use for long periods in a large number of patients.

To avoid wrong assumptions and deleterious decisions, the quest for better drugs to combat CF inflammation should be grounded on an adequate knowledge of its pathogenetic mechanisms. In this respect, the experience with the leukotriene (LT)B_4 receptor antagonist BIIL 284 gives a cautionary tale. Based on the strong evidence for the role of LTB_4 in driving PMN lung infiltration and activation, a phase IIb/III clinical trial enrolling 600 adults and children with CF was conducted. Unfortunately, the trial had to be prematurely interrupted because of severe adverse effects in adults, including increase in pulmonary exacerbations (Konstan et al., 2014). A take-home message from this experience is that in developing anti-inflammatory agents for CF, we should keep in mind the characteristics of this disease, where an adequate anti-microbial immune response should be preserved. Therefore, an alternative, perhaps more rational, approach might be to enhance the body's own mechanism to resolve inflammation.

SPECIALIZED PRORESOLVING LIPID MEDIATORS

Pioneering work by Serhan and coworkers demonstrated that resolution of inflammation is an *active process* regulated by specific mediators, including a class of small lipid molecules termed specialized proresolving lipid mediators (SPM). SPM stop excessive PMN infiltration and activation, counter proinflammatory signals, enhance the active clearance of pathogens and dead cells by MΦ, are organ protective and stimulate tissue regeneration, thus accelerating the resolution of inflammation and restitutio ad integrum (reviewed by Serhan and Levy, 2018). SPM are biosynthesized from essential polyunsaturated fatty acids (PUFA) such as arachidonic acid (AA), eicosapentaenoic (EPA), docosapentaenoic (DPA) or docosahexaenoic acid (DHA). The SPM genus includes: lipoxins (LX) from AA, E-series resolvins (RvE) from EPA, D-series Rv, protectins (PD), and maresins (MaR) from DHA and their congenerous SPM from DPA (Recchiuti et al., 2019). Recently, SPM derived by the conjugation of epoxy-DHA to glutathione (GSH) have been uncovered and denominated "SPM conjugated in tissue regeneration" (Dalli et al., 2015).

The rationale for the use of SPM to control CF inflammation originates by studies showing that inflammation resolution is defective in CF, contributing to the development of lung disease. Karp et al. found reduced concentrations of LXA_4 in BAL of CF children (Karp et al., 2004); our group demonstrated that CFTR loss-of-function dampens LX production during PLT:PMN interactions by a mechanism involving platelet 12-lipoxygenase (LO) dysfunction (Mattoscio et al., 2010). Defective LX-biosynthesis in CF was also recently reported (Ringholz et al., 2014). Along these lines, the RvD1:IL-8 ratio is diminished in sputum collected from individuals with CF compared to matched subjects without CF (Eickmeier et al., 2017; Isopi et al., 2020). In addition, we demonstrated that expression of ALX/FPR2, a receptor shared by LXA_4 and RvD1, is significantly lower in F508del/F508del bronchial cells and CF MΦ (Pierdomenico et al., 2017). Remarkably, the reduced ALX/FPR2 expression blunts antimicrobial and proresolution responses of normal and CF cells to LXA_4 and RvD1 (Pierdomenico et al., 2015; Pierdomenico et al., 2017).

Observation of defective SPM biosynthesis and downstream pathways in patients with CF provides the framework for innovative drugs that stimulate the generation of proresolving mediators in CF. Acebilustat (CTX-4430) is an oral inhibitor of LTA_4 hydrolase that turns off LTB_4 biosynthesis and increases LX formation. Results from phase I and II clinical trials with volunteers with mild to moderate CF, show that acebilustat significantly reduces sputum PMN number and neutrophil elastase levels in study participants (Elborn et al., 2017). A larger phase II trial has been conducted to identify the optimal patient population, dose, duration and endpoints for future acebilustat trials aimed at defining its efficacy in patients with CF (Elborn et al., 2018).

Lenabasum (JBT-101) is an oral agonist of leukocyte cannabinoid CB2 receptor that resolves experimental inflammation in mice by triggering LXA_4 biosynthesis (Zurier et al., 2009). A phase IIa clinical trial of lenabasum has been recently completed in CF (Chmiel et al., 2017). Volunteers in the lenabasum arm had significant lower concentrations in sputum IL-8 and a downward trend in sputum neutrophil, elastase, and IgG, as well as in the risk of pulmonary exacerbation compared to volunteers in the no lenabasum arm. A multicenter phase IIb trial is underway (NCT03451045). In a recent study, lenabasum significantly reduced the number of PMN in exudate and level of proinflammatory prostanoids and increased the biosynthesis of RvD1 and LXA_4 in human volunteers undergoing UV-killed *E. coli* skin injection (Motwani et al., 2018a).

SPM carry potent biological proresolving biactions. We reported that in wild type and *Cftr* knockout mice undergoing chronic *P. aeruginosa* infection, RvD1 reduces PMN influx shortening the time required to resolve inflammation, dampens bacterial load, and improves survival, weight recovery, and lung histopathology (Codagnone et al., 2018; Isopi et al., 2020). RvD1 also diminishes several cytokines and chemokines that are increased in CF airways including IL-8, IL-1β, and IL-17 and has additive effects when co-administered with ciprofloxacin at sub-optimal doses (Codagnone et al., 2018). Moreover, RvD1 enhances phagocytic clearance of *P. aeruginosa* in vivo and in vitro by human blood-derived and sputum MΦ and PMN from volunteers with CF (Isopi et al., 2020). In a mouse model of *P. aeruginosa* infection, Karp and coworkers also demonstrated that a LXA_4 stable analog reduces PMN recruitment and bacterial titer (Karp et al., 2004), while other studies have shown that SPM reduces polymicrobial sepsis (Spite et al., 2009), peritonitis (Chiang et al., 2012), and pneumonia by viral and bacterial co-infection (Wang et al., 2017), indicating that counter-regulation of excessive inflammation and activation of host defense against pathogens are pivotal SPM bioactions.

Many of the actions exerted by SPM to limit inflammation and infection, such as the enhancement of bacterial phagocytosis by leukocytes (Chiang et al., 2012; Colas et al., 2014; Colas et al., 2016; Pierdomenico et al., 2017; Codagnone et al., 2018) and the ability to skew MΦ from a proinflammatory to a proresolutive phenotype (Dalli and Serhan, 2012; Recchiuti et al., 2014; Pistorius et al., 2018; Matte et al., 2019), were also recapitulated with isolated human cells. We recently demonstrated that RvD1 treatment of MΦ from volunteers with CF infected in vitro results in a broad modification of the transcriptomic fingerprint. In fact, RvD1 downregulated genes associated with inflammation, NF-κB activation, and leukocyte infiltration such as chemokines (CCL5, IL-8 and CXCL1), surface molecules (CD14, CD40, CD80, CCR5), PGE_2 receptors (PTEGR) 2 and 4), and the 5-LO activating protein, which controls LTB_4 synthesis and MΦ activation. On the contrary, RvD1 upregulated genes that enhance MΦ phagocytosis and reduce the inflammatory response, like CD93, IL10 receptor α (IL10RA), CD93, and the Wnt family member 1 and 7B (WNT1/7B) (Isopi et al., 2020).

SPM also act on airway epithelial cells regulating mucociliary clearance. LXA_4 and RvD1 activate CFTR-independent Cl^- efflux and inhibit Na^+ reabsorption, thus restoring the airway surface hydration (ASL) in CF bronchial epithelia (Verriere et al., 2012; Al-Alawi et al., 2014; Higgins et al., 2016; Ringholz et al., 2018). In airway epithelia exposed to bacterial infection in vitro, LXA_4 and RvD1 also protect from cell injury, strengthen tight junctions and reduce IL-8 production (Grumbach et al., 2009; Higgins et al., 2016; Ringholz et al., 2018). In primary CF bronchial epithelial cells from F508del/F508del patients infected in vitro with *P. aeruginosa*, RvD1 upregulates the expression of genes that promote cell survival, such as tumor protein 63 (TP63), opioid receptor μ 1 (OPRM1), and aurora kinase B (AURKB), while it diminishes inflammatory genes, like CCL5 (Isopi et al., 2020).

SPM regulate inflammatory responses in the vasculature. LXA_4 and B_4 counter PMN chemotaxis triggered by LTB_4 (Papayianni et al., 1996). RvD1 reduces PMN-EC interactions and transmigration (Sun et al., 2007; Norling et al., 2012) and diminishes vascular permeability induced by IL-1β and edema formation in vivo (Codagnone et al., 2018); LXA_4 and RvD2 stimulate nitric oxide release that limits PMN adhesion to EC (Paul-Clark et al., 2004; Spite et al., 2009). Further, RvD4 modulates the formation of neutrophil extracellular traps that contribute to thrombosis and lung injury (Cherpokova et al., 2019), whereas RvE1 controls PLT/leukocyte interaction (Dona et al., 2008) and PLT aggregation (Fredman et al., 2010), which are dysregulated in people with CF and play significant pathogenetic roles in CF lung disease (Mattoscio et al., 2010; Ortiz-Muñoz et al., 2020).

Several clinical trials have demonstrated efficacy and safety of SPM in humans. In infants with eczema, a LXA_4 stable analog was as potent as steroid treatment in reducing disease severity, eczema area and clinical scores (Wu et al., 2013). LXA_4 proved superior efficacy to corticosteroids in improving lung function of asthmatic children (Kong et al., 2017). More recently, SPM stopped neutrophil infiltration in skin blisters raised in volunteers injected with UV-killed *E. coli* (Motwani et al., 2018b).

SPM act at multiple levels on cells and mechanisms involved in the pathophysiology of CF airway inflammation and activated resolution of inflammation and infection in preclinical and clinical studies, thus providing evidence for resolution pharmacology based on SPM in CF.

OTHER PRORESOLVING AGENTS POTENTIALLY RELEVANT FOR CF

Annexin A1

Annexin A1 (ANXA1) is a calcium and phospholipid binding protein, induced by glucocorticoids that inhibits phospholipase A2 (Flower and Blackwell, 1979). ANXA1 is detectable in biological fluids and is widely expressed in both circulating (particularly PMN and monocytes) and resident (epithelial, endothelial and mesangial cells, fibroblasts and synoviocytes) cells from where it is released upon activation (reviewed by Sheikh and Solito, 2018). It promotes resolution by activating the ALX/FPR2 receptor (Perretti et al., 2002), shared with LXA_4 and RvD1, placing this receptor at the crossroad of multiple proresolving pathways that can be altered in CF, where ALX/FPR2 expression is downregulated (Pierdomenico et al., 2017).

ANXA1 controls key proresolving mechanisms. It, in fact, limits PMN recruitment, while stimulating PMN apoptosis and clearance (reviewed by Sugimoto et al., 2016). It promotes M1 to M2 macrophage skewing (McArthur et al., 2020) and efferocytosis (Scannell et al., 2007). ANXA1 also downregulates proinflammatory cytokines and iNOS activity, while upregulating IL-10 expression (Ferlazzo et al., 2003). It stimulates tissue repair and reduces pulmonary fibrosis (Damazo et al., 2011). ANXA1 regulates platelet function in human and murine stroke, driving inflammation resolution (Senchenkova et al., 2019). This may be relevant in CF where platelet dysfunction drives lung hyperinflammation (Ortiz-Muñoz et al., 2020).

ANXA1 involvement in CF is documented by a number of reports. Downregulation of ANXA1 was observed in nasal epithelial cells from individuals with CF, as well as in lung and pancreas of *cftr* $^{-/-}$ mice (Bensalem et al., 2005). Moreover, degradation of ANXA1 in bronchoalveolar lavage fluids from subjects with CF has been reported (Tsao et al., 1998). Consistent with these findings, administration of the selective CFTR inhibitor CFTRinh-172 to mice exacerbated zymosan-induced acute peritonitis, which was corrected by the administration of ANXA1 or its peptido mimetic (Dalli et al., 2010). More recently, the downregulation of ANXA1 was observed in injured tendon of F508del, thereby contributing to sustain inflammation (Liu et al., 2018). Therefore, targeting ANXA1 defects or supplying ANXA1 or its active peptide derivatives may be relevant to control CF inflammation.

The Melanocortin System

The melanocortin system encompasses four peptide hormones, ACTH, α-MSH, β-MSH and γ-MSH, derived from post-translational processing of the precursor proopiomelanocortin (POMC), and two endogenous antagonists, agouti-related peptide (AgRP) and agouti signaling protein (ASIP) (Catania et al., 2004). ACTH is the best known melanocortin, because of its role in the hypothalamus-pituitary-adrenal axis and anti-inflammatory actions (Cone, 2006; Montero-Melendez, 2015).

Melanocortins activate five, high homologous, seven-transmembrane domains G protein-coupled receptors (MCR 1 to 5), some of which exert regulatory functions on the immune-inflammatory response (Patel et al., 2011). For instance, MCR1 is expressed by immune cells (monocytes, lymphocytes, neutrophils) (Brzoska et al., 2008) and carries anti-inflammatory and proresolution actions in ischemia-reperfusion (Leoni et al., 2008). MCR2 is activated only by ACTH and controls the synthesis of cortisol in the adrenal cortex (Xing et al., 2010), whereas MC3R has a relevant role in controlling lung inflammation (Getting et al., 2008) and ischemia-reperfusion (Leoni et al., 2008). MC5R is expressed also in immune cells and its activation is beneficial in immune disorders (Xu et al., 2020). Recently, we examined the proresolving signalling of MC1,3,4,5 receptors in human macrophages exposed to αMSH and some synthetic derivatives. ERK1/2 phosphorylation at any receptor was predominant to trigger efferocytosis and MC1R was the most relevant to downregulate cytokine release (Patruno et al., 2018).

The anti-inflammatory properties of the melanocortin system have been long known (reviewed by Wang et al., 2019). It is now recognized that ACTH exert proresolving actions, i.e. stimulation of efferocytosis, decrease in cytokine and chemokine accumulation, and increase in production of anti-inflammatory mediators, also independently by the hypothalamus-pituitary-adrenal circuit by targeting melanocortin receptors expressed by immune cells (Montero-Melendez, 2015). Moreover, similarly to SPM and ANXA1, melanocortins suppress the release of proinflammatory cytokines (Böhm et al., 1999; Patruno et al., 2018), inhibit PMN chemotaxis (Catania et al., 1996) and the NFkB pathway (Manna and Aggarwal, 1998). Melanocortins also inhibit the production of PGE_2 (Nicolaou et al., 2004) and nitric oxide (Star et al., 1995), induce fibroblast senescence (Montero-Melendez et al., 2020) and reverse pulmonary fibrosis (Xu et al., 2011).

The melanocortin system exerts relevant protective action in the respiratory district (Moscowitz et al., 2019). α-MSH downregulates the MUC5AC-TNFα-NFkB pathway in nasal

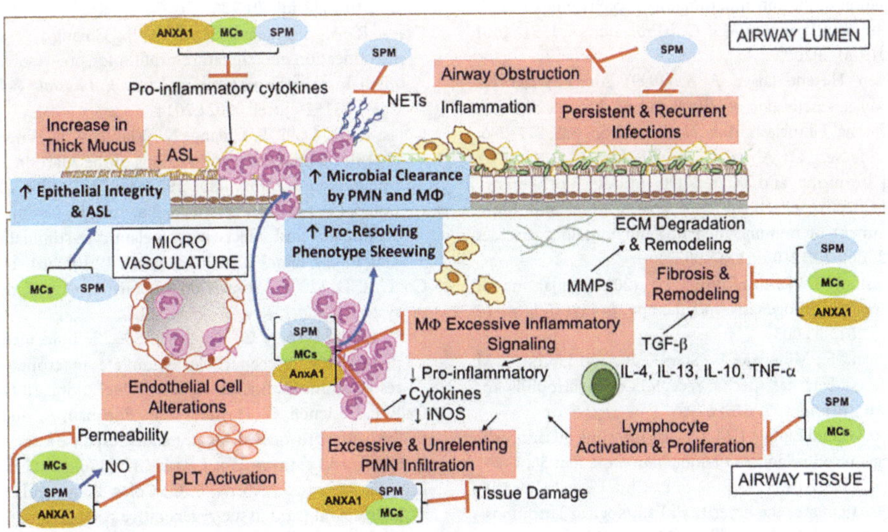

FIGURE 1 | Overlapping specialized proresolving lipid mediators (SPM), Annexin A1(ANXA1), and Melanocortin (MCs) bioactions, relevant to control cystic fibrosis (CF) airway inflammation. These molecules exert multipronged functions, encompassing anti-inflammatory (limitation of further PMN infiltration, reduction in cytokine production, and decrease in lymphocyte, EC, and PLT activation) and proresolution (enhancement of MΦ phagocytosis and bacterial clearance, promotion of tissue repair, restoration of epithelial barrier integrity) activities. See within text and references for further details.

epithelial cells (Lee et al., 2011) and diminishes BAL infiltrate in allergic lung inflammation (Raap et al., 2003). Similar to SPM and ANXA1, it limits acute lung injury (Deng et al., 2004; Colombo et al., 2007).

Despite the promising outlook of the melanocortin system as endogenous machinery that, similarly to SPM, promotes inflammation resolution little is known regarding this system in CF. In a study of genome-wide association and linkage, Wright and co-workers reported that mutations in the MCR3 are associated with the severity CF lung disease (Wright et al., 2011), suggesting that MCR3 acts as a modifier gene in CF. A reasonable, yet to be tested, hypothesis could be that dysfunctions in the melanocortin system may contribute to sustain inflammation in CF and that pharmacological modulation of this system may downtone CF inflammation. Data from our laboratory seem to be in line with this hypothesis. We recently evaluated MCR expression and bioactions of α-MSH and a synthetic selective MC1R agonist, on macrophages and PMN from volunteers with CF. We consistently observed that these molecules exert anti-inflammatory (inhibition of cytokine release) and proresolving (stimulation of efferocytosis and PMN apoptosis) activities in addition to promoting microbial clearance (Patruno et al., 2019). Although preliminary, these results indicate that the melanocortin system may represent a promising field of investigation within the context of CF.

Figure 1 shows the overlapping functions of SPM and proresolving peptides that are relevant in the pathogenesis of CF inflammation.

CONCLUSION

The modest efficacy of the current anti-inflammatory pharmacology for CF lung disease reflects our incomplete knowledge of the mechanisms underlying the development of the aberrant inflammation that occurs in CF and its correlation with recurrent infection. Clinical and experimental evidence indicates that a complete suppression of the inflammatory response may be detrimental in CF, where instead reprogramming of the immune response to promote resolution appears to represent a more rational strategy. The discovery of endogenous proresolving pathways and the evidence that proresolving mediators promote resolution of inflammation and bacterial clearance in preclinical and in vitro models of CF opens new and promising perspectives for the development of innovate pharmacology for CF lung disease.

AUTHOR CONTRIBUTIONS

AR and MR conceived the manuscript. AR, SP, and RP wrote the manuscript. MR revised the manuscript. All authors contributed to the article and approved the submitted version.

REFERENCES

Al-Alawi, M., Buchanan, P., Verriere, V., Higgins, G., McCabe, O., Costello, R. W., et al. (2014). Physiological Levels of Lipoxin A4 Inhibit ENaC and Restore Airway Surface Liquid Height in Cystic Fibrosis Bronchial Epithelium. *Physiol. Rep.* 2 (8), e12093. doi: 10.14814/phy2.12093

Bensalem, N., Ventura, A. P., Vallée, B., Lipecka, J., Tondelier, D., Davezac, N., et al. (2005). Down-regulation of the anti-inflammatory protein annexin A1 in cystic fibrosis knock-out mice and patients. *Mol. Cell. Proteomics* 4, 1591–1601. doi: 10.1074/mcp.M500019-MCP200

Böhm, M., Schulte, U., Kalden, H., and Luger, T. A. (1999). Alpha-Melanocyte-Stimulating Hormone Modulates Activation of NF-κB and AP-1 and Secretion of Interleukin-8 in Human Dermal Fibroblasts. *Ann. N. Y. Acad. Sci.* 885, 277–286.

Brzoska, T., Luger, T. A., Maaser, C., Abels, C., and Böhm, M. (2008). α-melanocyte-stimulating hormone and related tripeptides: Biochemistry, antiinflammatory and protective effects in vitro and in vivo, and future perspectives for the treatment of immune-mediated inflammatory diseases. *Endocr. Rev.* 29, 581–602. doi: 10.1210/er.2007-0027

Cantin, A. M., Hartl, D., Konstan, M. W., and Chmiel, J. F. (2015). Inflammation in cystic fibrosis lung disease: Pathogenesis and therapy. *J. Cyst. Fibros.* 14, 419–430. doi: 10.1016/j.jcf.2015.03.003

Catania, A., Rajora, N., Capsoni, F., Minonzio, F., Star, R. A., and Lipton, J. M. (1996). The neuropeptide α-MSH has specific receptors on neutrophils and reduces chemotaxis in vitro. *Peptides* 17, 675–679.

Catania, A., Gatti, S., Colombo, G., and Lipton, J. M. (2004). Targeting melanocortin receptors as a novel strategy to control inflammation. *Pharmacol. Rev.* 56, 1–29.

Cherpokova, D., Jouvene, C. C., Libreros, S., DeRoo, E. P., Chu, L., de la Rosa, X., et al. (2019). Resolvin D4 Attenuates the Severity of Pathological Thrombosis in Mice. *Blood* 134, 1458–1468. doi: 10.1182/blood.2018886317

Chiang, N., Fredman, G., Backhed, F., Oh, S. F., Vickery, T., Schmidt, B. A., et al. (2012). Infection Regulates Pro-Resolving Mediators That Lower Antibiotic Requirements. *Nature* 484, 524–528. doi: 10.1038/nature11042

Chmiel, J. F., Elborn, S., Constantine, S., and White, B. (2017). A double-blind, placebo-controlled phase 2 study in adults with cystic fibrosis of anabasum, A selective cannabinoid receptor Type 2 agonist. *Pediatr. Pulmonol.* S47, 317. doi: 10.1002/ppul.23837

Codagnone, M., Cianci, E., Lamolinara, A., Mari, V. C., Nespoli, A., Arita, M., et al. (2018). Resolvin D1 Enhances the Resolution of Lung Inflammation Caused by Long-term Pseudomonas aeruginosa Infection. *Mucosal Immunol.* 11, 35–49. doi: 10.1038/mi.2017.36

Colas, R. A., Shinohara, M., Dalli, J., Chiang, N., and Serhan, C. N. (2014). Identification and signature profiles for pro-resolving and inflammatory lipid mediators in human tissue. *Am. J. Physiol. Cell Physiol.* 307, C39–C54. doi: 10.1152/ajpcell.00024.2014

Colas, R. A., Dalli, J., Chiang, N., Vlasakov, I., Sanger, J. M., Riley, I. R., et al. (2016). Identification and Actions of the Maresin 1 Metabolome in Infectious Inflammation. *J. Immunol.* 197, 4444–4452. doi: 10.4049/jimmunol.1600837

Colombo, G., Gatti, S., Sordi, A., Turcatti, F., Carlin, A., Rossi, C., et al. (2007). Production and effects of α-melanocyte-stimulating hormone during acute lung injury. *Shock* 27, 326–333. doi: 10.1097/01.shk.0000239764.80033.7e

Cone, R. D. (2006). Studies on the physiological functions of the melanocortin system. *Endocr. Rev.* 27, 736–749.

Dalli, J., and Serhan, C. N. (2012). Specific lipid mediator signatures of human phagocytes: microparticles stimulate macrophage efferocytosis and pro-resolving mediators. *Blood* 120, e60–e72. doi: 10.1182/blood-2012-04-423525

Dalli, J., Rosignoli, G., Hayhoe, R. P., Edelman, A., and Perretti, M. (2010). CFTR inhibition provokes an inflammatory response associated with an imbalance of the annexin A1 pathway. *Am. J. Pathol.* 177, 176–186. doi: 10.2353/ajpath.2010.091149

Dalli, J., Ramon, S., Norris, P. C., Colas, R. A., and Serhan, C. N. (2015). Novel proresolving and tissue-regenerative resolvin and protectin sulfido-conjugated pathways. *FASEB J.* 29, 2120–2136. doi: 10.1096/fj.14-268441

Damazo, A. S., Sampaio, A. L., Nakata, C. M., Flower, R. J., Perretti, M., and Oliani, S. M. (2011). Endogenous annexin A1 counter-regulates bleomycin-induced lung fibrosis. *BMC Immunol.* 12, 59. doi: 10.1186/1471-2172-12-59

Del Porto, P., Cifani, N., Guarnieri, S., Di Domenico, E. G., Mariggiò, M. A., Spadaro, F., et al. (2011). Dysfunctional CFTR alters the bactericidal activity of human macrophages against Pseudomonas aeruginosa. *PLoS One* 6, e19970. doi: 10.1371/journal.pone.0019970

Deng, J., Hu, X., Yuen, P. S., and Star, R. A. (2004). α-Melanocyte-stimulating Hormone Inhibits Lung Injury after Renal Ischemia/Reperfusion. *Am. J. Respir. Crit. Care Med.* 169, 749–756. doi: 10.1164/rccm.200303-372OC

Dona, M., Fredman, G., Schwab, J. M., Chiang, N., Arita, M., Goodarzi, A., et al. (2008). Resolvin E1, an EPA-derived mediator in whole blood, selectively counterregulates leukocytes and platelets. *Blood* 112, 848 LP – 855. doi: 10.1182/blood-2007-11-122598

Eickmeier, O., Fussbroich, D., Mueller, K., Serve, F., Smaczny, C., Zielen, S., et al. (2017). Pro-resolving lipid mediator Resolvin D1 serves as a marker of lung disease in cystic fibrosis. *PLoS One* 12, e0171249. doi: 10.1371/journal.pone.0171249

Elborn, J. S., Horsley, A., MacGregor, G., Bilton, D., Grosswald, R., Ahuja, S., et al. (2017). Phase I Studies of Acebilustat: Biomarker Response and Safety in Patients with Cystic Fibrosis. *Clin. Trans. Sci.* 10, 28–34. doi: 10.1111/cts.12428

Elborn, J. S., Ahuja, S., Springman, E., Mershon, J., Grosswald, R., and Heltshe, S. (2018). EMPIRE-CF: A phase II randomized placebo-controlled trial of once-daily, oral acebilustat in adult patients with cystic fibrosis - Study design and patient demographics». *Contemp. Clin. Trials* 72, 86–94. doi: 10.1016/j.cct.2018.07.014

Ferlazzo, V., D'Agostino, P., Milano, S., Caruso, R., Feo, S., Cillari, E., et al. (2003). Anti-inflammatory effects of annexin-1: stimulation of IL-10 release and inhibition of nitric oxide synthesis. *Int. Immunopharmacol.* 3, 1363–1369. doi: 10.1016/S1567-5769(03)00133-4

Flower, R. J., and Blackwell, G. J. (1979). Anti-inflammatory steroids induce biosynthesis of a phospholipase A2 inhibitor which prevents prostaglandin generation. *Nature* 278, 456–459. doi: 10.1038/278456a0

Fredman, G., Van Dyke, T. E., and Serhan, C. N. (2010). Resolvin E1 regulates adenosine diphosphate activation of human platelets. *Arterioscler. Thromb. Vasc. Biol.* 30, 2005–2013. doi: 10.1161/ATVBAHA.110.209908

Getting, S. J., Riffo-Vasquez, Y., Pitchford, S., Kaneva, M., Grieco, P., Page, C. P., et al. (2008). A role for MC3R in modulating lung inflammation. *Pulm. Pharmacol. Ther.* 21, 866–873. doi: 10.1016/j.pupt.2008.09.004

Grumbach, Y., Quynh, N. V., Chiron, R., and Urbach, V. (2009). LXA4 Stimulates ZO-1 Expression and Transepithelial Electrical Resistance in Human Airway Epithelial (16HBE14o-) Cells. *Am. J. Physiol. Lung Cell Mol. Physiol.* 296, L101–L108. doi: 10.1152/ajplung.00018.2008

Heijerman, H. G. M., McKone, E. F., Downey, D. G., Van Braeckel, E., Rowe, S. M., Tullis, E., et al. (2019). Efficacy and safety of the elexacaftor plus tezacaftor plus ivacaftor combination regimen in people with cystic fibrosis homozygous for the F508del mutation: a double-blind, randomised, phase 3 trial. *Lancet* 394, 1940–1948. doi: 10.1016/S0140-6736(19)32597-8

Heltshe, S. L., Mayer-Hamblett, N., Burns, J. L., Khan, U., Baines, A., Ramsey, B. W., et al. (2015). Pseudomonas Aeruginosa in Cystic Fibrosis Patients with G551D-CFTR Treated with Ivacaftor. *Clin. Infect. Dis.* 60, 703–712. doi: 10.1093/cid/ciu944

Higgins, G., Fustero Torre, C., Tyrrell, J., McNally, P., Harvey, B. J., and Urbach, V. (2016). Lipoxin A4 Prevents Tight Junction Disruption and Delays the Colonization of Cystic Fibrosis Bronchial Epithelial Cells by Pseudomonas Aeruginosa. *Am. J. Physiol. Lung Cell. Mol. Physiol.* 310, L1053–L1061. doi: 10.1152/ajplung.00368.2015

Hisert, K. B., Heltshe, S. L., Pope, C., Jorth, P., Wu, X., Edwards, R. M., et al. (2017). Restoring Cystic Fibrosis Transmembrane Conductance Regulator Function Reduces Airway Bacteria and Inflammation in People with Cystic Fibrosis and Chronic Lung Infections. *Am. J. Resp. Crit. Care Med.* 195, 1617–1628. doi: 10.1164/rccm.201609-1954OC

Isopi, E., Mattoscio, D., Codagnone, M., Mari, V. C., Lamolinara, A., D'Aurora, M., et al. (2020). Resolvin D1 reduces lung infection and inflammation activating resolution in cystic fibrosis. *Front. Immunol.* 11:581. doi: 10.3389/fimmu.2020.00581

Karp, C. L., Flick, L. M., Park, K. W., Softic, S., Greer, T. M., Keledjian, R., et al. (2004). Defective lipoxin-mediated anti-inflammatory activity in the cystic fibrosis airway. *Nat. Immunol.* 5, 388–392. doi: 10.1038/ni1056

Khan, T. Z., Wagener, J. S., Bost, T., Martinez, J., Accurso, F. J., and Riches, D. W. (1995). Early pulmonary inflammation in infants with cystic fibrosis. *Am. J. Respir. Crit. Care Med.* 151, 1075–1082.

Kong, X., Wu, S. H., Zhang, L., and Chen, X. Q. (2017). Pilot Application of Lipoxin A4 Analog and Lipoxin A4 Receptor Agonist in Asthmatic Children with Acute Episodes. *Exp. Ther. Med.* 14, 2284–2290. doi: 10.3892/etm.2017.4787

Konstan, M. W., Byard, P. J., Hoppel, C. L., and Davis, P. (1995). Effect of High-Dose Ibuprofen in Patients with Cystic Fibrosis. *New Engl. J. Med.* 332, 848–854. doi: 10.1056/NEJM199503303321303

Konstan, M. W., Krenicky, J. E., Finney, M. R., Kirchner, H. L., Hilliard, K. A., Jay, B., et al. (2003). Effect of Ibuprofen on Neutrophil Migration in Vivo in Cystic Fibrosis and Healthy Subjects. *J. Pharmacol. Exp. Ther.* 306, 1086–1091. doi: 10.1124/jpet.103.052449

Konstan, M. W., Döring, G., Heltshe, S. L., Lands, L. C., Hilliard, K. A., Koker, P., et al. (2014). A Randomized Double Blind, Placebo Controlled Phase 2 Trial of BIIL 284 BS (an LTB4 Receptor Antagonist) for the Treatment of Lung Disease in Children and Adults with Cystic Fibrosis. *J. Cyst. Fibros.* 13, 148–155. doi: 10.1016/j.jcf.2013.12.009

Konstan, M. W., VanDevanter, D. R., Sawicki, G. S., Pasta, D. J., Foreman, A. J., Neiman, E. A., et al. (2018). Association of High-Dose Ibuprofen Use, Lung Function Decline, and Long-Term Survival in Children with Cystic Fibrosis. *Ann. Am. Thor. Soc.* 15, 485–493. doi: 10.1513/AnnalsATS.201706-486OC

Lee, S. N., Ryu, J. H., Joo, J. H., Choi, Y. H., Lee, H. J., Kim, Y. J., et al. (2011). α-Melanocyte-stimulating hormone inhibits tumor necrosis factor α-stimulated MUC5AC expression in human nasal epithelial cells. *Am. J. Respir. Cell. Mol. Biol.* 44, 716–724. doi: 10.1165/rcmb.2009-0420OC

Leoni, G., Patel, H. B., Sampaio, A. L., Gavins, F. N., Murray, J. F., Grieco, P., et al. (2008). Inflamed phenotype of the mesenteric microcirculation of melanocortin type 3 receptor-null mice after ischemia-reperfusion. *FASEB J.* 22, 4228–4238. doi: 10.1096/fj.08-113886

Liu, Y., Feng, L., Wang, H., Wang, Y. J., Chan, H. C., Jiang, X. H., et al. (2018). Identification of an Anti-Inflammation Protein, Annexin A1, in Tendon Derived Stem Cells (TDSCs) of Cystic Fibrosis Mice: A Comparative Proteomic Analysis. *Proteomics Clin. Appl.* 12, e1700162. doi: 10.1002/prca.201700162

Manna, S. K., and Aggarwal, B. B. (1998). Alpha-melanocyte-stimulating hormone inhibits the nuclear transcription factor NF-kappa B activation induced by various inflammatory agents. *J. Immunol.* 161, 2873–2880.

Matte, A., Recchiuti, A., Federti, E., Koehl, B., Mintz, T., El Nemer, W., et al. (2019). Resolution of sickle cell disease-associated inflammation and tissue damage with 17R-resolvin D1. *Blood* 133, 252–265. doi: 10.1182/blood-2018-07-865378

Mattoscio, D., Evangelista, V., De Cristofaro, R., Recchiuti, A., Pandolfi, A., Di Silvestre, S., et al. (2010). Cystic fibrosis transmembrane conductance regulator (CFTR) expression in human platelets: impact on mediators and mechanisms of the inflammatory response. *FASEB J.* 24, 3970–3980. doi: 10.1096/fj.10-159921

McArthur, S., Juban, G., Gobbetti, T., Desgeorges, T., Theret, M., Gondin, J., et al. (2020). Annexin A1 drives macrophage skewing to accelerate muscle regeneration through AMPK activation. *J. Clin. Invest.* 130, 1156–1167. doi: 10.1172/JCI124635

Middleton, P. G., Mall, M. A., Drevinek, P., Lands, L. C., McKone, E. F., Polinei, D., et al. (2019). Elexacaftor-tezacaftor-ivacaftor for CF with a single Phe508del allele. *N. Engl. J. Med.* 381, 1809–1819. doi: 10.1056/NEJMoa1908639

Montero-Melendez, T., Nagano, A., Chelala, C., Filer, A., Buckley, C. D., and Perretti, M. (2020). Therapeutic senescence via GPCR activation in synovial fibroblasts facilitates resolution of arthritis. *Nat. Commun.* 11, 745. doi: 10.1038/s41467-020-14421-x

Montero-Melendez, T. (2015). ACTH: The forgotten therapy. *Semin. Immunol.* 27, 216–226. doi: 10.1016/j.smim.2015.02.003

Moscowitz, A. E., Asif, H., Lindenmaier, L. B., Calzadilla, A., Zhang, C., and Mirsaeidi, M. (2019). The Importance of Melanocortin Receptors and Their Agonists in Pulmonary Disease. *Front. Med.* 6:145. doi: 10.3389/fmed.2019.00145

Motwani, M. P., Bennett, B., Norris, P. C., Maini, A. A., George, M. J., Newson, J., et al. (2018a). Potent Anti-Inflammatory and Pro-Resolving Effects of Anabasum in a Human Model of Self-Resolving Acute Inflammation. *Clin. Pharmacol. Ther.* 104, 675–686. doi: 10.1002/cpt.980

Motwani, M. P., Colas, R. A., George, M. J., Flint, J. D., Dalli, J., Richard-Loendt, A., et al. (2018b). Pro-resolving mediators promote resolution in a human skin model of UV-killed Escherichia coli-driven acute inflammation. *J.C.I. Insight* 3, e94463. doi: 10.1172/jci.insight.94463

Nicolaou, A., Estdale, S. E., Tsatmali, M., Herrero, D. P., and Thody, A. J. (2004). Prostaglandin production by melanocytic cells and the effect of α-melanocyte stimulating hormone. *FEBS Lett.* 570, 223–226. doi: 10.1016/j.febslet.2004.06.041

Norling, L. V., Dalli, J., Flower, R. J., Serhan, C. N., and Perretti, M. (2012). Resolvin D1 limits polymorphonuclear leukocyte recruitment to inflammatory loci: receptor-dependent actions. *Arterioscler. Thromb. Vasc. Biol.* 32 (8), 1970–1978. doi: 10.1161/ATVBAHA.112.249508

Ortiz-Muñoz, G., Yu, M. A., Lefrançais, E., Mallavia, B., Valet, C., Tian, J. J., et al. (2020). Cystic fibrosis transmembrane conductance regulator dysfunction in platelets drives lung hyperinflammation. *J. Clin. Invest.* 130, 2041–2053. doi: 10.1172/JCI129635

Painter, R. G., Valentine, V. G., Lanson, N. A. Jr, Leidal, K., Zhang, Q., Lombard, G., et al. (2006). CFTR Expression in human neutrophils and the phagolysosomal chlorination defect in cystic fibrosis. *Biochemistry* 45, 10260–10269. doi: 10.1021/bi060490t

Papayianni, A., Serhan, C. N., and Brady, H. R. (1996). Lipoxin A4 and B4 Inhibit Leukotriene-Stimulated Interactions of Human Neutrophils and Endothelial Cells. *J. Immunol.* 156, 264–272.

Patel, H. B., Montero-Melendez, T., Greco, K. V., and Perretti, M. (2011). Melanocortin receptors as novel effectors of macrophage responses in inflammation. *Front. Immunol.* 2:41. doi: 10.3389/fimmu.2011.00041

Patruno, S., Garrido-Mesa, J., Romano, M., Perretti, M., and Montero-Melendez, T. (2018). Ligand Bias and Its Association With Pro-resolving Actions of Melanocortin Drugs. *Front. Pharmacol.* 9:919. doi: 10.3389/fphar.2018.00919

Patruno, S., Pomilio, A., Recchiuti, A., and Romano, M. (2019). Proresolving and antimicrobial bioactions of melanocortins on CF cells. *Pedriatr. Pulmol.* 54, S339–S340. WOS:000484544000581.

Paul-Clark, M. J., Van Cao, T., Moradi-Bidhendi, N., Cooper, D., and Gilroy, D. W. (2004). 15-Epi-Lipoxin A4-Mediated Induction of Nitric Oxide Explains How Aspirin Inhibits Acute Inflammation. *J. Exp. Med.* 200, 69–78. doi: 10.1084/jem.20040566

Perretti, M., Chiang, N., La, M., Fierro, I. M., Marullo, S., Getting, S. J., et al. (2002). Endogenous lipid- and peptide-derived anti-inflammatory pathways generated with glucocorticoid and aspirin treatment activate the lipoxin A4 receptor. *Nat. Med.* 8, 1296–1302. doi: 10.1038/nm786

Pierdomenico, A. M., Recchiuti, A., Simiele, F., Codagnone, M., Mari, V. C., Davì, G., et al. (2015). MicroRNA-181b Regulates ALX/FPR2 Receptor Expression and Proresolution Signaling in Human Macrophages. *J. Biol. Chem.* 290, 3592–3600. doi: 10.1074/jbc.M114.592352

Pierdomenico, A. M., Patruno, S., Codagnone, M., Simiele, F., Mari, V. C., Plebani, R., et al. (2017). microRNA-181b is increased in cystic fibrosis cells and impairs lipoxin A4 receptor-dependent mechanisms of inflammation resolution and antimicrobial defense. *Sci. Rep.* 7, 13519. doi: 10.1038/s41598-017-14055-y

Pistorius, K., Souza, P. R., De Matteis, R., Austin-Williams, S., Primdahl, K. G., Vik, A., et al. (2018). PDn-3 DPA Pathway Regulates Human Monocyte Differentiation and Macrophage Function. *Cell Chem. Biol.* 25, 749–760.e9. doi: 10.1016/j.chembiol.2018.04.017

Plebani, R., Tripaldi, R., Lanuti, P., Recchiuti, A., Di Silvestre, S., Anile, M., et al. (2017). Establishment and long-term culture of human cystic fibrosis endothelial cells. *Lab. Invest.* 97, 1375–1384. doi: 10.1038/labinvest.2017.74

Raap, U., Brzoska, T., Sohl, S., Päth, G., Emmel, J., Herz, U., et al. (2003). α-Melanocyte-Stimulating Hormone Inhibits Allergic Airway Inflammation. *J. Immunol.* 171, 353–359.

Recchiuti, A., Codagnone, M., Pierdomenico, A. M., Rossi, C., Mari, V. C., Cianci, E., et al. (2014). Immunoresolving actions of oral resolvin D1 include selective regulation of the transcription machinery in resolution-phase mouse macrophages. *FASEB J.* 28, 3090–3102. doi: 10.1096/fj.13-248393

Recchiuti, A., Mattoscio, D., and Isopi, E. (2019). Roles, Actions, and Therapeutic Potential of Specialized Pro-resolving Lipid Mediators for the Treatment of Inflammation in Cystic Fibrosis. *Front. Pharmacol.* 10:252. doi: 10.3389/fphar.2019.00252

Ringholz, F. C., Buchanan, P. J., Clarke, D. T., Millar, R. G., McDermott, M., Linnane, B., et al. (2014). Reduced 15-Lipoxygenase 2 and Lipoxin A4/Leukotriene B4 Ratio in Children with Cystic Fibrosis. *Eur. Respir. J.* 44, 394–404. doi: 10.1183/09031936.00106013

Ringholz, F. C., Higgins, G., Hatton, A., Sassi, A., Moukachar, A., Fustero-Torre, C., et al. (2018). Resolvin D1 Regulates Epithelial Ion Transport and Inflammation in Cystic Fibrosis Airways. *J. Cyst. Fibros.* 17, 607–615. doi: 10.1016/j.jcf.2017.11.017

Rowe, S. M., Heltshe, S. L., Gonska, T., Donaldson, S. H., Borowitz, D., Daniel Gelfond, D., et al. (2014). Clinical Mechanism of the Cystic Fibrosis Transmembrane Conductance Regulator Potentiator Ivacaftor in G551D-Mediated Cystic Fibrosis. *Am. J. Resp. Crit. Care Med.* 190, 175–184. doi: 10.1164/rccm.201404-0703OC

Scannell, M., Flanagan, M. B., deStefani, A., Wynne, K. J., Cagney, G., Godson, C., et al. (2007). Annexin-1 and peptide derivatives are released by apoptotic cells and stimulate phagocytosis of apoptotic neutrophils by macrophages. *J. Immunol.* 178, 4595–4605.

Senchenkova, E. Y., Ansari, J., Becker, F., Vital, S. A., Al-Yafeai, Z., Sparkenbaugh, E. M., et al. (2019). Novel Role for the AnxA1-Fpr2/ALX Signaling Axis as a Key Regulator of Platelet Function to Promote Resolution of Inflammation. *Circulation* 140, 319–335. doi: 10.1161/CIRCULATIONAHA.118.039345

Serhan, C. N., and Levy, B. D. (2018). Resolvins in inflammation: emergence of the pro-resolving superfamily of mediators. *J. Clin. Invest.* 128, 2657–2669. doi: 10.1172/JCI97943

Sheikh, M. H., and Solito, E. (2018). Annexin A1: Uncovering the Many Talents of an Old Protein. *Int. J. Mol. Sci.* 19:1045. doi: 10.3390/ijms19041045

Sorio, C., Buffelli, M., Angiari, C., Ettorre, M., Johansson, J., Vezzalini, M., et al. (2011). Defective CFTR expression and function are detectable in blood monocytes: development of a new blood test for cystic fibrosis. *PLoS One* 6, e22212. doi: 10.1371/journal.pone.0022212

Spite, M., Norling, L. V., Summers, L., Yang, R., Cooper, D., Petasis, N. A., et al. (2009). Resolvin D2 is a potent regulator of leukocytes and controls microbial sepsis. *Nature* 461, 1287–1291. doi: 10.1038/nature08541

Star, R., Rajora, N., Huang, J., Stock, R. C., Catania, A., and Lipton, J. M. (1995). Evidence of autocrine modulation of macrophage nitric oxide synthase by alpha-melanocyte-stimulating hormone. *Proc. Natl. Acad. Sci. U.S.A.* 92, 8016–8020. doi: 10.1073/pnas.92.17.8016

Sugimoto, M. A., Vago, J. P., Teixeira, M. M., and Sousa, L. P. (2016). Annexin A1 and the Resolution of Inflammation: Modulation of Neutrophil Recruitment, Apoptosis, and Clearance. *J. Immunol. Res.* 2016, 8239258. doi: 10.1155/2016/8239258

Sun, Y. P., Oh, S. F., Uddin, J., Yang, R., Gotlinger, K., Campbell, E., et al. (2007). Resolvin D1 and Its Aspirin-Triggered 17R Epimer. Stereochemical Assignments, Anti-Inflammatory Properties, and Enzymatic Inactivation. *J. Biol. Chem.* 282, 9323–9334. doi: 10.1074/jbc.M609212200

Totani, L., Plebani, R., Piccoli, A., Di Silvestre, S., Lanuti, P., Recchiuti, A., et al. (2017). Mechanisms of endothelial cell dysfunction in cystic fibrosis. *Biochim. Biophys. Acta* 1863, 3243–3253. doi: 10.1016/j.bbadis.2017.08.011

Tsao, F. H., Meyer, K. C., Chen, X., Rosenthal, N. S., and Hu, J. (1998). Degradation of annexin I in bronchoalveolar lavage fluid from patients with cystic fibrosis. *Am. J. Resp. Cell Mol. Biol.* 18, 120–128. doi: 10.1165/ajrcmb.18.1.2808

Verriere, V., Higgins, G., Al-Alawi, M., Costello, R. W., McNally, P., Chiron, R., et al. (2012). Lipoxin A4 Stimulates Calcium-Activated Chloride Currents and Increases Airway Surface Liquid Height in Normal and Cystic Fibrosis Airway Epithelia. *PLoS One* 7, e37746. doi: 10.1371/journal.pone.0037746

Wang, H., Anthony, D., Yatmaz, S., Wijburg, O., Satzke, C., Levy, B. D., et al. (2017). Aspirin-triggered resolvin D1 reduces pneumococcal lung infection and inflammation in a viral and bacterial coinfection pneumonia model. *Clin. Sci. (Lond).* 131, 2347–2362. doi: 10.1042/CS20171006

Wang, W., Guo, D. Y., Lin, Y. J., and Tao, Y. X. (2019). Melanocortin Regulation of Inflammation. *Front. Endocrinol. (Lausanne).* 10:683. doi: 10.3389/fendo.2019.00683

Wright, F. A., Strug, L. J., Doshi, V. K., Commander, C. W., Blackman, S. M., Sun, L., et al. (2011). Genome-wide association and linkage identify modifier loci of lung disease severity in cystic fibrosis at 11p13 and 20q13.2. *Nat. Genet.* 43, 539–546. doi: 10.1038/ng.838

Wu, S. H., Chen, X. Q., Liu, B., Wu, H. J., and Dong, L. (2013). Efficacy and Safety of 15(R/S)-Methyl-Lipoxin A(4) in Topical Treatment of Infantile Eczema. *Br. J. Dermatol.* 168, 172–178. doi: 10.1111/j.1365-2133.2012.11177.x

Xing, Y., Parker, C. R., Edwards, M., and Rainey, W. E. (2010). ACTH is a potent regulator of gene expression in human adrenal cells. *J. Mol. Endocrinol.* 45, 59–68. doi: 10.1677/JME-10-0006

Xu, P. B., Mao, Y. F., Meng, H. B., Tian, Y. P., and Deng, X. M. (2011). STY39, a novel alphamelanocyte-stimulating hormone analogue, attenuates bleomycin-induced pulmonary inflammation and fibrosis in mice. *Shock* 35, 308–314. doi: 10.1097/SHK.0b013e3181f8f15e

Xu, Y., Guan, X., Zhou, R., and Gong, R. (2020). Melanocortin 5 receptor signaling pathway in health and disease. *Cell. Mol. Life Sci.* 4. doi: 10.1007/s00018-020-03511-0

Zurier, R. B., Sun, Y. P., George, K. L., Stebulis, J. A., Rossetti, R. G., Skulas, A., et al. (2009). Ajulemic acid, a synthetic cannabinoid, increases formation of the endogenous proresolving and anti-inflammatory eicosanoid, lipoxin A4. *FASEB J.* 23, 1503–1509. doi: 10.1096/fj.08-118323

6

Designing Clinical Trials for Anti-Inflammatory Therapies in Cystic Fibrosis

Lucy Perrem [1,2,3]* *and Felix Ratjen* [1,2,3]

[1] Division of Respiratory Medicine, The Hospital for Sick Children, Toronto, ON, Canada, [2] Department of Paediatrics, University of Toronto, Toronto, ON, Canada, [3] Translational Medicine Program, SickKids Research Institute, Toronto, ON, Canada

***Correspondence:**
Lucy Perrem
lucy.perrem@sickkids.ca

The inflammatory response in the CF airway begins early in the disease process and becomes persistent through life in most patients. Inflammation, which is predominantly neutrophilic, worsens airway obstruction and plays a critical role in the development of structural lung damage. While cystic fibrosis transmembrane regulator modulators will likely have a dramatic impact on the trajectory of CF lung disease over the coming years, addressing other important aspects of lung disease such as inflammation will nevertheless remain a priority. Considering the central role of neutrophils and their products in the inflammatory response, potential therapies should ultimately affect neutrophils and their products. The ideal anti-inflammatory therapy would exert a dual effect on the pro-inflammatory and pro-resolution arms of the inflammatory cascade, both of which contribute to dysregulated inflammation in CF. This review outlines the key factors to be considered in the design of clinical trials evaluating anti-inflammatory therapies in CF. Important lessons have been learned from previous clinical trials in this area and choosing the right efficacy endpoints is key to the success of any anti-inflammatory drug development program. Identifying and validating non-invasive biomarkers, novel imaging techniques and sensitive lung function tests capable of monitoring disease activity and therapeutic response are important areas of research and will be useful for the design of future anti-inflammatory drug trials.

Keywords: anti-inflammatories, cystic fibrosis, clinical trials, lung, airway inflammation

INTRODUCTION

Airway inflammation plays a critical role in the development of bronchiectasis in cystic fibrosis (CF) and contributes to the progressive decline in lung function (Pillarisetti et al., 2011; Sagel et al., 2012; Sly et al., 2013; Nichols and Chmiel, 2015). Inflammation typically beings early in the disease process and becomes persistent in most patients (Pillarisetti et al., 2011; Sagel et al., 2012; Sly et al., 2013; Nichols and Chmiel, 2015).

Abbreviations: CF, cystic fibrosis; CFTR, cystic fibrosis transmembrane regulator; NE, neutrophil elastase; MRI, magnetic resonance imaging; CT, computed tomography; PET, positron emission tomography; MBW, multiple breath washout; FEV1, forced expiratory volume in 1 s.

The inflammatory process in CF is predominantly driven by neutrophils (Cohen-Cymberknoh et al., 2013). Neutrophils are recruited into the airway in response to infection and then kill bacteria by releasing their contents including peroxidases and proteases (Watt et al., 2005). A key feature of inflammation in CF is that the response is excessive relative to the burden of infection due to a combination of increased influx and decreased clearance of pathogens and inflammatory cells (Nichols and Chmiel, 2015). Normally, once the intracellular contents are released, neutrophils undergo apoptosis by alveolar macrophages. However, in the CF airway, neutrophils undergo necrosis rather than apoptosis and this results in the release of damaging intracellular contents and chemoattractants and fuels further neutrophil influx (Watt et al., 2005; Cohen-Cymberknoh et al., 2016). The release of massive quantities of neutrophil elastase overwhelms the endogenous anti-proteases, such as anti-1 antitrypsin, needed to neutralize proteolytic activity, and this ultimately leads to the destruction of lung tissue (Birrer et al., 1994). The actions of neutrophil elastase also work to make the neutrophils in CF airways less effective at killing bacteria, partly due to cleavage of immunoglobulins and complement (McElvaney, 2016). This becomes a vicious cycle of neutrophilic inflammation, protease release, and oxidative stress which leads to tissue destruction and fibrosis of the lungs (Cohen-Cymberknoh et al., 2013).

Cystic fibrosis transmembrane regulator (CFTR) modulators are a new class of therapy that targets the basic genetic defect and could dramatically change the landscape of CF care. These drugs are potentially efficacious for approximately 90% of the CF population (Bell et al., 2020). However, despite the impressive improvements in lung function observed with ivacaftor in CF patients with gating mutations (Whiting et al., 2014), there is limited evidence that CFTR modulators impact inflammation. In a multicenter prospective cohort study in the post-approval setting, Rowe and co-workers found that patients on ivacaftor experienced significant improvements in forced expiratory volume in 1 second (FEV_1) and reductions in sweat chloride, but there were no significant changes in any sputum inflammatory markers (Rowe et al., 2014). In contrast, Hisert and co-workers evaluated the impact of ivacaftor on airway inflammation over a longer period of time and reported a significant reduction in sputum inflammatory markers including neutrophil elastase, IL-8 and IL-1b (Rowe et al., 2014). However, even in this study, most patients had ongoing chronic infection and inflammation, albeit at a lower level. A large observational study designed to evaluate the effects of the triple combination CFTR modulator (elexacaftor/tezacaftor/ivacaftor) may be able to more definitively establish how this class of drug impacts airway inflammation (Block et al., 2006).

Considering that the clinical response to CFTR modulators is variable, they are not universally available and, if bronchiectasis is already established, chronic infection and inflammation persist and lung function continues to decline (Sawicki et al., 2015), developing new therapies that target other aspects of CF lung disease remains a priority (Perrem and Ratjen, 2019). The purpose of this review is to outline key aspects to be considered in the design of clinical trials evaluating the efficacy of anti-inflammatory therapies.

WHAT IS THE IDEAL INFLAMMATORY PATHWAY TO TARGET?

The complexity of the inflammatory process in CF provides multiple potential targets for intervention. Due to the central role of neutrophils in the inflammatory process, effective anti-inflammatory therapies must target neutrophils or their products (Torphy et al., 2015).

The CF airway contains a broad spectrum of pro-inflammatory mediators, such as TNF-alpha, IL-1beta, IL-6, IL-8, IL-17, IL-33. GM-CSF, G-CSF, and HMGB-1 (Nichols and Chmiel, 2015). The downregulation of inflammation is also defective, with many studies demonstrating a deficiency in counter-regulatory molecules such as IL-10 and lipoxin-A4 (LXA4). The multiplicity of inflammatory pathways and inherent redundancy in the process makes it challenging to target specific components, both the pro-inflammatory and pro-resolving pathways offer potential targets for therapeutic interventions.

Longitudinal data from the Australian Respiratory Early Surveillance Team for Cystic Fibrosis (*AREST* CF) surveillance program demonstrated that free neutrophil elastase activity in bronchoalveolar lavage (BAL) fluid at 3 months of age was associated with bronchiectasis on computed tomography (CT) scan at 1 and 3 years of age (Sly et al., 2013). While it is unclear whether targeting a specific mediator of inflammation will be successful, given the intense burden of neutrophil elastase in CF and the predictive value of this biomarker, neutrophil elastase is a key target for anti-inflammatory therapy. Studies investigating alpha-1 antitrypsin therapy as a way to restore the protease-antiprotease balance in the CF airway have shown an improvement in neutrophil function, a reduction in inflammation, and augmentation on bacterial clearance (McElvaney et al., 1991; Birrer et al., 1994; Griese et al., 2007; McElvaney, 2016). This provides proof of concept that this approach could be successful in future clinical trials.

LESSONS LEARNED FROM PREVIOUS TRIALS

Previous studies investigating anti-inflammatory therapies have demonstrated the importance of choosing the right target and the right dose of active drug.

The major concern in undertaking trials with anti-inflammatory agents in CF is the potential that suppressing the inflammatory response in a chronically infected airway will impair host defense and exacerbate infections (Torphy et al., 2015). We learned these lessons from a large phase II clinical trial of an LTB4 receptor antagonist (BIIL 284 BS). The CF inflammatory response is mediated in part by LTB4, a key modulator of inflammation that attracts and activates neutrophils in the airway. Preclinical studies suggested that

LTB4-receptor inhibition could have positive clinical effects (Konstan et al., 1993) but the phase II BIL 284BS trial was terminated early because of increased pulmonary exacerbations in the adults treated with the study drug, combined with evidence of decreased pulmonary function and increased circulating neutrophils (Konstan et al., 2014). To understand the mechanisms underlying these negative results, subsequent studies in mice found that lower doses of the drug attenuated the inflammatory response without increasing infection, but high doses, like the dose used in the clinical trial, overly suppressed the inflammatory response and were associated with increased bacterial colony counts (Döring et al., 2014). Therefore, future trials evaluating anti-inflammatory drugs in the clinical trial setting should first have generated sufficient information about the possible harms of the drug. Preclinical studies or data available from studies investigating the same drug in other patient populations are essential to ensure a drug is safe for clinical trials in CF. **Table 1** describes how the study design and outcome measure will vary with the development phase when investigating anti-inflammatory therapies in cystic fibrosis.

ROLE OF BIOMARKERS

Given the important role of inflammation in CF lung disease, identifying biomarkers capable of monitoring disease activity or therapeutic response would be very useful (Tiddens et al., 2015). In clinical drug development, biomarkers can be used in early phase studies to demonstrate the biological safety and efficacy of new therapies, confirm the mechanism of action and inform dose selection (Muhlebach et al., 2016). Biomarkers can also be useful to compare results from preclinical and clinical studies (Torphy et al., 2015; Muhlebach et al., 2016). The relatively poor success rate in developing new anti-inflammatory therapies can, in part, be attributed to a lack of accurate, reproducible, noninvasive biomarkers that reflect the anti-inflammatory process (Martinez et al., 2011).

Lung-Derived Inflammatory Biomarkers

Bronchoalveolar lavage (BAL) is considered the gold standard for quantifying airway inflammation in the CF (Tiddens et al., 2015). However, the use of BAL longitudinally is limited by the invasiveness of the procedure. Sputum is an alternative way of obtaining material directly from the site of inflammation. For younger subjects or those with mild lung disease who cannot expectorate, sputum induction improves sample acquisition and biomarker measurements and are reasonably comparable with expectorated sputum (Sagel et al., 2001; Zemanick et al., 2015). However, both spontaneously expectorated and induced sputum are variable, making it difficult to track patients over time (Sagel et al., 2007; Chmiel et al., 2015).

The utility of sputum biomarkers of inflammation in CF clinical trials has been previously reviewed in detail, with findings from multiple studies supporting the association between pro-inflammatory cytokines and disease status in CF subjects (Sagel et al., 2007; Tiddens et al., 2015; Muhlebach et al., 2016). A secondary analysis of data from four randomized controlled trials, which included a diverse CF population, demonstrated that free neutrophil elastase and IL-8 were negatively correlated with FEV1. Neutrophil elastase, a key mediator of lung damage, was the inflammatory marker with the strongest relationship with FEV_1 (Mayer-Hamblett et al., 2007), correlating with FEV_1 both cross-sectionally and longitudinally. As neutrophil elastase correlates with bronchiectasis (DeBoer et al., 2014), tracks with and is predictive of future lung function decline (Mayer-Hamblett et al., 2007; Sagel et al., 2012), relates to treatment response and predicts time to next exacerbation (Ordoñez et al., 2003; Waters et al., 2015), it is currently considered the most informative sputum biomarker to monitor CF lung disease.

Another sputum biomarker with supportive longitudinal data is high-mobility group box-1 protein (HMGB-1); this inflammatory marker predicted subsequent pulmonary exacerbations and survival during 7 years of follow-up (Liou et al., 2001).

Despite these strong observational data, it is still not clear what magnitude of biomarker change that could be considered clinically meaningful in the interventional setting. Furthermore, for biomarkers to convincingly reflect the treatment effect of an investigational drug, multiple biomarkers should improve rather than just a single one. Chmiel and colleagues designed a placebo-controlled randomized trial to investigate whether sputum biomarkers could be used to screen candidate anti-inflammatory therapies over a short period of time (Chmiel et al., 2015). Results from a screening study such as this could provide a go-no-go decision on whether to proceed with a phase 2 trial. Given than high-dose ibuprofen is the only anti-inflammatory drug recommended for use in CF (Mogayzel et al., 2013), it was chosen to test this hypothesis. Ibuprofen is a non-steroidal anti-inflammatory drug that affects the cyclo-oxygenase pathway and results in the inhibition of prostaglandin synthesis and, at high doses, is associated with a reduction in neutrophil migration into the lung (Konstan et al., 2003). However, in this proof of concept study, there was no significant change in key inflammatory markers, including neutrophil elastase, over a 28-day trial period. It is conceivable that a longer trial is required to see a decrease in inflammatory markers in a chronically infected airway; alternatively, ibuprofen may not have been the ideal drug to test the hypothesis.

Blood-Based Inflammatory Markers

Blood-based markers are relatively non-invasive, are easily standardized and can be obtained from subjects of any age and disease severity. Although the data linking blood-based inflammatory markers to clinical outcomes is less extensive than for sputum and BAL markers, systemic inflammatory biomarkers correlate with important clinical events including pulmonary exacerbations and lung function decline (Proesmans et al., 2011; Shoki et al., 2013; Reid et al., 2015; Quon et al., 2016).

A clinical trial of school-age children with CF uninfected with *Pseudomonas aeruginosa* investigated the responsiveness of a panel of systemic inflammatory markers to treatment with azithromycin

(Ratjen et al., 2012). Azithromycin, a macrolide antibiotic, is presumed to exert its proinflammatory effect in the CF airway by reducing proinflammatory cytokine production by cells such as neutrophils, monocytes, and bronchial epithelial cells; although its precise mechanism of action remains unclear (Parnham et al., 2005). The trial by Ratjen and co-workers demonstrated that circulating neutrophil counts, C-reactive protein, serum amyloid A, and calprotectin all significantly reduced within 28-days of treatment. Furthermore, reductions in these inflammatory markers were correlated with improvements in lung function and weight gain, providing indirect evidence that these changes were associated with clinically meaningful outcomes. A secondary analysis of this study data showed that early changes in serum calprotectin levels after the first 28 days of azithromycin treatment were predictive of pulmonary exacerbation risk by day 168 (Dong et al., 2019). This demonstrates that early changes in biomarkers have the potential to predict meaningful longer-term outcomes and could be useful outcome measures in interventional trials.

CAPTURING THE EFFECT ON LUNG DISEASE

Spirometry

Reduced FEV_1, derived from spirometry, is strongly linked with increased morbidity and mortality and is, therefore, a key outcome measure in CF clinical studies (Kerem et al., 1992). Unlike drugs targeting other aspects of CF lung disease (e.g., CFTR modulators and mucoactive drugs) which have shown improvements in FEV_1 within 14 to 28 days (Fuchs et al., 1994; Ramsey et al., 2011), trials evaluating anti-inflammatory drugs have not reported immediate effects on lung function (Perrem and Ratjen, 2019). However, failure to show short-term improvements in expiratory flows airway resistance does not necessarily predict long-term benefits in lung function decline. This was demonstrated by trials investigating ibuprofen, a non-steroidal anti-inflammatory drug that reduces neutrophil influx into the lung a at higher dose (Mogayzel et al., 2013). High dose ibuprofen does not improve FEV_1, but data from two prospective clinical trials that included 226 participants, showed that the use of ibuprofen twice daily slows the decline of FEV_1 (Konstan et al., 2007; Lands et al., 2007; Lands and Stanojevic, 2019). A recent observational study also demonstrated that this beneficial effect of high-dose ibuprofen translates to improved survival (Konstan et al., 2018). Ibuprofen, therefore, provides proof of concept that targeting inflammation might improve outcomes for patients with CF, but that short-term benefits in lung function may not be seen. However, this does not exclude the possibility that a more potent anti-inflammatory compound could potentially achieve this. Interventional studies using lung function decline as an endpoint would need to be conducted over multiple years with large sample sizes size and few drug development programs would be willing to take this route. This highlights the need to identify sensitive biomarkers that can more rapidly screen candidate drugs and be used as surrogate endpoints in phase II trials reducing the failure of drugs in phase III.

A *post hoc* analysis of data from the ibuprofen trial from Konstan et al. showed a slower rate of annual decline in lung function in the ibuprofen group in younger children than in those 13 years and older (Konstan et al., 2018). The findings were consistent for all lung function outcomes (FEV_1, FVC, and FEF 25%–75%) and suggest that ibuprofen is more efficacious when used in individuals with mild CF lung disease. It is also possible that it is the trajectory of lung function and not just baseline FEV_1 that influences response to therapy. Future trials should consider stratifying patients not only based on the severity of lung disease but also on the trajectory of lung function over time.

Multiple Breath Washout Test

With more CF patients categorized as early lung disease with FEV_1 in the normal range, there is an urgent need for more sensitive outcome measures (Tiddens et al., 2015). The lung clearance index (LCI), derived from the multiple breath washout (MBW) test, reflects ventilation inhomogeneity with higher values indicating more severe lung disease. LCI is a reliable, valid, and responsive functional test and is now an established outcome measure in interventional trials (Kent et al., 2014). LCI also correlates with markers of systemic inflammation(Horsley et al., 2013; O'Neill et al., 2018), including CRP and calprotectin, and with the extent of airway inflammation (Ramsey et al., 2017). The LCI has been shown to detect treatment effects to medications such as hypertonic saline in trials involving both preschool (Subbarao et al., 2013; Ratjen et al., 2019) and school-age CF subjects with preserved spirometry (Amin et al., 2010; Amin et al., 2011; Davies et al., 2013; Ratjen et al., 2017), where a change in FEV_1 with treatment was not detected. The published treatment effects for LCI range from less than 1 units (0.6 for hypertonic saline, 0.9 units for dornase alfa) (Amin et al., 2011; Stanojevic and Ratjen, 2016) up to 2.2 units for ivacaftor in patients with CFTR gating mutations (Davies et al., 2013). LCI has not yet been incorporated into the design of a clinical trial for an anti-inflammatory therapy but the enhanced sensitivity to detect treatment effects compared to FEV_1 may potentially facilitate anti-inflammatory trials in the future.

Pulmonary Exacerbations

Pulmonary exacerbations are important clinical events in the disease process and directly contribute to the progression of lung disease (Sanders et al., 2010; Heltshe et al., 2016; Stanojevic et al., 2017; van Horck et al., 2018). Therefore, pulmonary exacerbations also serve as meaningful clinical efficacy endpoints in interventional trials. Multiple clinical trials investigating different classes of CF medications, such as CFTR modulators (Davies et al., 2013; Ratjen et al., 2018) dornase alfa (Fuchs et al., 1994), hypertonic saline (Elkins and Dentice, 2020), and tobramycin (Ramsey et al., 1999) have shown a reduction in pulmonary exacerbations compared with placebo. Given the role of inflammation in pulmonary exacerbations, targeting the inflammatory process should logically result in a reduction in pulmonary exacerbations but this has not yet been proven in phase III trials. Furthermore, given the improved overall state of health in CF, powering a study to pulmonary exacerbation endpoints, particularly in patients with mild lung disease, require large numbers of subjects, and longer follow-up times to demonstrate a treatment effect. With respect to pulmonary exacerbations, it is unclear as to what is the best definition and surrogate outcome measure — risk, frequency, or time to the next pulmonary exacerbation event. Studies using pulmonary exacerbations as an endpoint could reduce the number of patients required by limiting recruitment to individuals with a recent history of exacerbations as this has predictive value for future events (Block et al., 2006). This concept has been implemented in the design of a phase 2 study investigating lenabasum (Chmiel and Elborn); a drug that acts as a selective agonist of the cannabinoid receptor on type 2 immune cells and exerts anti-inflammatory and pro-resolution effects without suppressing the immune system (Motwani et al., 2018).

The ideal timing to initiate anti-inflammatory therapies is unclear, whether they would be most efficacious if initiated when a patient is clinically stable or during a pulmonary exacerbation when the inflammatory process is at its peak. A pilot randomized controlled trial investigating the short-term use of oral prednisone in CF patients presenting with pulmonary exacerbations demonstrated a modest improvement in lung function (Dovey et al., 2007). The PIPE study is an ongoing multisite randomized placebo-controlled trial that is investigating the efficacy of oral prednisone as an adjunctive therapy during pulmonary exacerbations. If successful, this study design could provide a model for evaluating other anti-inflammatory therapies in the future (Prednisone in Cystic Fibrosis Pulmonary Exacerbations - Full Text View - ClinicalTrials.gov).

Other Outcome Measures

Various types of imaging techniques are now available to determine the presence and extent of lung disease in patients with CF, including CT and chest magnetic resonance imaging (MRI) (Tiddens et al., 2015). Studies have demonstrated that infection, inflammation, and abnormal chest CT findings are already present in a significant proportion of asymptomatic infants with CF at 3-months of age (Sly et al., 2009) and that these early structural changes are progressive (Mott et al., 2012). On the other end of the spectrum, in CF patients screened for lung transplantation, those with a higher volume of infection/inflammation-like changes were shown to have a higher risk of dying on the waiting list (Loeve et al., 2009). Furthermore, individuals with more extensive structural lung disease on CT experience more pulmonary exacerbations (Brody et al., 2005; Loeve et al., 2011).

While chest CT scans are sensitive at detecting structural changes, the evolution of these changes over time is slow, with bronchiectasis deteriorating at about 1.5% per year on serial CT scans in CF patients(De Jong et al., 2006). Therefore, trials using the development of bronchiectasis on CT as the primary endpoint would take multiple years and/or large numbers of subjects (De Jong et al., 2006; Owens et al., 2011).

Pulmonary MRI can now provide high-resolution images that are sensitive to early disease and specific to inflammation in cystic fibrosis (CF) lung disease (Amin and Ratjen, 2008; Tiddens et al., 2015; Ciet et al., 2017; Woods et al., 2019). Unlike CT, MRI does not use ionizing radiation, and this is particularly advantageous in children and when scans need to be repeated within a relatively short time period (Amin and Ratjen, 2008; Tiddens et al., 2015). MRI techniques can track changes in lung function longitudinally and quantify treatment response (Rayment et al., 2018; Santyr et al., 2019; Woods et al., 2019). Proton density and T_1/T_2 contrast images can be obtained within a single breath-hold, providing a depiction of structural abnormalities and active inflammation. Hyperpolarized-gas MRI, increasingly using ^{129}Xe, is now becoming more widespread and has been demonstrated to have high sensitivity to early airway obstruction in CF and could have utility as an endpoint in future clinical trials, particularly in the acute setting of pulmonary exacerbations.

Another promising non-invasive imaging technique that provides information about the level of inflammation is positron emission tomography (PET) with [18]fluorodeoxyglucose ([18] FDG; FDG-PET). 18F-FDG is taken up by activated neutrophils, macrophages, and lymphocytes so in contrast to other imaging techniques, FDG-PET scans assess CF airway inflammation directly. Several observational studies have shown that 18F-FDG uptake can determine the location and intensity of pulmonary inflammation and, combined with CT, PET can be used to assess anatomy and structures. (Labiris et al., 2003; Chen et al., 2006; Klein et al., 2009; Amin et al., 2012). A study by Amin and co-workers, demonstrated that FDG PET/CT depicts changes in inflammation in the lung after intravenous antibiotics for a pulmonary exacerbation, with the PET signal correlating with the burden of sputum neutrophils (Amin et al., 2012). Data from this study support the utility of FDG PET/CT as an outcome measure in treatment studies, although it is not yet a validated outcome for use in interventional trials.

CFTR MODULATORS AND ANTI-INFLAMMATORY THERAPIES

Time will tell how increasing CFTR modulator access will affect future anti-inflammatory therapeutic development. The positive effects of CFTR modulators on the progression of CF lung disease are undoubtedly positive but this will make the issues of endpoints for anti-inflammatory trials event more challenging.

Acebilustat is an inhibitor of leukotriene A4 hydrolase (LTA4H), an enzyme that catalyzes the rate-limiting step in the formation of leukotriene B4 (LTB4), a potent chemoattractant and activator of inflammatory immune cells including neutrophils (Rao et al., 2010). This anti-inflammatory drug is also proposed to work by shunting substrates down the metabolic pathway to produce the pro-resolving mediator LXA4 (Tobin et al., 2010). In the Acebilustat phase IIb trial, the observed reduction in pulmonary exacerbations during the 48-week study period was also observed in the subgroup of patients taking CFTR modulators (Griese et al., 2007). This suggests that patients taking modulators may receive additional benefit from anti-inflammatory drugs. It would be important for future trials to take this into account and stratify groups based on whether subjects are taking CFTR modulators.

TABLE 1 | The study design and outcome measure will vary with the development phase of an anti-inflammatory therapy.

Phase of development	Population	Duration	Outcome measures	Example
Preclinical study	Animal models In vitro assays	Days	**Safety** Lack of negative effect on airway infection	CFTR-deficient mouse model to investigate infection susceptibilities associated with study drug (Bonfield, 2020)
Phase I	Healthy volunteers or Non-CF patients	≤3 months	**Safety and pharmacokinetics**	Phase 1 study of acebilistat in CF patients and healthy volunteers (Elborn et al., 2017)
Phase IIa	CF adults	8–12 weeks	**Biomarkers** **e.g. sputum NE, IL-6, IL-8** **serum CRP, calprotectin** Trends in a reduction in PEx *New imaging techniques e.g. MRI, PET-CT* *Functional tests e.g. MBW*	Phase II randomized placebo-controlled trial of acebilustat 48-week study Primary endpoint: change in FEV1pp and safety outcomes Secondary outcomes: PEx rate, time to first PEx and biomarkers of inflammation (Elborn et al., 2018)
Phase IIb/III	CF adolescents and adults	≥6 months	**PEx rate** FEV1 decline *Evolution of bronchiectasis on CT*	Phase IIb placebo-controlled trial of lenabasum in cystic fibrosis. 28-week study Primary outcome: PEx rate Secondary outcomes: time to first PEx; PEx rate using secondary PEx definition; change in CFQ-R Respiratory domain score; Change in FEV1pp; Adverse events (Trial to Evaluate Efficacy and Safety of Lenabasum in Cystic Fibrosis—Full Text View—ClinicalTrials.gov)
Alternative study design	CF adolescents and adults	Treatment during PEx	**FEV1 change with treatment** **FEV1 recovery post treatment** Biomarkers	Randomized placebo-controlled trial Of prednisone in cystic fibrosis PEx Primary outcome the proportion of subjects who achieve >90% of baseline FEV1% predicted at day 14 of IV antibiotic treatment (Prednisone in Cystic Fibrosis Pulmonary Exacerbations - Full Text View - ClinicalTrials.gov)

NE, neutrophil elastase; CRP, C-reactive protein; CFQ-R, Cystic Fibrosis Questionnaire- Revised; MRI, magnetic resonance imaging; PET-CT positron emission tomography – computed tomography; PEx; pulmonary exacerbation; FEV1pp, FEV_1 percent predicted; MBW, multiple breath washout.
Key outcome measures in bold, potential future outcome measures in italics.

CONCLUSION

Designing trials of anti-inflammatory therapies in CF faces specific challenges different from other drug development programs. Demonstrating safety data from preclinical studies, choosing appropriate and realistic efficacy endpoints and integrating sensitive imaging and lung function outcomes into future trials are important considerations. These measures will increase the likelihood that potentially efficacious therapies are not abandoned prematurely and that efficacy can be conclusively demonstrated in studies that can be completed in reasonable time frames.

AUTHOR CONTRIBUTIONS

Both authors conceptualized the content of the review. LP wrote the first draft and FR reviewed and edited the final manuscript.

REFERENCES

Amin, R., and Ratjen, F. (2008). MRI: the next frontier for cystic fibrosis clinicians? *Expert Rev. Respir. Med.* 2, 179–182. doi: 10.1586/17476348.2.2.179

Amin, R., Subbarao, P., Jabar, A., Balkovec, S., Jensen, R., Kerrigan, S., et al. (2010). Hypertonic saline improves the LCI in paediatric patients with CF with normal lung function. *Thorax* 65, 379–383. doi: 10.1136/thx.2009.125831

Amin, R., Subbarao, P., Lou, W., Jabar, A., Balkovec, S., Jensen, R., et al. (2011). The effect of dornase alfa on ventilation inhomogeneity in patients with cystic fibrosis. *Eur. Respir. J.* 37, 806–812. doi: 10.1183/09031936.00072510

Amin, R., Charron, M., Grinblat, L., Shammas, A., Grasemann, H., Graniel, K., et al. (2012). Cystic fibrosis: Detecting changes in airway inflammation with FDG PET/CT. *Radiology* 264, 868–875. doi: 10.1148/radiol.12111873

Bell, S. C., Mall, M. A., Gutierrez, H., Macek, M., Madge, S., Davies, J. C., et al. (2020). The future of cystic fibrosis care: a global perspective. *Lancet Respir. Med.* 8, 65–124. doi: 10.1016/S2213-2600(19)30337-6

Birrer, P., McElvaney, N. G., Rüdeberg, A., Sommer, C. W., Liechti-Gallati, S., Kraemer, R., et al. (1994). Protease-antiprotease imbalance in the lungs of children with cystic fibrosis. *Am. J. Respir. Crit. Care Med.* 150, 207–213. doi: 10.1164/ajrccm.150.1.7912987

Block, J. K., Vandemheen, K. L., Tullis, E., Fergusson, D., Doucette, S., Haase, D., et al. (2006). Predictors of pulmonary exacerbations in patients with cystic fibrosis infected with multi-resistant bacteria. *Thorax* 61, 969–974. doi: 10.1136/thx.2006.061366

Bonfield, T. L. (2020). Preclinical modeling for therapeutic development in cystic fibrosis. *Am. J. Respir. Crit. Care Med.* 201, 267–268. doi: 10.1164/rccm.201910-2056ED

Brody, A. S., Sucharew, H., Campbell, J. D., Millard, S. P., Molina, P. L., Klein, J. S., et al. (2005). Computed tomography correlates with pulmonary exacerbations in children with cystic fibrosis. *Am. J. Respir. Crit. Care Med.* 172, 1128–1132. doi: 10.1164/rccm.200407-989OC

Chen, D. L., Ferkol, T. W., Mintun, M. A., Pittman, J. E., Rosenbluth, D. B., and Schuster, D. P. (2006). Quantifying pulmonary inflammation in cystic fibrosis with positron emission tomography. *Am. J. Respir. Crit. Care Med.* 173, 1363–1369. doi: 10.1164/rccm.200506-934OC

Chmiel, J., and Elborn, S. *A Multicenter, Randomized, Double-Blind, Placebo-Controlled Phase 2 Trial to Evaluate Efficacy and Safety of Lenabasum in Cystic Fibrosis.* Available at: https://clinicaltrials.gov/ct2/show/NCT03451045 (Accessed March 26, 2019).

Chmiel, J. F., Konstan, M. W., Accurso, F. J., Lymp, J., Mayer-Hamblett, N., VanDevanter, D. R., et al. (2015). Use of ibuprofen to assess inflammatory biomarkers in induced sputum: Implications for clinical trials in cystic fibrosis. *J. Cyst. Fibros.* 14, 720–726. doi: 10.1016/j.jcf.2015.03.007

Ciet, P., Bertolo, S., Ros, M., Andrinopoulou, E. R., Tavano, V., Lucca, F., et al. (2017). Detection and monitoring of lung inflammation in cystic fibrosis during respiratory tract exacerbation using diffusion-weighted magnetic resonance imaging. *Eur. Respir. J.* 50, 1601437. doi: 10.1183/13993003.01437-2016

Cohen-Cymberknoh, M., Kerem, E., Ferkol, T., and Elizur, A. (2013). Airway inflammation in cystic fibrosis: molecular mechanisms and clinical implications. *Thorax* 68, 1157–1162. doi: 10.1136/thoraxjnl-2013-203204

Cohen-Cymberknoh, M., Gilead, N., Gartner, S., Rovira, S., Blau, H., Mussaffi, H., et al. (2016). Eradication failure of newly acquired Pseudomonas aeruginosa isolates in cystic fibrosis. *J. Cyst. Fibros.* 15, 776–782. doi: 10.1016/j.jcf.2016.04.006

Davies, J., Sheridan, H., Bell, N., Cunningham, S., Davis, S. D., Elborn, J. S., et al. (2013). Assessment of clinical response to ivacaftor with lung clearance index in cystic fibrosis patients with a G551D-CFTR mutation and preserved spirometry: A randomised controlled trial. *Lancet Respir. Med.* 1, 630–638. doi: 10.1016/S2213-2600(13)70182-6

De Jong, P. A., Lindblad, A., Rubin, L., Hop, W. C. J., De Jongste, J. C., Brink, M., et al. (2006). Progression of lung disease on computed tomography and pulmonary function tests in children and adults with cystic fibrosis. *Thorax* 61, 80–85. doi: 10.1136/thx.2005.045146

DeBoer, E. M., Swiercz, W., Heltshe, S. L., Anthony, M. M., Szefler, P., Klein, R., et al. (2014). Automated ct scan scores of bronchiectasis and air trapping in cystic fibrosis. *Chest* 145, 593–603. doi: 10.1378/chest.13-0588

Dong, K., Singh, A., Ng, R. T., Sin, D. D., Tebbutt, S. J., Ratjen, F., et al. (2019). "Proteomic Profiling to Identify Blood Biomarkers Predictive of Response to Azithromycin in Children and Adolescents With Cystic Fibrosis," in *Chest* (Elsevier Inc), 667–673. doi: 10.1016/j.chest.2019.05.017

Döring, G., Bragonzi, A., Paroni, M., Aktürk, F.-F., Cigana, C., Schmidt, A., et al. (2014). BIIL 284 reduces neutrophils numbers but increases P. aeruginosa bacteraemia and inflammation in mouse lungs. *J. Cyst. Fibros.* 13, 156. doi: 10.1016/J.JCF.2013.10.007

Dovey, M., Aitken, M. L., Emerson, J., McNamara, S., Waltz, D. A., and Gibson, R. L. (2007). Oral corticosteroid therapy in cystic fibrosis patients hospitalized for pulmonary exacerbation: A pilot study. *Chest* 132, 1212–1218. doi: 10.1378/chest.07-0843

Elborn, J. S., Bhatt, L., Grosswald, R., Ahuja, S., and Springman, E. B. (2017). Phase I Studies of Acebilustat: Pharmacokinetics, Pharmacodynamics, Food Effect, and CYP3A Induction. *Clin. Transl. Sci.* 10, 20–27. doi: 10.1111/cts.12426

Elborn, J. S., Ahuja, S., Springman, E., Mershon, J., Grosswald, R., and Rowe, S. M. (2018). EMPIRE-CF: A phase II randomized placebo-controlled trial of once-daily, oral acebilustat in adult patients with cystic fibrosis – Study design and patient demographics. *Contemp. Clin. Trials* 72, 86–94. doi: 10.1016/j.cct.2018.07.014

Elkins, M., and Dentice, R. (2020). Timing of hypertonic saline inhalation for cystic fibrosis. *Cochrane Database Syst. Rev.* 2020. doi: 10.1002/14651858.CD008816.pub4

Fuchs, H. J., Borowitz, D. S., Christiansen, D. H., Morris, E. M., Nash, M. L., Ramsey, B. W., et al. (1994). Effect of Aerosolized Recombinant Human DNase on Exacerbations of Respiratory Symptoms and on Pulmonary Function in Patients with Cystic Fibrosis. *N. Engl. J. Med.* 331, 637–642. doi: 10.1056/NEJM199409083311003

Griese, M., Latzin, P., Kappler, M., Weckerle, K., Heinzimaier, T., Bernhardt, T., et al. (2007). α1-Antitrypsin inhalation reduces airway inflammation in cystic fibrosis patients. *Eur. Respir. J.* 29, 240–250. doi: 10.1183/09031936.00047306

Heltshe, S. L., Goss, C. H., Thompson, V., Sagel, S. D., Sanders, D. B., Marshall, B. C., et al. (2016). Short-term and long-term response to pulmonary exacerbation treatment in cystic fibrosis. *Thorax* 71, 223–229. doi: 10.1136/thoraxjnl-2014-206750

Horsley, A. A. R., Davies, J. C. J., Gray, R. R. D., Macleod, K. A., Donovan, J., Aziz, Z. A., et al. (2013). Changes in physiological, functional and structural markers of cystic fibrosis lung disease with treatment of a pulmonary exacerbation. *Thorax* 68, 532–539. doi: 10.1136/thoraxjnl-2012-202538

Kent, L., Reix, P., Innes, J. A., Zielen, S., Le Bourgeois, M., Braggion, C., et al. (2014). Lung clearance index: evidence for use in clinical trials in cystic fibrosis. *J. Cyst. Fibros.* 13, 123–138. doi: 10.1016/j.jcf.2013.09.005

Kerem, E., Reisman, J., Corey, M., Canny, G. J., and Levison, H. (1992). Prediction of mortality in patients with cystic fibrosis. *N. Engl. J. Med.* 326, 1187–1191. doi: 10.1056/NEJM199204303261804

Klein, M., Cohen-Cymberknoh, M., Armoni, S., Shoseyov, D., Chisin, R., Orevi, M., et al. (2009). 18F-fluorodeoxyglucose-PET/CT imaging of lungs in patients with cystic fibrosis. *Chest* 136, 1220–1228. doi: 10.1378/chest.09-0610

Konstan, M. W., Walenga, R. W., Hilliard, K. A., and Hilliard, J. B. (1993). Leukotriene B4 markedly elevated in the epithelial lining fluid of patients with cystic fibrosis. *Am. Rev. Respir. Dis.* 148, 896–901. doi: 10.1164/ajrccm/148.4_Pt_1.896

Konstan, M. W., Krenicky, J. E., Finney, M. R., Kirchner, H. L., Hilliard, K. A., Hilliard, J. B., et al. (2003). Effect of ibuprofen on neutrophil migration in vivo in cystic fibrosis and healthy subjects. *J. Pharmacol. Exp. Ther.* 306, 1086–1091. doi: 10.1124/jpet.103.052449

Konstan, M. W., Schluchter, M. D., Xue, W., and Davis, P. B. (2007). Clinical use of Ibuprofen is associated with slower FEV1 decline in children with cystic fibrosis. *Am. J. Respir. Crit. Care Med.* 176, 1084–1089. doi: 10.1164/rccm.200702-181OC

Konstan, M. W., Döring, G., Heltshe, S. L., Lands, L. C., Hilliard, K. A., Koker, P., et al. (2014). A randomized double blind, placebo controlled phase 2 trial of BIIL 284 BS (an LTB4 receptor antagonist) for the treatment of lung disease in children and adults with cystic fibrosis. *J. Cyst. Fibros.* 13, 148–155. doi: 10.1016/j.jcf.2013.12.009

Konstan, M. W., VanDevanter, D. R., Sawicki, G. S., Pasta, D. J., Foreman, A. J., Neiman, E. A., et al. (2018). Association of High-Dose Ibuprofen Use, Lung Function Decline, and Long-Term Survival in Children with Cystic Fibrosis. *Ann. Am. Thorac. Soc* 15, 485–493. doi: 10.1513/AnnalsATS.201706-486OC

Labiris, N. R., Nahmias, C., Freitag, A. P., Thompson, M. L., and Dolovich, M. B. (2003). Uptake of 18fluorodeoxyglucose in the cystic fibrosis lung: A measure of lung inflammation? *Eur. Respir. J.* 21, 848–854. doi: 10.1183/09031936.03.00065102

Lands, L. C., and Stanojevic, S. (2019). Oral non-steroidal anti-inflammatory drug therapy for lung disease in cystic fibrosis. *Cochrane Database Syst. Rev.* 2019. doi: 10.1002/14651858.CD001505.pub5

Lands, L. C., Milner, R., Cantin, A. M., Manson, D., and Corey, M. (2007). High-dose ibuprofen in cystic fibrosis: Canadian safety and effectiveness trial. *J. Pediatr.* 151, 249–254. doi: 10.1016/j.jpeds.2007.04.009

Liou, T. G., Adler, F. R., Fitzsimmons, S. C., Cahill, B. C., Hibbs, J. R., and Marshall, B. C. (2001). Predictive 5-year survivorship model of cystic fibrosis. *Am. J. Epidemiol.* 153, 345–352. doi: 10.1093/aje/153.4.345

Loeve, M., van Hal, P. T. W., Robinson, P., de Jong, P. A., Lequin, M. H., Hop, W. C., et al. (2009). The spectrum of structural abnormalities on CT scans from patients with CF with severe advanced lung disease. *Thorax* 64, 876–882. doi: 10.1136/thx.2008.110908

Loeve, M., Gerbrands, K., Hop, W. C., Rosenfeld, M., Hartmann, I. C., and Tiddens, H. A. (2011). Bronchiectasis and pulmonary exacerbations in children and young adults with cystic fibrosis. *Chest* 140, 178–185. doi: 10.1378/chest.10-1152

Martinez, F. J., Donohue, J. F., and Rennard, S.II (2011). The future of chronic obstructive pulmonary disease treatment - Difficulties of and barriers to drug development. *Lancet* 378, 1027–1037. doi: 10.1016/S0140-6736(11)61047-7

Mayer-Hamblett, N., Aitken, M. L., Accurso, F. J., Kronmal, R. A., Konstan, M. W., Burns, J. L., et al. (2007). Association between pulmonary function and sputum biomarkers in cystic fibrosis. *Am. J. Respir. Crit. Care Med.* 175, 822–828. doi: 10.1164/rccm.200609-1354OC

McElvaney, N. G., Hubbard, R. C., Birrer, P., Crystal, R. G., Chernick, M. S., Frank, M. M., et al. (1991). Aerosol α1 -antitrypsin treatment for cystic fibrosis. *Lancet* 337, 392–394. doi: 10.1016/0140-6736(91)91167-S

McElvaney, N. G. (2016). "Alpha-1 antitrypsin therapy in cystic fibrosis and the lung disease associated with alpha-1 antitrypsin deficiency," in *Annals of the American Thoracic Society* (American Thoracic Society), S191–S196. doi: 10.1513/AnnalsATS.201504-245KV

Mogayzel, P. J., Naureckas, E. T., Robinson, K. A., Mueller, G., Hadjiliadis, D., Hoag, J. B., et al. (2013). Cystic fibrosis pulmonary guidelines: Chronic medications for maintenance of lung health. *Am. J. Respir. Crit. Care Med.* 187, 680–689. doi: 10.1164/rccm.201207-1160OE

Mott, L. S., Park, J., Murray, C. P., Gangell, C. L., De Klerk, N. H., Robinson, P. J., et al. (2012). Progression of early structural lung disease in young children with cystic fibrosis assessed using CT. *Thorax* 67, 509–516. doi: 10.1136/thoraxjnl-2011-200912

Motwani, M. P., Bennett, F., Norris, P. C., Maini, A. A., George, M. J., Newson, J., et al. (2018). Potent Anti-Inflammatory and Pro-Resolving Effects of Anabasum in a Human Model of Self-Resolving Acute Inflammation. *Clin. Pharmacol. Ther.* 104, 675–686. doi: 10.1002/cpt.980

Muhlebach, M. S., Clancy, J. P., Heltshe, S. L., Ziady, A., Kelley, T., Accurso, F., et al. (2016). Biomarkers for cystic fibrosis drug development. *J. Cyst. Fibros.* 15, 714–723. doi: 10.1016/j.jcf.2016.10.009

Nichols, D. P., and Chmiel, J. F. (2015). Inflammation and its genesis in cystic fibrosis. *Pediatr. Pulmonol.* 50, S39–S56. doi: 10.1002/ppul.23242

Ordoñez, C. L., Henig, N. R., Mayer-Hamblett, N., Accurso, F. J., Burns, J. L., Chmiel, J. F., et al. (2003). Inflammatory and Microbiologic Markers in Induced Sputum after Intravenous Antibiotics in Cystic Fibrosis. *Am. J. Respir. Crit. Care Med.* 168, 1471–1475. doi: 10.1164/rccm.200306-731OC

O'Neill, K., Bradley, J. M., Reid, A., Downey, D. G., Rendall, J., McCaughan, J., et al. (2018). Airway infection, systemic inflammation and lung clearance index in children and adults with cystic fibrosis. *Eur. Respir. J.* 51, 1701704. doi: 10.1183/13993003.01704-2017

Owens, C. M., Aurora, P., Stanojevic, S., Bush, A., Wade, A., Oliver, C., et al. (2011). Lung clearance index and HRCT are complementary markers of lung abnormalities in young children with CF. *Thorax* 66, 481–488. doi: 10.1136/thx.2010.150375

Parnham, M. J., Čulić, O., Eraković, V., Munić, V., Popović-Grle, S., Barišić, K., et al. (2005). Modulation of neutrophil and inflammation markers in chronic obstructive pulmonary disease by short-term azithromycin treatment. *Eur. J. Pharmacol.* 517, 132–143. doi: 10.1016/j.ejphar.2005.05.023

Perrem, L., and Ratjen, F. (2019). Anti-inflammatories and mucociliary clearance therapies in the age of CFTR modulators. *Pediatr. Pulmonol.* 54 Suppl 3, S46–S55. doi: 10.1002/ppul.24364

Pillarisetti, N., Williamson, E., Linnane, B., Skoric, B., Robertson, C. F., Robinson, P., et al. (2011). Infection, Inflammation, and Lung Function Decline in Infants with Cystic Fibrosis. *Am. J. Respir. Crit. Care Med.* 184, 75–81. doi: 10.1164/rccm.201011-1892OC

Prednisone in Cystic Fibrosis Pulmonary Exacerbations *Full Text View - ClinicalTrials.gov*. Available at: https://clinicaltrials.gov/ct2/show/NCT03070522 (Accessed August 10, 2020).

Proesmans, M., Els, C., Vermeulen, F., and De Boeck, K. (2011). Change in IgG and evolution of lung function in children with cystic fibrosis. *J. Cyst. Fibros.* 10, 128–131. doi: 10.1016/j.jcf.2010.12.004

Quon, B. S., Dai, D. L. Y., Hollander, Z., Ng, R. T., Tebbutt, S. J., Man, S. F. P., et al. (2016). Discovery of novel plasma protein biomarkers to predict imminent cystic fibrosis pulmonary exacerbations using multiple reaction monitoring mass spectrometry. *Thorax* 71, 216–222. doi: 10.1136/thoraxjnl-2014-206710

Ramsey, B. W., Pepe, M. S., Quan, J. M., Otto, K. L., Montgomery, A. B., Williams-Warren, J., et al. (1999). Intermittent Administration of Inhaled Tobramycin in Patients with Cystic Fibrosis. *N. Engl. J. Med.* 340, 23–30. doi: 10.1056/NEJM199901073400104

Ramsey, B. W., Davies, J., McElvaney, N. G., Tullis, E., Bell, S. C., Dřevínek, P., et al. (2011). A CFTR Potentiator in Patients with Cystic Fibrosis and the *G551D* Mutation. *N. Engl. J. Med.* 365, 1663–1672. doi: 10.1056/NEJMoa1105185

Ramsey, K., Foong, R., and Grdosic, J. (2017). Multiple breath washout outcomes are sensitive to inflammation and infection in children with cystic fibrosis. *Ann. Am. Thorac. Soc.* 14, 1436–1442. doi: 10.1513/AnnalsATS.201611-935OC

Rao, N. L., Riley, J. P., Banie, H., Xue, X., Sun, B., Crawford, S., et al. (2010). Leukotriene A_4 Hydrolase Inhibition Attenuates Allergic Airway Inflammation and Hyperresponsiveness. *Am. J. Respir. Crit. Care Med.* 181, 899–907. doi: 10.1164/rccm.200807-1158OC

Ratjen, F., Saiman, L., Mayer-Hamblett, N., Lands, L. C., Kloster, M., Thompson, V., et al. (2012). Effect of Azithromycin on Systemic Markers of Inflammation in Patients With Cystic Fibrosis Uninfected With Pseudomonas aeruginosa. *Chest* 142, 1259–1266. doi: 10.1378/chest.12-0628

Ratjen, F., Hug, C., Marigowda, G., Tian, S., Huang, X., Stanojevic, S., et al. (2017). Efficacy and safety of lumacaftor and ivacaftor in patients aged 6–11 years with cystic fibrosis homozygous for F508del-CFTR: a randomised, placebo-controlled phase 3 trial. *Lancet Respir. Med.* 5, 557–567. doi: 10.1016/S2213-2600(17)30215-1

Ratjen, F., Davis, S. D., Stanojevic, S., Kronmal, R. A., Hinckley Stukovsky, K. D., Jorgensen, N., et al. (2019). Inhaled hypertonic saline in preschool children with cystic fibrosis (SHIP): a multicentre, randomised, double-blind, placebo-controlled trial. *Lancet Respir. Med.* 9, 802–809. doi: 10.1016/S2213-2600(19)30187-0

Rayment, J. H., Stanojevic, S., Davis, S. D., Retsch-Bogart, G., and Ratjen, F. (2018). Lung clearance index to monitor treatment response in pulmonary exacerbations in preschool children with cystic fibrosis. *Thorax* 73, 451–458. doi: 10.1136/thoraxjnl-2017-210979

Reid, P. A., McAllister, D. A., Boyd, A. C., Innes, J. A., Porteous, D., Greening, A. P., et al. (2015). Measurement of serum calprotectin in stable patients predicts exacerbation and lung function decline in cystic fibrosis. *Am. J. Respir. Crit. Care Med.* 191, 233–236. doi: 10.1164/rccm.201407-1365LE

Rowe, S. M., Heltshe, S. L., Gonska, T., Donaldson, S. H., Borowitz, D., Gelfond, D., et al. (2014). Clinical Mechanism of the Cystic Fibrosis Transmembrane Conductance Regulator Potentiator Ivacaftor in G551D-mediated Cystic Fibrosis. *Am. J. Respir. Crit. Care Med.* 190, 175–184. doi: 10.1164/rccm.201404-0703OC

Sagel, S. D., Kapsner, R., Osberg, I., Sontag, M. K., and Accurso, F. J. (2001). Airway inflammation in children with cystic fibrosis and healthy children assessed by sputum induction. *Am. J. Respir. Crit. Care Med.* 164, 1425–1431. doi: 10.1164/ajrccm.164.8.2104075

Sagel, S. D., Chmiel, J. F., and Konstan, M. W. (2007). "Sputum biomarkers of inflammation in cystic fibrosis lung disease," in *Proceedings of the American Thoracic Society* (Proc Am Thorac Soc), 406–417. doi: 10.1513/pats.200703-044BR

Sagel, S. D., Wagner, B. D., Anthony, M. M., Emmett, P., and Zemanick, E. T. (2012). Sputum Biomarkers of Inflammation and Lung Function Decline in Children with Cystic Fibrosis. *Am. J. Respir. Crit. Care Med.* 186, 857–865. doi: 10.1164/rccm.201203-0507OC

Sanders, D. B., Bittner, R. C. L., Rosenfeld, M., Hoffman, L. R., Redding, G. J., and Goss, C. H. (2010). Failure to recover to baseline pulmonary function after cystic fibrosis pulmonary exacerbation. *Am. J. Respir. Crit. Care Med.* 182, 627–632. doi: 10.1164/rccm.200909-1421OC

Santyr, G., Kanhere, N., Morgado, F., Rayment, J. H., Ratjen, F., and Couch, M. J. (2019). Hyperpolarized Gas Magnetic Resonance Imaging of Pediatric Cystic Fibrosis Lung Disease. *Acad. Radiol.* 26, 344–354. doi: 10.1016/j.acra.2018.04.024

Sawicki, G. S., McKone, E. F., Pasta, D. J., Millar, S. J., Wagener, J. S., Johnson, C. A., et al. (2015). Sustained Benefit from Ivacaftor Demonstrated by Combining Clinical Trial and Cystic Fibrosis Patient Registry Data. *Am. J. Respir. Crit. Care Med.* 192, 836–842. doi: 10.1164/rccm.201503-0578OC

Shoki, A. H., Mayer-Hamblett, N., Wilcox, P. G., Sin, D. D., and Quon, B. S. (2013). Systematic review of blood biomarkers in cystic fibrosis pulmonary exacerbations. *Chest* 144, 1659–1670. doi: 10.1378/chest.13-0693

Sly, P. D., Brennan, S., Gangell, C., de Klerk, N., Murray, C., Mott, L., et al. (2009). Lung Disease at Diagnosis in Infants with Cystic Fibrosis Detected by Newborn Screening. *Am. J. Respir. Crit. Care Med.* 180, 146–152. doi: 10.1164/rccm.200901-0069OC

Sly, P. D., Gangell, C. L., Chen, L., Ware, R. S., Ranganathan, S., Mott, L. S., et al. (2013). Risk Factors for Bronchiectasis in Children with Cystic Fibrosis. *NEJM. Org. N Engl. J. Med.* 21, 1963–1970. doi: 10.1056/NEJMoa1301725

Stanojevic, S., and Ratjen, F. (2016). Physiologic endpoints for clinical studies for cystic fibrosis. *J. Cyst. Fibros.* 15, 416–423. doi: 10.1016/j.jcf.2016.05.014

Stanojevic, S., McDonald, A., Waters, V., MacDonald, S., Horton, E., Tullis, E., et al. (2017). Effect of pulmonary exacerbations treated with oral antibiotics on clinical outcomes in cystic fibrosis. *Thorax* 72, 327–332. doi: 10.1136/thoraxjnl-2016-208450

Subbarao, P., Stanojevic, S., Brown, M., Jensen, R., Rosenfeld, M., Davis, S., et al. (2013). Lung Clearance Index as an Outcome Measure for Clinical Trials in Young Children with Cystic Fibrosis A Pilot Study Using Inhaled Hypertonic Saline. *Am. J. Respir. Crit. Care Med.* 188, 456–460. doi: 10.1164/rccm.201302-0219OC

Tiddens, H. A. W. M., Puderbach, M., Venegas, J. G., Ratjen, F., Donaldson, S. H., Davis, S. D., et al. (2015). Novel outcome measures for clinical trials in cystic fibrosis. *Pediatr. Pulmonol.* 50, 302–315. doi: 10.1002/ppul.23146

Tobin, D. M., Vary, J. C., Ray, J. P., Walsh, G. S., Dunstan, S. J., Bang, N. D., et al. (2010). The lta4h Locus Modulates Susceptibility to Mycobacterial Infection in Zebrafish and Humans. *Cell* 140, 717–730. doi: 10.1016/J.CELL.2010.02.013

Torphy, T. J., Allen, J., Cantin, A. M., Konstan, M. W., Accurso, F. J., Joseloff, E., et al. (2015). "Considerations for the conduct of clinical trials with antiinflammatory agents in cystic fibrosis: A cystic fibrosis foundation workshop report," in *Annals of the American Thoracic Society* (American Thoracic Society), 1398–1406. doi: 10.1513/AnnalsATS.201506-361OT

Trial to Evaluate Efficacy and Safety of Lenabasum in Cystic Fibrosis *Full Text View - ClinicalTrials.gov*. Available at: https://clinicaltrials.gov/ct2/show/NCT03451045 (Accessed August 13, 2020).

van Horck, M., van de Kant, K., Winkens, B., Wesseling, G., Gulmans, V., Hendriks, H., et al. (2018). Risk factors for lung disease progression in children with cystic fibrosis. *Eur. Respir. J.* 51, 1702509. doi: 10.1183/13993003.02509-2017

Waters, V. J., Stanojevic, S., Sonneveld, N., Klingel, M., Grasemann, H., Yau, Y. C. W., et al. (2015). Factors associated with response to treatment of pulmonary exacerbations in cystic fibrosis patients. *J. Cyst. Fibros.* 14, 755–762. doi: 10.1016/j.jcf.2015.01.007

Watt, A. P., Courtney, J., Moore, J., Ennis, M., and Elborn, J. S. (2005). Neutrophil cell death, activation and bacterial infection in cystic fibrosis. *Thorax* 60, 659–664. doi: 10.1136/thx.2004.038240

Whiting, P., Maiwenn, Al, Burgers, L., Westwood, M., Ryder, S., Hoogendoorn, M., et al. (2014). Ivacaftor for the treatment of patients with cystic fibrosis and the G551D mutation: A systematic review and cost-effectiveness analysis. *Health Technol. Assess. (Rockv).* 18, 1–106. doi: 10.3310/hta18180

Woods, J. C., Wild, J. M., Wielpütz, M. O., Clancy, J. P., Hatabu, H., Kauczor, H., et al. (2019). Current state of the art MRI for the longitudinal assessment of cystic fibrosis. *J. Magn. Reson. Imaging* 10.1002, jmri.27030. doi: 10.1002/jmri.27030

Zemanick, E. T., Wagner, B. D., Robertson, C. E., Stevens, M. J., Szefler, S. J., Accurso, F. J., et al. (2015). Assessment of airway microbiota and inflammation in cystic fibrosis using multiple sampling methods. *Ann. Am. Thorac. Soc* 12, 221–229. doi: 10.1513/AnnalsATS.201407-310OC

7

Protective Effects of *Pterostilbene* on Lipopolysaccharide-Induced Acute Lung Injury in Mice by Inhibiting NF-κB and Activating Nrf2/HO-1 Signaling Pathways

Yong Zhang[1†], Zhen Han[1†], Aimin Jiang[1], Di Wu[1], Shuangqiu Li[1], Ziyi Liu[1], Zhengkai Wei[2], Zhengtao Yang[2] and Changming Guo[1*]*

[1]College of Veterinary Medicine, Jilin University, Changchun, China, [2]College of Life Sciences and Engineering, Foshan University, Foshan, China

***Correspondence:**
Zhengtao Yang
yangzhengtao01@sina.com
Changming Guo
guochm1980@163.com

†These authors have contributed equally to this work

Pterostilbene (PTER) is a kind of stilbene compound with biological activity isolated from plants such as red sandalwood, blueberry and grape. It has anti-tumor, anti-bacterial, anti-oxidation and other pharmacological activities. However, the underlying mechanism of the protective effect of PTER on lipopolysaccharide (LPS)-induced acute lung injury (ALI) remained not clarified. In this study, LPS was used to establish a mouse model of ALI. Bronchoalveolar lavage fluid (BALF) was collected for inflammatory cells, and the wet-to-dry weight ratio of the lungs was measured. The activities of myeloperoxidase (MPO), antioxidant indexes such as superoxide dismutase (SOD), catalase (CAT), glutathione peroxidase (GSH-Px) and oxidation index such as malondialdehyde (MDA) in lung tissues of mice were measured by the corresponding kits. The levels of Cyclooxygenase-2 (COX-2), inducible nitric oxide synthase (iNOS), TNF-α, IL-6 and IL-1β in lung tissues of mice were detected by quantitative real-time polymerase chain reaction (qRT-PCR). The activities of Nrf2, HO-1, p-p65 and *p*-IκB were determined by western blotting. The results showed that the model of LPS-induced ALI was successfully replicated, and it was found that PTER could significantly improve the pathological degree of ALI such as sustained the integrity of the lung tissue structure, alleviated pulmonary interstitial edema and alveolar wall thickening, reduced infiltrated inflammatory cells. PTER could decrease the number of inflammatory cells and obviously inhibit the increase of W/D ratio caused by LPS. PTER could also significantly reduce LPS-induced MPO and MDA, and increase LPS-decreased SOD, CAT and GSH-Px in the lungs. In addition, it was also found that PTER has the ability to decrease LPS-induced production of COX-2, iNOS, TNF-α, IL-6 and IL-1β. The underlying mechanism involved in the protective effect of PTER on ALI were via activating Nrf2 and HO-1, and inhibiting the phosphorylation of p65 and IκB. These results suggested that PTER can protect LPS-induced ALI in mice by inhibiting inflammatory response and oxidative stress, which provided evidence that PTER may be a potential therapeutic candidate for LPS-induced ALI intervention.

Keywords: pterostilbene, lipopolysaccharide, acute lung injury, inflammatory response, oxidative stress

INTRODUCTION

Acute lung injury (ALI) is a respiratory disease characterized by a large number of inflammatory cell infiltration, damage to alveolar epithelial cells and capillary endothelial cells, destruction of alveolar structure, pulmonary interstitial edema, marked thickening of alveolar walls, and acute hypoxic respiratory insufficiency. ALI can be caused by many factors including pulmonary infection caused by viruses, bacteria, fungi, inhalation injury caused by high concentration of oxygen and other harmful gases, seawater and other liquids, lung and chest wall trauma, sepsis and so on (Confalonieri et al., 2017; Matthay et al., 2017). If the condition is aggravated, it can further develop into Acute respiratory distress syndrome (ARDS) (Ware and Matthay, 2000). Due to the complex pathogenesis of the disease, it has not yet been fully elucidated, and there is no effective prevention and treatment method. For human patients, respiratory support technology (mainly including: small tidal volume ventilation, positive end expiratory pressure, prone position ventilation, high frequency oscillatory ventilation, extracorporeal lung membrane technology and so on) is currently the most important treatment for ALI in clinical practice (Amato et al., 1998). Some drugs, such as glucocorticoids and ulinastatin, have therapeutic effects on ALI, but they are not widely recommended in clinic due to more adverse reactions (Liu et al., 2013). For livestock and poultry, ALI is mostly caused by dirty and humid environment, mildew, dirty air, overcrowding and poor ventilation in livestock houses. The morbidity and mortality of livestock and poultry remain high, causing significant economic losses to the livestock industry, and seriously hindering the development of the livestock industry.

Nuclear factor-κB (NF-κB), as a transcription factor in organism, plays an important role in physiological and pathological processes, such as regulating inflammatory response and apoptosis (Wei et al., 2015; Wang J. et al., 2019). For example, classical inflammatory cytokines, TNF-α, IL-6 and IL-1β are regulated by NF-κB. Cyclooxygenase-2 (COX-2) and inducible nitric oxide synthase (iNOS) interact with and interact with NF-κB. Activation of the NF-κB signaling pathway can induce the expression of COX-2 and iNOS. These induced gene products can further participate in inflammation and immune response, and play an important role in physiological and pathological conditions (Fan et al., 2018). Lots of experiments have confirmed that under the stimulation of inflammatory factors such as lipopolysaccharide (LPS), NF-κB can be transferred from cytoplasm to nucleus, from inactive state to active structure, thus initiating gene transcription of various inflammatory mediators and chemokines at the transcriptional level, thus intensifying the degree and duration of inflammation (Huang et al., 2016). Nrf2 is a key factor in oxidative stress. Its activation energy regulates a variety of downstream antioxidant enzymes (such as HO-1, SOD, CAT, and GSH-Px) to eliminate excessive free radicals in the body, thereby reducing the degree and duration of oxidative stress (Zhao et al., 2014). Therefore, ALI can be prevented or treated in both anti-oxidative stress and anti-inflammatory by activating Nrf2 and inhibiting NF-κB signaling pathway.

Pure natural plant products have attracted wide attention for their remarkable efficacy and relatively low toxicity in the treatment of ALI. Therefore, the treatment of ALI with pure natural plant products is a valuable research direction and has great application prospects. *Pterostilbene* (3,5-Dimethoxy-4′-hydroxystilbene; **Figure 1A**) is a kind of stilbene compound extracted from small berries such as blueberries and grapes (Wang and Sang, 2018). It has been found that PTER has many biological effects such as anti-inflammatory (Paul et al., 2009) and anti-oxidative (Perecko et al., 2010) effects. Previous studies have shown that PTER and its compounds have protective effects against LPS-induced ALI (Park et al., 2018). However, the underlying mechanism involved in the protective effect of PTER on ALI are not completely clear. This study was designed to investigate the effects of PTER on LPS-induced ALI and to elucidate its molecular mechanisms.

MATERIALS AND METHODS

Chemicals and Reagents

PTER (SP9570, purity ≥98%) was purchased from Beijing Solarbio Science and Technology Co., Ltd. (Beijing, China). LPS (L2880, purity >97%) was purchased from the Sigma Chemical Co. (St. Louis, MO, United States). MPO (A044-1–1), SOD (A001-3–2), CAT (A007-1–1), GSH-Px (A005-1–2) and MDA (A003-1–2) Assay Kit and were purchased from Nanjing Jiancheng Bioengineering Institute (Nanjing, China). TNF-α, IL-6, IL-1β, COX-2 and iNOS primers were purchased from Sangon Biotech Co., Ltd. (Shanghai, China). p-p65 rabbit polyclonal antibody (A13599) was acquired from Boster Biological Technology co.ltd. p65 rabbit polyclonal antibody (BS9879M), *p*-IκB rabbit polyclonal antibody (BS4105), IκB rabbit polyclonal antibody (BS3601), Nrf2 rabbit polyclonal antibody (BS1258) and HO-1 rabbit polyclonal antibody (BS6626) were acquired from Bioworld Technology, Inc (Minnesota, United States). Actin-β polyclonal antibody (YT0099) was acquired from ImmunoWay Biotechnology Company (Plano, TX, United States). All other chemicals were at the reagent level.

Animals

Male BALB/c mice (4 weeks old; weight 18–20 g) were obtained from Liaoning Changsheng Biotechnology Co., Ltd (Liaoning, China). The initial weight of mice was shown in **Figure 1B**. Before the experiment, all mice were kept in a controlled environment with ambient temperature at 24 ± 1°C and humidity at 60 ± 5%, and a 12 h light/dark cycle was guaranteed. The mice were free to eat and drink, and adapted to the environment for one week. All the animal experiments were performed in accordance with the Animal Welfare and Research Ethics Committee at Jilin University (approval ID 20111106-2).

Establishment of Acute Lung Injury in Mice

All the mice were randomly divided into six groups (n = 6 per group). The six groups are Control group, LPS-induced ALI model group, LPS + PTER (10, 20, and 40 mg/kg) groups and LPS + DEX group. All the mice were fasted for 8 h, but they could

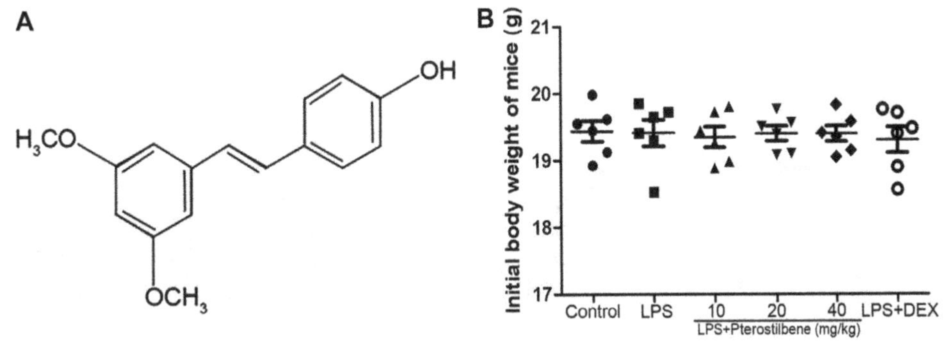

FIGURE 1 | (A) Chemical structure of PTER. **(B)** Initial weight of mice.

drink water freely. Before the establishment of the model of LPS-induced ALI, the LPS + PTER (10, 20, and 40 mg/kg) groups were given corresponding PTER concentrations, the mice of the LPS + DEX group were given DEX (5 mg/kg) and the Control group and the LPS-induce ALI model group were given equal volume of 0.9% NaCl solution. All the above administration methods were intraperitoneal injection (i.p.). 1 h later, all groups of mice were inhaled with a little of ether to make them slightly anesthetized. Except for the Control group, 10 μg LPS in 50 μl of 0.9% NaCl solution were injected into the nasal cavity of all groups of mice. And the mice of the Control group were given 50 μl of 0.9% NaCl solution in the same way. After treating the mice with LPS for 7 h, the mice were sacrificed by bloodletting and their lung tissues were collected.

Cell Count and Protein Concentration of Bronchoalveolar Lavage Fluid in Mice

After the mice were sacrificed, the skin of the larynx was cut to expose the trachea, the catheter was inserted into the trachea from the mouth, and the trachea and the catheter were tied tightly with a surgical thread. Slowly rinsed with PBS solution three times, 500 μl each time, 1.5 ml in total, the washing fluid was BALF, and then the collected BALF was centrifuged at 4°C 3 000 rpm for 10 min, the supernatant was used to determine the protein concentration by BCA method, and the resulting precipitate was resuspended in PBS solution. The number of total cells, neutrophils and macrophages was measured with a blood cell analyzer instrument (Japan Photoelectric MEK-7222 K Whole Blood Cell Analyzer).

Measurement of Wet-To-Dry Ratio of the Lungs

The whole lungs were removed, washed with PBS solution for three times, and then the water on the surface of the lungs was dried with absorbent paper and weighed immediately, that is, the wet weight. Then they were put into the incubator, baked at 80°C for 48 h, and then weighed again, that is, the dry weight, and then the ratio of wet weight to dry weight (W/D) was calculated.

Histopathological Analysis

The right lungs were removed and placed in 10% formaldehyde solution and fixed for 24 h. Then, the lung tissues were treated with different concentrations of alcohol to dehydrate and wrapped in paraffin. Finally, the obtained lung tissue sections were stained with hematoxylin and eosin, and the histopathological changes of the lung tissues were observed with an optical microscope, and the images were collected.

Superoxide Dismutase, Catalase, Glutathione Peroxidase, and Malondialdehyde Analysis

According to the manufacturer's protocols, the GSH-Px, CAT, SOD and MDA contents in lung tissues of mice were determined by GSH-Px, CAT, SOD and MDA assay kits.

Quantitative Real-Time Polymerase Chain Reaction Analysis Cytokines in Lung Tissue

This experiment was designed to detect the expression of RNA of COX-2, iNOS, TNF-α, IL-6 and IL-1β in lung tissue as previous described (Wei et al., 2015). Total RNA was extracted from lung tissues of mice in each group by Trizol reagent. Then the extracted RNA was reverse transcribed into cDNA. qRT-PCR was carried out with a 7,500 real-time PCR system (Applied

TABLE 1 | Primers used in this study.

Primer name	Nucleotide sequence (5'-3')
TNF-α forward	ACGGGCTTTACCTCATCTACTC
TNF-α reverse	GCTCTTGATGGCAGACAGG
IL-6 forward	AGTTGTGCAATGGCAATTCTGA
IL-6 reverse	CCCCAGCATCGAAGGTAGA
IL-1β forward	AGGTGGTGTCGGTCATCGT
IL-1β reverse	GCTCTCTGTCCTGGAGTTTGC
COX-2 forwad	ATTCCAAACCAGCAGACTCATA
COX-2 reverse	CTTGAGTTTGAAGTGGTAACCG
iNOS forward	TGCCACGGACGAGACGGATAG
iNOS reverse	CTCTTCAAGCACCTCCAGGAACG
GAPDH forward	TCAACGGGAAGCTCACTGG
GAPDH reverse	CCCCAGCATCGAAGGTAGA

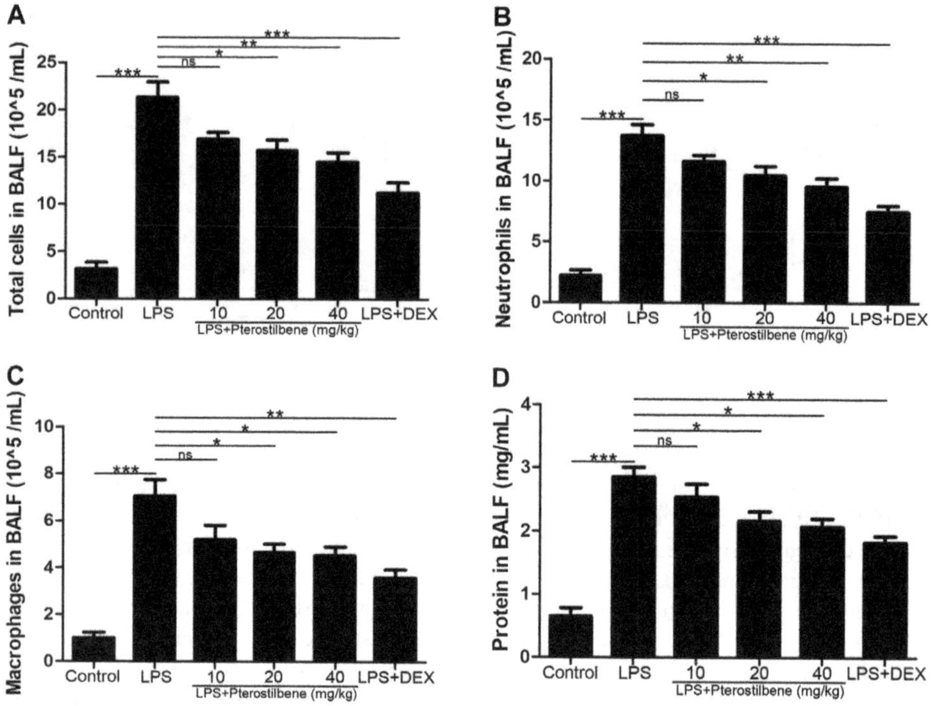

FIGURE 2 | PTER reduced LPS-induced the number of inflammatory cells and protein concentration in BALF. **(A)** Total cells in BALF. **(B)** Neutrophils in BALF. **(C)** Macrophages in BALF. **(D)** Protein concentration in BALF. Values are presented as mean ± SEM (*n* = 6). *p* values of <0.05 were considered significant (**p* < 0.05; ***p* < 0.01; ****p* < 0.001; "ns" means not significant).

Biosystems, Carlsbad, CA). Primers were obtained from Sangon Biotech Co., Ltd. (Shanghai, China) and were listed in **Table 1**.

Western Blot Analysis

According to the manufacturer's protocols as previous described (Wei et al., 2018b; Liu et al., 2019; Wei et al., 2019), the total protein in the lung tissues were extracted with tissue total protein lysis buffer. The concentration of total protein was determined by BCA method. The obtained total protein samples were separated by SDS-polyacrylamide gel electrophoresis (SDS-PAGE) and transferred to polyvinylidene difluoride (PVDF) membranes. Then the PVDF membranes were put into TBST solution containing 5% skimmed milk powder and blocked for 3 h at room temperature. Then the PVDF membranes were incubated overnight with the corresponding antibody at 4°C. The PVDF membranes were washed with TBST solution and then incubated at room temperature for 2 h with appropriate horseradish peroxidase (HRP)-conjugated secondary antibodies. Then the PVDF membranes were washed with TBST solution. Finally, the PVDF membranes were treated with Immobilon Western Chemiluminescent HRP Substrate, the proteins were observed by enhanced chemiluminescence (ECL) under Western Blotting Detection System (Amersham Life Science, United Kingdom). We used ImageJ software to analyze strips.

Statistical Analysis

The experimental data were analyzed by GraphPad Prism 5.0 software, and the results were expressed by mean ± SEM (Standard Error of Mean). In data analysis, one-way ANOVA was used to compare the data between groups, and LSD was used to make multiple comparisons. $p < 0.05$ or $p < 0.01$ showed significant or extremely significant statistical differences, respectively.

RESULTS

Pterostilbene Reduced Lipopolysaccharide-Induced the Number of Inflammatory Cells and Protein Concentration in Bronchoalveolar Lavage Fluid

In order to confirm the effect of PTER on inflammatory cells in BALF with LPS-induced ALI, BALF was collected to count the number of total cells, neutrophils and macrophages. Compared with control group, the number of total cells (**Figure 2A**), neutrophils (**Figure 2B**), and macrophages (**Figure 2C**) in BALF in the LPS-induced model group increased significantly, while PTER pretreatment reduced the infiltration of these inflammatory cells into the lung tissue. Moreover, compared with control group, the protein concentration in BALF in the LPS-induced model group increased significantly, while PTER pretreatment reduced the protein concentration in BALF (**Figure 2D**). These results suggested that PTER could inhibit the migration of inflammatory cells to lung tissue, thereby reducing LPS-induced inflammatory responses of in ALI.

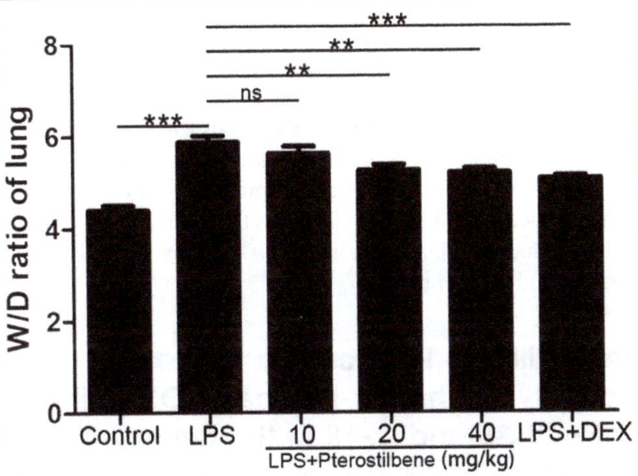

FIGURE 3 | PTER reduced LPS-increased W/D ratio of the lungs. Values are presented as mean ± SEM (n = 6). p values of <0.05 were considered significant (**p < 0.01; ***p < 0.001; "ns" means not significant).

Pterostilbene Reduced Lipopolysaccharide–Increased W/D Ratio of the Lungs

The W/D ratio of the lungs can reflect the degree of edema in LPS-induced ALI model in mice. As shown in **Figure 3**, compared with control group, the W/D ratio increased significantly after LPS stimulation. After DEX treatment, the increase in W/D ratio caused by LPS stimulation was significantly inhibited. When the PTER concentration was 10 mg/kg, it had no obvious inhibitory effect on the increase of W/D value caused by LPS, and when the concentration of PTER increased to 20 and 40 mg/kg, it could obviously inhibit the increase of W/D ratio caused by LPS. The result showed that PTER could significantly reduce the degree of the lungs edema in LPS-induced ALI model in mice.

Pterostilbene Attenuated Lipopolysaccharide-Induced Histopathological Changes in the Lungs

The lung tissues of mice were stained with H&E to observe the pathological changes, and the protective effect of PTER on LPS-induced ALI was revealed intuitively. Compared with control group (**Figure 4A**), the lung tissue of mice in LPS-induced ALI model group (**Figure 4B**) showed obvious and unique pathological changes, such as smaller alveolar cavity, alveolar structure destruction, thicker alveolar septum, congestion and edema of alveolar wall, and a large number of inflammatory cell infiltration. Compared with the LPS-induced ALI model group, the lung tissue structure of mice in LPS + PTER (10, 20, and 40 mg/kg) group (**Figures 4C–E**) and LPS + DEX group (**Figure 4F**) tended to be normal, pulmonary interstitial edema and alveolar wall thickening were alleviated, inflammation was reduced, and inflammatory cells were decreased. These results suggest that PTER has a protective effect on LPS-induced ALI in a dose-dependent manner.

Pterostilbene Reduced Lipopolysaccharide-Induced Myeloperoxidase in the Lungs

MPO activity is an effective indicator of neutrophil influx into lung tissue. As shown in **Figure 5**, LPS significantly increased MPO activity in the lungs of mice. Compared with LPS model group, PTER (10, 20, and 40 mg/kg) and DEX decreased MPO activity. These data suggested that PTER can reduce the activity of MPO in the lungs of mice in a dose-dependent manner.

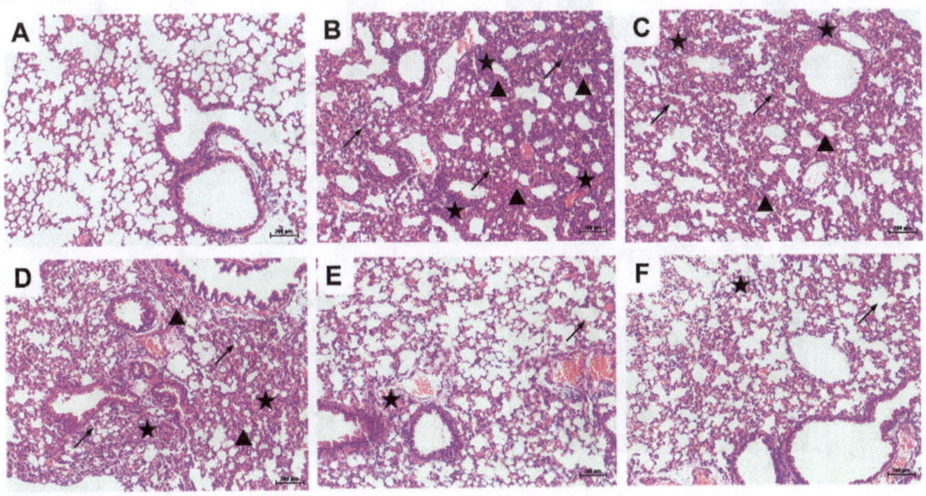

FIGURE 4 | PTER attenuated LPS-induced histopathological changes in the lungs (100×). Mice treated with **(A)** 0.9% NaCl solution **(B)** LPS + 0.9% NaCl solution **(C)** LPS + PTER 10 mg/kg **(D)** LPS + PTER 20 mg/kg **(E)** LPS + PTER 40 mg/kg **(F)** LPS + DEX 5 mg/kg. The stars show a large number of inflammatory cells infiltrating, the triangles show thickening of alveolar septum, and the arrows show destruction of alveolar structure.

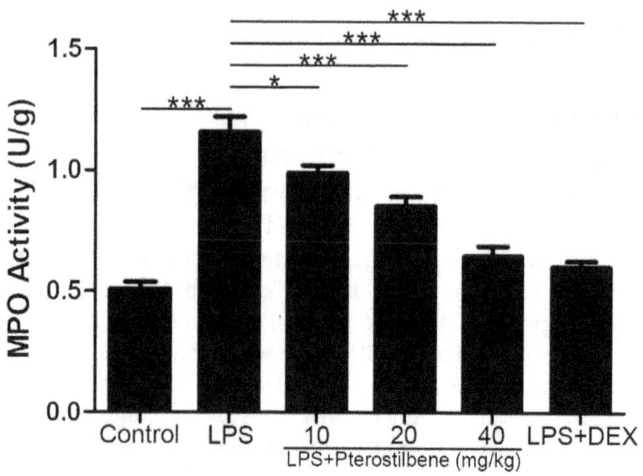

FIGURE 5 | PTER reduced LPS-induced MPO in the lungs. Values are presented as mean ± SEM (n = 6). p values of <0.05 were considered significant ($^*p < 0.05$; $^{***}p < 0.001$).

Pterostilbene Increased Superoxide Dismutase, Catalase, Glutathione Peroxidase, and Induced Malondialdehyde in the Lungs

MDA is an important indicator of oxidative stress, and SOD, CAT, and GSH-Px are important indicators of antioxidant stress. Through the determination of these indicators, it was verified that PTER can protect LPS-induced ALI in mice through anti-oxidative stress. The results showed that MDA increased significantly in mice exposed to LPS. MDA levels in LPS + PTER (10, 20, and 40 mg/kg) group and LPS + DEX group were significantly lower than those in LPS-induced ALI model groups (**Figure 6D**). In addition, LPS stimulation reduced the activities of SOD, CAT and GSH-Px. Treatment with PTER (10, 20 and 40 mg/kg) and DEX significantly increased SOD, CAT and GSH-Px levels in lung tissue of mice (**Figures 6A–C**). The results showed that PTER could protect mice from LPS-induced ALI by reducing MDA, increasing SOD, CAT and GSH-Px in a dose-dependent manner.

Pterostilbene Reduced Lipopolysaccharide-Induced COX-2, iNOS, TNF-α, IL-6 and IL-1β in the Lungs

Inflammatory cytokines and oxidative stress are involved in the initiation and expansion of inflammation and persist in LPS-induced ALI. We measured the levels of cytokines in lung tissue of mice by qRT-PCR.

In terms of oxidative stress, the result showed that compared with control group, LPS significantly increased the production of two important pro-inflammatory enzymes COX-2 and iNOS in lung tissue. In addition, PTER significantly inhibited COX-2 and iNOS induced by LPS (**Figures 7A, B**), which confirmed its good anti- oxidative stress activity *in vivo*. The results showed that PTER could protect mice from LPS-induced ALI by inhibiting the release of COX-2 and iNOS in a dose-dependent manner.

In terms of inflammation, the result showed that compared with control group, LPS significantly increased TNF-α, IL-6 and IL-1β in lung tissue. On the other hand, PTER significantly reduced the secretion of cytokines TNF-α, IL-6 and IL-1β

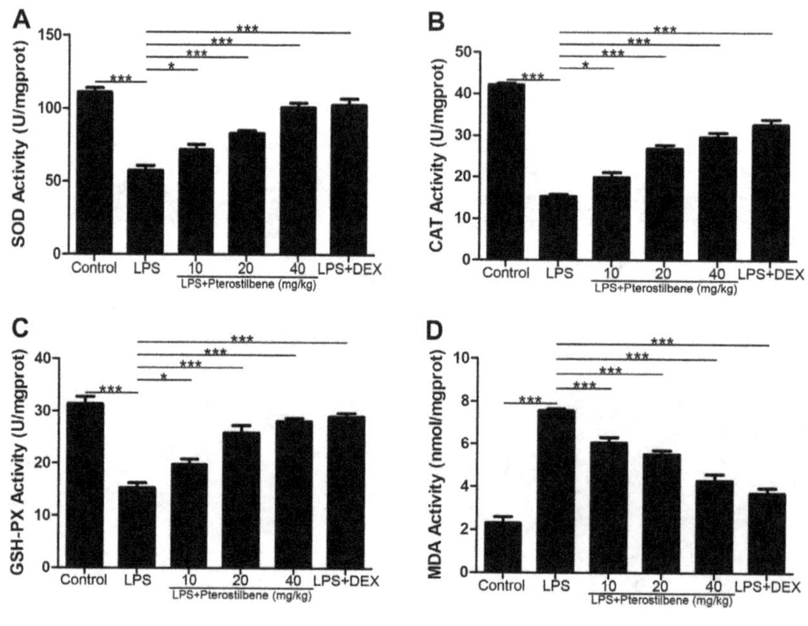

FIGURE 6 | PTER increased SOD, CAT, and GSH-Px and reduced MDA in the lungs. **(A)** SOD activity of lung tissues in mice. **(B)** CAT activity of lung tissues in mice. **(C)** GSH-Px activity of lung tissues in mice **(D)** MDA activity of lung tissues in mice. Values are presented as mean ± SEM (n = 6). p values of <0.05 were considered significant ($^*p < 0.05$; $^{***}p < 0.001$).

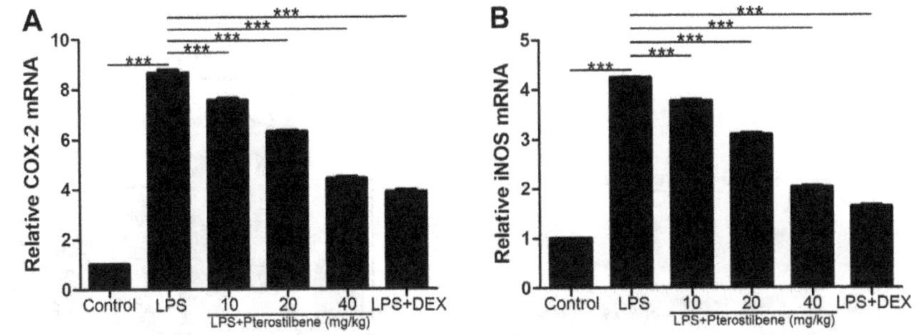

FIGURE 7 | PTER reduced LPS-induced COX-2 and iNOS in the lungs. The relative **(A)** COX-2 and **(B)** iNOS expressions of lung tissues in mice were evaluated by qRT-PCR. Values are presented as mean ± SEM (n = 6). p values of <0.05 were considered significant (***$p < 0.001$).

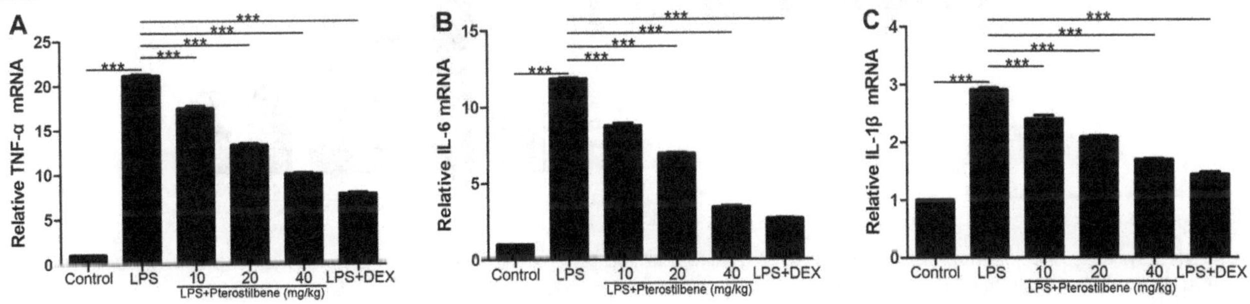

FIGURE 8 | PTER reduced LPS-induced TNF-α, IL-6 and IL-1β in the lungs. The relative **(A)** TNF-α **(B)** IL-6 and **(C)** IL-1β expressions of lung tissues in mice were evaluated by qRT-PCR. Values are presented as mean ± SEM (n = 6). p values of <0.05 were considered significant (***$p < 0.001$).

induced by LPS (**Figures 8A–C**), which confirmed its good anti-inflammatory activity *in vivo*. The results showed that PTER could protect mice from LPS-induced ALI by inhibiting the release of TNF-α, IL-6 and IL-1β in a dose-dependent manner.

Pterostilbene Inhibited the Protein Expressions of NF-κB Signaling Pathway in the Lungs

NF-κB signaling pathway has long been considered as a typical inflammatory signaling pathway. As shown in **Figure 9**, compared with control group, LPS-induced ALI model group significantly promoted the expression of p-p65 and *p*-IκB. Compared with LPS-induced ALI model group, LPS + PTER (10, 20, and 40 mg/kg) group and LPS + DEX group significantly inhibited the expression of p-p65 and *p*-IκB, and the degree of inhibition increased with the increase of PTER concentration in a dose-dependent manner. The results showed that the protective effect of PTER on LPS-induced ALI in mice was related to inhibition of p-p65 and *p*-IκB expression.

Pterostilbene Activated the Protein Expressions of Nrf2/HO-1 Signaling Pathway in the Lungs

Nrf2 is an activator of the antioxidant response element ARE and is considered to be the core transcription factor regulating the antioxidant stress response. As shown in **Figure 10**, compared with control group, the expression of Nrf2 and HO-1 in lung tissue of LPS-induced ALI model group was significantly lower. Compared with LPS-induced ALI model group, the expression of Nrf2 and HO-1 in lung tissue of LPS + PTER (10, 20, and 40 mg/kg) group and LPS + DEX group increased significantly in a dose-dependent manner with the increase of PTER concentration. The results showed that the protective effect of PTER on LPS-induced ALI in mice was related to up-regulation of Nrf2 and HO-1 expression.

DISCUSSION

ALI is a serious respiratory disease in animal feeding process, which seriously threatens the life safety of sick livestock and poultry. LPS is a component of the cell wall of Gram-negative bacteria and it is also an important stimulator triggering inflammation in the body (Bhattacharyya et al., 2004). Intranasal instillation of LPS is a classical and widely used method to construct ALI model (Hsu et al., 2015; Huang et al., 2015). This method can better simulate the pathological process of ALI, control the degree of ALI, only cause local severe injury, and will not cause systemic inflammatory response and organ failure (Santos et al., 2018). Recently, a study has confirmed that PTER can protect female mice in this ALI model (Yang et al.,

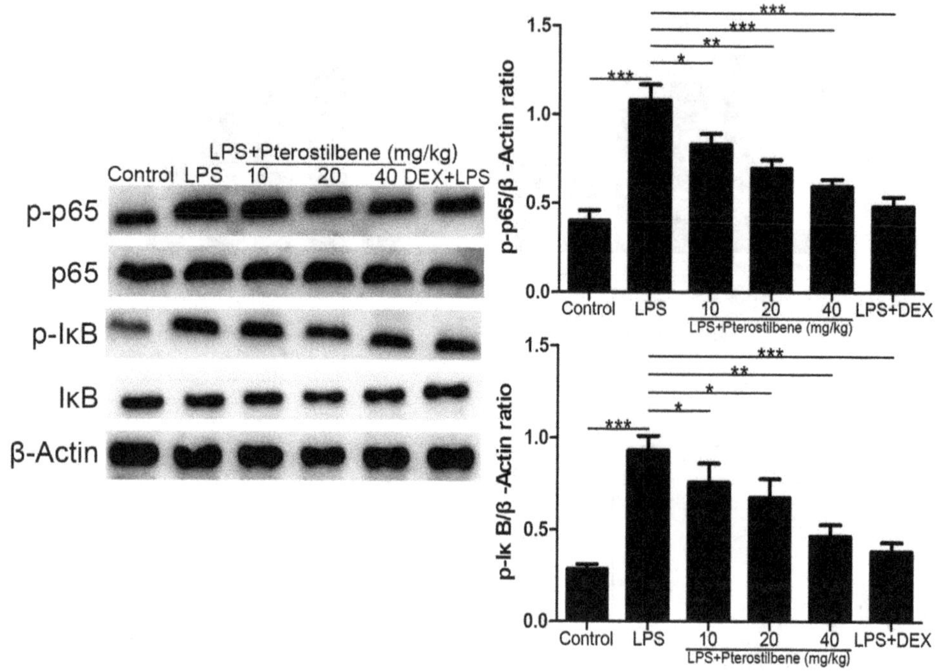

FIGURE 9 | PTER inhibited the protein expressions of NF-κB signaling pathway in the lungs. Values are presented as mean ± SEM (n = 6). p values of <0.05 were considered significant (*p < 0.05; **p < 0.01; ***p < 0.001).

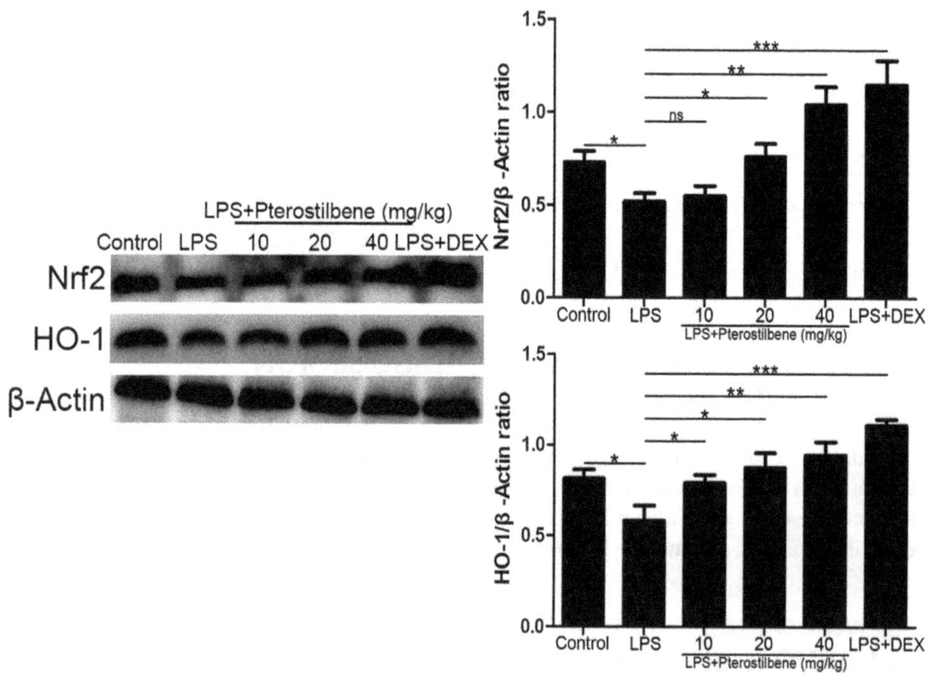

FIGURE 10 | PTER activated the protein expressions of Nrf2/HO-1 signaling pathway in the lungs. Values are presented as mean ± SEM (n = 6). p values of <0.05 were considered significant (*p < 0.05; **p < 0.01; ***p < 0.001; "ns" means not significant).

2020). However, the protective effect of PTER in male mice has not been fully investigated. Therefore, adult male mice are used in this study to establish ALI model and evaluate the protective effect of *pterostilbene* in male mice.

Dexamethasone (DEX) is a synthetic glucocorticoid that has been widely used to reduce various inflammatory reactions and has significant effects. However, under normal circumstances, the hormone content in the body is extremely small, which can regulate metabolism, growth and development and other physiological activities. Once the body ingests hormones for a long time, it will inevitably have some toxic and side effects on the body. For example, long-term use of DEX can easily lead to osteoporosis, abnormal mental symptoms, disorder of material metabolism and water and salt metabolism of the body. After DEX is stopped, it will also produce such adverse symptoms as anorexia, vomiting, fatigue, muscle and joint pain. PTER is derived from small berry plants and belongs to natural structural compounds. It has anti-inflammatory and anti-oxidant effects, and has the advantages of small toxic and side effects, low drug resistance, and not easy to remain. Previous experiments had proved that PTER had protective effect on ALI (Park et al., 2018), but the underlying mechanism is still unclear. The purpose of this study is to reveal the specific protective mechanism of PTER on ALI. At the same time, this experiment also set up LPS + DEX group, compared the protective effect of PTER with that of DEX, in order to evaluate the protective effect of PTER on LPS-induced ALI. With the development of new drugs, it is essential to appropriately transfer the dosage of the drugs from one animal species to another. In this study, we explored the protective mechanism of PTER on LPS-induced ALI in mice at these concentrations (10, 20, and 40 mg/kg). According to the concentrations of PTER in mice, we can calculate the effective concentrations of PTER in poultry, livestock and other economic animals, even in human body through the drug dose conversion formula between different animals, which can provide reference and basis for the use concentrations of PTER in veterinary and human clinical treatment of ALI, which has certain reference value and significance. For humans, the conversion formula is as follows: Human Equivalent Dose (HED) = Animal dose (mg/kg) × [Animal *Km*/Human *Km*]. *Km* factor = Animal weight/Animal body surface area. *Km* Mouse *Km* = 3, Human *Km* = 37 (Reagan-Shaw et al., 2008). In this study, the most effective concentration in mice is 40 mg/kg, so it can be calculated that HED = 40 mg/kg × 3/37 = 3.24 mg/kg. The formula is also applicable to the conversion of drug dosage between different animals.

In the process of drug research and development, its drug metabolism in the body is very important. Through the study of its metabolism, many pharmacokinetic data can be understood and obtained to prepare for large-scale clinical research. The chemical structure of *pterostilbene* contains two benzene rings and one conjugated double bond, which has good UV absorption. UV absorption detector is generally used for *in vitro* analysis, and MS method with higher sensitivity is selected for *in vivo* analysis. Shao et al. (2010) gave *pterostilbene* solution (200 mg/kg-1, DMSO) to mice by gavage. Urine was collected 24 h later. The metabolites of *pterostilbene* in mouse urine were studied by LC/APCI-MS/MS method. It has been found that nine new metabolites of *pterostilbene* have been identified by MSn which are sulfated or glucuronized metabolites, such as *pterostilbene* glucuronide, *pterostilbene* sulfate, mono-demethylated *pterostilbene* glucuronide, mono-demethylated *pterostilbene* sulfate, mono-hydroxylated *pterostilbene*, mono-hydroxylated *pterostilbene* glucuronide, mono-hydroxylated *pterostilbene* sulfate, and mono-hydroxylated *pterostilbene* glucuronide sulfate. Lin et al. (2009) conducted a pharmacokinetic study on intravenous and oral *pterostilbene* in SD rats and found that the half-life and clearance rate of *pterostilbene* intravenously were (96.6 ± 23.7) min and (37.0 ± 2.5) min. The bioavailability of the drug is (72.5 ± 4.7) %, which may be due to the first pass effect reducing the blood content of *pterostilbene*. Remsberg et al. (2008) analyzed the pharmacokinetics of *pterostilbene* in rats. After fasting for 12 h, the rats were injected intravenously with *pterostilbene* at 20 mg/kg. Regular blood samples are collected through intubation. *Pterostilbene* was quickly removed from the serum (t 1/2 = 1.73 h). Within 30 min, the concentration of *pterostilbene* dropped from about 100 μg/ml to about 2 μg/ml. Glucuronate appeared in the earliest sample, that is, 1 min, about 6 μg/ml. Glucuronic acid increases slightly at about 1–2 h, indicating enterohepatic circulation. The methods they used to determine the concentration of *pterostilbene* and its metabolites were high performance liquid chromatography tandem mass spectrometry (LC-MS/MS). But the conditions of our laboratory could not finish the experiments of levels of *pterostilbene* and its metabolites in plasma/serum/tissue (lungs), we only discussed it here.

LPS-induced ALI can cause pulmonary edema, the volume and weight of lung tissue increase, which is one of the main characteristics of acute lung injury (Zhang et al., 2009). The W/D value of lung tissue was calculated to objectively evaluate the degree of pulmonary edema. The higher the W/D value, the more serious the pulmonary edema. In addition, in LPS. In addition, in LPS induced ALI, a large number of neutrophils to the lung tissue and participate in the inflammatory reaction. By counting the total cells, neutrophils and macrophages in the BALF, it was more fully confirmed that PTER reduced the number of neutrophils in the inflammatory site, which indicated that PTER could inhibit the migration of neutrophils to lung tissue, thereby reducing the inflammatory injury of lung tissue.

ROS plays a dual role in the biological activities of organisms (Wei et al., 2018a; Wei et al., 2018c; Wang C. et al., 2019; Yan et al., 2020). In the low physiological state, it can be used as a signaling molecule to participate in processes such as cell division, apoptosis and immune response (Han et al., 2019). The removal of excess ROS by related enzymes maintains this relatively stable state. Under pathological conditions, ROS clearance is inhibited and causes accumulation in cells. Hydroxyl radicals can react with purine, pyrimidine and deoxyribose skeletons in DNA molecules, destroying DNA structure, and oxidative damage to unsaturated fatty acids Oxide MDA. ROS also oxidizes cysteine and methionine residues in protein structures, resulting in the formation of reversible disulfide bonds between protein sulfhydryl groups and GSH, affecting the binding of GSH to electrophiles. An oxidative stress reaction occurred. ROS in the body are mainly cleared by antioxidant enzymes, including SOD, CAT and GSH-Px. After being reduced to H_2O_2 by SOD, it continues to generate H_2O under the action of CAT and GSH-Px, and is excreted from the body, thereby eliminating ROS and protecting the body from oxidative attack. SOD is the only enzyme in the body that can remove O_2^-. It plays an important role in cell protection. The level of oxidative stress can be reflected by these indicators: MPO is a marker of neutrophil aggregation, which itself and a large number of oxidants derived from MPO can cause tissue damage (Xie et al., 2018). MDA is a product of lipid peroxidation, which is often used to reflect the level of oxidative stress (Jiang et al., 2016). SOD, CAT and GSH-Px are three important antioxidants in the body, which will be consumed heavily under oxidative stress (Manca et al., 1991; Annapurna et al., 2013). Therefore, we measured the above indicators in the experiment. The results showed that PTER had good antioxidant activity in LPS-induced ALI model: PTER significantly inhibited the production of MPO and MDA in lung tissue of LPS-induced mice, and significantly increased the contents of SOD, CAT, and GSH-Px.

In response to oxidative stress damage, the body has developed a complex oxidative stress response system. One of the defense mechanisms is the antioxidant response element ARE, which is a *cis*-enhancing element in the upstream of phase II detoxification enzymes and a variety of antioxidant protein/enzyme genes. Recent studies have found that nuclear transcription-related factor Nrf2 is an activator of ARE, and is considered to be the core transcription factor regulating antioxidant stress response (Zhang et al., 2017). It is a receptor of exogenous toxic substances and oxidative stress. It is closely related to the occurrence and development of inflammation, respiratory diseases, malignant tumors, precancerous lesions and cardiovascular diseases (Kansanen et al., 2013; Milani et al., 2013). Normally, Nrf2 binds to Keap1, a specific receptor in the cytoplasm, in the form of heterodimer, which is activated under oxidative stress, decouples with Keap1, translocates into the nucleus, binds to ARE, and then activates the transcription of ARE-mediated target genes and promotes the release of SOD, CAT, and GSH-Px to increase cell resistance to oxidative stress (Kitaoka et al., 2013; Gan and Johnson, 2014). Many Nrf2-related target genes such as HO-1 are expressed in the lungs. HO-1, also known as heat shock protein 32, is an endogenous antioxidant enzyme that attracts much attention. Studies have shown that HO-1 and related products of heme metabolism can play an antioxidant stress role. Targeted activation of HO-1 can prevent the occurrence and development of ALI (Park et al., 2018). In this study, the expression of Nrf2 and HO-1 in lung tissue of mice 7 h after ALI model was established, and the role and signaling pathways of oxidative stress in the pathogenesis of ALI were analyzed. The results showed that the expression of Nrf2 and HO-1 in lung tissue of the LPS-induced model group was lower than that of the Control group. It is suggested that oxidative stress may reduce the expression of antioxidant protein HO-1 by interfering with Nrf2-ARE signaling pathway, thus reducing the resistance of lung cells to oxidative stress and leading to ALI.

Nuclear factor NF-κB signaling pathway has long been considered as a typical inflammatory signaling pathway. Because it regulates gene expression of inflammatory factors, chemokines and adhesion molecules, it is often used as a key target of anti-inflammatory drug intervention in experiments (Shen et al., 2009). NF-κB is widely distributed in organisms. It can regulate the growth, differentiation, inflammation and apoptosis of all cells. Numerous experiments have proved that the NF-κB signaling pathway can indeed regulate the production of pro-inflammatory cytokines and induce leukocyte aggregation (Li et al., 2018). Through feedback mechanism, it can continuously activate leukocytes to induce systemic inflammatory response, and directly affect the intensity and duration of inflammatory response. It has also been shown that the apoptotic function of NF-κB can prevent the spread of inflammation by promoting leukocyte apoptosis, maintaining the survival of epithelial cells and the integrity of mucosal barrier (Andonegui et al., 2002). Future research needs to assess the different roles of NF-κB and their respective cellular signaling pathways in different disease states, and to intervene effectively with this goal, which may open up new ideas for the treatment of inflammatory diseases. Inflammation is usually considered as the main adaptive response. In classical inflammatory signaling pathways, NF-κB can be stimulated by extracellular pathogenic factors, such as endotoxin (LPS), oxygen free radicals, radiation and other stimulating factors (Yang et al., 2012), which can induce the activation of NF-κB signaling pathway, change the conformation of NF-κB in resting state, dissociate from complex state, transfer from cytoplasm to nucleus, and correspond to it in nucleus. The specific binding of κB loci on the gene regulates the expression of genes related to inflammatory mediators (Perkins, 2007). After the activation of the NF-κB signaling pathway, it can enhance the transcription of TNF-α, IL-6 and IL-1β genes. With the increase in the production and release of TNF-α, IL-6 and IL-1β, the NF-κB signaling pathway is activated again, resulting in further amplification of the initial inflammatory signal, exacerbating body damage and microcirculation disorders, ALI can aggravate the conversion to ARDS. COX-2 and iNOS are two important signaling protein molecules in the NF-κB signaling pathway. Under physiological conditions, the activity of iNOS and COX-2 in most tissues is almost not expressed; both can be rapidly induced and expressed under pathological conditions. The promoter sequence of COX-2 contains a specific binding sequence of NF-κB, which can promote the transcription of COX-2 gene after binding to NF-κB. iNOS and COX-2 coordinate with each other, directly damage the DNA and protein of cells, and play an important role in activating NF-κB. At present, many *in vivo* and *in vitro* experiments have shown that PTER can play a powerful anti-inflammatory role by inhibiting the NF-κB signaling pathway, which can mediate the regulation of a variety of inflammatory mediators, including COX-2, iNOS, TNF-α, IL-6 and IL-1β and so on (Cichocki et al., 2008; Zhang and Zhang, 2016; Yao et al., 2018). It was found that p-p65 and *p*-IκB proteins in lung tissue of ALI mice were significantly higher than those in blank group. Inhibiting the activity of NF-κB signaling pathway by PTER could significantly reduce the degree of inflammatory reaction in lung tissue, indicating that controlling the NF-κB signaling pathway is an important link in preventing ALI and preventing disease progression. Therefore, inhibiting the NF-κB signaling pathway is a feasible way to prevent ALI.

In conclusion, our study has shown that PTER can significantly protect LPS-induced ALI in mice, significantly inhibit LPS-caused histopathological changes, the number of inflammatory cells in BALF, and the increase of W/D ratio. PTER can improve the antioxidant capacity of lung tissue and reduce the inflammatory cytokines induced by LPS, and play a protective in LPS-induced ALI through regulating Nrf2/HO-1 and NF-κB signaling pathways. All these results indicate that PTER may be a drug to prevent ALI and has broad prospects.

ETHICS STATEMENT

The animal study was reviewed and approved by Animal Welfare and Research Ethics Committee at Jilin University.

AUTHOR CONTRIBUTIONS

YZ, ZH, AJ, DW, SL, and ZL assisted in carrying out the experiment. YZ wrote the manuscript. ZW, ZY, and CG helped with the design of experimental ideas and the revision of manuscripts.

REFERENCES

Amato, M. B., Barbas, C. S., Medeiros, D. M., Magaldi, R. B., Schettino, G. P., Lorenzi-Filho, G., et al. (1998). Effect of a protective-ventilation strategy on mortality in the acute respiratory distress syndrome. *N. Engl. J. Med.* 338 (6), 347–354. doi:10.1056/nejm199802053380602

Andonegui, G., Goyert, S. M., and Kubes, P. (2002). Lipopolysaccharide-induced leukocyte-endothelial cell interactions: a role for CD14 versus toll-like receptor 4 within microvessels. *J. Immunol.* 169 (4), 2111–2119. doi:10.4049/jimmunol.169.4.2111

Annapurna, A., Ansari, M. A., and Manjunath, P. M. (2013). Partial role of multiple pathways in infarct size limiting effect of quercetin and rutin against cerebral ischemia reperfusion injury in rats. *Eur. Rev. Med. Pharmacol. Sci.* 17 (4), 491–500

Bhattacharyya, J., Biswas, S., and Datta, A. G. (2004). Mode of action of endotoxin: role of free radicals and antioxidants. *Curr. Med. Chem.* 11 (3), 359–368. doi:10.2174/0929867043456098

Cichocki, M., Paluszczak, J., Szaefer, H., Piechowiak, A., Rimando, A. M., and Baer-Dubowska, W. (2008). Pterostilbene is equally potent as resveratrol in inhibiting 12-O-tetradecanoylphorbol-13-acetate activated NFkappaB, AP-1, COX-2, and iNOS in mouse epidermis. *Mol. Nutr. Food Res.* 52, S62–S70. doi:10.1002/mnfr.200700466

Confalonieri, M., Salton, F., and Fabiano, F. (2017). Acute respiratory distress syndrome. *Eur. Respir. Rev.* 26 (144), 160116. doi:10.1183/16000617.0116-2016

Fan, L., Fan, Y., Liu, L., Tao, W., Shan, X., Dong, Y., et al. (2018). Chelerythrine attenuates the inflammation of lipopolysaccharide-induced acute lung inflammation through NF-κB signaling pathway mediated by Nrf2. *Front. Pharmacol.* 9, 1047. doi:10.3389/fphar.2018.01047

Gan, L., and Johnson, J. A. (2014). Oxidative damage and the Nrf2-ARE pathway in neurodegenerative diseases. *Biochim. Biophys. Acta.* 1842 (8), 1208–1218. doi:10.1016/j.bbadis.2013.12.011

Han, Z., Zhang, Y., Wang, C., Liu, X., Jiang, A., Liu, Z., et al. (2019). Ochratoxin A-triggered chicken heterophil extracellular traps release through reactive oxygen species production dependent on activation of NADPH oxidase, ERK, and p38 MAPK signaling pathways. *J. Agric. Food Chem.* 67 (40), 11230–11235. doi:10.1021/acs.jafc.9b03155

Hsu, A. T., Barrett, C. D., DeBusk, G. M., Ellson, C. D., Gautam, S., Talmor, D. S., et al. (2015). Kinetics and role of plasma matrix metalloproteinase-9 expression in acute lung injury and the acute respiratory distress syndrome. *Shock* 44 (2), 128–136. doi:10.1097/shk.0000000000000386

Huang, X., Liu, Y., Lu, Y., and Ma, C. (2015). Anti-inflammatory effects of eugenol on lipopolysaccharide-induced inflammatory reaction in acute lung injury via regulating inflammation and redox status. *Int. Immunopharm.* 26 (1), 265–271. doi:10.1016/j.intimp.2015.03.026

Huang, W. C., Lai, C. L., Liang, Y. T., Hung, H. C., Liu, H. C., and Liou, C. J. (2016). Phloretin attenuates LPS-induced acute lung injury in mice via modulation of the NF-κB and MAPK pathways. *Int. Immunopharm.* 40, 98–105. doi:10.1016/j.intimp.2016.08.035

Jiang, W., Luo, F., Lu, Q., Liu, J., Li, P., Wang, X., et al. (2016). The protective effect of Trillin LPS-induced acute lung injury by the regulations of inflammation and oxidative state. *Chem. Biol. Interact.* 243, 127–134. doi:10.1016/j.cbi.2015.09.010

Kansanen, E., Kuosmanen, S. M., Leinonen, H., and Levonen, A. L. (2013). The Keap1-Nrf2 pathway: mechanisms of activation and dysregulation in cancer. *Redox Biol.* 1 (1), 45–49. doi:10.1016/j.redox.2012.10.001

Kitaoka, Y., Ogborn, D. I., Nilsson, M. I., Mocellin, N. J., MacNeil, L. G., and Tarnopolsky, M. A. (2013). Oxidative stress and Nrf2 signaling in McArdle disease. *Mol. Genet. Metabol.* 110 (3), 297–302. doi:10.1016/j.ymgme.2013.06.022

Li, W., Zhao, R., Wang, X., Liu, F., Zhao, J., Yao, Q., et al. (2018). Nobiletin-ameliorated lipopolysaccharide-induced inflammation in acute lung injury by suppression of NF-κB pathway in vivo and vitro. *Inflammation* 41 (3), 996–1007. doi:10.1007/s10753-018-0753-3

Lin, H. S., Yue, B. D., and Ho, P. C. (2009). Determination of pterostilbene in rat plasma by a simple HPLC-UV method and its application in pre-clinical pharmacokinetic study. *Biomed. Chromatogr.* 23 (12), 1308–1315. doi:10.1002/bmc.1254

Liu, Z., Yang, Z., Fu, Y., Li, F., Liang, D., Zhou, E., et al. (2013). Protective effect of gossypol on lipopolysaccharide-induced acute lung injury in mice. *Inflamm. Res.* 62 (5), 499–506. doi:10.1007/s00011-013-0603-6

Liu, X., Wang, Y., Wu, D., Li, S., Wang, C., Han, Z., et al. (2019). Magnolol prevents acute alcoholic liver damage by activating PI3K/Nrf2/PPARγ and inhibiting NLRP3 signaling pathway. *Front. Pharmacol.* 10, 1459. doi:10.3389/fphar.2019.01459

Manca, D., Ricard, A. C., Trottier, B., and Chevalier, G. (1991). Studies on lipid peroxidation in rat tissues following administration of low and moderate doses of cadmium chloride. *Toxicology* 67 (3), 303–323. doi:10.1016/0300-483x(91)90030-5

Matthay, M. A., McAuley, D. F., and Ware, L. B. (2017). Clinical trials in acute respiratory distress syndrome: challenges and opportunities. *Lancet Respir. Med.* 5 (6), 524–534. doi:10.1016/s2213-2600(17)30188-1

Milani, P., Ambrosi, G., Gammoh, O., Blandini, F., and Cereda, C. (2013). SOD1 and DJ-1 converge at Nrf2 pathway: a clue for antioxidant therapeutic potential in neurodegeneration. *Oxid. Med. Cell. Longev.* 2013, 836760. doi:10.1155/2013/836760

Park, J., Chen, Y., Zheng, M., Ryu, J., Cho, G. J., Surh, Y. J., et al. (2018). Pterostilbene 4'-β-Glucoside attenuates LPS-induced acute lung injury via induction of heme oxygenase-1. *Oxid. Med. Cell. Longev.* 2018, 2747018. doi:10.1155/2018/2747018

Paul, S., Rimando, A. M., Lee, H. J., Ji, Y., Reddy, B. S., and Suh, N. (2009). Anti-inflammatory action of pterostilbene is mediated through the p38 mitogen-activated protein kinase pathway in colon cancer cells. *Canc. Prev. Res.* 2 (7), 650–657. doi:10.1158/1940-6207.capr-08-0224

Perecko, T., Drabikova, K., Rackova, L., Ciz, M., Podborska, M., Lojek, A., et al. (2010). Molecular targets of the natural antioxidant pterostilbene: effect on protein kinase C, caspase-3 and apoptosis in human neutrophils *in vitro*. *Neuroendocrinol. Lett.* 31, 84–90

Perkins, N. D. (2007). Integrating cell-signalling pathways with NF-kappaB and IKK function. *Nat. Rev. Mol. Cell Biol.* 8 (1), 49 62. doi:10.1038/nrm2083

Reagan-Shaw, S., Nihal, M., and Ahmad, N. (2008). Dose translation from animal to human studies revisited. *Faseb. J.* 22 (3), 659–661. doi:10.1096/fj.07-9574LSF

Remsberg, C. M., Yáñez, J. A., Ohgami, Y., Vega-Villa, K. R., Rimando, A. M., and Davies, N. M. (2008). Pharmacometrics of pterostilbene: preclinical pharmacokinetics and metabolism, anticancer, antiinflammatory, antioxidant and analgesic activity. *Phytother. Res.* 22 (2), 169–179. doi:10.1002/ptr.2277

Santos, L., Rodrigues, G. B., Mota, F. V. B., França, M. E. R., de Souza Barbosa, K. P., Oliveira, W. H., et al. (2018). New thiazolidinedione LPSF/GQ-2 inhibits NFκB and MAPK activation in LPS-induced acute lung inflammation. *Int. Immunopharm.* 57, 91–101. doi:10.1016/j.intimp.2018.02.011

Shen, W., Gan, J., Xu, S., Jiang, G., and Wu, H. (2009). Penehyclidine hydrochloride attenuates LPS-induced acute lung injury involvement of NF-kappaB pathway. *Pharmacol. Res.* 60 (4), 296–302. doi:10.1016/j.phrs.2009.04.007

Shao, X., Chen, X., Badmaev, V., Ho, C. T., and Sang, S. (2010). Structural identification of mouse urinary metabolites of pterostilbene using liquid chromatography/tandem mass spectrometry. *Rapid Commun. Mass Spectrom.* 24 (12), 1770–1778. doi:10.1002/rcm.4579

Wang, C., Liu, X., Han, Z., Zhang, X., Wang, J., Wang, K., et al. (2019). Nanosilver induces the formation of neutrophil extracellular traps in mouse neutrophil granulocytes. *Ecotoxicol. Environ. Saf.* 183, 109508. doi:10.1016/j.ecoenv.2019.109508

Wang, J., Fan, S. M., and Zhang, J. (2019). Epigallocatechin-3-gallate ameliorates lipopolysaccharide-induced acute lung injury by suppression of TLR4/NF-κB signaling activation. *Braz. J. Med. Biol. Res.* 52 (7), e8092. doi:10.1590/1414-431x20198092

Wang, P., and Sang, S. (2018). Metabolism and pharmacokinetics of resveratrol and pterostilbene. *Biofactors* 44 (1), 16–25. doi:10.1002/biof.1410

Ware, L. B., and Matthay, M. A. (2000). The acute respiratory distress syndrome. *N. Engl. J. Med.* 342 (18), 1334–1349. doi:10.1056/nejm200005043421806

Wei, Z., He, X., Kou, J., Wang, J., Chen, L., Yao, M., et al. (2015). Renoprotective mechanisms of morin in cisplatin-induced kidney injury. *Int. Immunopharm.* 28 (1), 500–506. doi:10.1016/j.intimp.2015.07.009

Wei, Z., Wang, J., Wang, Y., Wang, C., Liu, X., Han, Z., et al. (2019). Effects of neutrophil extracellular traps on bovine mammary epithelial cells *in vitro*. *Front. Immunol.* 10, 1003. doi:10.3389/fimmu.2019.01003

Wei, Z., Wang, Y., Zhang, X., Wang, X., Gong, P., Li, J., et al. (2018a). Bovine macrophage-derived extracellular traps act as early effectors against the abortive parasite Neospora caninum. *Vet. Parasitol.* 258, 1–7. doi:10.1016/j.vetpar.2018.06.002

Wei, Z., Zhang, X., Wang, J., Wang, Y., Yang, Z., and Fu, Y. (2018b). The formation of canine neutrophil extracellular traps induced by sodium arsenic in polymorphonuclear neutrophils. *Chemosphere* 196, 297–302. doi:10.1016/j.chemosphere.2017.12.175

Wei, Z., Zhang, X., Wang, Y., Wang, J., Fu, Y., and Yang, Z. (2018c). Nickel (II) nitrate hexahydrate triggered canine neutrophil extracellular traps release *in vitro*. *Chemosphere* 208, 117–121. doi:10.1016/j.chemosphere.2018.05.184

Xie, R., Yang, Y., Zhu, Y., Gao, L., Jiang, X., Sun, J., et al. (2018). Microparticles in red cell concentrates prime polymorphonuclear neutrophils and cause acute lung injury in a two-event mouse model. *Int. Immunopharm.* 55, 98–104. doi:10.1016/j.intimp.2017.11.029

Yan, S., Resta, T. C., and Jernigan, N. L. (2020). Vasoconstrictor mechanisms in chronic hypoxia-induced pulmonary hypertension: role of oxidant signaling. *Antioxidants* 9 (10). doi:10.3390/antiox9100999

Yang, H., Hua, C., Yang, X., Fan, X., Song, H., Peng, L., et al. (2020). Pterostilbene prevents LPS-induced early pulmonary fibrosis by suppressing oxidative stress, inflammation and apoptosis *in vivo*. *Food Funct.* 11 (5), 4471–4484. doi:10.1039/c9fo02521a

Yang, R., Yang, L., Shen, X., Cheng, W., Zhao, B., Ali, K. H., et al. (2012). Suppression of NF-κB pathway by crocetin contributes to attenuation of lipopolysaccharide-induced acute lung injury in mice. *Eur. J. Pharmacol.* 674 (2-3), 391–396. doi:10.1016/j.ejphar.2011.08.029

Yao, Y., Liu, K., Zhao, Y., Hu, X., and Wang, M. (2018). Pterostilbene and 4'-methoxyresveratrol inhibited lipopolysaccharide-induced inflammatory response in RAW264.7 macrophages. *Molecules* 23 (5). doi:10.3390/molecules23051148

Zhang, X., Song, K., Xiong, H., Li, H., Chu, X., and Deng, X. (2009). Protective effect of florfenicol on acute lung injury induced by lipopolysaccharide in mice. *Int. Immunopharm.* 9 (13-14), 1525–1529. doi:10.1016/j.intimp.2009.09.007

Zhang, Y., Wei, Z., Liu, W., Wang, J., He, X., Huang, H., et al. (2017). Melatonin protects against arsenic trioxide-induced liver injury by the upregulation of Nrf2 expression through the activation of PI3K/AKT pathway. *Oncotarget* 8 (3), 3773–3780. doi:10.18632/oncotarget.13931

Zhang, Y., and Zhang, Y. (2016). Pterostilbene, a novel natural plant conduct, inhibits high fat-induced atherosclerosis inflammation via NF-κB signaling pathway in Toll-like receptor 5 (TLR5) deficient mice. *Biomed. Pharmacother.* 81, 345–355. doi:10.1016/j.biopha.2016.04.031

Zhao, F., Li, K., Zhao, L., Liu, J., Suo, Q., Zhao, J., et al. (2014). Effect of Nrf2 on rat ovarian tissues against atrazine-induced anti-oxidative response. *Int. J. Clin. Exp. Pathol.* 7 (6), 2780–2789

8

Enhancing Cystic Fibrosis Immune Regulation

Anna M. van Heeckeren[1], *Morgan T. Sutton*[1,2,3,4,5,6], *David R. Fletcher*[1,4,5], *Craig A. Hodges*[1,5], *Arnold I. Caplan*[2,3,4] *and Tracey L. Bonfield*[1,2,3,4,5]*

[1]Pediatrics, Case Western Reserve University School of Medicine, Cleveland, OH, United States, [2]Department of Biology, Case Western Reserve University School of Medicine, Cleveland, OH, United States, [3]Skeletal Research Center, Case Western Reserve University School of Medicine, Cleveland, OH, United States, [4]National Center for Regenerative Medicine, Case Western Reserve University School of Medicine, Cleveland, OH, United States, [5]Departments of Genetics and Genome Sciences, Case Western Reserve University School of Medicine, Cleveland, OH, United States, [6]St. Jude Children's Research Hospital Graduate School of Biomedical Sciences, Memphis, TN, United States

***Correspondence:**
Tracey L. Bonfield
Tracey.Bonfield@case.edu

In cystic fibrosis (CF), sustained infection and exuberant inflammation results in debilitating and often fatal lung disease. Advancement in CF therapeutics has provided successful treatment regimens for a variety of clinical consequences in CF; however effective means to treat the pulmonary infection and inflammation continues to be problematic. Even with the successful development of small molecule cystic fibrosis transmembrane conductance regulator (CFTR) correctors and potentiators, there is only a modest effect on established infection and inflammation in CF patients. In the pursuit of therapeutics to treat inflammation, the conundrum to address is how to overcome the inflammatory response without jeopardizing the required immunity to manage pathogens and prevent infection. The key therapeutic would have the capacity to dull the inflammatory response, while sustaining the ability to manage infections. Advances in cell-based therapy have opened up the avenue for dynamic and versatile immune interventions that may support this requirement. Cell based therapy has the capacity to augment the patient's own ability to manage their inflammatory status while at the same time sustaining anti-pathogen immunity. The studies highlighted in this manuscript outline the potential use of cell-based therapy for CF. The data demonstrate that 1) total bone marrow aspirates containing *Cftr* sufficient hematopoietic and mesenchymal stem cells (hMSCs) provide *Cftr* deficient mice >50% improvement in survival and improved management of infection and inflammation; 2) myeloid cells can provide sufficient *Cftr* to provide pre-clinical anti-inflammatory and antimicrobial benefit; 3) hMSCs provide significant improvement in survival and management of infection and inflammation in CF; 4) the combined interaction between macrophages and hMSCs can potentially enhance anti-inflammatory and antimicrobial support through manipulating PPARγ. These data support the development of optimized cell-based therapeutics to enhance CF patient's own immune repertoire and capacity to maintain the balance between inflammation and pathogen management.

Keywords: bone marrow transplantation, hematopoietic cells, macrophages, mesenchymal stem cells, immune support, infection, inflammation, cystic fibrosis

INTRODUCTION

The question of immune sufficiency in CF has been the focus of scrutiny for many years due to the inability to resolve bacterial infections and the overzealous inflammatory response (Bruscia and Bonfield 2016a; Ralhan et al., 2016). CF patients are inefficient at managing chronic pulmonary infections with pathogens such as *Pseudomonas aeruginosa*, *Mycobacterium abscessus*, *Mycobacterium avium*, *Aspergillus fumigatus* and *Burkholderia cepacia*, all pathogens generally found in scenarios of immune insufficiency (Knutsen and Slavin, 2011; Nichols and Chmiel, 2015; Roesch et al., 2018; Bell et al., 2019; Martiniano et al., 2019). Susceptibility to infection in CF has been associated with defective mucociliary clearance, mucus plugging, epithelial cell pro-inflammatory sensitivity and the inability for innate immune cells to reach or effectively interact with the inciting pathogens (Ma et al., 2018; Bell et al., 2019). Treatment for CF has advanced with successful CFTR modulators, inhaled saline, improved antibiotics, active elastase inhibitors, nutrition, supportive care and chest clearance techniques (Elborn, 2016; Spielberg and Clancy, 2016). Unfortunately, these advances in care do not resolve the inflammation and infection that has already been established in CF patients (McElvaney et al., 2018; West and Flume, 2018). Further, the balance between immunosuppression for chronic lung inflammation and prevention of infection have been more elusive with patients living longer and the dynamic changes associated with disease progression and shifts in the species of inciting pathogens (Clancy et al., 2019; Egan, 2020). Therapeutics that could improve the immune inefficiencies in CF have the potential to provide patients with additional gain toward management of infection and inflammation resulting in improved clinical outcomes. Finally, chronic diseases that are associated with chronic inflammation are impacted by aging and immuno-senescence (Pawelec, 2017; Fulop et al., 2018) suggesting that providing a means of refreshing CF immunity may aide in maintaining minimal morbidity and mortality until a cure for CF is ultimately achieved (Aiello et al., 2019; Bezzerri et al., 2019).

Immune dysregulation and inefficient management of infection, whether intrinsic or resultant from CF disease pathophysiology is important to understand and treat therapeutically. The CF literature has several references to therapeutic strategies focusing on specific immune cells such as: neutrophils, monocyte/macrophages, T lymphocytes, dendritic cells and airway epithelial cells (Bruscia and Bonfield, 2016a; Ralhan et al., 2016). Many of these studies have utilized the strengths of the CF knockout mouse infection model to mimic CF infection and inflammation (Soltys et al., 2002; Heeckeren et al., 2006; Bruscia et al., 2009). In CF, the cystic fibrosis transmembrane conductance regulator (*Cftr*) knockout (KO) mouse has provided important insight into avenues for immune cell based interventions with better understanding of the roles epithelial cells, macrophages and T-cells (Hodges et al., 2011; Bonfield et al., 2012; Ng et al., 2014). As is the case of most animal models of human disease, the CF mouse model does not recapitulate all aspects of human CF, however, even with these criticisms, the CF mouse has played an essential role in understanding the inflammatory response to pathogens and for the development of the other more complex CF animal models (Stotland et al., 2000; Bragonzi, 2010; Fan et al., 2018; Rosen et al., 2018; Hodges and Conlon, 2019). This manuscript will combine historical non-congenic and congenic transplantation studies along with more recent cell specific knockout models and human mesenchymal stem cells (hMSCs) to test the hypothesis that immune supportive therapy can provide clinical benefit in CF.

MATERIALS AND METHODS

Mice

All procedures involving mice were reviewed and approved by Case Western Reserve University, Institutional Animal Care and Use Committee. $Cftr^{tm1Unc}$ mice were obtained from The Jackson Laboratory (Stock#002196) ((Snouwaert et al., 1992) and bred by the Case Western Reserve University Cystic Fibrosis Mouse Models Core. Creation of the conditional alleles $Cftr^{fl10}$ and $Cftr^{invfl10}$ as well as the LysMCre-control (WT) are described elsewhere (Hodges et al., 2008; Hodges et al., 2011; Bonfield et al., 2012). Genotyping of the mice was completed by PCR analysis using DNA extracts from tissue. To detect the $Cftr^{fl10}$ allele (408 bp) and the *KO* allele (148 bp), primers P1 (5′ GTAGGG GCTCGCTCTTCTTT-3′), P2 (5′-GTACCCGGCATAATCCAA GA-3′), and P3 (5′-AGCCCCTCGAGGGACCTAAT-3′) were used. To detect the $Cftr^{invfl10}$ allele (563 bp) and the knock-in (*KI*) allele, primers P1, P2, and P4 (5′- CACCCACTCCAGCTTAAT CC-3′) were used. PCR reactions were completed using 30 cycles of 95°C for 30 s, 55°C for 30 s, and 72°C for 30 s. The bone marrow transplantation studies were all done with B6.129P-2 $Cftr^{tm1Unc}$ ($Cftr^{tm1Unc}$, null) and the appropriate littermate controls. The different murine models are listed in **Table 1**.

Preparation of Bone Marrow Cells for Transplant Studies

Bone marrow aspirates were obtained from the femur and tibia as described previously (Bonfield et al., 2008). Bone marrow recipient mice were provided with antibiotics (sulfatrim suspension of sulfamethoxazole and trimethoprim, USP 200 mg/40 mg per 5 ml, cherry flavor; Henry Schein 4207716) in the drinking water (20 ml sulfatrim to 1 L of water; 0.8 mg/ml sulfamethoxazole and 0.016 mg/ml trimethoprim) starting two weeks before irradiation with a single dose of 8 Gy of Ce^{137} and the same day total bone marrow cells were injected into the tail vein (~10^6 cells/100 µl RPMI; 0.1 ml/mouse). These mice were maintained on water containing antibiotics for another 4 weeks followed by autoclaved water. The mouse strain in which bone marrow cells are harvested will be listed first, the recipient mice will be designated after the arrow (example: WT → CF, WT bone marrow aspirates were harvested and injected into CF mice).

Pseudomonas aeruginosa Lung Infection

Transplanted mice were infected with *P. aeruginosa* laden agarose beads, three months after bone marrow reconstitution (van Heeckeren et al., 1997; Bonfield et al., 2012; Hsu et al., 2016).

TABLE 1 | Nomenclature of murine models.

Genotype	Description
B6.129P2-Cftr^{tm1Unc}	Cftr deficient everywhere (CF)
C57BL/6J	Cftr is expressed everywhere (WT)
Cftr^{fl10}	Floxed KO control. Cftr is everywhere (like WT)
Cftr^{invfl10}	Floxed KI control. Cftr is nowhere (like a cftr null, CF)
Cftr^{fl10} + LysMCre	Floxed KO everywhere but myeloid lineage (KO)
Cftr^{invfl10} + LysMCre	Floxed KI. Cftr deficient everywhere but the myeloid lineage (KI)

TABLE 2 | Key to murine model clinical outcomes.

Score	Histologic findings	Clinical scores	Gross lung pathology
0	Within normal limits	Healthy appearance and activity	Within normal limits
1	Presence of inflammatory cells	Scruffy appearance	Darker red
2	Presence of interstitial inflammation and fibrotic foci	Scruffy and dehydrated	Few nodules
3	Interstitial and alveolar inflammation, fibrosis	Scruffy, dehydrated and decreased activity	Several nodules, <25% consolidation
4	N/A	Scruffy, dehydrated and minimal activity	Numerous nodules 25–50% consolidation
5	N/A	Moribund or dead	Numerous nodules>50% consolidation

Mice were assessed clinically once daily for 3 or 10 days for coat quality, posture, ability to right themselves after being placed in lateral recumbence, ambulation and body weight utilizing a standardized clinical score profile outlined in **Table 2**. Post-mortem was completed during the study and at the termination on any mouse that succumbed during the study to determine cause of death.

Bronchoalveolar Lavage (BAL)

Mice were injected subcutaneously with a lethal dose of ketamine (80 mg/kg) and xylazine (10 mg/kg) (Hsu et al., 2016; Bonfield et al., 2012). The lungs were exposed followed by inserting a cannula through the trachea into the bronchi with a BAL wash of 1 × 1 ml aliquot of warm PBS. The BAL was evaluated for total and cell type (differential) cell counts with cytokine analysis. In the case of culturing the cells for gene expression, 3 × 1 ml aliquots of warm PBS were instilled in the lung.

Bone Marrow Derived Macrophages (BMDM)

BMDM were isolated as previously described (Bonfield et al., 2008) and counted for viability (trypan blue exclusion) followed by culture for 7–10 days with L929 support medium containing macrophage colony stimulating factor.

Cytokine Analysis

Cytokines TNF-α, IL-1β, IL-6, MIP-2 and KC, by Luminex according to the manufacturer's recommendations (R&D Systems, Minneapolis, MN). Cytokine concentrations were normalized to units/ml of epithelial lining fluid (ELF).

Human Mesenchymal Stem Cells (hMSCs)

Human bone marrow derived hMSCs were obtained in collaboration with Dr. Arnold Caplan's laboratory under (IRB# 09-90-195) and validated according to stringent guidelines previously outlined (Lennon and Caplan 2006; Crapnell et al., 2013). hMSCs supernatants (containing 5% fetal bovine serum) were obtained from hMSC cell cultures that were grown in the absence of antibiotics at confluence for 72 h. Conditions using the supernatants utilized 1:1 dilution of the hMSC supernatant with the bone marrow derived medium required for appropriate growth (Sutton et al., 2017).

Human Sputum Cell Preparations

All samples were obtained with informed consent and compliance by the Case Western Reserve University/Rainbow Babies and Children's Hospitals IRB approval (IRB#11-67-200). CF sputum was processed and cells were obtained using standardized procedures (Matuska et al., 2016). Induced sputum was provided by the CFF Integrated Cytology Core which supports TDN trials. Controls (n = 3, HC) were obtained from healthy volunteers in the Case Western Reserve University community.

RT-PCR

BAL, sputum BMDM or hMSCs were processed for messenger ribonucleic acid (mRNA) followed by complementary deoxyribonucleic acid (cDNA) synthesis for chemokine gene expression using RT-PCR. Quality of mRNA and cDNA was assessed through nanodrop spectrophotometry (optimal threshold 260–280 nm). Validation was done through use of a reference gene peptidyl prolyl isomerase (hPPIA) for human samples or GAPDH for mouse cells. The expression of interleukin 6 (IL-6), tumor necrosis factor alpha (TNFα), peroxisome proliferator activator receptor gamma (PPARγ) was compared to the expression of hPPIA. All PCR samples were compared to hPPIA expression for fold change in each target gene threshold cycle (dCT).

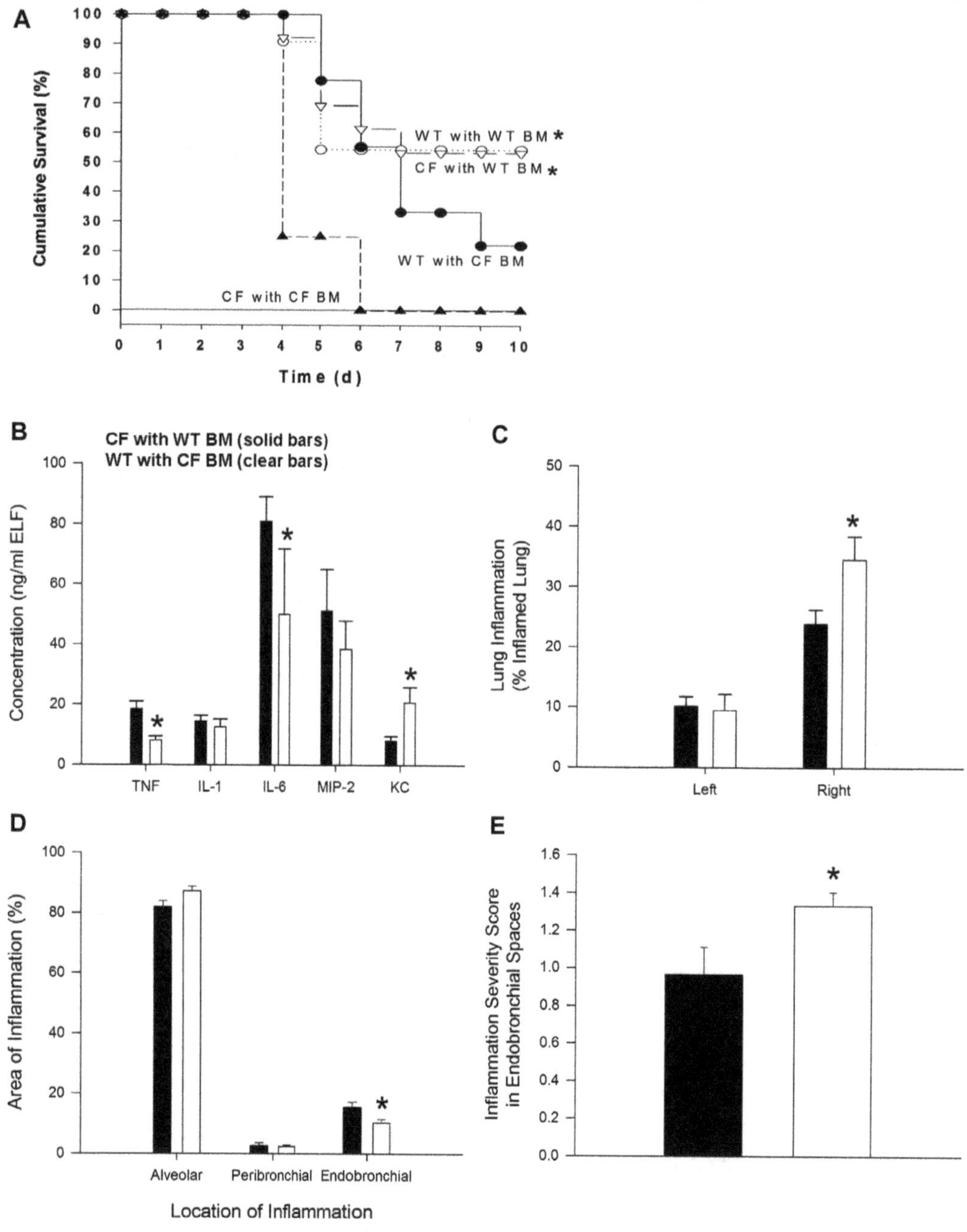

FIGURE 1 | Bone marrow non-congenic chimeras and response to chronic *P. aeruginosa infection*. CF→CF (closed triangles), WT→CF (open triangles; closed bars), CF→WT (closed circles; clear bars) and WT→WT (open circles) mice were inoculated with *P. aeruginosa*-laden agarose beads on Day 0, three months following bone marrow reconstitution. Mice were monitored daily following infection. Moribund mice were euthanized for humane reasons and included as if spontaneous death had occurred. **(A)** Significantly different survival rates on Day 10 between the four possible groups ($p = 0.03$; Fisher's exact test) where donors and recipients were males. Significantly different survival rates on Day 10 with improvement in survival of CF animals with WT BM and decrease survival of WT mice with CF BM compared to survival of CF animals and WT animals without BM four possible groups ($p = 0.0284$; Fisher's exact test). **(B)** BAL fluid was collected from one subset of WT→CF (N = 11), CF→WT (N = 10) mice sacrificed three days after *P. aeruginosa* challenge for cytokine and chemokine analysis. *Significantly different from CF → WT mice ($p \leq 0.03$; Wilcoxon test). **(C)** Following BAL fluid collection in mice represented in **Figure 1C**, the areas of inflammation in the left and right lungs were evaluated using point counting. *Significantly different from CF → WT mice ($p \leq 0.01$; Wilcoxon test). **(D)** The area of the location of the inflammation in the right lung is shown. *Significantly different from CF → WT mice ($p = 0.03$; Wilcoxon test). **(E)** The severity of the inflammation within the endobronchial spaces of the right lung is shown. *Significantly different from CF → WT mice ($p = 0.04$; Wilcoxon test). Data in the bar graphs are shown as the means ± SEM.

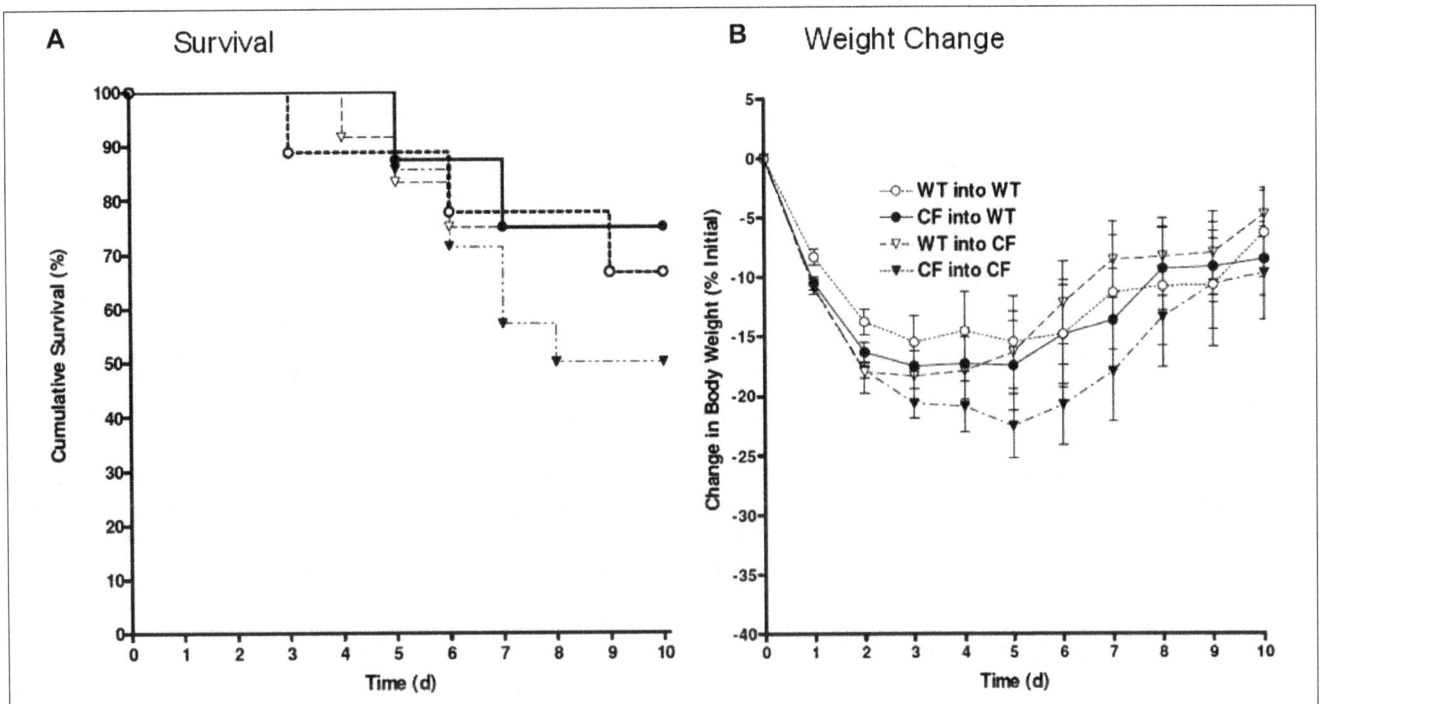

FIGURE 2 | Bone marrow congenic chimeras and response to chronic *P. aeruginosa* infection. Bone marrow chimeras were generated using congenic CF (*Cftr*^{tm1Unc}) mice and litter mate controls. Mice were >6 generations on the C57Bl/6 background. Mice were irradiated and given bone marrow by retro-orbital administration. None of our animals died using this protocol suggesting efficiency of engraftment. CF mice given CF bone marrow showed the least ability to survive, averaging around 50% survival (black triangles, n = 12). *Cftr*^{tm1Unc} null mice given wild type bone marrow (open triangles, n = 10) had 76% survival. WT mice given CF (closed circles, n = 12) had 80% survival. WT mice given WT bone marrow (open circles, n = 10) had 76% survival. WT mice infected without transplantation had 94 ± 6% survival compared to 50 ± 13% survival of CF mice infected without transplantation. Weight changes **(B)** are consistent survival **(A)**.

Statistics

Statistical analysis was performed using GraphPad Prism (version 6.5–8.0). Data are shown as means ± standard deviation, unless indicated otherwise. Comparisons of survival at a specified time (e.g., 10-days) were made using Fisher's exact test. Two-group comparisons for continuous data were made using one-way ANOVA and Student's t-test or the Kruskal-Wallis and Wilcoxon rank sum tests. The Bonferroni correction was used when making pairwise comparisons among 3 or more groups. When pooling data from more than one experiment, the data was evaluated using a two-way ANOVA, or using the nonparametric van Elteren test with each experiment as a stratifying factor. Analyses of log or square-root transformation were utilized to compare between experimental conditions at a single point with paired t-tests and slopes over time (van Heeckeren and Schluchter, 2002). In the chronic infection models, survival curves were compared using stratified log-rank tests, cell treatment as the as the strata. Pathology (e.g., bacterial load, white blood cell counts, and cytokines) was log-transformed as necessary to compared between groups or conditions using one or two-way ANOVA, treating donors as experimental blocks. Differential counts are expressed as percentages will be transformed using logit or arcsin (square root) transformations to stabilize variances to meet normality assumptions. All significance was defined by the 95% confidence interval at $p \leq 0.05$.

RESULTS

Bone Marrow Transplantation and *Pseudomonas aeruginosa* Infection in *Cftr* Deficient Mice

Bone marrow transplantation studies were done with non-congenic (**Figure 1**) and congenic (**Figure 2**) *Cftr* deficient (CF) mice and wild type (WT) controls. WT or CF mice were irradiated, and reconstituted with an intravenous infusion of either male or female autologous total bone marrow aspirates in sex-mismatched groups to follow the model and treatment regime. WT aspirates were infused into WT recipients (WT → WT) and CF aspirates were infused into CF recipients (CF → CF). To assess whether the irradiation and/or transplant sex mismatched procedures caused baseline changes of radiation pneumonitis or other effects, lung inflammation and survival 3 months after the transplant mice were infected with *P. aeruginosa* (average of 3.24 × 10^4 CFU/mouse embedded into 10^3 microns in diameter agarose beads) and followed for out to 10 days. There was no significant difference between counts of BAL inflammatory cells in the different transplant paradigms in the male to female transplants, with no statistically significant histologic inflammation scores between the groups (**Supplementary Table S1A**). These results suggested only minimal lung inflammatory changes due to the irradiation and transplant schemes and sex-mismatched transplant conditions (**Supplementary Table S1B**).

In the next series of studies, bone marrow transplant studies were conducted between the different mouse genotypes: WT → WT, CF → CF, WT → CF and CF → WT (bone marrow source → recipient). After 3 months mice were infected with agarose beads embedded with *P. aeruginosa*. There were no differences in the WT → WT and CF → CF groups, from the non-transplanted WT and CF infected mice respectively. WT → WT mice had a higher survival rate than CF → CF (55% vs. 0% respectively, p = 0.02). Improved survival and inflammation occurred when CF mice received WT bone marrow (WT → CF) compared to CF receiving CF (CF → CF) whereas decreased survival and inflammation occurred when WT mice received CF bone marrow (CF → WT) (**Figure 1A**; $p < 0.03$; logistic regression model). WT → CF mice had a survival rate indistinguishable from that of WT → WT mice (54 vs. 55% respectively), a significant improvement from the CF → CF transplant series (0% by day 6, $p = 0.02$). CF → WT mice (22% survival) had an intermediate response between CF → CF (0%) mice and WT → WT mice (55%), suggesting a CF specific hematopoietic impact on the transplantation.

To monitor changes in inflammation, BAL cytokines and cellular infiltrate types were quantified. TNF-α and IL-6 were decreased in the WT → CF (open bars) with statistically higher levels of KC compared to the CF → WT (**Figure 1B**, $p < 0.05$, dark bars). Absolute and differential cell counts were not significantly different between the two groups, except for the neutrophil levels (**Supplementary Tables S2A,S2B**). In evaluating the histological differences, there was more inflammation in the WT → CF (opened bars) than the CF → WT (dark bars). The predominance of inflammation in the right lobe is likely due to the trans-tracheal administration of the agarose beads embedded with *P. aeruginosa* is instilled in the right lobe, inducing inflammation in that area (**Figure 1C**). Histological evaluation demonstrated that although the endobronchial inflammation was greater in the WT → CF mice (**Figures 1D,E**), the total severity score of lung infection induced inflammation was higher in the CF → WT mice. This is likely due to the heterogeneity in the endobronchial sections and the impact of mix-matched HLA on the inflammation post-implant.

Congenic Bone Marrow CFTR Expression Alters the Severity of the Pulmonary Response to Chronic Lung Infection with *Pseudomonas aeruginosa*

In these studies, the bone marrow chimera studies were repeated using the same transplantation combinations outlined in **Figure 1** but utilizing congenic CF and WT mice. The survival kinetics and weight profile of the studies (10–12 congenic animals/group) are outlined in **Figure 2**. Only 50% of the congenic CF mice transplanted with CF bone marrow (CF → CF) survived whereas 66% of the CF mice transplanted with WT bone marrow (WT → CF) survived (**Figure 2A**). WT mice given congenic CF bone marrow (CF → WT) had 76% survival, similar to 66% survival of WT mice transplanted with WT bone marrow. Although not done at the same time due to the sheer size of the experiments, WT mice chronically infected *P. aeruginosa* without transplantation traditionally have a 94 ± 6% survival compared to 50 ± 13% survival of infected congenic CF mice, in the absence of transplantation (van Heeckeren et al., 1997; Bonfield et al., 2012; Hsu et al., 2016). The survival post-infection with and without treatment was tracked through daily weight loss kinetics (**Figure 2B**), which tracked with the survival.

To determine the neutrophilic response to infection in the lung post-transplantation, broncho-alveolar lavage was performed on surviving mice followed by an assessment of total cell count and cell type. Transplantation of the CF animals with CF bone marrow (CF → CF) had similar levels of neutrophils to the CF animals in the non-treated group (**Table 3**, 343 ± 21 vs. 330 ± 121, respectively). Reconstitution of the CF animals with WT bone marrow (WT → CF) trended toward a decreased in both absolute and relative numbers of neutrophils in the BAL (343.6 ± 20.9 to 300.2 ± 52.6 absolute neutrophils, $p = 0.08$; 69.8 ± 5.5 to 61.9 ± 4.04 relative neutrophils, $p = 0.06$). There was a 23% and 4% increase in alveolar macrophages and lymphocytes; respectively which was not significantly different between the transplant groups. Reconstitution of the WT mice with CF bone marrow (CF → WT), however, did result in a 47% increase in BAL neutrophils (113.5 ± 21.6 to 167.9 ± 41.4, $p < 0.05$) as a response to infection with *P. aeruginosa* consistent with the non-congenic studies.

Myeloid Knock-Out and Knock-In Models

Murine models in which we specifically knocked-out *Cftr* in all myeloid cells had increased mortality, neutrophil recruitment and inefficient resolution of *P. aeruginosa* infection (Bonfield et al., 2012). To compliment the myeloid *Cftr* KO mice, we developed the *Cftr* knock-in (KI) model (**Figure 3**). The myeloid specific KO ($Cftr^{fl10}$ + LysM Cre,) has *Cftr* everywhere but the myeloid compartment (**Table 1**). The myeloid specific KI ($Cftr^{Invfl10}$ + LysM Cre) has *Cftr* expression in the myeloid compartment with *Cftr* deficient everywhere else. The WT ($Cftr^{+/+}$) mice have *Cftr* in all the tissues which express the gene. All of these mice are congenic on a C57BL/6J background. The *Cftr* allele schematic is shown in **Figure 3A**, demonstrating the placement of the Cre-lox sites for recombination to generate the *Cftr* KO or KI myeloid mouse models. Genotype verification of the mice is shown in **Figure 3B**. DNA amplification was directed toward the region surrounding exon 10 gene of *Cftr* from various tissues of mice homozygous for $Cftr^{fl10}$ or $Cftr^{invfl10}$ with and without LysMCre to generate the KO or KI. Mice carrying the $Cftr^{fl10}$ allele display no deletion of exon 10 (408 bp) but with LysMCre they display at least some of the deleted exon 10 product (148 bp, KO) in all tissues including bone marrow derived macrophages (M), bone marrow (BM), BAL cells (B), lung (Lu), kidney (Ki) and Liver (Li) due to the presence of myeloid cells throughout the body. Mice carrying the $Cftr^{invfll10}$ allele display the inverted exon 10 (563 bp) but with LysMCre display inversion of at least some the allele (408 bp, KI) leading to functional CFTR in all tissues including bone marrow derived

TABLE 3 | Transplantation in congenic mice.

Experiment	Neutrophils		Alveolar macrophages		Lymphocytes
	Absolute (× 10^3)	Relative	Absolute (× 10^3)	Relative	Absolute (^{a}× 10^3)
WT → WT (n = 6)	113 ± 22	52 ± 5	183 ± 135	38 ± 12	6 ± 2
CF → WT (n = 6)	168 ± 41	60 ± 12	171 ± 64	46 ± 4	5 ± 2
CF → CF (n = 7)	344 ± 21	70 ± 6	107 ± 18	29 ± 4	6 ± 2
WT → CF (n = 8)	300 ± 53	62 ± 4	133 ± 48	34 ± 6	12 ± 3
CF (n = 9)	331 ± 121	80 ± 4	68 ± 7	20 ± 4	1 ± 1
WT (n = 5)	67 ± 27	59 ± 8	25 ± 7	39 ± 8	2 ± 1

[a]*× 10^3/ml of bronchoalveolar lavage fluid;* [a]*in at least 3 fields of 100 cells each.*

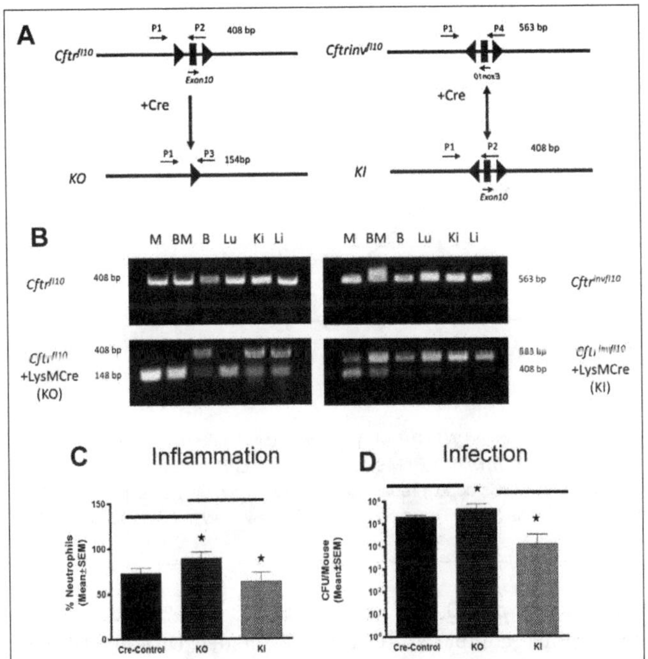

FIGURE 3 | Myeloid specific *Cftr* KO and KI and response to chronic infection. **(A)** Schematic of the *Cftr*^{fl10} or *Cftr*^{invfl10} alleles with and without Cre recombinase present. Primers P1-P4 were used to detect the different alleles (specifics in the methods section). The *Cftr*^{fl10} conversion to the KO allele is a one way reaction whereas the *Cftr*^{invfl10} conversion to the KI allele is bidirectional. **(B)** DNA amplification of the region surrounding exon 10 from various tissues of mice homozygous for *Cftr*^{fl10} or *Cftr*^{invfl10} with and without LysMCre. Mice carrying the *Cftr*^{fl10} allele display no deletion of exon 10 (408 bp) but with LysMCre display at least some of the deleted product KI (148 bp) in bone marrow derived macrophages (M), bone marrow (BM), BAL cells **(B)**, lung (Lu), kidney (Ki) and Liver (Li). Mice carrying the *Cftr*^{invfl10} allele display the inverted exon 10 (563 bp) but with LysMCre display inversion of at least some of the KI allele (408 b+p) **(C,D)** Mice were infected with *P. aeruginosa* and followed for 10 days. Myeloid specific KI (n = 6) and KO (n = 6) models were compared with the WT control (n = 5) mice and each other for BAL neutrophil numbers **(C)** and *P. aeruginosa* CFUs **(D)**. The KO had significantly elevated neutrophils ($p \leq 0.05$) and more bacteria ($p \leq 0.05$) in the BAL than the WT control, whereas the KI model had comparable levels of neutrophils and bacteria. The KI levels of neutrophils and CFUs were significantly less than the KO model ($p \leq 0.05$).

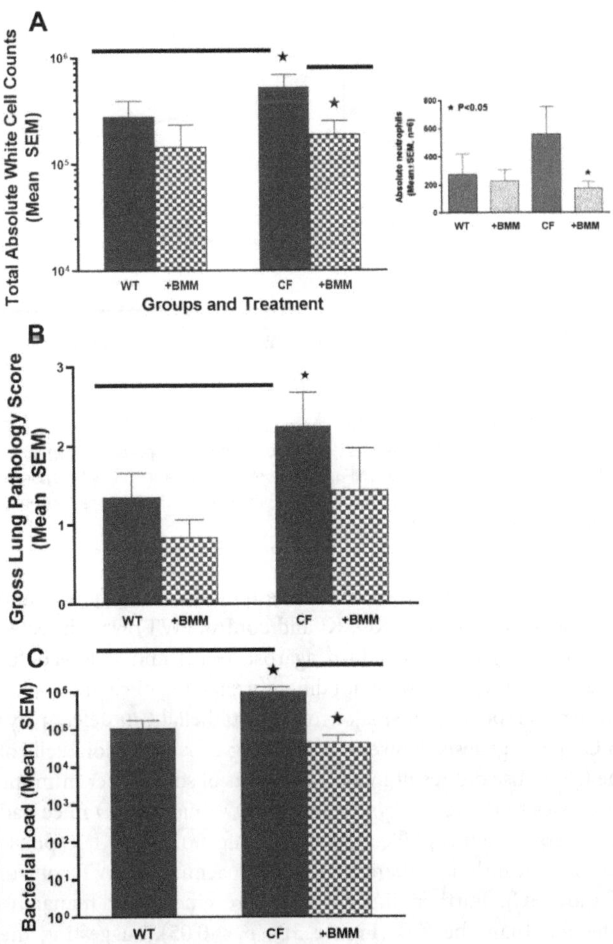

FIGURE 4 | Exogenous WT BMDM decrease lung inflammation and infection *in vivo*. CF mice (n = 12) and WT controls (n = 10) were chronically infected with *P. aeruginosa* and followed for up to 10 days. Mice were infused with 10^6 WT BMDM at day 1 post-infection. Animals were euthanized and evaluated for **(A)** white cell count, including a decrease in neutrophils (insert), **(B)** gross lung pathology and **(C)** *P. aeruginosa* infection burden. Treatment with bone marrow derived macrophages resulted in significantly (*) decreased recruitment of white blood cells improved gross lung pathology score and bacterial burden ($p < 0.05$).

macrophages (M) andbone marrow (BM), BAL cells (B), lung (Lu), kidney (Ki) and Liver (Li). The *Cftr*^{fl10} allele can be completely converted to the deleted allele (148 bp) but due to the reversible nature of the *Cftr*^{invfl10} allele the inverted allele (563 bp) will always be present and the active allele (408 bp) will never be 100%.

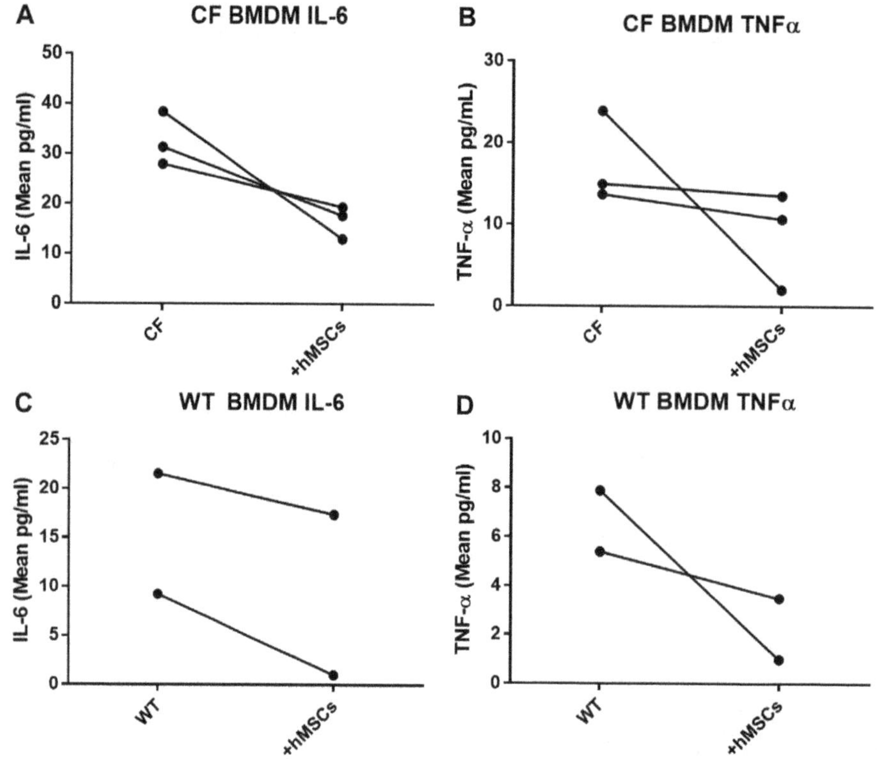

FIGURE 5 | hMSCs improve BMDM Inflammatory Response to Pathogens. CF BMDM (n = 3) preparations and WT BMDM (n = 2) treated with LPS demonstrated IL-6 and TNFα secretion. This was used as to explore the suppressive capacity of three different bone marrow donor hMSC supernatants. LPS stimulated CF and WT BMDM produce both IL-6 and TNFα. Treatment of the different BMDM preparations with the different hMSCs donor preparations resulted in cumulative decreased IL-6 ($p \leq 0.05$) and TNFα ($p \leq 0.05$) regardless of whether the BMDM were derived from CF **(A,B)** *or* WT mice **(C,D)**. This is consistent with previously published data (Leyendecker et al., 2018).

To investigate the response of these myeloid specific KO and KI models to infection, KO, KI and control (WT) were infected with *P. aeruginosa* embedded agarose beads and followed for 10 days. The KI mice were not different than CF mice in terms of survival, supporting the major role the epithelial *Cftr* defect plays in CF pathogenesis. However, correcting *Cftr* in myeloid cells of the CF mouse did result in improvements of some other immune responses to the *P. aeruginosa* infection. While the KO mice had an excessive neutrophilic response to infection, the KI response was significantly less than the KO approaching the WT control (**Figure 3C**). Further, the KI was more efficient at managing infection than the KO (**Figure 3D**, $p \leq 0.05$), suggesting the prominence of the macrophage in the inefficiency of managing infections in a *Cftr* deficient environment.

Macrophage Cell Based Therapy

Taking advantage of congenic mouse models and the ability to deliver autologous myeloid cells without immunosuppression, the next series of studies were done to evaluate the potential of providing immune support with exogenously delivered WT macrophages. In these studies, autologous 10^6 WT BMDM were administered to either WT mice or CF mice infected 24 h previously with *P. aeruginosa* embedded agarose beads (**Figure 4**). Infusing WT BMDM into infected CF mice, significantly reduced the numbers of white blood cells (**Figure 4A**, $p < 0.05$), which includes a 30% reduction in neutrophils compared to the CF model without BMDM treatment (insert, $p < 0.05$). Treatment of the infected CF model with WT BMDM also improve lung consolidation and pathology (**Figure 4B**, $p < 0.05$) and the capacity to manage the *P. aeruginosa* infection (**Figure 4C**, $p < 0.05$). There was no major effect of the BMDM on the infected WT mice model.

Mesenchymal Stem Cell Therapy

In providing immune support, we investigated the impact of hMSCs on LPS stimulated BMDM (**Figure 5**). BMDM from CF (**Figures 5A,B**) and WT (**Figures 5C,D**) mice were cultured in the presence and absence of LPS to induce an inflammatory response as monitored by the secretion of TNFα and IL-6 in response to LPS. The BMDM cultures stimulated with LPS were evaluated with and without the addition of hMSC conditioned in three different studies using conditioned medium derived from 3 different donor hMSC preparations. The hMSCs conditioned medium significantly suppressed LPS induced IL-6 and TNF-α secretion relative to the LPS treated control without hMSC treatment regardless of whether the BMDM were derived from CF or WT mice ($p \leq 0.05$, n = 3). Each of the hMSC preparations had the capacity to suppress the LPS induced IL-6 and TNFα secretion; however there was significant variability in

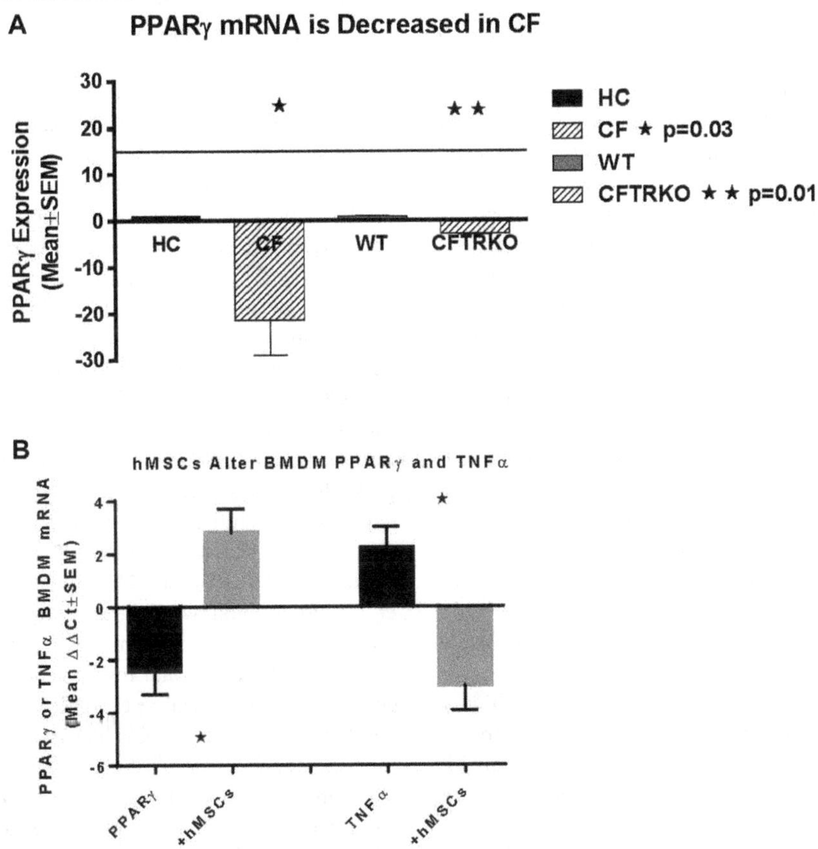

FIGURE 6 | hMSC Effect on PPARγ and TNFα expression. BMDM from CF patients and CF mice were evaluated for PPARγ **(A)**. Sputum was obtained from CF patients (n = 3) and compared to healthy control (n = 3), demonstrating deficient PPARγ ($p \leq 0.05$). BMDM from *Cftr* deficient mice also had deficient expression of PPARγ ($p \leq 0.05$). **(B)** BMDM were stimulated with LPS and processed for PPARγ and TNFα gene expression demonstrating a decreased of PPARγ ($p \leq 0.05$) and increased TNFα ($p \leq 0.05$) relative to the unstiluated control of PPARγ and TNFα (2.1 ± 0.07 dCT and 1.7 ± 1.0 dCt respectively, n = 3) at baseline. The same culture conditions were done in the presence of hMSC condition medium. hMSC supernatants increased PPARγ and decreased TNFα ($p \leq 0.05$) above the baseline controls.

the suppressive effect of the individual donor hMSC supernatants.

Since hMSCs have the ability to facilitate the changes in the LPS induced BMDM IL-6 and TNFα production, the next series of studies explored the impact of the hMSCs on macrophage IL-6 and TNFα gene expression. Peroxisome proliferator activator receptor gamma (PPARγ) is an important regulator of the macrophage pro-inflammatory responses to infection regulating TNFα and IL-6 production (Knethen and Brune, 2002; Korbecki et al., 2019). PPARγ is deficient in CF patient sputum and BMDM from *Cftr* deficient mice exposed to LPS compared to healthy controls (HC) (**Figure 6A**, $p \leq 0.05$ for sputum and *Cftr* deficient BAL cells). hMSC supernatants can alter the BMDM activity by recovering PPARγ expression decreasing TNFα expression (**Figure 6B**, $p \leq 0.05$).

DISCUSSION

In the past 20 years, improved CF clinical care and innovation in therapeutic development has significantly improved the quality and duration of life for the majority of CF patients. However, the main cause of morbidity and mortality in CF continues to be the chronic pulmonary infection and the associated on-going inflammation (Elborn, 2016; Ma et al., 2018). In addition, there continues to be a subset of patients which are not eligible for modulator therapy either due to their specific CFTR mutation or relative intolerance to the drugs (Bell et al., 2019; Clancy et al., 2019; Egan, 2020). CF patients with established inflammation and infection, individuals not able to benefit from small molecule modulator therapy, would benefit from supportive immune therapy to enhance control over the miss-matched inflammation/infection conundrum in CF. Further, immune support would also be beneficial when considering the longer life expectancy and sustainability for patients, which become complicated with pathogen resistance, and immune-senescence (Fischer et al., 2013; Bezzerri et al., 2019).

The studies in this manuscript describe the benefit of *Cftr* sufficient bone marrow aspirates, bone marrow derived macrophages (BMDM) and bone marrow derived hMSCs in providing immune support in CF. The data highlight how supplementation of *Cftr* deficient murine models with WT total bone marrow aspirates, WT BMDM or hMSCs improved pathogen and inflammation resolution. The models also demonstrated that the WT cell-based products provided improvements in managing weight loss, survival, and lung neutrophil recruitment and cytokine profiles. The non-congenic studies demonstrate the therapeutic potency of providing CFTR sufficient hematopoietic/mesenchymal sources. The congenic studies implicate the concept of bone marrow corrective technology to boost the capacity to regulate the response to infection and management of inflammation. The development of the myeloid specific KO and KI mouse models demonstrates that hematopoietic compartment plays an essential role in managing the host immune response in CF, and promotes the idea of hematopoietic correction using CRISPR/Cas9, Talen's or zinc fingers (Phang et al., 2013; Marangi and Pistritto, 2018; Cabrini, 2019).

The question remains as to the nature of macrophages in CF management of both infection and the host response. The macrophage is an important contributor to how the inflammatory response is initiated, sustained and resolved. Macrophages also have considerable plasticity, which could be enhanced toward targeted therapeutic impact in specific clinical settings of inflammation with or without the presence of infecting pathogens (Morales-Nebreda et al., 2015; Funes et al., 2018; Tarique et al., 2018). Macrophages are highly sensitive to their environment resulting in subtle changes in membrane proteins, which can shift their function (Bonfield, 2015; Bruscia and Bonfield, 2016b). These observations become important in the era of modulator therapy, which provides significant clinical benefit to patients who are eligible and responsive to treatment, including improved macrophage function (Zhang et al., 2018; Clancy et al., 2019; Hisert et al., 2020). Even with the modulator benefits, patients continue to have concurrent issues with infection and inflammation, as well as battles with the residual lung damage that has occurred during the pre-modulator phase of therapeutic accessibility (Burgener and Moss, 2018). The tissue specific contribution of macrophages in the context of CF is evident by the literature associated with functional contribution to CF pathophysiology (Worgall et al., 2002; Assani et al., 2017; Di Pietro et al., 2017). Currently, modulator therapy aids in the management of CFTR dysfunction in greater than 90% of patients with CF, leaving 10% of patients that will continue to struggle with the disease while sustainable treatment options are pursued (McElvaney et al., 2018; Egan, 2020). With the advent of hematopoietic supplementation, it could be that early support with autologous-based therapeutics might provide enough added immune support to minimize the pulmonary damage associated with chronic exposure to pathogens and the inflammatory response. To continue to pursue this line of therapeutic support, future studies are needed to interrogate lung macrophage phenotype relative to CF infection and inflammation and to discern the direct mechanisms for the therapeutic benefit highlighted in this manuscript.

A major caveat for macrophage based therapy is the inability to utilize the patient's own cells (Canan et al., 2014; Stahl and Brown, 2015; Morgan et al., 2018) and the potential for graft vs. host disease (GvHD) with allogeneic sources requiring immunosuppression (Bashyam, 2007). The era of gene editing technology has provided the opportunity to consider developing corrected autologous patient macrophages for BMDM delivery. The potential of this technology is in its infancy is not ready for clinical application in scenarios like CF, especially since BMDM corrective therapy would not provide a curative outcome. Further, it would be essential to discern any changes in BMDM function or off target effects that might occur with gene editing technology (Papasavva et al., 2019). Further, one of the major hurdles in implementing gene correction is the efficiency of site directed editing in scenarios of low levels of expression of CFTR in hematopoietic cells (Abdulrahman et al., 2011; Zhang et al., 2018). Whole bone marrow aspirates, hMSC and *Cftr* sufficient macrophages provide clear implications for therapeutic development of immune support in managing CF lung infection and inflammation based upon the data we have presented in this manuscript. These observations are consistent with previous studies that have also pursued immune supportive therapeutic directives (Weiss, 2008; Bruscia et al., 2009; Bonfield et al., 2012; Sutton et al., 2017; Duchesneau et al., 2020; Zhang et al., 2020). Follow-up studies will focus on delivering CF macrophages or hMSCs in the preclinical model and further investigate the functional insufficiency of CF derived cells. The goal will be to determine the efficiencyof the CF origin of the autologous cells on the CF like manifestation observed in the murine model of the CF lung infection and inflammation-like pathophysiology. A future study will be delivering the myeloid specific Cftr KO and KI macrophages to either WT or CF mice, which again will continue to define how macrophages can be utilized to improve the care of patients with CF. Many of these studies could then be translated to more expensive complex models like the ferret or pig, to determine the effect of the cell therapy on other aspects of CF pathophysiology that are not bridged by the mouse models.

hMSCs are immune evasive therefore having greater versatility over gene corrective BMDM (Auletta et al., 2015; Leyendecker et al., 2018). hMSCs can be delivered as an allogeneic source with patients not requiring immunosuppression to prevent GvHD (Auletta et al., 2015; Leyendecker et al., 2018). hMSCs treatment has been the foundation of cell-based therapeutic approaches to inflammation in a variety of diseases globally without adverse reaction, and with significant clinical response (Caplan 2017; Leyendecker et al., 2018). We have shown *in vitro*, *in vivo* and *ex vivo* clinical models that hMSCs can provide therapeutic benefit in CF through attenuating inflammation and aiding in infection resolution similar to the efficiency of macrophages (Bonfield et al., 2013). Further, we have published that hMSC treatment is antibiotic "saving" through their antimicrobial potency decreasing the required dose of antibiotics for eradication of bacteria (Bonfield et al., 2013; Sutton et al., 2016). In our "First in CF" Phase I clinical trial we have also been able to demonstrate their safety (Roesch et al., 2019). hMSCs can alter macrophage response to pathogens enabling better control of the overactive inflammatory response to infection (**Figure** 7), consistent. Cell-based approaches have the capacity to enhance current therapeutic availability strategies for CF through aiding the patient's own

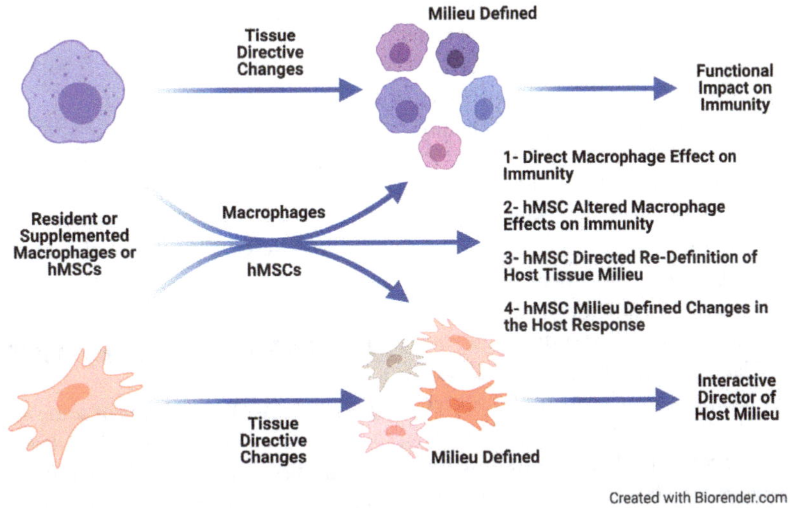

FIGURE 7 | Immune supportive therapy model for cystic fibrosis. Patients with CF early become infected with pathogens which contributed to the triad of infection → inflammation → lung-damage. The lung damage continues to create a pulmonary milieu that is susceptible to infection, so the triad continues resulting in the vicious circle of that is pathologic in CF. The feasibility of providing immune support focusing on hMSCs and BMDM which could be harnessed to skew the balance of the host response to infection and establishing chronic inflammation. Macrophages and hMSCs both have their potential roles in providing clinical efficacy and potency, but the key is likely how they interact *in vivo*. Macrophages defining the hMSC phenotype due to the milieu elicited and the contribution of the functionally tissue cued hMSCs to support the resolution toward homeostasis and tissue recovery. The hematopoietic approach would minimize the CFTR induced damage to the lung and other tissue, while at the same time promoting the patient's management of their internal milieu. CRISPR/Cas9, the advent of iPSC cells and other gene editing technologies opens the door toward the potential adding corrective immune support in CF.

immune capacity to regulate the inflammatory response and exposure to pathogens. CF patients are living longer,and, whether due to the chronicity of their disease or intrinsic pathophysiology, immune-senescence is likely (Pawelec, 2017; Fulop et al., 2018). Immune support may be ideal in the prevention of immune-senescence.

The concept of cell therapy for the treatment of CF lung infection and inflammation is complex, particularly with the dynamic nature of the "drug" in the form of macrophages, hMSCs or both (Hodges and Conlon, 2019). Fortunately, cell-based approaches have been described in other diseases such as alveolar proteinosis (Suzuki et al., 2014), Niemen Pick disease (Schuchman and Desnick, 2017) acute respiratory distress syndrome (Horie et al., 2018), interstitial pulmonary fibrosis (Bonfield and Caplan, 2010), bronchopulmonary dysplasia (Cerny et al., 2008), rheumatoid arthritis (Jorgensen, 2010) and others (Lachmann et al., 2014; Morrison et al., 2017; Khoury et al., 2020; Verma et al., 2020). Bone marrow supplementation or hMSC therapy is not corrective longitudinally, but would enhance the capacity of patients to manage their own immune environment. Supporting CFTR corrective approaches and managing more difficult mutations and other systemic pathologies associated with CF disease would be major benefactors of hMSCs treatment and clinical care. The immune evasiveness of hMSCs has been demonstrated in greater than 900 clinical trials currently on-going globally with no major adverse effects (clinicaltrials.gov). Many patients in these trials have effectively tolerated and benefited from multiple infusions which speaks to the safety as well as the capacity to have the option for repetitive care during exacerbations of disease (Murphy et al., 2013; Caplan, 2018).

Another benefit in hMSC cell based therapy is related to the impact hMSCs have on macrophages (Al-Rubaie et al., 2018; Leyendecker et al., 2018). hMSCs are engulfed by macrophages (*in vitro* and *in vivo*), resulting in a change in the macrophage phenotype (Morrison et al., 2017; Yin et al., 2017; Philipp et al., 2018; Harrell et al., 2019). It might be that treating CF patients with hMSCs will have a direct hMSC effect (anti-inflammatory and antimicrobial) but also an indirect effect on optimizing macrophage immune function. These studies still need to be vetted, but provide support for hMSC therapeutics as an option of supplemental care in CF. The added advantage of hMSC enhancement of antibiotic potency is also very attractive in patients who constantly suffer from chronic colonization with bacteria (Bonfield et al., 2013). hMSCs would not be a stand-alone therapy in CF, but would be given in the context of on-going treatment such as modulators, antibiotics, anti-oxidants, anti-mucolytic and the whole host of other drugs available for patient treatment schemes. These treatment algorithms would not require pre-treatment of the hMSCs, but would be considered a co-therapeutic with the patient's traditional clinical regimen. Manipulating either macrophages or hMSCs for optimization strategies is complex but would bridge manipulated cell therapy for the unique application in CF. The capacity for manipulated cell-based therapeutic approaches is a bit more tenuous to get FDA approval, requiring innovative ways to demonstrate the safety and efficacy in the setting of CF (Philipp et al., 2018; Saeedi et al., 2019). An important aspect of hMSC therapy should focus on hMSC product development and the assurance of the optimal antimicrobial and anti-inflammatory potency in scenarios of pathogens consistent with CF infection. The concept of choosing the right hMSC donor preparation has the potential to enhance the beneficial response of the immune supportive therapy, which is also the foundation of much of our research focus currently (Caplan 2018; Sutton and Bonfield 2014; Bonfield et al., 2019).

The advancement of small molecule correctors and potentiators has made substantial contributions to the management of CF lung disease and extending patient survival (Bell et al., 2019; Clancy et al., 2019; Egan 2020). The potentiators and correctors appear to also limit the degree of insidious inflammation associated with CF lung disease; however, the success of this aspect is probably years out for defining the ultimate clinical impact on disease. As with all chronic inflammatory diseases, immunity can be impacted by chronicity of disease and the contribution of immune dysregulation based upon sustained inflammatory sequelae (Walsh, 2006; Zuo et al., 2019). The initiation of the inflammation/infection vicious circle and the inability to "turn-off" established inflammation will continue to be an issue in the foreseeable future until a cure is assured. The modulators are not curative for CF, they address the need for functional CFTR, but it is still pharmacological and short-lived, requiring a daily regimen for sustained optimal physiological dosed over time. The long-term impact and effectiveness of the small molecule drugs remains to be determined necessitating the continued pursuit of other treatment modalities. Immune support has the capacity to enhance the duration and sustainability of current therapeutics by providing patients with an extra boost to manage their own immunity. Cell based immune therapies are not curative in CF, implicating that to sustained benefit patients might require a couple doses a year (Murphy et al., 2013; Caplan, 2018). Harnessing hematopoietic stores for "efficient" management of inflammation is not a difficult vision, given the success in other diseases (Horwitz et al., 2001; Loebinger et al., 2008; Doerschuk, 2015; Sallese et al., 2017). The age of personalized medicine, hMSCs, cell based hematopoietic support, and immune correction is an opportunity to minimize disease and improve the overall health of CF patients as the pursuit of a cure for all patients with the disease is sought.

ETHICS STATEMENT

The animal study was reviewed and approved by the Case Western Reserve Institutional Animal Care and Use Committee.

AUTHOR CONTRIBUTIONS

AH- wrote earlier versions of some aspects of the manuscript and facilitated some of the initial studies. MS- wrote and did many of the studies outlined in the manuscript. DF- facilitated and did many of the studies and data evaluation, CH- generated the mice, and provided insight into the manuscript perspectives, AC- provided insight and funds for the mesenchymal stem cells studies, and contributed to the manuscript. TB- Wrote the manuscript, provide funds for the studies, technically did many of the studies, mentored other aspects of the study.

ACKNOWLEDGMENTS

There are many people that have been involved with this work over the years. The CF Animal Core with Pamela Davis under the direction of AH: Nicole Brown, R. Christiaan van Heeckeren, Sarah Frischmann, Alma Wilson. The current CF Animal Core under the direction of CH: Dana Valerio, Alma Wilson, Molly Schneider. The Bonfield laboratory support: Mary Koloze-Nolan, Nejimol Joy, Christiaan van Heeckeren, DF, MS and Ariana Kian (Hathaway Brown High School SREP Program). There were also collaborators of earlier drafts of manuscripts in the earlier studies with AH, which may have contributed to discussions of data that are not part of this manuscript: Daniel P. Hsu, Daniel Weiss, Scott A. Fulton, Roberto Loi, Aura Perez, Nicholas P. Ziats, Wei Xue, Mark Schluchter. Cystic Fibrosis Mouse Model Resource Center: Cystic Fibrosis Foundation: HODGES19R (CH).

REFERENCES

Abdulrahman, B. A., Khweek, A. A., Akhter, A., Caution, K., Kotrange, S., Abdelaziz, D. H., et al. (2011). Autophagy stimulation by rapamycin suppresses lung inflammation and infection by Burkholderia cenocepacia in a model of cystic fibrosis. *Autophagy* 7 (11), 1359–1370. doi:10.4161/auto.7.11.17660

Aiello, A., Farzaneh, F., Candore, G., Caruso, C., Davinelli, S., Gambino, C. M., et al. (2019). Immunosenescence and its hallmarks: how to oppose aging strategically? A review of potential options for therapeutic intervention. *Front. Immunol.* 10, 2247. doi:10.3389/fimmu.2019.02247

Al-Rubaie, Ali., Wise, A. F., Sozo, F., De Matteo, R., Samuel, C. S., Harding, R., et al. (2018). The therapeutic effect of mesenchymal stem cells on pulmonary myeloid cells following neonatal hyperoxic lung injury in mice. *Respir. Res.* 19 (1), 114. doi:10.1186/s12931-018-0816-x

Assani, K., Shrestha, C. L., Robledo-Avila, F., Rajaram, M. V., Partida-Sanchez, S., Schlesinger, L. S., et al. (2017). Human cystic fibrosis macrophages have defective calcium-dependent protein kinase C activation of the NADPH oxidase, an effect augmented byBurkholderia cenocepacia. *J. Immunol.* 198 (5), 1985–1994. doi:10.4049/jimmunol.1502609

Auletta, J. J., Eid, S. K., Wuttisarnwattana, P., Silva, I., Metheny, L., Keller, M. D., et al. (2015). Human mesenchymal stromal cells attenuate graft-versus-host disease and maintain graft-versus-leukemia activity following experimental allogeneic bone marrow transplantation. *Stem Cells* 33 (2), 601–614. doi:10.1002/stem.1867

Bashyam, H. (2007). Crossing barriers in transplantation. *J. Exp. Med.* 204 (3), 459. doi:10.1084/jem.2043fta

Bell, S. C., Mall, M. A., Gutierrez, H., Macek, M., Madge, S., Davies, J. C., et al. (2019). The future of cystic fibrosis care: a global perspective. *Lancet Respir. Med.* 8 (1), 65–124. doi:10.1016/S2213-2600(19)30337-6

Bezzerri, V., Piacenza, F., Caporelli, N., Malavolta, M., Provinciali, M., and Cipolli, M. (2019). Is cellular senescence involved in cystic fibrosis? *Respir. Res.* 20 (1), 32. doi:10.1186/s12931-019-0993-2

Bonfield, T. L. (2015). Macrophage dysfunction in cystic fibrosis: a therapeutic target to enhance self-immunity. *Am. J. Respir. Crit. Care Med.* 192, 1406–1407. doi:10.1164/rccm.201509-1811ED

Bonfield, T. L., and Caplan, A. I. (2010). Adult mesenchymal stem cells: an innovative therapeutic for lung diseases. *Discov. Med.* 9 (47), 337–345.

Bonfield, T. L., Hodges, C. A., Cotton, C. U., and Drumm, M. L. (2012). Absence of the cystic fibrosis transmembrane regulator (cftr) from myeloid-derived cells slows resolution of inflammation and infection. *J. Leukoc. Biol.* 92, 1938–3673. doi:10.1189/jlb.0412188

Bonfield, T. L., Roesch, E., Lazarus, H., Reese, J., Chmiel, J. F., and Caplan, A. I. (2019). Mesenchymal stem cell donor selection for the "first in CF" phase I clinical trial. *Pediatr.* 54, S155–S480. doi:10.1002/ppul.22495

Bonfield, T. L., Lennon, D., Ghosh, S. K., DiMarino, A. M., Weinberg, A., and Caplan, A. I. (2013). Cell based therapy aides in infection and inflammation resolution in the murine model of cystic fibrosis lung disease. *SCD* 3, 139–153. doi:10.4236/scd.2013.32019

Bonfield, T. L., Thomassen, M. J., Farver, C. F., Abraham, S., Koloze, M. T., Zhang, X., et al. (2008). Peroxisome proliferator-activated receptor-γ regulates the expression of alveolar macrophage macrophage colony-stimulating factor. *J. Immunol.* 181 (1), 235. doi:10.4049/jimmunol.181.1.235

Bragonzi, A. (2010). Murine models of acute and chronic lung infection with cystic fibrosis pathogens. *Int. J. Med. Microbiol.* 300 (8), 584–593. doi:10.1016/j.ijmm.2010.08.012

Bruscia, E. M., and Bonfield, T. L. (2016a). Innate and adaptive immunity in cystic fibrosis. *Clin. Chest Med.* 37 (1), 17–29. doi:10.1016/j.ccm.2015.11.010

Bruscia, E. M., and Bonfield, T. L. (2016b). Cystic fibrosis lung immunity: the role of the macrophage. *J. Innate Immun.* 8, 550. doi:10.1159/000446825

Bruscia, E. M., Zhang, P.-X., Ferreira, E., Caputo, C., Emerson, J. W., Tuck, D., et al. (2009). Macrophages directly contribute to the exaggerated inflammatory response in cystic fibrosis transmembrane conductance Regulator−/−Mice. *Am. J. Respir. Cel Mol Biol* 40 (3), 295–304. doi:10.1165/rcmb.2008-0170oc

Burgener, E. B., and Moss, R. B. (2018). "Cystic fibrosis transmembrane conductance regulator modulators: precision medicine in cystic fibrosis," in *Current opinion in pediatrics* (Philadelphia, PA: Lippincott Williams and Wilkins). doi:10.1097/MOP.0000000000000627

Cabrini, G. (2019). Innovative therapies for cystic fibrosis: the road from treatment to cure. *Mol. Diagn. Ther.* 23 (2), 263–279. doi:10.1007/s40291-018-0372-6

Canan, C. H., Gokhale, N. S., Carruthers, B., Lafuse, W. P., Schlesinger, L. S., Torrelles, J. B., et al. (2014). Characterization of lung inflammation and its impact on macrophage function in aging. *J. Leukoc. Biol.* 96 (3), 473–480. doi:10.1189/jlb.4a0214-093rr

Caplan, A. I. (2018). Cell-based therapies: the nonresponder. *Stem Cel. Trans. Med.* 7 (11), 762–766. doi:10.1002/sctm.18-0074

Caplan, A. I. (2017). Mesenchymal stem cells: time to change the name! *Stem Cel. Trans. Med.* 6 (6), 1445–1451. doi:10.1002/sctm.17-0051

Cerny, L., Torday, J. S., and Rehan, V. K. (2008). Prevention and treatment of bronchopulmonary dysplasia: contemporary status and future outlook. *Lung* 186, 75–89. doi:10.1007/s00408-007-9069-z

Clancy, J. P., Cotton, C. U., Donaldson, S. H., Solomo, G. M., VanDevanter, D. R., Boyle, M. P., et al. (2019). CFTR modulator theratyping: current status, gaps and future directions. *J. Cyst. Fibr.* 18 (1), 22–34. doi:10.1016/j.jcf.2018.05.004

Crapnell, K., Blaesius, R., Hastings, A., Lennon, D. P., Caplan, A. I., and Bruder, S. P. (2013). Growth, differentiation capacity, and function of mesenchymal stem cells expanded in serum-free medium developed via combinatorial screening. *Exp.Cell Res.* 319 (10), 1409–1418. doi:10.1016/j.yexcr.2013.04.004

Di Pietro, C., Zhang, P.-X., O'Rourke, T. K., Murray, T. S., Wang, L., Britto, C. J., et al. (2017). Ezrin links CFTR to TLR4 signaling to orchestrate anti-bacterial immune response in macrophages. *Scientific Rep.* 7 (1), 10882. doi:10.1038/s41598-017-11012-7

Doerschuk, C. M. (2015). Pulmonary alveolar proteinosis and macrophage transplantation. *New Engl. J. Med.* 372 (18). doi:10.1056/nejmcibr1413035

Duchesneau, P., Waddell, T. K., and Karoubi, G. (2020). Cell-based therapeutic approaches for cystic fibrosis. *Int. J. Mol. Sci.* 21 (15), 5219. doi:10.3390/ijms21155219

Egan, M. E. 2020. Emerging technologies for cystic fibrosis transmembrane conductance regulator (CFTR) restoration in all people with CF. *Ped. Pulmonol.* 56, S32–S39. doi:10.1002/ppul.24965

Elborn, J. S. (2016). Cystic fibrosis. *Lancet* 388 (10059), 2519–2531. doi:10.1016/S0140-6736(16)00576-6

Fan, Z., Perisse, I. V., Cotton, C. U., Regouski, M., Meng, Q., Domb, C., et al. (2018). A sheep model of cystic fibrosis generated by CRISPR/Cas9 disruption of the CFTR gene. *JCI Insight* 3 (19), 123529. doi:10.1172/jci.insight.123529

Fischer, B. M., Wong, J. K., Degan, S., Kummarapurugu, A. B., Zheng, S., Haridass, P., et al. (2013). Increased expression of senescence markers in cystic fibrosis airways. *Am. J. Physiology-Lung Cell Mol. Physiol.* 304 (6), L394. doi:10.1152/ajplung.00091.2012

Fulop, T., Witkowski, J. M., Olivieri, F., and Larbi, A. (2018). The integration of inflammaging in age-related diseases. *Semin. Immunol.* 40, 17–35. doi:10.1016/j.smim.2018.09.003

Funes, S. C., Rios, M., Escobar-Vera, J., Alexis, M., and Kalergis, A. M. (2018). Implications of macrophage polarization in autoimmunity. *Immunology* 154 (2), 186–195. doi:10.1111/imm.12910

Harrell, C. R., Markovic, B. S., Fellabaum, C., Arsenijevic, A., and Volarevic, V. (2019). Mesenchymal stem cell-based therapy of osteoarthritis: current knowledge and future perspectives. *Biomed. Pharmacother.* 109, 2318–2326. doi:10.1016/j.biopha.2018.11.099

Heeckeren, A. M., Schluchter, M. D., Xue, W., and Davis, P. B. (2006). Response to acute lung infection with mucoid Pseudomonas aeruginosa in cystic fibrosis mice. *Am. J. Respir. Crit. Care Med.* 173 (3), 288–296. doi:10.1164/rccm.200506-917OC

Hisert, K. B., Birkland, T. P., Kelly, Q. S., Long, M. E., Grogan, B., Carter, S., et al. (2020). CFTR modulator therapy enhances peripheral blood monocyte contributions to immune responses in people with cystic fibrosis. *Front. Pharmacol.* 11, 1219. doi:10.3389/fphar.2020.01219

Hodges, C. A., Cotton, C. U., Palmert, M. R., and Drumm, M. L. (2008). Generation of a conditional null allele forCftrin mice. *Genesis* 46 (10), 546–552. doi:10.1002/dvg.2043310.1002/dvg.20433

Hodges, C. A., and Conlon, R. A. (2019). Delivering on the promise of gene editing for cystic fibrosis. *Genes Dis.* 6 (2), 97–108. doi:10.1016/j.gendis.2018.11.005

Hodges, C. A., Grady, B. R., Mishra, K., Cotton, C. U., and Drumm, M. L. (2011). Cystic fibrosis growth retardation is not correlated with loss of cftr in the intestinal epithelium. *Am. J. Physiol. Gastrointest. Liver Physiol.* 301 (3), G528–G536. doi:10.1152/ajpgi.00052.2011

Horie, S., Gonzalez, H. E., Laffey, J. G., and Masterson, C. H. (2018). Cell therapy in acute respiratory distress syndrome. *J. Thorac. Dis.* 10 (9), 5607–5620. doi:10.21037/jtd.2018.08.28

Horwitz, E. M., Prockop, D. J., Gordon, P. L., Koo, W. W., Fitzpatrick, L. A., Neel, M. D., et al. (2001). Clinical responses to bone marrow transplantation in children with severe osteogenesis imperfecta. *Blood* 97 (5), 1227–1231. doi:10.1182/blood.v97.5.1227

Hsu, D., Taylor, P., Fletcher, D., van Heeckeren, R., Eastman, J., van Heeckeren, A., et al. (2016). Interleukin-17 pathophysiology and therapeutic intervention in cystic fibrosis lung infection and inflammation. *Infect. Immun.* 84 (9), 2410–2421. doi:10.1128/iai.00284-16

Jorgensen, C. (2010). Mesenchymal stem cells in arthritis: role of bone marrow microenvironment. *Arthritis Res.Ther.* 12, 1478–6362. doi:10.1186/ar3105

Khoury, M., Cuenca, J., Cruz, F. F., Figueroa, F. E., Rocco, P. R. M., and Weiss, D. J. (2020). Current status of cell-based therapies for respiratory virus infections: applicability to COVID-19. *Eur. Respir. J.* 55 (6), 2000858. doi:10.1183/13993003.00858-2020

Knethen, A., and Brune, B. (2002). Activation of peroxisome proliferator-activated receptor _g_ by nitric oxide in monocytes/macrophages down-regulates P47_phox_ and attenuates the respiratory burst. *J. Immunol.* 169, 2619–2626. doi:10.4049/jimmunol.169.5.2619

Knutsen, A. P., and Slavin, R. G. (2011). Allergic bronchopulmonary aspergillosis in asthma and cystic fibrosis. *Clin.Dev.Immunol.* 2011, 843763. doi:10.1155/2011/843763

Korbecki, J., Bobiński, R., and Dutka, M. (2019). Self-regulation of the inflammatory response by peroxisome proliferator-activated receptors. *Inflamm. Res.* 68 (6), 443–458. doi:10.1007/s00011-019-01231-1

Lachmann, N., Happle, C., Ackermann, M., Lüttge, D., Wetzke, M., Merkert, S., et al. (2014). Gene correction of human induced pluripotent stem cells repairs the cellular phenotype in pulmonary alveolar proteinosis. *Am. J. Respir. Crit. Care Med.* 189 (2), 167. doi:10.1164/rccm.201306-1012OC

Lennon, D. P., and Caplan, A. I. (2006). Isolation of human marrow-derived mesenchymal stem cells. *Exp. Hematol.* 34 (11), 1604–1605. doi:10.1016/j.exphem.2006.07.014

Leyendecker, A., Pinheiro, C. C. G., Amano, M. T., and Bueno, D. F. (2018). The use of human mesenchymal stem cells as therapeutic agents for the *in Vivo* treatment of immune-related diseases: a systematic review. *Front. Immunol.* 9, 2056. doi:10.3389/fimmu.2018.02056

Loebinger, M. R., Aguilar, S., and Janes, S. M. (2008). Therapeutic potential of stem cells in lung disease: progress and pitfalls. *Clin.Sci.* 114 (2), 99–108. doi:10.1042/cs20070073

Ma, J. T., Tang, C., Kang, L., Voynow, J. A., and Rubin, B. K. (2018). Cystic fibrosis sputum rheology correlates with both acute and longitudinal changes in lung function. *Chest* 154 (2), 370–377. doi:10.1016/j.chest.2018.03.005

Marangi, M., and Pistritto, G. (2018). Innovative therapeutic strategies for cystic fibrosis: moving forward to CRISPR technique. *Front. Pharmacol.* 9, 396. doi:10.3389/fphar.2018.00396

Martiniano, S. L., Nick, J. A., and Daley, C. L. (2019). Nontuberculous mycobacterial infections in cystic fibrosis. *Thorac. Surg. Clin.* 29 (1), 95–108. doi:10.1016/j.thorsurg.2018.09.008

Matuska, B., Comhair, S., Farver, C., Chmiel, J., Midura, R. J., Bonfield, T., et al. (2016). Pathological hyaluronan matrices in cystic fibrosis airways and secretions. *Am. J. Respir. Cel Mol Biol* 55 (4), 576–585. doi:10.1165/rcmb.2015-0358oc

McElvaney, O. J., Gunaratnam, C., McElvaney, O. F., Bagwe, I., Reeves, E. P., and McElvaney, N. G. (2018). Emerging pharmacotherapies in cystic fibrosis. *Expert Rev. Respir. Med.* 12 (10), 843–855. doi:10.1080/17476348.2018.1512409

Morales-Nebreda, L., Misharin, A. V., Perlman, H., and Scott Budinger, G. R. (2015). The heterogeneity of lung macrophages in the susceptibility to disease. *Eur. Respir. Rev.* 24 (137), 505–509. doi:10.1183/16000617.0031-2015

Morgan, D. J., Casulli, J., Chew, C., Connolly, E., Lui, S., Brand, O. J., et al. (2018). Innate immune cell suppression and the link with secondary lung bacterial pneumonia. *Front. Immunol.* 9, 2943. doi:10.3389/fimmu.2018.02943

Morrison, T. J., Jackson, M. V., Cunningham, E. K., Kissenpfennig, A., McAuley, D. F., O'Kane, C. M., et al. (2017). Mesenchymal stromal cells modulate macrophages in clinically relevant lung injury models by extracellular vesicle mitochondrial transfer. *Am. J. Respir. Crit. Care Med.* 196 (10), 1275–1286. doi:10.1164/rccm.201701-0170oc

Murphy, M. B., Moncivais, K., and Caplan, A. I. (2013). Mesenchymal stem cells: environmentally responsive therapeutics for regenerative medicine. *Exp. Mol. Med.* 45 (11), e54. doi:10.1038/emm.2013.94

Ng, H. P., Zhou, Y., Song, K., Hodges, C. A., Drumm, M. L., and Wang, G. (2014). Neutrophil-mediated phagocytic host defense defect in myeloid cftr-inactivated mice. *PLoS One* 9 (9), e106813. doi:10.1371/journal.pone.0106813

Nichols, D. P., and Chmiel, J. F. (2015). Inflammation and its genesis in cystic fibrosis. *Pediatr. Pulmonol.* 50 (Suppl. 40), S39–S56. doi:10.1002/ppul.23242

Papasavva, P., Kleanthous, M., and Lederer, C. W. (2019). Rare opportunities: CRISPR/Cas-Based therapy development for rare genetic diseases. *Mol. Diagn. Ther.* 23 (2), 201–222. doi:10.1007/s40291-019-00392-3

Pawelec, G. (2017). Does the human immune system ever really become "senescent?" *F1000Res* 6, 1323. doi:10.12688/f1000research.11297.1

Phang, R. Z., Tay, F. C., Goh, S. L., Lau, C. H., Zhu, H., Tan, W. K., et al. (2013). Zinc finger nuclease-expressing baculoviral vectors mediate targeted genome integration of reprogramming factor genes to facilitate the generation of human induced pluripotent stem cells. *Stem Cells Transl.Med.* 2, 2157–6564. doi:10.5966/sctm.2013-0043

Philipp, D., Suhr, L., Wahlers, T., Choi, Y.-H., and Paunel-Görgülü, A. (2018). Preconditioning of bone marrow-derived mesenchymal stem cells highly strengthens their potential to promote IL-6-dependent M2b polarization. *Stem Cel Res. Ther.* 9 (1), 286. doi:10.1186/s13287-018-1039-2

Ralhan, A., Laval, J., Lelis, F., Ballbach, M., Grund, C., Hector, A., et al. (2016). Current concepts and controversies in innate immunity of cystic fibrosis lung disease. *J. Innate Immun.* 8 (6), 531–540. doi:10.1183/13993003.congress-2016.pa4858

Roesch, E. A., Nichols, D. P., and Chmiel, J. F. (2018). Inflammation in cystic fibrosis: an update. *Pediatr. Pulmonol* 53 (S3), S30–S50. doi:10.1002/ppul.24129

Roesch, E., Bonfield, T. L., Lazarus, H., Resse, J., Hillard, K., Hirth, B., et al. (2019). Poster session. *Pediatr. Pulmonol* 54 (Suppl. 2), S155–S480. doi:10.1002/ppul.22495

Rosen, B. H., Evans, T. I. A., Moll, S. R., Gray, J. S., Liang, B., Sun, X., et al. (2018). Infection is not required for mucoinflammatory lung disease in CFTR-knockout ferrets. *Am. J. Respir. Crit. Care Med.* 197 (10), 1308–1318. doi:10.1164/rccm.201708-1616oc

Saeedi, P., Halabian, R., and Fooladi, A. A. I. (2019). Antimicrobial effects of mesenchymal stem cells primed by modified LPS on bacterial clearance in sepsis. *J. Cel. Physiol.* 234 (4), 4970–4986. doi:10.1002/jcp.27298

Sallese, A., Suzuki, T., McCarthy, C., Bridges, J., Filuta, A., Arumugam, P., et al. (2017). Targeting cholesterol homeostasis in lung diseases. *Scientific Rep.* 7 (1). doi:10.1038/s41598-017-10879-w

Schuchman, E. H., and Desnick, R. J. (2017). Types A and B niemann-pick disease. *Mol. Genet. Metab.* 120 (1–2), 27–33. doi:10.1016/j.ymgme.2016.12.008

Snouwaert, J. N., Brigman, K. K., Latour, A. M., Malouf, N. N., Boucher, R. C., Smithies, O., et al. (1992). An animal model for cystic fibrosis made by gene targeting. *Science* 257 (5073), 1083–1088. doi:10.1126/science.257.5073.1083

Soltys, J., Bonfield, T., Chmiel, J., and Berger, M. (2002). Functional IL-10 deficiency in the lung of cystic fibrosis (cftr−/−) and IL-10 knockout mice causes increased expression and function of B7 costimulatory molecules on alveolar macrophages. *J. Immunol.* 168 (4), 1903–1910. doi:10.4049/jimmunol.168.4.1903

Spielberg, D. R., and Clancy, J. P. (2016). Cystic fibrosis and its management through established and emerging therapies. *Annu. Rev. Genom. Hum. Genet.* 17, 155–175. doi:10.1146/annurev-genom-090314-050024

Stahl, E. C., and Brown, B. N. (2015). Cell therapy strategies to combat immunosenescence. *Organogenesis* 11 (4), 159–172. doi:10.1080/15476278.2015.1120046

Stotland, P. K., Radzioch, D., and Stevenson, M. M. (2000). Mouse models of chronic lung infection with *Pseudomonas aeruginosa*: models for the study of cystic fibrosis. *Pediatr. Pulmonol* 30, 413–424. doi:10.1002/1099-0496

Sutton, M. T., Fletcher, D., Episalla, N., Auster, L., Folz, M., Roy, V., et al. (2017). Mesenchymal stem cell soluble mediators and cystic fibrosis. *J. Stem Cel Res. Ther.* 7 (9), 400. doi:10.4172/2157-7633.1000400

Sutton, M. T., Fletcher, D., Ghosh, S. K., Weinberg, A., van Heeckeren, R., Kaur, S., et al. (2016). Antimicrobial properties of mesenchymal stem cells: therapeutic potential for cystic fibrosis infection, and treatment. *Stem Cell Int.* 2016, 5303048. doi:10.1155/2016/5303048

Sutton, M. T., and Bonfield, T. L. (2014). Stem cells: innovations in clinical applications. *Stem Cell Int.* 2014 516278. doi:10.1155/2014/516278

Suzuki, T., Arumugam, P., Sakagami, T., Lachmann, N., Chalk, C., Anthony, S., et al. (2014). Pulmonary macrophage transplantation therapy. *Nature* 514 (7253). doi:10.1038/nature13807

Tarique, A. A., Sly, P. D., Cardenas, D. G., Luo, L., Stow, J. L., Bell, S. C., et al. (2018). Differential expression of genes and receptors in monocytes from patients with cystic fibrosis. *J. Cystic Fibr.* 18 (3), 342–348. doi:10.1016/j.jcf.2018.07.012

Verma, Y. K., Verma, R., Tyagi, N., Behl, A., Kumar, S., and Gangenahalli, G. U. (2020). COVID-19 and its therapeutics: special emphasis on mesenchymal stem cells based therapy. *Stem Cel Rev. Rep.* 17 (1), 113–131. doi:10.1007/s12015-020-10037-2

van Heeckeren, A. M., and Schluchter, M. D. (2002). Murine models of chronic *Pseudomonas* aeruginosa lung infection. *Lab. Anim.* 36 (3), 291–312. doi:10.1258/002367702320162405

van Heeckeren, A., Walenga, R., Konstan, M. W., Bonfield, T., Davis, P. B., and Ferkol, T. (1997). Excessive inflammatory response of cystic fibrosis mice to bronchopulmonary infection with Pseudomonas aeruginosa. *J. Clin. Invest.* 100 (11), 2810–2815. doi:10.1172/jci119828

Walsh, G. M. (2006). Targeting airway inflammation: novel therapies for the treatment of asthma. *Curr.Med.Chem.* 13, 3105–3111. doi:10.2174/092986706778201594

Weiss, D. J. (2008). Stem cells and cell therapies for cystic fibrosis and other lung diseases. *Pulm. Pharmacol. Ther.* 21 (4), 588–594. doi:10.1016/j.pupt.2007.11.004

West, N. E., and Flume, P. A. (2018). Unmet needs in cystic fibrosis: the next steps in improving outcomes. *Expert Rev. Respir. Med.* 12 (7), 585–593. doi:10.1080/17476348.2018.1483723

Worgall, S., Martushova, K., Busch, A., Lande, L., and Crystal, R. G. (2002). Apoptosis induced by *Pseudomonas aeruginosa* in antigen presenting cells is diminished by genetic modification with CD40 ligand. *Pediatr. Res.* 52 (5), 636–644. doi:10.1203/00006450-200211000-00006

Yin, Y., Wu, R. X., He, X. T., Xu, X. Y., Wang, J., and Chen, F. M. (2017). Influences of age-related changes in mesenchymal stem cells on macrophages during *in-vitro* culture. *Stem Cel Res. Ther.* 8 (1), 153. doi:10.1186/s13287-017-0608-0

Zhang, S., Shrestha, C. L., and Kopp, B. T. (2018). Cystic fibrosis transmembrane conductance regulator (CFTR) modulators have differential effects on cystic fibrosis macrophage function. *Scientific Rep.* 8 (1), 17066. doi:10.1038/s41598-018-35151-7

Zhang, S., Shrestha, C. L., Wisniewski, B. L., Pham, H., Hou, X., Li, W., et al. (2020). Consequences of CRISPR-cas9-mediated CFTR knockout in human macrophages. *Front. Immunol.* 11, 1871. doi:10.3389/fimmu.2020.01871

Zuo, L., Prather, E. R., Stetskiv, M., Garrison, D. E., Meade, J. R., Peace, T. I., et al. (2019). Inflammaging and oxidative stress in human diseases: from molecular mechanisms to novel treatments. *Ijms* 20 (18), 4472. doi:10.3390/ijms20184472

9

Targeting IgG Autoantibodies for Improved Cytotoxicity of Bactericidal Permeability Increasing Protein in Cystic Fibrosis

Karen McQuillan, Fatma Gargoum, Mark P. Murphy, Oliver J. McElvaney, Noel G. McElvaney[†] and Emer P. Reeves[†]*

Irish Centre for Genetic Lung Disease, Department of Medicine, Royal College of Surgeons in Ireland, Education and Research Centre, Beaumont Hospital, Dublin, Ireland

Correspondence:
Emer P. Reeves
emerreeves@rcsi.ie

[†]These authors share senior authorship

In people with cystic fibrosis (PWCF), inflammation with concurrent infection occurs from a young age and significantly influences lung disease progression. Studies indicate that neutrophils are important effector cells in the pathogenesis of CF and in the development of anti-neutrophil cytoplasmic autoantibodies (ANCA). ANCA specific for bactericidal permeability increasing protein (BPI-ANCA) are detected in people with CF, and correlate with infection with *Pseudomonas aeruginosa*. The aim of this study was to determine the signaling mechanism leading to increased BPI release by CF neutrophils, while identifying IgG class BPI-ANCA in CF airways samples as the cause for impaired antimicrobial activity of BPI against *P. aeruginosa.* Plasma and/or bronchoalveolar lavage fluid (BAL) was collected from PWCF ($n = 40$), CF receiving ivacaftor therapy ($n = 10$), non-CF patient cohorts ($n = 7$) and healthy controls ($n = 38$). Plasma and BAL BPI and BPI-ANCA were measured by ELISA and GTP-bound Rac2 detected using an *in vitro* assay. The antibacterial effect of all treatments tested was determined by colony forming units enumeration. Levels of BPI are significantly increased in plasma ($p = 0.007$) and BALF ($p < 0.0001$) of PWCF. The signaling mechanism leading to increased degranulation and exocytosis of BPI by CF neutrophils ($p = 0.02$) involved enhancement of Rac2 GTP-loading ($p = 0.03$). The full-length BPI protein was detectable in all CF BAL samples and patients displayed ANCA with BPI specificity. IgG class autoantibodies were purified from CF BAL complexed to BPI (n=5), with IgG autoantibody cross-linking of antigen preventing BPI induced *P. aeruginosa* killing ($p < 0.0001$). Results indicate that the immune-mediated diminished antimicrobial defense, attributed to anti-BPI-IgG, necessitates the formation of a drug/immune complex intermediate that can maintain cytotoxic effects of BPI towards Gram-negative pathogens, with the potential to transform the current treatment of CF airways disease.

Keywords: cystic fibrosis, neutrophils, bactericidal permeability increasing protein, IgG class autoantibodies, *Pseudomonas aeruginosa*

INTRODUCTION

Cystic Fibrosis (CF) is an autosomal recessive pleiotropic disorder caused by mutations in the gene encoding the CF transmembrane conductance regulator (CFTR) chloride channel (Riordan et al., 1989; Rommens et al., 1989). Over 2000 CFTR mutations have been identified that result in disturbed synthesis or function of the CFTR protein, leading to the development of specialized therapies targeting the basic defect (Mcelvaney et al., 2018). The most common mutation is deletion of phenylalanine at position 508 (*Phe508del*) which is present in one or both alleles in approximately 90% of PWCF (Riordan, 2008). CF related symptoms, although variable from patient to patient, are present early in life and increase in severity with age, with respiratory manifestations impacting on morbidity and mortality. CFTR absence or malfunction causes defective ion transport, reduction in airway surface liquid (ASL) volumes and persistent mucus hypersecretion. Inflammation is further amplified by bacterial infections, initially *Haemophilus influenza* and *Staphylococcus aureus* in infants, and later *Pseudomonas aeruginosa*, with early eradication with anti-pseudomonal antibiotics demonstrating significant improvements in FEV_1, reductions in exacerbations (Ramsey et al., 1999; Konstan et al., 2011) and in bacterial density (Mccoy et al., 2008). Accordingly, in the adult CF population, *S. aureus* infections without the presence of *P. aeruginosa*, is a marker of milder lung disease (Ahlgren et al., 2015). Conversely, a greater rate of decline of lung function has been recorded in young people with *P. aeruginosa* lung infection compared to infants with no infection detected (Pillarisetti et al., 2011).

Sustained neutrophil recruitment and neutrophil dominated inflammation are hallmarks of CF airways disease progression, yet paradoxically, recruited cells fail to kill invading bacteria, with chronic infection with mucoid, alginate-producing strains of *P. aeruginosa* a major cause of mortality. Primary granules of neutrophils contain a battery of antimicrobial mediators, including the potent cytotoxic bactericidal permeability increasing protein (BPI) that targets gram-negative bacteria such as *Pseudomonas*. BPI is a bipartite molecule with distinct domain functionality, involving anti-bacterial and endotoxin neutralization properties of *N*- and *C*-terminal domains, respectively. The remarkable ability of *P. aeruginosa* to colonize the CF airways despite the presence of BPI is not fully understood. A rise in anti-neutrophil cytoplasmic antibodies (ANCA) with BPI specificity have been identified in PWCF (Sediva et al., 1998; Mahadeva et al., 1999), varying from 17.9% to 83% positivity (Iwuji et al., 2019), with a strong correlation between IgA and IgG BPI-ANCA and reduced lung function recorded (Carlsson et al., 2007). Although anti-BPI IgA has been detected in CF bronchoalveolar lavage (BAL), strikingly, *in vitro* anti-BPI-IgG inhibits the antibiotic function of BPI (Schinke et al., 2004). This prompted us to investigate the *in vivo* concept that BPI present in CF airways is immune complexed to anti-BPI-IgG, and this direct interaction inhibits anti-*Pseudomonas* activity.

MATERIALS AND METHODS

Chemicals and Reagents

All chemicals and reagents were of the highest purity available and were purchased from Sigma-Aldrich Ireland unless indicated otherwise.

Study Design

PWCF were recruited from the Beaumont Hospital Cystic Fibrosis Clinic. Ethical approval was received from the Beaumont Hospital Ethics Board (REC reference 14/98) and informed consent obtained from all study participants. Demographic details of PWCF are listed in **Tables 1** and **2**. The CF-ABLE score is a predictive score for determining outcome in CF, validated against the CF registry of Ireland (Mccarthy et al., 2013). Scores range from 0 to 7, with a higher score predicting a worse outcome. The CF-ABLE score of recruited patients was 3.68 ± 2.11 (**Table 1**). To assess the effect of ivacaftor therapy on plasma levels of BPI autoantibodies, clinically stable CF patients, homozygous or heterozygous for the *Gly551Asp CFTR* variant, receiving 150 mg ivacaftor twice daily (n = 10) were recruited (**Table 2**). Details regarding healthy controls (HC), patients with non-cystic fibrosis bronchiectasis (NCFB) or

TABLE 1 | Demographic details of PWCF recruited to this study.

Clinical demographic parameter	CF participants
Total number	28
Age in years	27.7 ± 5.02
Male	16
Female	12
Homozygous for *Phe508del*	11
At least one *Phe508del* copy	25
FEV_1	42.01 ± 21.92
BMI	20.06 ± 2.55
CF-ABLE score	3.68 ± 2.11
P. aeruginosa colonization at time of sample	19
P. aeruginosa colonization within last 5 years	28

Data are presented as number or mean ± standard deviation.
Phe508del, CFTR gene mutation; FEV_1, forced expiratory volume in 1 s (% predicted); BMI, body mass index (kg/m^2); P. aeruginosa, Pseudomonas aeruginosa.

TABLE 2 | Demographic details of the CF cohort receiving ivacaftor therapy.

Patient	CFTR mutation	FEV_1Pre-therapy (% predicted)	FEV_1Post-therapy (% predicted)
1	*Phe508del/Gly551Asp*	45	56
2	*Phe508del/Gly551Asp*	25	31
3	*Phe508del/Gly551Asp*	53	71
4	*Phe508del/Gly551Asp*	45	64
5	*Phe508del/Gly551Asp*	93	86
6	*Phe508del/Gly551Asp*	56	27
7	*Phe508del/Gly551Asp*	57	95
8	*Gly551Asp/G542X*	24	24
9	*Gly551Asp/G542X*	45	40
10	*Gly551Asp/Gly551Asp*	30	36

FEV_1, forced expiratory volume in one second.

chronic obstructive pulmonary disease (COPD) are available in **Table 3**.

Preparation of Blood and Airways Samples

Blood samples were collected in 7.5-ml heparinized S-monovette tubes (10 U/ml; Sarstedt, Germany) and centrifuged at 350×*g* for 5 min at room temperature. Plasma was aliquoted for immediate use or stored at -80°C. Peripheral blood neutrophils were isolated using a previously described method, (Reeves et al., 2002) with all steps performed at room temperature. Purity of isolated neutrophils was validated by flow cytometric analysis using a monoclonal antibody against CD16b (Saeki et al., 2009; Bergin et al., 2014) and neutrophil viability was assessed by trypan blue exclusion assays. Bronchoalveolar lavage (BAL) samples were obtained from PWCF (**Table 4**). BAL was performed and samples processed as previously published (Rennard et al., 1998). Briefly, 100 ml of buffered saline was instilled into the right middle lobe or lingula and harvested. BAL was filtered through sterile gauze and then centrifugation at 462 x *g* for 10 min at 4°C. Cell-free supernatants were aliquoted and stored at −80°C for subsequent analysis.

Gel Electrophoresis and Western Blot Analyses

Samples were subjected to SDS-PAGE under denaturing and non-denaturing conditions using the NativePAGE™ Novex® Bis-Tris gel system (Invitrogen™) following the manufacturer's instructions. After Electrophoresis, gels were stained with Coomassie® Brilliant blue G250 for visualization of proteins or transferred to 0.2 µM PVDF membrane (Roche) by western blotting. Blots were incubated with 0.2 µg/ml mouse monoclonal anti-BPI specific antibody (Santa Cruz Biotech Inc.), 0.01 mM rabbit polyclonal anti-Rac2 specific antibody (Cell Signalling Technology- Rac 1/2/3 antibody) or 1.0 µg/ml of monoclonal anti-actin antibody (Millipore, UK). The secondary antibodies used were HRP-linked rabbit anti-mouse and goat anti-rabbit IgG (Cell Signalling Technology). Immunoreactivity was detected using Immobilon™ Western Chemiluminescent HRP-substrate (Millipore) solution and a G-Box Chemie XL (Syngene) and analyzed using GeneSnap and GeneTools software.

TABLE 3 | Characteristics of healthy controls, patients with chronic obstructive pulmonary disease or patients with non-cystic fibrosis bronchiectasis recruited to this study.

Clinical demographic parameter	NCFB	COPD	HC
Total number	5	2	38
Age in years	68.53 ± 11.4	48	32.38 ± 4.6
FEV_1	50.66 ± 15.22	64.5	101.33 ± 7.6
BMI	28.31 ± 5.5	25.91	25.84 ± 2.16

Data are presented as number or mean ± standard deviation.
NCFB, non-cystic fibrosis bronchiectasis; COPD, chronic obstructive pulmonary disease; HC, healthy control; FEV_1, forced expiratory volume in one second; BMI, body mass index (kg/m^2).

TABLE 4 | Demographic details of PWCF who donated BAL and plasma samples for LPS experiments.

Clinical demographic parameter	CF cohort (*Phe508del*)
Total number	12
Age in years	29.6 ± 5.61
Male	6
Female	6
Homozygous for *Phe508del*	12
FEV_1	45.71 ± 17.92
BMI	20.88 ± 2.61
CF-ABLE score	3.72 ± 2.11
P. aeruginosa colonization	12

Data are presented as number or mean ± standard deviation.
Phe508del, CFTR gene mutation; FEV_1, forced expiratory volume in 1 s (% predicted); BMI, body mass index (kg/m^2); P. aeruginosa, Pseudomonas aeruginosa.

Quantification of LPS, BPI, or BPI ANCA Levels

Lipopolysaccharide (LPS) was quantified in plasma and BAL of PWCF (**Table 4**) using an LPS ELISA (Cusabio: catalog number CSB-E09945h). BPI levels were quantified using the Human BPI ELISA kit (Hycult® Biotech: catalog number HK314-01). Anti-BPI (IgG) levels were evaluated using the Human anti-BPI ELISA kit (Orgentec: catalog number ORG 523). Plate readings were recorded using a Spectra Max M3 plate reader. All ELISA experiments were undertaken in accordance with the manufacturer's instructions.

Neutrophil Rac2 Activation and Degranulation Assays

The Rac activation kit (Abcam: catalog number ab139586) was used to isolate active GTP-bound Rac from neutrophil lysates. This kit utilizes the selective interaction of the Cdc42/Rac interactive binding domain (CRIB) of the effector p21 activated kinase-1 (PAK-1) with the active RacGTP conformation. Anti-Rac2 antibody was used to detect total and active GTP-bound Rac2 in neutrophil lysates by Western blotting. For neutrophil degranulation assays, cells (1 x 10^7/ml) were either unstimulated or stimulated with TNF-α (1 ng/ml) and fMLP (100 ng/ml) at 37°C and 100 µl aliquots removed at 0, 5, 10 or 20 min and added to 4 volumes of ice cold PBS containing protease inhibitors (Nα-tosyl-L-lysine chloromethyl ketone hydrochloride (10 µg/ml), phenylmethanesulfonyl fluoride (1 µg/ml), pepstatin A (10 µg/ml), and leupeptin (10 µg/ml)). Cell free supernatants were harvested following centrifugation at 500×*g* for 5 min at 4°C and analyzed for degranulated BPI by Western blotting. The use of equal cell numbers (2 × 10^7/ml) in each reaction was demonstrated by identical immune band intensity of actin in Western blots of whole cell lysates of cells used per reaction.

Purification of IgG BPI-ANCA

Starting BAL (100µl) supplemented with protease inhibitors (as listed above) was incubated with Protein G Sepharose 4 Fast Flow (GE Healthcare) (30µl packed bed) and gently rotated for 1 h at 4°C. Protein G Sepharose 4 Fast Flow comprises immobilized recombinant protein G that binds to the Fc region of IgG. Reactions were centrifuged at 12,000 x g for 1 min and the unbound supernatant harvested. The Protein G

Sepharose pellet was washed x 6 in 1 ml pre-chilled PBS containing protease inhibitors before addition of 2× Laemmli Sample Buffer with or without 1 mM DTT. Samples were boiled at 98°C for 3 min and subjected to SDS-PAGE and stained with Coomassie blue to visualize proteins or Western blotted for BPI. In a subset of experiments, BPI autoantibodies were purified as previously described (Bergin et al., 2014), concentrated using an Amicon® Ultra-30K Centrifugal filter device, and protein concentration determined using a Nanodrop™ 8000, prior to use in bactericidal assays.

BPI Anti-*Pseudomonas* Assays

Luria-Bertani (LB) broth was inoculated with a single bacterial colony of *P. aeruginosa* strain PAO1 and incubated overnight at 220 rpm at 37°C (Brunswick™ Excels® E25 shaker incubator). Bacteria were sub-cultured into fresh LB broth and incubated until mid-logarithmic phase was reached (Bergsson et al., 2009). After culturing the bacteria were washed x 3 in PBS and resuspended at a density of 1 x 10^8/ml. For BPI bactericidal assays, PAO1 was re-suspended in 0, 1, 2.5, 5, 10, 20 or 40 µg/ml of human neutrophil purified BPI (Athens Research) in PBS pH 7.5 at 37°C. An aliquot was removed at 32 min into ice cold LB broth and samples were diluted and plated in triplicate on LB agar plates and incubated overnight at 37°C. Colony forming units (c.f.u.) were counted, and the percentage survival was quantified by setting the number of c.f.u. with no BPI at 100% survival. Experiments were repeated in PBS set at pH 5.5, 6.5 or 7.5 in the presence of 10 µg/ml BPI for 10 min. Alternatively, bacteria were suspended in PBS pH 7.5 with BPI (10 µg/ml) in the presence of glycosaminoglycans (GAG) (heparin sulphate, chondroitin sulphate and hyaluronic acid (1 mg/ml of each)) for 2, 4 or 8 min. BPI inhibitory assays employed a rabbit *N*-terminal directed anti-BPI antibody (Sigma Aldrich: catalog number B2188) or CF purified anti-BPI IgG. BPI (10 µg/ml) was incubated in the presence or absence of antibody (10 µg/ml) for 20 min prior to use.

Statistical Analysis

All data were analyzed using GraphPad Prism version 7 (La Jolla, CA, USA). Unless stated otherwise, data are expressed as mean ± SEM and p values were determined by Students t-test. One-way or two-way ANOVA was used to determine statistical significance when comparing three or more groups tested with one or two factors, respectively. A p value of ≤ 0.05 was deemed statistically significant following Bonferroni or Tukey *post-hoc* multiple comparision tests as indicated.

RESULTS

Elevated Levels of BPI Are Present in the Plasma and BAL of People With CF Colonized With *P. aeruginosa*

PWCF were recruited from the Beaumont Hospital Cystic Fibrosis Clinic (**Table 4**). Patients had a mean % FEV_1 of 45.71 ± 17.92 and CF-ABLE score of 3.72 ± 2.11. Patients were colonized with *P. aeruginosa* at the time of sampling or in the preceding 5 years. Confirming bacterial colonization, plasma (n=12, R^2 = 0.61, p=0.003) and BAL (n=12, R^2 = 0.86, p=0.0006) levels of LPS correlated directly with severity of CF airways disease, as determined by the CF-ABLE score (**Figures 1A, B**).

To investigate whether cytotoxicity of neutrophil BPI is limited against *P. aeruginosa* due to proteolysis, we first determined the levels and structural integrity of extracellular BPI protein *in vivo*. Plasma and BAL samples were obtained from PWCF, healthy controls (HC), or non-CF bronchiectasis (NCFB) patients for comparison. Quantification of BPI by ELISA revealed that plasma from PWCF contained significantly higher levels of soluble BPI than that measured in HC plasma (24.2 ± 3.9 ng/ml and 11.2 ± 2.6 ng/ml respectively, p=0.007) (**Figure 1C**). To further evaluate BPI levels *in vivo*, ELISA analysis of BAL was performed (**Figure 1D**). Results revealed that CF BAL had a greater than 100-fold increase in concentration of BPI when compared to HC BAL (4.6 ± 0.5 and 0.04 ± 0.03µg/ml respectively, p<0.0001) and a 5-fold increase compared to BAL from NCFB patients (0.8 ± 0.5µg/ml, p<0.001).

As increased levels of proteolytic activity can degrade structural and immune proteins present in the CF airways (Birrer et al., 1994; Margaroli et al., 2018), we next assessed the integrity of BPI and its ability to remain intact within the CF lung. Western blot was employed to detect BPI in CF BAL, and also NCFB, HC or COPD BAL samples for comparison. In CF BAL, although detected at various intensities, an immunoband for BPI of the correct molecular mass of 55 kDa was detected in all samples (**Figure 1E**). BPI was minimally detected in NCFB BAL and undetectable in COPD or HC BAL samples. The molecular mass of the protein and specificity of the BPI primary antibody employed was confirmed in control experiments employing secondary antibody only (**Figure 1E**, lower panel). Collectively these results indicate increased levels of extracellular BPI in the blood circulation and airways of PWCF, posing the question of whether CF neutrophils release significantly greater quantities of BPI, and the mechanism thereof.

Increased Rac2 Activation in CF Neutrophils

Previous studies have revealed a disparity in CF neutrophil degranulation of primary granule components including increased release of myeloperoxidase (MPO) and neutrophil elastase (NE) (Koller et al., 1995; Taggart et al., 2000). Following the finding of increased levels of BPI in plasma and BAL of PWCF, the level of BPI released by CF neutrophils was compared to HC cells. Within this set of experiments, a combination of TNF-α (1 ng) and fMLP (100 ng) was the chosen stimulus to trigger granule release. In unstimulated, and upon activation, release of BPI from primary granules was detected in the extracellular supernatant by immunoblotting and protein levels evaluated by densitometry. The level of BPI released by unstimulated CF neutrophils (p=0.02), and after 20 min stimulation (p=0.02), was significantly greater than HC cells (**Figure 2A**). The Rho

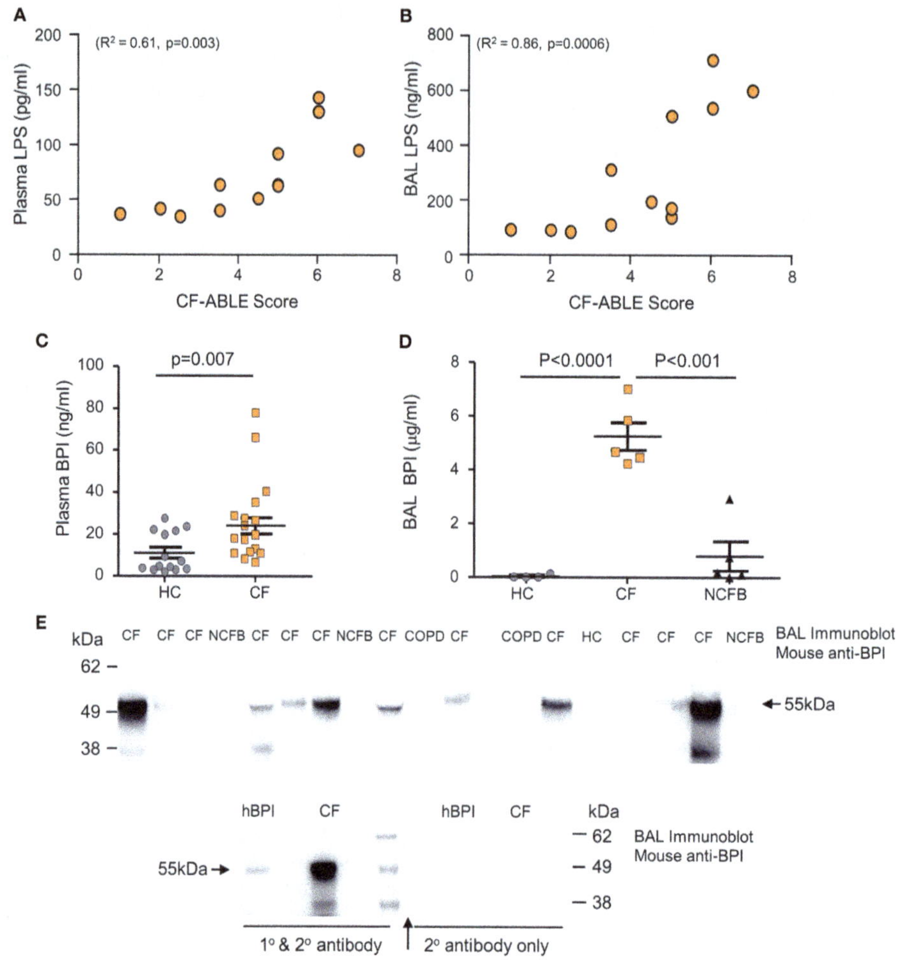

FIGURE 1 | Elevated levels of BPI present in plasma and BAL of people with CF. **(A, B)** LPS levels in CF plasma and BAL correlated with CF-ABLE score. Quantification of an association between variables was achieved by Spearman correlation. **(C, D)** Comparative analysis of BPI present in plasma or BAL of *Phe508del* homozygous PWCF (CF), healthy controls (HC) or NCFB patients was performed by ELISA. **(C)** BPI levels were significantly increased in plasma of CF compared to HC (n=22 and n=14 subjects per group, respectively, p=0.007, Mann Whitney U-test). **(D)** BAL levels of BPI were significantly increased in CF (n=5) compared to HC (n=4) or NCFB patients (n=5) (p<0.0001, One-way ANOVA, followed by Bonferroni post-hoc test for selected groups). **(E)** BAL samples from HC, CF, NCFB or COPD were subjected to SDS-PAGE and Western blot analysis for BPI. An immuno-band of increased intensity for BPI was detected in CF BAL samples (top panels). Lower panel, a control immunoblot to ensure BPI specificity. The blot was halved, with one half probed with secondary antibody only with no BPI immune-bands visible (↑ indicates where blot was cut). Human BPI (hBPI) was used as a positive control. All measurements are means ± SEM from biological replicates.

GTPase Rac2 has been implicated in control of primary granule degranulation (Abdel-Latif et al., 2004), and therefore the levels of GTP-bound Rac2 in CF neutrophils was compared to healthy control cells. Using a GST-PAK-CRIB isolation method, GTP-bound Rac2 was precipitated from whole cell lysates, with subsequent total and active GTP-bound Rac2 content detected by immunoblotting. Results revealed a significant 2.5-fold increase in the level of GTP-bound Rac2 in unstimulated CF neutrophils compared to control cells (p=0.03) (**Figure 2B**). Collectively, these results illustrate increased Rac2 activation and increased secretion of BPI by CF cells, and thus the cause for impaired BPI activity in the CF airways was next explored.

The Bactericidal Action of BPI Is Increased at Low pH and Unaffected by High Glycosaminoglycan Content of the CF Airways

The potent cytotoxicity of BPI is confined to gram negative bacteria (Elsbach and Weiss, 1993). As BPI protein was identified within the CF airways, and all recruited patients were colonized by *P. aeruginosa*, we explored parameters that may impede the antibacterial effect of BPI against *Pseudomonas* in the CF airways. In initial *in vitro* experiments, bacteria were exposed to increasing concentrations of BPI (1 to 40 μg/ml). A statistically significant reduction in survival was visible upon exposure to the physiologically relevant CF BAL concentration of 10 μg/ml BPI

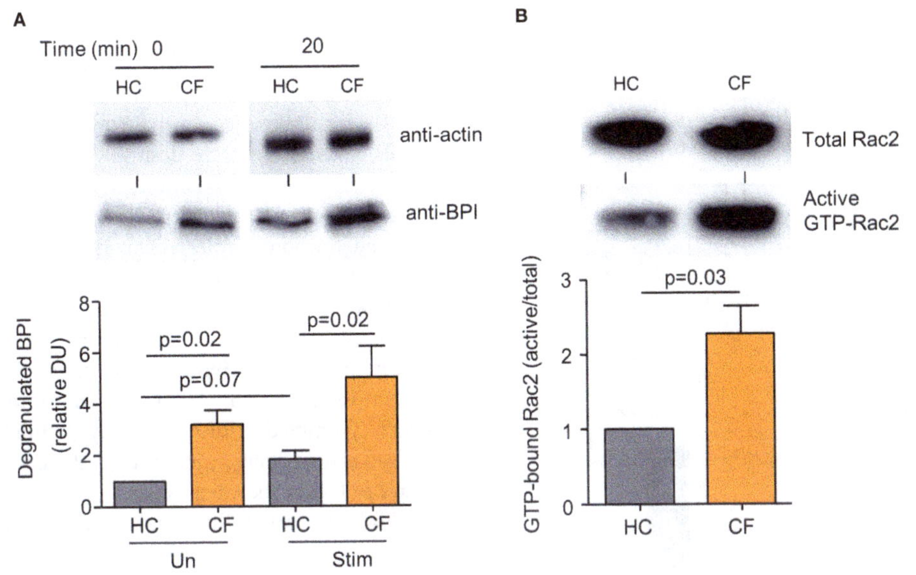

FIGURE 2 | Increased degranulation of BPI from CF neutrophils. **(A)** Neutrophils from *Phe508del* homozygous PWCF (CF) or healthy controls (HC) remained unstimulated (Un) or were stimulated (Stim) with TNF-α (1 ng)/fMLP (100 ng) (2 × 10^7 cells/mL) for 20 min and extracellular supernatants immunoblotted for degranulated BPI. Values presented as densitometry units (DU) and normalized to time zero of unstimulated HC cells. Levels of BPI released from unstimulated and stimulated CF cells was significantly greater than that of HC (p=0.02, n=5 subjects per group, Student's t test). **(B)** Active GTP bound Rac2 (GTP-Rac2) was extracted from whole cell lysates of CF and HC neutrophils. GTP-Rac2 immuno-bands were normalized to total Rac2 levels and the HC value and expressed as a % of total Rac2. Significantly increased levels of GTP-Rac2 were detected in CF samples (p=0.03, Student's t test, n=5 subjects per group). In **(A)** immuno-blots of whole cell lysates probed for actin determined equal protein loading, confirming equal cell numbers per reaction and representative blot images are shown. Each measurement is the mean ± SEM from biological replicates.

($p<0.0001$) (**Figure 3A**), thus consolidating the need to understand the cause for impaired BPI killing of *P. aeruginosa in vivo*.

Studies in humans and CF cell lines indicate that pH of ASL is reduced in the absence of CFTR function (Smith and Welsh, 1992; Coakley et al., 2003; Abou Alaiwa et al., 2014a), and the more acidic pH diminished the effect of ASL antimicrobials including LL-37 and β-defensin-3 (Abou Alaiwa et al., 2014b). In contrast, results of the current study demonstrate that BPI (10 μg/ml) caused a significant reduction in *P. aeruginosa* survival at pH 7.5, 6.5 and 5.5, with the greatest reduction (~20% survival) observed at pH 5.5 ($p<0.0001$) (**Figure 3B**). Moreover, through interactions with negatively charged glycosaminoglycans (GAGs) present within the CF lung, it has been demonstrated that the antimicrobial activity of LL-37 is inactivated (Bergsson et al., 2009). In the current study, however, pre-exposure of BPI (10μg/ml) to a mixture of GAGs including heparan sulfate, chondroitin sulfate, and hyaluronic acid used at a 1:10 (w:w) ratio had no effect on BPI-induced bacterial killing across a time course of 2- 8 min (**Figure 3C**). Taken together, these data suggest that the antipseudomonal effect of BPI is unperturbed by factors known to inactivate antimicrobials in the CF airways.

IgG Autoantibodies Present in the CF Airways Inhibit BPI Antimicrobial Activity

As a consequence of increased neutrophil degranulation and high plasma levels of BPI, the potential for the development of autoantibodies in adult PWCF was evaluated. A comparison of anti-BPI IgG-class autoantibodies in plasma from PWCF and HC was performed (**Figure 4A**). By employing a predetermined threshold level for positivity previously described as 10 U/ml, all 28 PWCF tested proved positive for autoantibodies against BPI, with recorded levels significantly higher than that observed for HC donors ($p<0.0001$). Using ELISA, we evaluated the effect of ivacaftor therapy on plasma levels of anti-BPI autoantibodies. Results revealed that the levels of anti-BPI autoantibodies in plasma of PWCF heterozygous for the *Gly551Asp* mutation who were receiving ivacaftor for 2 years was significantly increased compared to HC (p=0.0001) but similar to PWCF not receiving therapy (p=0.39) (**Figure 4B**), thus confirming ongoing inflammation. Increased anti-BPI autoantibodies in plasma of PWCF is in line with previous reports (Zhao et al., 1996; Mahadeva et al., 1999), but to date, the presence with subsequent consequence of anti-BPI IgG antibodies in the CF lung has not been fully studied. Thus to first confirm that IgG antibodies are in CF airway samples, protein G sepharose was employed which has a high binding capacity for human IgG, but not IgA. Post incubation of protein G sepharose with CF BAL, immuno-precipitated protein was subjected to SDS-PAGE. The 150-kDa IgG protein was confirmed by Coomassie blue staining, which showed a single band under nonreducing conditions and two bands corresponding to the heavy and light chains after reduction by inclusion of DTT (**Figure 4C**).

To evaluate whether IgG-autoantibodies are present cross-linked to BPI in the CF lung, protein G sepharose precipitated reactions were subjected to Western blot analysis and probed for BPI. The antibody used for Western blotting was a mouse monoclonal

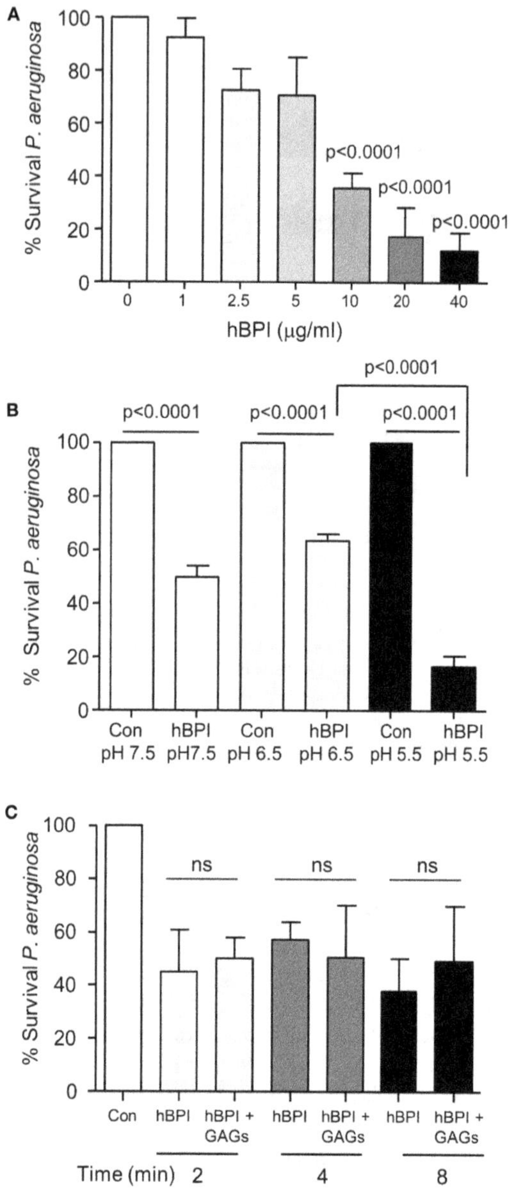

FIGURE 3 | Bactericidal activity of BPI is unaffected by the pH and GAGs present in the CF airways. **(A)** Survival of *P. aeruginosa* (1×10^8 c.f.u./ml) after 20 min incubation with BPI (1-40μg/ml). Data expressed as percentage survival of the untreated bacterial count. Bacterial survival was significantly decreased following treatment with 10, 20 or 40 μg/ml BPI (n=4 separate experiments, p<0.0001, One-way ANOVA test, followed by Bonferroni post-hoc test for selected groups). **(B)** To determine the effect of pH on the bactericidal effect of BPI, *P. aeruginosa* (1×10^8 c.f.u./ml) was incubated at 37°C in 0·01 M phosphate buffer pH 7.5, 6·5 or 5·5 with or without BPI (10 μg/ml). Reduction in survival of *P. aeruginosa* by BPI at pH 5·5 compared to 6·5 was found to be significant (n=4 separate experiments, p<0.0001, two-way ANOVA test followed by Tukeys' post-hoc test on unadjusted cfu data). **(C)** Bactericidal effect of BPI in the presence or absence of GAGs was determined by suspending *P. aeruginosa* (1×10^8 c.f.u./ml) in phosphate buffer (pH 7·5) with BPI (10 μg/ml) with or without GAGs (1:10 (w/w) ratio) for 2, 4, or 8 min. No significant difference (ns) was recorded at any time point tested (n=3, two-way ANOVA test, followed by Tukeys' post-hoc test on unadjusted cfu data).

antibody directed against residues 227-254, which links the *N*- (1-229) and *C*-terminal domain (251-456) of BPI. For each Western blot the starting BAL sample prior to the addition of protein G sepharose (St), the unbound protein material (Un), and the protein that bound the G sepharose is shown (Bd) (**Figure 4C**). Human BPI (hBPI) was used as a positive control (55 kDa). Immuno-band signals of the correct size positively identified BPI in reactions of protein G sepharose bound IgG from CF BAL (Bd fractions) (**Figure 4D**, 3 of 5 biological repeats presented). Positive signal in unbound fraction may represent free BPI or BPI bound to IgA ANCA, the latter known to be present in CF (Theprungsirikul et al., 2020), while the lesser signal intensity of bound and unbound fractions with respect to starting materials is a probable result of loss during wash steps. Hence, we have employed this setup as a qualitative approach. A control immunoblot to ensure BPI specificity omitted primary antibody (bottom panel). Collectively, this set of experiments indicates that neutrophil-released BPI is bound to IgG in the CF airways.

Next, the possibility that autoantibody cross-linking of antigen could prevent BPI-induced *Pseudomonas* killing was examined. A bactericidal assay was carried out using 10 μg/ml of BPI in the presence and absence of equimolar anti-BPI antibody. The reduction in survival visible upon exposure of bacteria to BPI was significantly inhibited by inclusion of a commercially available *N*-terminal directed anti-BPI antibody (**Figure 5**). In addition, experiments exploring the effect of anti-BPI autoantibodies purified from CF samples revealed that purified autoantibodies mediated inactivation of BPI, resulting in a significant 2.5-fold increase in bacterial survival (p<0.0001) (**Figure 5**). From this set of experiments, we conclude that IgG class autoantibodies directed against BPI present in airway samples of PWCF, can target antigen and inhibit BPI bacterial killing.

DISCUSSION

Airway neutrophilia is common in PWCF and recruited neutrophils release large quantities of antimicrobial proteins and peptides from their cytoplasmic granules into surrounding delicate lung tissues. Moreover, *P. aeruginosa* dwelling in the airway can secrete factors that antagonise neutrophils, such as rhamnolipid or pyocyanin, that promote release of antimicrobials through direct lysis or induction of cell death (Allen et al., 2005; Jensen et al., 2007). Released antimicrobials are not fully effective at microbial clearance, and these granule proteins accrue to an extent that prompts the loss of self-tolerance and development of ANCA. BPI is present in the CF airway at high levels compared to healthy airways, and BPI-ANCA are present in the airways of a large proportion of people with CF (Schinke et al., 2004). In this study, we demonstrate that IgG class autoantibodies against BPI are antigen complexed in the CF lung, thereby inhibiting BPI anti-*Pseudomonas* cytotoxic activity. We additionally demonstrate that CF adults retain BPI ANCA seropositivity for at least two years following commencement on therapy with the CFTR modulator, ivacaftor.

Despite nomenclature describing their antigens as cytoplasmic, it is striking that the set of common ANCA antigens are each components of neutrophil primary granules, with MPO,

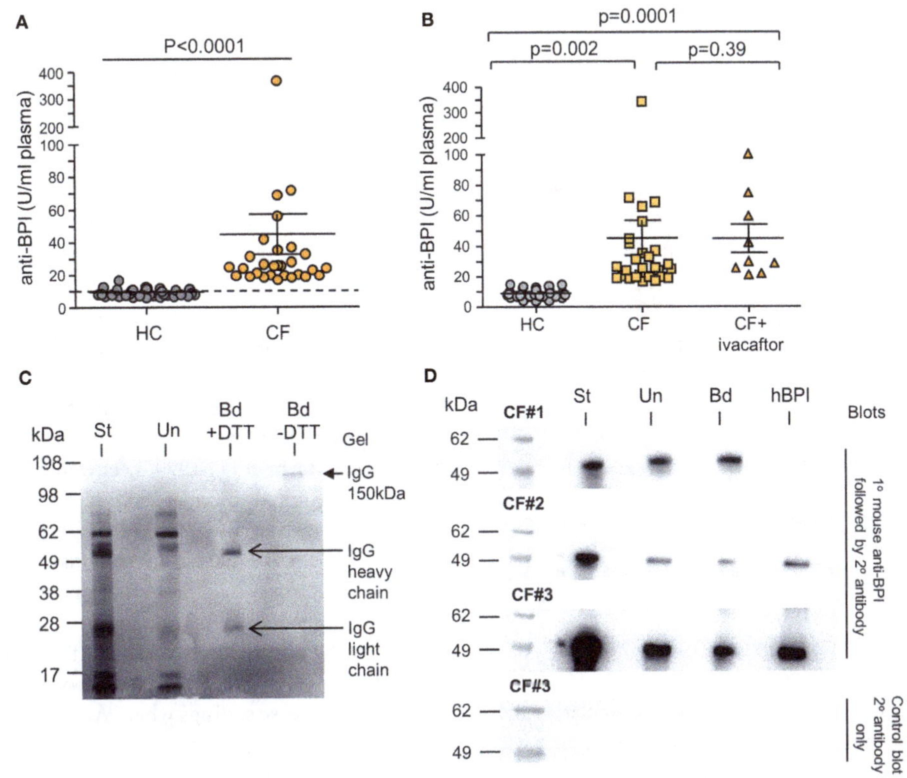

FIGURE 4 | Increased levels of plasma autoantibodies and IgG-bound BPI in CF airway samples. **(A)** IgG autoantibodies against BPI were quantified in plasma of PWCF (CF, n=30) or healthy controls (HC, n=37). A significant increase in the titre of BPI autoantibodies were detected in CF (p<0.0001, Mann-Whitney U test). Positivity was set as 10 U/ml as indicated by the hatched line. All CF samples were positive for BPI autoantibodies. Increased circulating IgG BPI antibody level in CF individuals determined by ELISA. **(B)** Plasma samples from HC (n=38), CF (n=28) and CF individuals receiving ivacaftor treatment (n=10). No difference in levels of circulating anti-BPI IgG autoantibodies between CF and CF individuals receiving ivacaftor treatment (p=0.39). **(C)** Representative Coomassie blue stained SDS gel of purified IgG from CF BAL. Protein G Sepharose was used to isolate IgG from BAL of *Phe508del* homozygous PWCF. Starting BAL sample (St), unbound material (Un) or purified bound IgG (Bd) with or without DTT reduction are presented. Purified IgG (150 kDa, closed arrow), and the heavy (50 kDa) and light chains (25 kDa) of IgG are indicated (open arrows) (1 representative images of n = 5 biological repeats). **(D)** Protein G Sepharose was used to isolate IgG-BPI complexes from CF BAL. Reactions were analyzed by immunoblotting for BPI positivity using a mouse monoclonal anti-BPI antibody. Starting BAL sample (St), unbound material (Un) or IgG-bound BPI (Bd) are presented. Human BPI (hBPI) was used as a positive control (55 kDa). A control immunoblot to ensure BPI specificity omitted primary antibody (right hand panel), with no immune-band apparent. 3 representative images of n=5 biological repeats.

proteinase 3 (PR3) and BPI being the most commonly described. CF neutrophils have been shown to have impaired degranulation processes, as greater levels of primary granule components including NE (Taggart et al., 2000) and MPO (Koller et al., 1995) were identified in the extracellular environment following stimulation of circulating CF cells. Excessive MPO levels have positively correlated with airflow obstruction and sputum production in *Phe508del* homozygous CF patients (Garner et al., 2004), in addition to augmenting oxidative damage to epithelial cells (Cantin et al., 1987; Cantin and Woods, 1993). Moreover, NE released upon dysregulated degranulation is the major destructive protease in the CF lung causing break down of the structural proteins, elastin, collagen and proteoglycans (Janoff et al., 1979; Cavarra et al., 1996). For this reason, the release of primary granules is tightly controlled by the small GTP-binding protein Rac2 (Abdel-Latif et al., 2004). In the current study increased GTP-bound Rac2 activation was observed, controlling BPI degranulation, leading to increased levels of extracellular BPI in both plasma and airway samples of PWCF. Despite this however, elevated BPI does not translate to clearance of *P. aeruginosa*. *In vitro*, we and others have demonstrated that *P. aeruginosa* is susceptible to BPI killing. We utilized strain PA01, a useful target microbe in this context as its innate resistance to BPI is high, attributable to *Pseudomonas* elastase (Skopelja et al., 2016). While *P. aeruginosa* can adapt to the CF airway over time, this does not explain the ability of environmental isolates to colonise people with CF, nor does it account for the observation that clinical, even mucoid, isolates of *P. aeruginosa* remain susceptible to BPI *ex vivo* (Aichele et al., 2006). Moreover, conditions that prevail in the CF lung milieu including low pH (Tate et al., 2002), and high concentrations of GAGs (Reeves et al., 2011), do not impair the cytotoxic effect of BPI, indeed, low pH supports increased BPI activity, as has previously been reported (Mannion et al., 1990). To our knowledge, the effect of BPI against *P. aeruginosa* present in an established biofilm is underexplored. We have shown BPI to be effective when combined in a mixture of glycosaminoglycans. Inasmuch as there is a superficial similarity between *Pseudomonas*

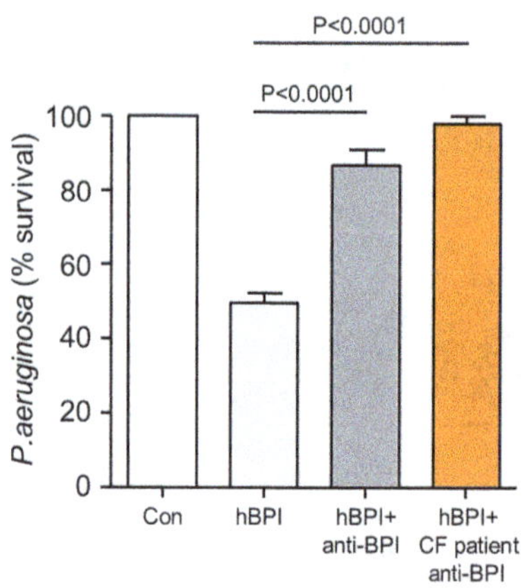

FIGURE 5 | Autoantibodies in CF airway samples are associated with decreased BPI bacterial killing. Survival of *P. aeruginosa* (1×10^8 c.f.u./ml) after incubation with BPI (10 µg/ml) in the presence or absence of 10µg/ml patient purified BPI autoantibodies or commercial anti-BPI antibody. Bacterial killing was significantly inhibited by CF BPI autoantibodies ($p<0.0001$, n = 4 separate experiments, One-way ANOVA test, followed by Bonferroni post-hoc test for selected groups).

alginate and our studied glycosaminoglycans, particularly their polyanionic character, it could be possible that BPI interacting with alginate would remain effective. Such positive antimicrobial effects of BPI supported early investigations into the potential therapeutic use of a recombinant amino-terminal fragment of human BPI in treatment of meningococcaemia (Giroir et al., 1997), and a randomized trial in children with severe meningococcal sepsis (Levin et al., 2000). These results and published observations raised the fundamental question of why BPI, present in high concentrations in the CF airway, fails to kill invading bacteria.

We have demonstrated that a proportion of extracellular BPI in the CF airway exists complexed to IgG autoantibodies. Incidence of BPI-directed ANCA in CF is particularly high in comparison to ANCAs against other neutrophil primary granule proteins such as MPO or NE, considering that these proteins are more abundant in neutrophil primary granules than BPI. For example, BPI ANCA positivity greatly exceeds that of PR3 ANCA in CF (Lachenal et al., 2009). The opsonizing capability of BPI may mean it is present in phagolysosomes during the disintegration of microbes that results in antigen presentation. It has also been proposed to result from the ability of BPI to deliver LPS-bacterial blebs to dendritic cells, thereby serving as a link between innate and adaptive immunity and a greater likelihood of self-reactive neo-epitope formation during antigen processing (Schultz et al., 2007). Our results demonstrate the presence of IgG class BPI ANCA in CF BAL samples. This result contrasts previous studies demonstrating fragmentation of IgG respiratory opsonins in the CF airways (Fick et al., 1984) and the identification of IgA rather than IgG in CF BAL (Theprungsirikul et al., 2020). An explanation for this disparity may in part be provided by the use of an alternative purification approach involving Protein G Sepharose in the current study, with full length IgG successfully identified in CF BAL.

Although studies have reported an increased incidence of BPI autoantibodies in PWCF for some time now (Zhao et al., 1996; Mahadeva et al., 1999), their actual role in inhibiting BPI mediated killing has received mixed reports. Some studies suggest that the BPI-ANCA present in the circulation are primarily raised against the C- terminal domain of the protein and thus do not inhibit killing (Dunn et al., 1999; Schultz et al., 2000), while others have noted that purified CF ANCA do in fact inhibit its bactericidal action (Sediva et al., 2003; Schultz et al., 2004). Our data illustrate the diminished antimicrobial potency of BPI against *P. aeruginosa* when complexed to IgG-class autoantibodies. Moreover, our data demonstrate that high levels of LPS present in CF BAL correlate with disease severity, and this raises the query of the consequence of BPI : IgG complexation. To further explain this point, BPI binding of LPS impedes delivery to CD14, thereby reducing immune cell activation (Marra et al., 1990; Leeuwenberg et al., 1994). Further studies are required to understand whether this anti-inflammatory role of BPI may possibly be impacted upon by IgG autoantibodies in the CF lung. To summarize, airway inflammation is exacerbated in PWCF through pro-inflammatory signaling resulting from higher bacterial burden and IgG-BPI immune complexes. As such, there is an unmet therapeutic need to disrupt these immune complexes or to limit the development of such antibodies.

In other disease settings where ANCA positivity is prominent, such as granulomatosis with polyangiitis, therapy with corticosteroids and rituximab are common, and reduce immune exertion and circulating B cell numbers, respectively. Indeed, a number of biologics targeting immune cells or their secreted components continue to be trialed in such conditions with some success (Basu et al., 2018). However, these ANCA-associated conditions do not co-present with chronic infection, and immunosuppressive therapy in chronically infected PWCF may not be advisable (King and Harper, 2017). Therefore, a targeted approach to abate BPI-ANCA development or function in CF would promote the endogenous antimicrobial BPI activity without off-target effects against the immune system.

One such tactic could include the use of small molecules. At the most basic level, provision of exogenous BPI to the airway could overwhelm ANCA interference while providing an additional antimicrobial effect. Such an approach might suit as adjunct therapy during pulmonary exacerbations, where the need for antibiotics is greatest. However, the potency of BPI when administered to patients who produce high levels of neutralizing anti-BPI antibodies needs to be explored. Our data show that, while BPI immune complexes exist in the airway, there may also be free BPI. Therefore, the protein is not immediately disabled. However, repeated dosing with BPI could also enhance BPI-ANCA production, diminishing BPI potency and exacerbating immune complex-mediated inflammation. Potentially, this may be alleviated by the use of small molecule decoys, peptidomimetics of BPI structural motifs, to neutralise the corresponding ANCAs (Vanpatten et al., 2016).

A second approach could include the use of anti-idiotype antibodies. The formation of antibodies that themselves target antibodies is a strategy that could be exploited to lessen the effect of ANCAs in CF. That said, the cost and complexity of developing a polyclonal anti-idiotype antibody against ANCAs could be prohibitive (Kohler et al., 2019). A third approach could include tolerogenic dendritic cell replacement therapy. Recent advancements in our understanding of the regulatory complexity of the immune system have enabled us to exert finer control over induction of specific components. Utilisation of tolerogenic dendritic cells (DCs) provide a highly relevant example. Pre-clinical work has shown that such cells can be programmed to suppress the function of T cells that would otherwise raise adaptive immunity against individual antigens such as BPI or MPO. Mice instilled with MPO-presenting tolerogenic DCs showed markedly reduced proliferation of MPO-specific T cells and, consequently, lesser glomerular injury (Odobasic et al., 2019). Extrapolation of this approach to PWCF could allow for suppression of the patients' T cell contingent that promotes an anti-BPI adaptive response. DC therapy in CF has not been explored clinically. Pre-clinical investigations have previously shown that murine dendritic cells, exposed to *P. aeruginosa*, could be used to immunise recipient mice (Worgall et al., 2001), however, this approach has not been pursued in patients.

Looking to the future, we have entered an era of CFTR potentiators and correctors that can restore much of the function of the majority of CFTR variants. With improved airflow and normalized airway surface liquid composition, inflammation is reduced and airway remodeling minimized. Triple therapy of CFTR modulators - elexacaftor, tezacaftor and ivacaftor (together, Trikafta) - has recently been reported to provide significant improvements to airway function and extension of exacerbation-free periods of PWCF, further improving that provided by dual therapy (Middleton et al., 2019). Interestingly, our study found no significant difference in levels of anti-BPI autoantibodies in plasma of adult PWCF with the *Gly551Asp* mutation receiving ivacaftor therapy compared to PWCF with different mutations. In this regard, we compared anti-BPI seropositivity in PWCF (N=28) who were corrector treatment naïve with those who had been receiving ivacaftor for the preceding two years (N=10). Prior to treatment, lung function was comparable between cohorts (FEV_1 42 ± 22 vs 53 ± 25, respectively). The continued presence of autoantibodies in adult PWCF with the *Gly551Asp* mutation receiving ivacaftor therapy would suggest that the problem lies, not with CFTR dysfunction, but with the underlying irreversible chronically infected and inflamed bronchiectatic airways present in our CF adult cohort. As approval for CF modulator therapies continues to be granted to younger cohorts, who will receive these treatments before the onset of structural changes in their airways (Ridley and Condren, 2020) this may be less a problem in the future. In such cohorts, it is possible that BPI ANCA will not emerge, as airway inflammatory burden will not manifest to the same extent. Regarding late juvenile or adult PWCF in whom bronchiectatic changes are already established, there is an important gap in our knowledge: following long-term administration of corrector therapy, along with anti-inflammatories, whether the titre of BPI ANCA (IgA or IgG) may decline is unclear. This metric will be important to assess considering the future of *Pseudomonas* in CF.

It has been shown that ANCA titres lower during resolution of infection in non-CF settings (Ohtami et al., 2001). Accordingly, it is possible that if *P. aeruginosa* can be eradicated from the airways of PWCF that ANCA titres would lower, thereby reducing immune complex-mediated inflammation. The use of BPI as a therapeutic may be hindered if it is not effective at killing biofilm dwelling *P. aeruginosa*, hence strategies to improve biofilm disruption and *P. aeruginosa* eradication remain crucial. More broadly, BPI levels and titres of BPI ANCA reflect an overall severity of disease. We have previously introduced a combined metric, the CF-ABLE score, to codify this severity with respect to prognosis of death or transplant (Mccarthy et al., 2013). Through its use in clinical research, airway fluid NE and IL-1β have been shown to associate linearly with poor FEV_1 and at the same time with worsening CF-ABLE score (Mcelvaney et al., 2019a; Mcelvaney et al., 2019b). It is known that higher BPI-ANCA titres correlate with lower lung function in PWCF with chronic *P. aeruginosa* infection (Carlsson et al., 2003). Further evidence is provided by a prospective 10-year study of whether IgA-BPI-ANCA positivity associates with prognosis in *P. aeruginosa*-infected CF patients (Lindberg et al., 2012). This study demonstrated that risk of mortality after 10 years is substantially greater in patients that have IgA-BPI-ANCA. Therefore, it is possible that a CF-ABLE score above 5, which itself predicts death or transplant in 4 years, would associate with high titres of BPI-ANCA.

This is an exciting field of investigation, and with the use of ivacaftor now from 6 months of age and the newest CFTR modulator combination therapy Trikafta for PWCF aged 12 years, it will be of major interest to discern whether these individuals will develop autoantibodies against products of activated neutrophils as they move from childhood to adolescence, and adolescence to adulthood. Equally, as measures to control chronic inflammation in CF develop, it will be important to understand whether this can confer a seronegative status on ANCA positive patients.

ETHICS STATEMENT

The studies involving human participants were reviewed and approved by Ethical approval was received from the Beaumont Hospital Ethics Board (REC reference # 14/98) and informed consent obtained from all study participants. The patients/participants provided their written informed consent to participate in this study.

AUTHOR CONTRIBUTIONS

KM, FG, MM and OM performed experiments, analyzed and interpreted the data. ER, KM, MM and NM are responsible for study design and wrote the manuscript.

ACKNOWLEDGMENTS

We thank the patients and healthy volunteers who graciously participated in this study.

REFERENCES

Abdel-Latif, D., Steward, M., Macdonald, D. L., Francis, G. A., Dinauer, M. C., and Lacy, P. (2004). Rac2 is critical for neutrophil primary granule exocytosis. *Blood* 104, 832–839. doi: 10.1182/blood-2003-07-2624

Abou Alaiwa, M. H., Beer, A. M., Pezzulo, A. A., Launspach, J. L., Horan, R. A., Stoltz, D. A., et al. (2014a). Neonates with cystic fibrosis have a reduced nasal liquid pH; a small pilot study. *J. Cyst Fibros* 13, 373–377. doi: 10.1016/j.jcf.2013.12.006

Abou Alaiwa, M. H., Reznikov, L. R., Gansemer, N. D., Sheets, K. A., Horswill, A. R., Stoltz, D. A., et al. (2014b). pH modulates the activity and synergism of the airway surface liquid antimicrobials beta-defensin-3 and LL-37. *Proc. Natl. Acad. Sci. U. S. A.* 111, 18703–18708. doi: 10.1073/pnas.1422091112

Ahlgren, H. G., Benedetti, A., Landry, J. S., Bernier, J., Matouk, E., Radzioch, D., et al. (2015). Clinical outcomes associated with Staphylococcus aureus and Pseudomonas aeruginosa airway infections in adult cystic fibrosis patients. *BMC Pulm Med.* 15, 67. doi: 10.1186/s12890-015-0062-7

Aichele, D., Schnare, M., Saake, M., Röllinghoff, M., and Gessner, A. (2006). Expression and antimicrobial function of bactericidal permeability-increasing protein in cystic fibrosis patients. *Infection Immun.* 74, 4708–4714. doi: 10.1128/IAI.02066-05

Allen, L., Dockrell, D. H., Pattery, T., Lee, D. G., Cornelis, P., Hellewell, P. G., et al. (2005). Pyocyanin Production by *Pseudomonas aeruginosa* Induces Neutrophil Apoptosis and Impairs Neutrophil-Mediated Host Defenses In Vivo. *J. Immunol.* 174, 3643–3649. doi: 10.4049/jimmunol.174.6.3643

Basu, N., Karabayas, M., and Pusey, C. (2018). Prognosis and future developments in vasculitis. *Best Pract. Res. Clin. Rheumatol.* 32, 148–165. doi: 10.1016/j.berh.2018.08.011

Bergin, D. A., Reeves, E. P., Hurley, K., Wolfe, R., Jameel, R., Fitzgerald, S., et al. (2014). The circulating proteinase inhibitor alpha-1 antitrypsin regulates neutrophil degranulation and autoimmunity. *Sci. Transl. Med.* 6, 217ra211. doi: 10.1126/scitranslmed.3007116

Bergsson, G., Reeves, E. P., Mcnally, P., Chotirmall, S. H., Greene, C. M., Greally, P., et al. (2009). LL-37 complexation with glycosaminoglycans in cystic fibrosis lungs inhibits antimicrobial activity, which can be restored by hypertonic saline. *J. Immunol.* 183, 543–551. doi: 10.4049/jimmunol.0803959

Birrer, P., Mcelvaney, N. G., Rudeberg, A., Sommer, C. W., Liechti-Gallati, S., Kraemer, R., et al. (1994). Protease-antiprotease imbalance in the lungs of children with cystic fibrosis. *Am. J. Respir. Crit. Care Med.* 150, 207–213. doi: 10.1164/ajrccm.150.1.7912987

Cantin, A., and Woods, D. E. (1993). Protection by antibiotics against myeloperoxidase-dependent cytotoxicity to lung epithelial cells in vitro. *J. Clin. Invest.* 91, 38–45. doi: 10.1172/JCI116196

Cantin, A. M., North, S. L., Fells, G. A., Hubbard, R. C., and Crystal, R. G. (1987). Oxidant-mediated epithelial cell injury in idiopathic pulmonary fibrosis. *J. Clin. Invest.* 79, 1665–1673. doi: 10.1172/JCI113005

Carlsson, M., Eriksson, L., Erwander, I., Wieslander, J., and Segelmark, M. (2003). Pseudomonas-induced lung damage in cystic fibrosis correlates to bactericidal-permeability increasing protein (BPI)-autoantibodies. *Clin. Exp. Rheumatol.* 21, S95–100.

Carlsson, M., Eriksson, L., Pressler, T., Kornfalt, R., Mared, L., Meyer, P., et al. (2007). Autoantibody response to BPI predict disease severity and outcome in cystic fibrosis. *J. Cyst Fibros* 6, 228–233. doi: 10.1016/j.jcf.2006.10.005

Cavarra, E., Martorana, P. A., Gambelli, F., De Santi, M., Van Even, P., and Lungarella, G. (1996). Neutrophil recruitment into the lungs is associated with increased lung elastase burden, decreased lung elastin, and emphysema in alpha 1 proteinase inhibitor-deficient mice. *Lab. Invest.* 75, 273–280.

Coakley, R. D., Grubb, B. R., Paradiso, A. M., Gatzy, J. T., Johnson, L. G., Kreda, S. M., et al. (2003). Abnormal surface liquid pH regulation by cultured cystic fibrosis bronchial epithelium. *Proc. Natl. Acad. Sci. U. S. A.* 100, 16083–16088. doi: 10.1073/pnas.2634339100

Dunn, A. C., Walmsley, R. S., Dedrick, R. L., Wakefield, A. J., and Lockwood, C. M. (1999). Anti-neutrophil cytoplasmic autoantibodies (ANCA) to bactericidal/permeability-increasing (BPI) protein recognize the carboxyl terminal domain. *J. Infect.* 39, 81–87. doi: 10.1016/S0163-4453(99)90107-X

Elsbach, P., and Weiss, J. (1993). The bactericidal/permeability-increasing protein (BPI), a potent element in host-defense against gram-negative bacteria and lipopolysaccharide. *Immunobiology* 187, 417–429. doi: 10.1016/S0171-2985(11)80354-2

Fick, R. B.Jr., Naegel, G. P., Squier, S. U., Wood, R. E., Gee, J. B., and Reynolds, H. Y. (1984). Proteins of the cystic fibrosis respiratory tract. Fragmented immunoglobulin G opsonic antibody causing defective opsonophagocytosis. *J. Clin. Invest.* 74, 236–248. doi: 10.1172/JCI111407

Garner, H. P., Phillips, J. R., Herron, J. G., Severson, S. J., Milla, C. E., and Regelmann, W. E. (2004). Peroxidase activity within circulating neutrophils correlates with pulmonary phenotype in cystic fibrosis. *J. Lab. Clin. Med.* 144, 127–133. doi: 10.1016/j.lab.2004.04.010

Giroir, B. P., Quint, P. A., Barton, P., Kirsch, E. A., Kitchen, L., Goldstein, B., et al. (1997). Preliminary evaluation of recombinant amino-terminal fragment of human bactericidal/permeability-increasing protein in children with severe meningococcal sepsis. *Lancet* 350, 1439–1443. doi: 10.1016/S0140-6736(97)06468-4

Iwuji, K., Larumbe-Zabala, E., Bijlani, S., Nugent, K., Kanu, A., Manning, E., et al. (2019). Prevalence of Bactericidal/Permeability-Increasing Protein Autoantibodies in Cystic Fibrosis Patients: Systematic Review and Meta-Analysis. *Pediatr. Allergy Immunol. Pulmonol.* 32, 45–51. doi: 10.1089/ped.2018.0970

Janoff, A., White, R., Carp, H., Harel, S., Dearing, R., and Lee, D. (1979). Lung injury induced by leukocytic proteases. *Am. J. Pathol.* 97, 111–136.

Jensen, P.Ø., Bjarnsholt, T., Phipps, R., Rasmussen, T. B., Calum, H., Christoffersen, L., et al. (2007). Rapid necrotic killing of polymorphonuclear leukocytes is caused by quorum-sensing-controlled production of rhamnolipid by Pseudomonas aeruginosa. *Microbiology* 153, 1329–1338. doi: 10.1099/mic.0.2006/003863-0

King, C., and Harper, L. (2017). Avoidance of Harm From Treatment for ANCA-Associated Vasculitis. *Curr. Treatm .Opt. Rheumatol.* 3, 230–243. doi: 10.1007/s40674-017-0082-y

Kohler, H., Pashov, A., and Kieber-Emmons, T. (2019). The Promise of Anti-idiotype Revisited. *Front. Immunol.* 10, 808. doi: 10.3389/fimmu.2019.00808

Koller, D. Y., Urbanek, R., and Gotz, M. (1995). Increased degranulation of eosinophil and neutrophil granulocytes in cystic fibrosis. *Am. J. Respir. Crit. Care Med.* 152, 629–633. doi: 10.1164/ajrccm.152.2.7633718

Konstan, M. W., Geller, D. E., Minic, P., Brockhaus, F., Zhang, J., and Angyalosi, G. (2011). Tobramycin inhalation powder for P. aeruginosa infection in cystic fibrosis: The EVOLVE trial. *Pediatr. Pulmonol.* 46, 230–238. doi: 10.1002/ppul.21356

Lachenal, F., Nkana, K., Nove-Josserand, R., Fabien, N., and Durieu, I. (2009). Prevalence and clinical significance of auto-antibodies in adults with cystic fibrosis. *Eur. Respiratory J.* 34, 1079–1085. doi: 10.1183/09031936.00006009

Leeuwenberg, J. F., Dentener, M. A., and Buurman, W. A. (1994). Lipopolysaccharide LPS-mediated soluble TNF receptor release and TNF receptor expression by monocytes. Role of CD14, LPS binding protein, and bactericidal/permeability-increasing protein. *J. Immunol.* 152, 5070–5076.

Levin, M., Quint, P. A., Goldstein, B., Barton, P., Bradley, J. S., Shemie, S. D., et al. (2000). Recombinant bactericidal/permeability-increasing protein (rBPI21) as adjunctive treatment for children with severe meningococcal sepsis: a randomised trial. rBPI21 Meningococcal Sepsis Study Group. *Lancet* 356, 961–967. doi: 10.1016/S0140-6736(00)02712-4

Lindberg, U., Carlsson, M., Löfdahl, C.-G., and Segelmark, M. (2012). BPI-ANCA and long-term prognosis among 46 adult CF patients: a prospective 10-year follow-up study. *Clin. Dev. Immunol.* 2012, 370107–370107. doi: 10.1155/2012/370107

Mahadeva, R., Dunn, A. C., Westerbeek, R. C., Sharples, L., Whitehouse, D. B., Carroll, N. R., et al. (1999). Anti-neutrophil cytoplasmic antibodies (ANCA) against bactericidal/permeability-increasing protein (BPI) and cystic fibrosis lung disease. *Clin. Exp. Immunol.* 117, 561–567. doi: 10.1046/j.1365-2249.1999.01006.x

Mannion, B. A., Weiss, J., and Elsbach, P. (1990). Separation of sublethal and lethal effects of the bactericidal/permeability increasing protein on Escherichia coli. *J. Clin. Invest.* 85, 853–860. doi: 10.1172/JCI114512

Margaroli, C., Garratt, L. W., Horati, H., Dittrich, A. S., Rosenow, T., Montgomery, S. T., et al. (2018). Elastase Exocytosis by Airway Neutrophils Associates with Early Lung Damage in Cystic Fibrosis Children. *Am. J. Respir. Crit. Care Med.* 199, 873–881. doi: 10.1164/rccm.201803-0442OC

Marra, M. N., Wilde, C. G., Griffith, J. E., Snable, J. L., and Scott, R. W. (1990). Bactericidal/permeability-increasing protein has endotoxin-neutralizing activity. *J. Immunol.* 144, 662–666.

Mccarthy, C., Dimitrov, B. D., Meurling, I. J., Gunaratnam, C., and Mcelvaney, N. G. (2013). The CF-ABLE score: a novel clinical prediction rule for prognosis in patients with cystic fibrosis. *Chest* 143, 1358–1364. doi: 10.1378/chest.12-2022

Mccoy, K. S., Quittner, A. L., Oermann, C. M., Gibson, R. L., Retsch-Bogart, G. Z., and Montgomery, A. B. (2008). Inhaled aztreonam lysine for chronic airway Pseudomonas aeruginosa in cystic fibrosis. *Am. J. Respir. Crit. Care Med.* 178, 921–928. doi: 10.1164/rccm.200712-1804OC

Mcelvaney, O. J., Gunaratnam, C., Mcelvaney, O. F., Bagwe, I., Reeves, E. P., and Mcelvaney, N. G. (2018). Emerging pharmacotherapies in cystic fibrosis. *Expert Rev. Respir. Med.* 12, 843–855. doi: 10.1080/17476348.2018.1512409

Mcelvaney, O. J., Gunaratnam, C., Reeves, E. P., and Mcelvaney, N. G. (2019a). A specialized method of sputum collection and processing for therapeutic interventions in cystic fibrosis. *J. Cyst Fibros* 18, 203–211. doi: 10.1016/j.jcf.2018.06.001

Mcelvaney, O. J., Zaslona, Z., Becker-Flegler, K., Palsson-Mcdermott, E. M., Boland, F., Gunaratnam, C., et al. (2019b). Specific Inhibition of the NLRP3 Inflammasome as an Antiinflammatory Strategy in Cystic Fibrosis. *Am. J. Respir. Crit. Care Med.* 200, 1381–1391. doi: 10.1164/rccm.201905-1013OC

Middleton, P. G., Mall, M. A., Drevinek, P., Lands, L. C., Mckone, E. F., Polineni, D., et al. (2019). Elexacaftor-Tezacaftor-Ivacaftor for Cystic Fibrosis with a Single Phe508del Allele. *N Engl. J. Med.* 381, 1809–1819. doi: 10.1056/NEJMoa1908639

Odobasic, D., Oudin, V., Ito, K., Gan, P. Y., Kitching, A. R., and Holdsworth, S. R. (2019). Tolerogenic Dendritic Cells Attenuate Experimental Autoimmune Antimyeloperoxidase Glomerulonephritis. *J. Am. Soc. Nephrol.* 30, 2140–2157. doi: 10.1681/ASN.2019030236

Ohtami, S., Kobayashi, O., and Ohtami, H. (2001). Analysis of intractable factors in chronic airway infections: role of the autoimmunity induced by BPI-ANCA. *J. Infection Chemotherapy* 7, 228–238. doi: 10.1007/s101560170018

Pillarisetti, N., Williamson, E., Linnane, B., Skoric, B., Robertson, C. F., Robinson, P., et al. (2011). Infection, inflammation, and lung function decline in infants with cystic fibrosis. *Am. J. Respir. Crit. Care Med.* 184, 75–81. doi: 10.1164/rccm.201011-1892OC

Ramsey, B. W., Pepe, M. S., Quan, J. M., Otto, K. L., Montgomery, A. B., Williams-Warren, J., et al. (1999). Intermittent administration of inhaled tobramycin in patients with cystic fibrosis. Cystic Fibrosis Inhaled Tobramycin Study Group. *N Engl. J. Med.* 340, 23–30. doi: 10.1056/NEJM199901073400104

Reeves, E. P., Lu, H., Jacobs, H. L., Messina, C. G., Bolsover, S., Gabella, G., et al. (2002). Killing activity of neutrophils is mediated through activation of proteases by K+ flux. *Nature* 416, 291–297. doi: 10.1038/416291a

Reeves, E. P., Bergin, D. A., Murray, M. A., and Mcelvaney, N. G. (2011). The involvement of glycosaminoglycans in airway disease associated with cystic fibrosis. *ScientificWorldJournal* 11, 959–971. doi: 10.1100/tsw.2011.81

Rennard, S. I., Aalbers, R., Bleecker, E., Klech, H., Rosenwasser, L., Olivieri, D., et al. (1998). Bronchoalveolar lavage: performance, sampling procedure, processing and assessment. *Eur. Respir. J. Suppl.* 26, 13S–15S.

Ridley, K., and Condren, M. (2020). Elexacaftor-Tezacaftor-Ivacaftor: The First Triple-Combination Cystic Fibrosis Transmembrane Conductance Regulator Modulating Therapy. *J. Pediatr. Pharmacol. Ther. JPPT Off. J. PPAG* 25, 192–197. doi: 10.5863/1551-6776-25.3.192

Riordan, J. R., Rommens, J. M., Kerem, B., Alon, N., Rozmahel, R., Grzelczak, Z., et al. (1989). Identification of the cystic fibrosis gene: cloning and characterization of complementary DNA. *Science* 245, 1066–1073. doi: 10.1126/science.2475911

Riordan, J. R. (2008). CFTR function and prospects for therapy. *Annu. Rev. Biochem.* 77, 701–726. doi: 10.1146/annurev.biochem.75.103004.142532

Rommens, J. M., Iannuzzi, M. C., Kerem, B., Drumm, M. L., Melmer, G., Dean, M., et al. (1989). Identification of the cystic fibrosis gene: chromosome walking and jumping. *Science* 245, 1059–1065. doi: 10.1126/science.2772657

Saeki, K., Saeki, K., Nakahara, M., Matsuyama, S., Nakamura, N., Yogiashi, Y., et al. (2009). A feeder-free and efficient production of functional neutrophils from human embryonic stem cells. *Stem Cells* 27, 59–67. doi: 10.1634/stemcells.2007-0980

Schinke, S., Fellermann, K., Herlyn, K., Reichel, P. H., Fundke, R., Stange, E. F., et al. (2004). Autoantibodies against the bactericidal/permeability-increasing protein from inflammatory bowel disease patients can impair the antibiotic activity of bactericidal/permeability-increasing protein. *Inflammation Bowel Dis.* 10, 763–770. doi: 10.1097/00054725-200411000-00011

Schultz, H., Csernok, E., Schuster, A., Schmitz, T. S., Ernst, M., and Gross, W. L. (2000). Anti-neutrophil cytoplasmic antibodies directed against the bactericidal/permeability-increasing protein (BPI) in pediatric cystic fibrosis patients do not recognize N-terminal regions important for the anti-microbial and lipopolysaccharide-binding activity of BPI. *Pediatr. Allergy Immunol.* 11, 64–70. doi: 10.1034/j.1399-3038.2000.00069.x

Schultz, H., Schinke, S., Mosler, K., Herlyn, K., Schuster, A., and Gross, W. L. (2004). BPI-ANCA of pediatric cystic fibrosis patients can impair BPI-mediated killing of E. coli DH5alpha in vitro. *Pediatr. Pulmonol* 37, 158–164. doi: 10.1002/ppul.10416

Schultz, H., Hume, J., Zhang, D. S., Gioannini, T. L., and Weiss, J. P. (2007). A novel role for the bactericidal/permeability increasing protein in interactions of gram-negative bacterial outer membrane blebs with dendritic cells. *J. Immunol.* 179, 2477–2484. doi: 10.4049/jimmunol.179.4.2477

Sediva, A., Bartunkova, J., Kolarova, I., Hrusak, O., Vavrova, V., Macek, M.Jr., et al. (1998). Antineutrophil cytoplasmic autoantibodies (ANCA) in children with cystic fibrosis. *J. Autoimmun* 11, 185–190. doi: 10.1006/jaut.1997.0186

Sediva, A., Bartunkova, J., Bartosova, J., Jennette, C., Falk, R. J., and Jethwa, H. S. (2003). Antineutrophil cytoplasmic antibodies directed against bactericidal/permeability-increasing protein detected in children with cystic fibrosis inhibit neutrophil-mediated killing of Pseudomonas aeruginosa. *Microbes Infect.* 5, 27–30. doi: 10.1016/S1286-4579(02)00049-7

Skopelja, S., Hamilton, B. J., Jones, J. D., Yang, M.-L., Mamula, M., Ashare, A., et al. (2016). The role for neutrophil extracellular traps in cystic fibrosis autoimmunity. *JCI insight* 1, e88912–e88912. doi: 10.1172/jci.insight.88912

Smith, J. J., and Welsh, M. J. (1992). cAMP stimulates bicarbonate secretion across normal, but not cystic fibrosis airway epithelia. *J. Clin. Invest.* 89, 1148–1153. doi: 10.1172/JCI115696

Taggart, C., Coakley, R. J., Greally, P., Canny, G., O'neill, S. J., and Mcelvaney, N. G. (2000). Increased elastase release by CF neutrophils is mediated by tumor necrosis factor-alpha and interleukin-8. *Am. J. Physiol. Lung Cell Mol. Physiol.* 278, L33–L41. doi: 10.1152/ajplung.2000.278.1.L33

Tate, S., Macgregor, G., Davis, M., Innes, J. A., and Greening, A. P. (2002). Airways in cystic fibrosis are acidified: detection by exhaled breath condensate. *Thorax* 57, 926–929. doi: 10.1136/thorax.57.11.926

Theprungsirikul, J., Skopelja-Gardner, S., Meagher, R. E., Clancy, J. P., Zemanick, E. T., Ashare, A., et al (2020). Dissociation of systemic and mucosal autoimmunity in cystic fibrosis. *J. Cyst Fibros.* 19, 196–202. doi: 10.1016/j.jcf.2019.06.006

Vanpatten, S., Sun, S., He, M., Cheng, K. F., Altiti, A., Papatheodorou, A., et al. (2016). Amending HIV Drugs: A Novel Small-Molecule Approach To Target Lupus Anti-DNA Antibodies. *J. Med. Chem.* 59, 8859–8867. doi: 10.1021/acs.jmedchem.6b00694

Worgall, S., Kikuchi, T., Singh, R., Martushova, K., Lande, L., and Crystal, R. G. (2001). Protection against Pulmonary Infection with *Pseudomonas aeruginosa* following Immunization with *P. aeruginosa* Pulsed Dendritic Cells. *Infection Immun.* 69, 4521–4527. doi: 10.1128/IAI.69.7.4521-4527.2001

10

Enhanced Expression of Human Epididymis Protein 4 (HE4) Reflecting Pro-Inflammatory Status is Regulated by CFTR in Cystic Fibrosis Bronchial Epithelial Cells

Zsolt Bene[1,2,3], *Zsolt Fejes*[1,3], *Tibor Gabor Szanto*[4], *Ferenc Fenyvesi*[5], *Judit Váradi*[5], *Luka A. Clarke*[6], *Gyorgy Panyi*[4], *Milan Macek Jr.*[7], *Margarida D. Amaral*[6], *István Balogh*[1,8] *and Béla Nagy Jr.*[1,3]*

[1]Department of Laboratory Medicine, Faculty of Medicine, University of Debrecen, Debrecen, Hungary, [2]Department of Pediatrics, Faculty of Medicine, University of Debrecen, Debrecen, Hungary, [3]Kálmán Laki Doctoral School of Biomedical and Clinical Sciences, Faculty of Medicine, University of Debrecen, Debrecen, Hungary, [4]Department of Biophysics and Cell Biology, Faculty of Medicine, University of Debrecen, Debrecen, Hungary, [5]Department of Pharmaceutical Technology, Faculty of Pharmacy, University of Debrecen, Debrecen, Hungary, [6]Faculty of Sciences, BioISI-Biosystems and Integrative Sciences Institute, University of Lisboa, Lisboa, Portugal, [7]Department of Biology and Medical Genetics, Charles University—2nd Faculty of Medicine and Motol University Hospital, Prague, Czech, [8]Division of Clinical Genetics, Department of Laboratory Medicine, Faculty of Medicine, University of Debrecen, Debrecen, Hungary

***Correspondence:**
Béla Nagy Jr.
nagy.bela@med.unideb.hu

Decreased human epididymis protein 4 (HE4) plasma levels were reported in cystic fibrosis (CF) patients under CFTR potentiator *ivacaftor* therapy, which inversely correlated with lung function improvement. In this study, we investigated whether HE4 expression was affected via modulation of CFTR function in CF bronchial epithelial (CFBE) cells *in vitro*. HE4 protein levels were measured in the supernatants of CFBE 41o⁻ cells expressing F508del-CFTR or wild-type CFTR (wt-CFTR) after administration of *lumacaftor/ivacaftor* or *tezacaftor/ivacaftor*, while HE4 expression in CFBE 41o⁻ cells were also analyzed following application of adenylate cyclase activators Forskolin/IBMX or $CFTR_{inh172}$. The effect of all of these compounds on CFTR function was monitored by the whole-cell patch-clamp technique. Induced HE4 expression was studied with interleukin-6 (IL-6) in F508del-CFTR CFBE 41o⁻ cells under TNF-α stimulation for 1 h up to 1 week in duration. In parallel, plasma HE4 was determined in CF subjects homozygous for *p.Phe508del-CFTR* mutation receiving *lumacaftor/ivacaftor* (Orkambi®) therapy. NF-κB-mediated signaling was observed via the nuclear translocation of p65 subunit by fluorescence microscopy together with the analysis of IL-6 expression by an immunoassay. In addition, HE4 expression was examined after NF-κB pathway inhibitor BAY 11-7082 treatment with or without CFTR modulators. CFTR modulators partially restored the activity of F508del-CFTR and reduced HE4 concentration was found in F508del-CFTR CFBE 41o⁻ cells that

Abbreviations: CF, cystic fibrosis; CFBE, cystic fibrosis bronchial epithelial cell; CFFT, Cystic Fibrosis Foundation Therapeutics; CFTR, CF transmembrane conductance regulator; FEV_1, forced expiratory volume in 1 second; HE4, human epididymis protein 4; IL-6, interleukin-6; LPS, lipopolysaccharide; NF-κB, nuclear factor-kappa B; PBMCs, peripheral blood mononuclear cells; PEx, pulmonary exacerbation; RT, room temperature; SLPI, Secretory Leukocyte Protease Inhibitor; TNF-α, tumor necrosis factor α; WFDC, whey acidic protein four-disulfide-core; wt-CFTR, wild-type CFTR.

was close to what we observed in CFBE $41o^-$ cells with wt-CFTR. These data were in agreement with decreased plasma HE4 concentrations in CF patients treated with Orkambi®. Furthermore, CFTR inhibitor induced elevated HE4 levels, while CFTR activator Forskolin/IBMX downregulated HE4 in the cell cultures and these effects were more pronounced in the presence of CFTR modulators. Higher activation level of baseline and TNF-α stimulated NF-κB pathway was detected in F508del-CFTR vs. wt-CFTR CFBE $41o^-$ cells that was substantially reduced by CFTR modulators based on lower p65 nuclear positivity and IL-6 levels. Finally, HE4 expression was upregulated by TNF-α with elevated IL-6, and both protein levels were suppressed by combined administration of NF-κB pathway inhibitor and CFTR modulators in CFBE $41o^-$ cells. In conclusion, CFTR dysfunction contributes to abnormal HE4 expression via NF-κB in CF.

Keywords: cystic fibrosis, inflammation, bronchial epithelial cell, HE4, CFTR modulator

INTRODUCTION

Cystic fibrosis (CF; MIM:219700) is a monogenic disorder that is caused by pathogenic variants in the *cystic fibrosis transmembrane conductance regulator (CFTR)* gene (MIM: 602421). CFTR protein is a chloride/bicarbonate channel, which regulates fluid transport across the apical membrane at various epithelial surfaces comprising e.g., the sweat gland, lumen of the bronchial tree and pancreatic exocrine ducts (Rowe et al., 2005). More than 2,000 variants have been identified in the *CFTR* gene with the major *p. Phe508del-CFTR* allele accounting for approximately 80% of all CF-causing alleles. CFTR dysfunction leads to impaired ion transport across epithelial surfaces resulting in airway dehydration and thick mucus secretion associated with chronic respiratory bronchial inflammation/obstruction that is further compounded by chronic lung colonization with pathognomonic bacteria, such as *P. aeruginosa* (Rowe et al., 2005). Neutrophil infiltration with high intrapulmonary protease levels (e.g., neutrophil elastase) and excess of proinflammatory cytokines, such as interleukin 6 (IL-6) are associated with "hyperinflammation" in the CF lung leading to the progressive damage of the bronchial tree (Nixon et al., 1998; Cantin et al., 2015).

The human epididymis protein 4 (HE4) is encoded by the *WFDC2* gene (MIM:617,548). Its enhanced expression was first detected in the lower, chronically inflamed CF airways according to immunohistochemistry findings (Bingle et al., 2006). Moreover, *WFDC2* was reported to be among the upregulated genes in the native CF nasal epithelium (Clarke et al., 2013). Since then, elevated serum HE4 concentration was positively associated with the overall disease severity of CF and the degree of pulmonary dysfunction in unrelated patient cohorts (Nagy et al., 2016). Additionally, HE4 mRNA levels were significantly higher in CF vs. non-CF airway biopsy specimens (Nagy et al., 2016).

Recently, CF patients treated with CFTR potentiator *ivacaftor* (IVA) and carrying at least one Class III *CFTR* CF-causing mutation (*p.Gly551Asp*) had lower plasma HE4 concentrations, which also inversely correlated with the improvement of their spirometry parameters (Nagy et al., 2019). Based on these preliminary results, serum or plasma HE4 concentration represents a novel biomarker that may be of value for routine monitoring of CFTR modulating therapy in CF (Bene et al., 2020).

However, the mechanism of abnormal HE4 expression in CF lung epithelial cells has not been investigated as yet. The link between CFTR dysfunction and chronic airway inflammation has been analyzed by former *in vitro* studies (Vij et al., 2009; Hunter et al., 2010). These data indicated that wild-type CFTR (wt-CFTR) has inherent anti-inflammatory properties that suppress baseline and stimulated NF-κB mediated inflammatory signaling in bronchial epithelial cells, while in CF abnormal CFTR function contributes to generally increased inflammation via disrupted suppression of the NF-κB pathway (Vij et al., 2009; Hunter et al., 2010). Similarly, aberrant *CFTR* expression and thus CFTR function reduce the ability of myeloid cells to successfully resolve infection and inflammation (Bonfield et al., 2012).

Introduction of CFTR modulator therapy renders a highly effective therapeutic modality which directly targets the basic CFTR defect and thus substantially improves the overall clinical course of CF (De Boeck and Amaral, 2016). In terms of the effect of CFTR modulators on cellular level of inflammatory processes, *lumacaftor/ivacaftor* (Orkambi®, LUM/IVA) treatment restores CFTR dependent chloride efflux (Favia et al., 2020) and decreases IL-18 and tumor necrosis factor α (TNF-α) expression in peripheral blood mononuclear cells (PBMCs) when measured in patients homozygous for the *p. Phe508del-CFTR* allele (Jarosz-Griffiths et al., 2020). This treatment with LUM/IVA also enhanced airway epithelial repair and thus improved transepithelial resistance, irrespective of the presence of *P. aeruginosa* (Adam et al., 2018). Similarly, *tezacaftor/ivacaftor* (Symdeko®, TEZ/IVA) downregulates serum IL-1β level at 3 months following its patient administration (Jarosz-Griffiths et al., 2020). Finally, in our recent clinical study, treatment with *ivacaftor* resulted in significantly lower plasma HE4 concentrations in three independent cohorts of CF patients already at 1 month following initiation of therapy (Nagy et al., 2019).

Currently, it is not clear whether HE4 expression is "directly" regulated by CFTR and thus could be influenced by CFTR modulators *in vitro* using human CF bronchial epithelial

(CFBE) cells as a model cell culture system. Therefore, the major aims of this study are i) to determine HE4 level in the supernatants of cystic fibrosis bronchial epithelial (CFBE) 41o$^-$ cells expressing F508del-CFTR or wt-CFTR after *in vitro* administration of clinically relevant concentrations of CFTR modulators as well as CFTR activators and inhibitor; ii) to analyze HE4 concentrations in plasma samples drawn from CF subjects receiving Orkambi®; and iii) to investigate the role of NF-κB pathway in HE4 expression in association with impaired CFTR function and pro-inflammatory signaling in CF. To the best of our knowledge, such comprehensive approaches have not been applied thus far.

MATERIALS AND METHODS

Reagents

CFTR correctors *lumacaftor* (VX-809, LUM) (S1565) and *tezacaftor* (VX-661, TEZ) (S7059), CFTR potentiator *ivacaftor* (VX-770, IVA) (S1144), voltage-independent selective CFTR inhibitor $CFTR_{inh172}$ (S7139), CFTR activator Forskolin (FSK, S2449), and NF-κB pathway inhibitor BAY 11-7082 (S2913) were purchased from Selleck Chemicals (Houston, TX, United States). cAMP phosphodiesterase inhibitor IBMX (3-isobuthyl-1-methylxanthine, I5879) was ordered from Sigma-Aldrich (St. Louis, MO, United States). Except for recombinant TNF-α (Gibco, Carlsbad, CA, United States), all reagents were dissolved in dimethyl sulfoxide (DMSO, Sigma-Aldrich).

Cell Culture

CFBE 41o$^-$ cells cultures stably expressing F508del-CFTR or wt-CFTR were grown in Minimum Essential Medium Eagle (EMEM) with Earle's BSS (EBSS) and 1% L-glutamine (Lonza, Walkersville, MD, United States), 10% fetal bovine serum (FBS, Sigma-Aldrich) and 5 μg/ml Puromycin (Sigma-Aldrich) at 37°C, 5% CO_2 (Nagy et al., 2016). These cells were obtained from Dr J. P. Clancy's lab (Cincinnati Children's Hospital Medical Center, OH, United States). CFBE cells were seeded in 6-well plates (250.000 cells per well/sample). Supernatants for the analysis of HE4 and IL-6 protein levels were collected after CFBE cells were treated with TNF-α or phosphate buffer solution PBS, (i.e. at baseline) and combined CFTR modulators: corrector *lumacaftor* (3 μM) with potentiator *ivacaftor* (10 μM) (LUM/IVA) or corrector *tezacaftor* (5 μM) with *ivacaftor* (10 μM) (TEZ/IVA) or DMSO vehicle alone (thus representing the baseline) were administered for 24 h. For the activation of CFTR function, FSK (10 μM) with IBMX (100 μM) (FSK/IBMX) were added to both types of CFBE cells, while CFTR inhibition was carried out by $CFTR_{inh172}$ (20 μM) in wt-CFTR CFBE cells vs. control samples with DMSO with or without CFTR modulators for 24 h. CFTR modulators were applied under similar experimental conditions as in comparable *in vitro* studies (Hunter et al., 2010; Wang et al., 2016; Pranke et al., 2017; Kmit et al., 2019). To investigate the role of NF-κB pathway in HE4 expression *in vitro*, BAY 11-7082 (5 μM) or DMSO (baseline) was used for 24 h to inhibit pro-inflammatory signaling in both unstimulated and TNF-α activated CFBE cells both in the presence or absence of LUM/IVA or TEZ/IVA molecules.

Electrophysiology

Cl^- currents in CFBE 41o$^-$ cells were measured in the whole-cell patch-clamp configuration similar to former publications (Boinot et al., 2014; Billet et al., 2017). The external (bath) solution contained 145 mM NaCl, 4 mM CsCl, 1 mM $CaCl_2$, 1 mM $MgCl_2$, 5 mM D-glucose, and 10 mM HEPES (pH 7.4 titrated with NaOH, 315 mOsm). The intracellular (pipette) solution contained 113 mM L-aspartic acid, 113 mM CsOH, 27 mM CsCl, 1 mM NaCl, 1 mM $MgCl_2$, 1 mM ethylene glycol tetraacetic acid (EGTA), 10 mM HEPES, and 3 mM Mg-ATP (pH 7.2 titrated with CsOH, 285 mOsm). Mg-ATP was freshly diluted into the intracellular solution every hour. The intracellular solution was stored on ice before usage. FSK/IBMX and $CFTR_{inh-172}$ were freshly diluted into the extracellular solution before the start of the experiments, respectively. Micropipettes were pulled in four stages by using a Flaming Brown automatic pipette puller (Sutter Instruments, San Rafael, CA, United States) from Borosilicate Standard Wall with Filament aluminum-silicate glass (GC150-TF10, Harvard Apparatus Co., Holliston, MA, United States) with tip diameters between 0.5 and 1 μm and heat polished to a tip resistance ranging typically 3–10 MΩ in the bath solution. All measurements were carried out by using Axopatch 200B amplifier connected to a personal computer using Axon Digidata 1,550 A data acquisition hardware, respectively (Molecular Devices Inc., Sunnyvale, CA, United States). The holding potential was maintained at −40 mV throughout the experiments, and two voltage-clamp protocols were used to measure whole-cell CFTR currents. First, a single depolarization from −40 to 0 mV was applied every 5 s for 4–5 min to monitor the current evolution and to confirm the absence of significant leak current. For determining the current–voltage (I–V) relationship the cells were held at a holding potential of −40 mV and depolarized to test potentials between −80 and +80 mV in steps of 20 mV increments every 10 s. Experiments were done at room temperature (RT) ranging between 20 and 24°C. Data were analyzed using the pClamp10.5 software package (Molecular Devices Inc.). Before analysis, current traces were digitally filtered with a three-point boxcar smoothing filter. Prior to analysis, current traces were corrected for ohmic leak.

Total mRNA Extraction

Total mRNA from CFBE cell culture samples was isolated by TRI reagent (Molecular Research Center Inc., Cincinnati, OH, United States) according to the manufacturer's recommendations. The purity and the concentration of separated mRNA samples were verified by a NanoDrop 2000 spectrophotometer (Thermo Scientific, Wilmington, DE, United States). Extracted mRNA samples were stored at −80°C before further analysis.

Real-Time Quantitative PCR Analysis

Complementary DNA (cDNA) synthesis was performed with High Capacity cDNA Reverse Transcription kit (Applied Biosystems, Vilnius, Lithuania) according to the manufacturer's protocol on extracted mRNA samples. The initial amount of RNA was 1,000 ng per reaction. Real-time quantitative PCR (RT-qPCR) was performed on a LightCycler 480 qPCR instrument (Roche Diagnostics,

Mannheim, Germany) with LightCycler 480 SYBR Green I Master mix (Roche Diagnostics) including *WFDC2*-specific oligonucleotide primers (10 μM, Integrated DNA Technologies, Leuven, Belgium). The reactions were incubated at 95°C for 10 min, followed by 40 cycles of 95°C for 10 s and 60°C for 1 min. All measurements were run in triplicate. For normalization, we used the reference gene *RPLPO (36B4)*. HE4 expression in TNF-α stimulated CFBE cells was monitored from 1 h up to 1 week vs. the baseline (using PBS) via measuring mRNA concentrations, while induced cellular activation was followed by IL6-, IL8- and IL1B-specific mRNA levels. Sequences of the primers for respective cDNA amplification are listed in **Supplementary Table S1**.

Immunofluorescence Staining and Fluorescent Microscopy

Detection of the NF-κB pathway activation in CFBE 41o$^-$ cells with or without CFTR dysfunction was initially visualized via p65 nuclear immunofluorescence staining based on the method drawn from our previous study (Fejes et al., 2018) with some modifications. For this purpose, F508del-CFTR and wt-CFTR CFBE cells were cultured in 12-well plates on sterile glass microscope slides at a density of 5×10^4 cells/slide for 2 days. Cells were then treated with TNF-α (100 ng/mL) or vehicle (PBS, baseline) for 4 h. When the impact of CFTR modulator treatment on activation level of NF-κB pathway was studied, CFBE cells were preincubated with *lumacaftor* (3 μM) with *ivacaftor* (10 μM) or *tezacaftor* (5 μM) with *ivacaftor* (10 μM) or DMSO (baseline) for 24 h, and with TNF-α (100 ng/ml) or PBS (baseline) was added for 4 h. After these pretreatments, cells were fixed with ice-cold methanol-acetone (50 v/v %) for 10 min. Non-specific antibody binding sites were blocked with fetal bovine serum (FBS, Sigma-Aldrich) for 15 min. For primary labeling of NF-κB p65 subunit, polyclonal rabbit anti-human p65 antibody (100 μg/ml, Sigma-Aldrich) was used for 1 h followed by secondary staining with Alexa Fluor 488-conjugated goat-anti-rabbit IgG (5 μg/ml, Sigma-Aldrich) for 1 h. Cell nuclei were labeled with 4′,6-diamidino-2-phenylindole (DAPI, Invitrogen, Carlsbad, CA, United States), and samples were observed by Zeiss Axio Scope. A1 fluorescent microscope (HBO 100 lamp) (Carl Zeiss Microimaging GmbH, Goettingen, Germany). DAPI: excitation at 365 nm, emission BP filter 445/50 nm; fluorescein: excitation of BP filter at 470/40 nm, emission BP filter 525/50 nm. Images were analyzed with ZEN 2012 v.1.1.0.0. software (Carl Zeiss Microimaging GmbH). The ratio of nuclear and perinuclear (cytosol) fluorescence intensity was calculated for NF-κB p65 staining. The specificity of immunostaining was checked by incubating the cells with the secondary antibody only, and where very limited background staining was seen.

CF Patients

Ten CF patients with the classical and stable form of the disease and being homozygous for the *p. Phe508del-CFTR* pathogenic variant (5 females and 5 males, mean age of 16.1 ± 4.8 years) were randomly selected from a pre-existing cohort in order to measure plasma HE4 levels in samples obtained at 1 month of Orkambi® administration (Vertex Pharmaceuticals, Boston, MA, United States) (**Supplementary Table S2**). These subjects formerly participated in the PROSPECT study (ClinicalTrials.gov identifier: NCT0247731), and samples were requested from Cystic Fibrosis Foundation Therapeutics (CFFT) Biorepository (Bethesda, MD, United States). Mean value of baseline forced expiratory volume in 1 s (FEV_1% predicted) of these subjects was 74.6 ± 16.6%. Before treatment, mean sweat chloride concentration was 101.2 ± 9.2 mmol/L, while the mean change of sweat chloride was −19.6 mmol/L. Aliquots of their blood samples were obtained through venous puncture, and were centrifuged, then stored at −80°C. K_3-EDTA anticoagulated plasma aliquots were transferred from CFFT for HE4 analysis by international courier service on dry ice to the Department of Laboratory Medicine, University of Debrecen, Hungary.

Laboratory Analyses

Chemiluminescent microparticle immunoassay (Architect-i1000SR®, Abbott Diagnostics, Wiesbaden, Germany) was used to analyze protein levels of HE4 in the supernatants obtained from CFBE cell cultures following different research treatments as indicated above. In addition, HE4 plasma concentrations were measured before treatment and after LUM/IVA treatment with the same immunoassay that we used on our previous cohorts (Nagy et al., 2019). IL-6 levels were measured by electro-chemiluminescent immunoassay on a Cobas c 411 instrument (Roche Diagnostics). These measurements were performed in an analyst-blinded mode in all studied cases in order to avoid any potential operator-related bias.

Ethics Statement

This study was approved by the Regional Ethics Committee of the University of Debrecen (permit number: 4813-2017) in accordance with the World Medical Association Declaration of Helsinki—Ethical Principles for Medical Research Involving Human Subjects.

Statistical Analysis

The Kolmogorov-Smirnov test was used for the evaluation of the normality of the data. Data are expressed in mean ± SD or SEM, where applicable. Unpaired *t*-test or Mann-Whitney *U* test was performed to compare two groups of data, while comparison of multiple groups was performed using the ANOVA with Bonferroni's multiple comparisons test. For comparison of plasma HE4 levels before and under CFTR modulator treatment, paired *t*-test was utilized. The $p < 0.05$ probability level was regarded as being statistically significant. Analyses were performed using GraphPad Prism, version 6.01 (GraphPad Software, La Jolla, CA, United States).

RESULTS

CFTR Modulators Partially Rescue F508del-CFTR Cl$^-$ Currents in CFBE 41o$^-$ cells

In order to demonstrate that the CFTR modulators applied in this study restore CFTR function in airway epithelial cells *in vitro*, we treated human CFBE 41O-cell cultures expressing F508del-CFTR with

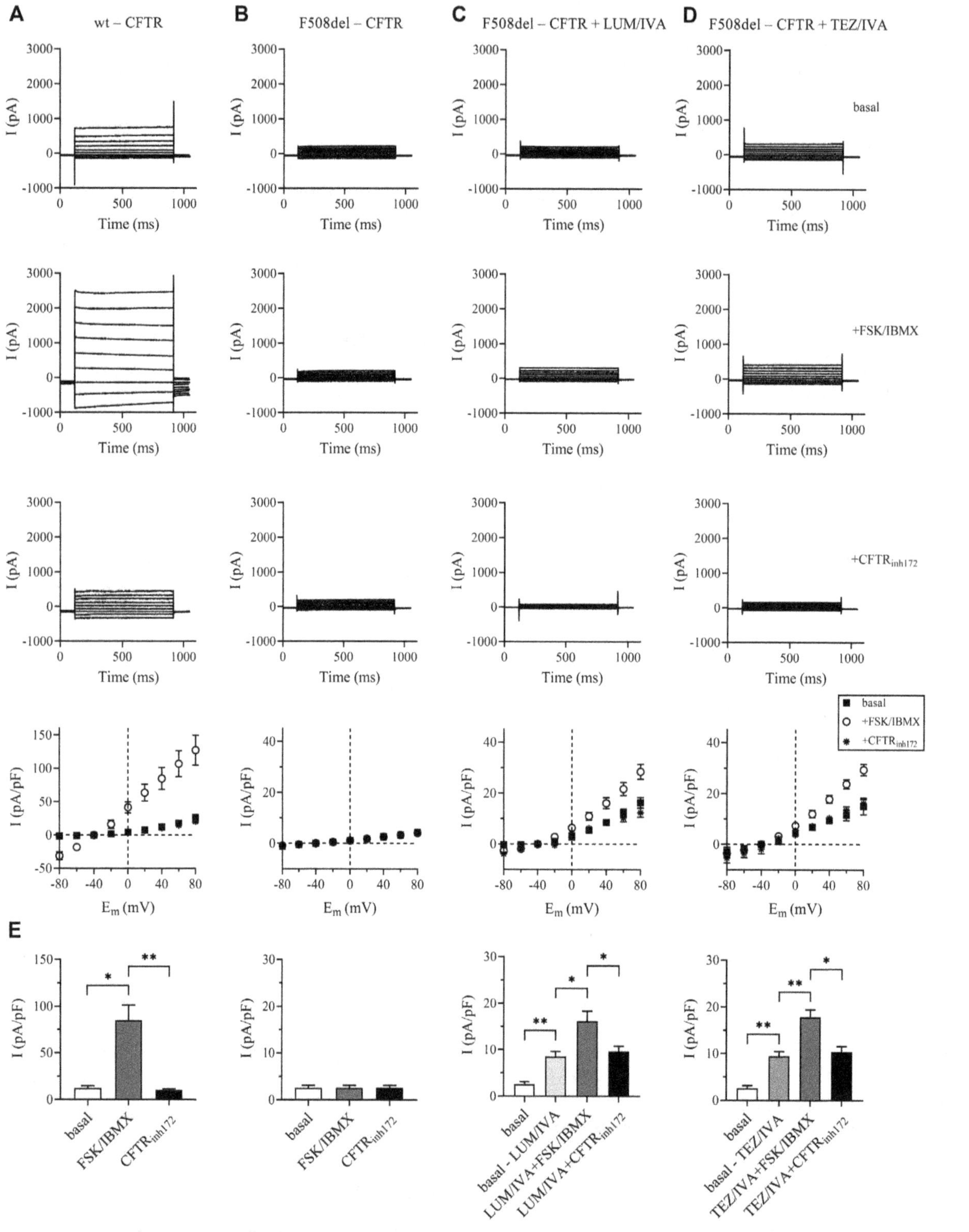

FIGURE 1 | Rescue of functional F508del-CFTR Cl^- currents in LUM/IVA and TEZ/IVA-treated CFBE 41o⁻ cells. Representative traces of whole-cell Cl^- currents were elicited by stepping from a holding potential of −40 mV to series test potentials ranging from −80 to +80 mV with 20-mV increments every 10 s in CFBE 41o⁻ cells expressing the wild-type CFTR [wt-CFTR, column **(A)**], the F508del-CFTR [F508del-CFTR, column **(B)**], or in cells expressing the deletion mutant CFTR but treated for 24 h with LUM/IVA [3/10 µM, column **(C)**], or TEZ/IVA [5/10 µM, column **(D)**]. Currents were measured at RT. Top traces: basal current, in the absence of FSK/IBMX stimulation; middle traces: after ~2 min stimulation by FSK/IBMX (10/100 µM); bottom traces: in the presence of FSK/IBMX and 20 µM of the CFTR inhibitor

(Continued)

FIGURE 1 | $CFTR_{inh172}$. The bottom panels show the peak current density-voltage relationships (pA/pF, mean ± SEM, n = 3–5) in the absence of FSK/IBMX (basal, filled squares), upon stimulation by FSK/IBMX (open circles) and in the presence of FSK/IBMX and 20 μM $CFTR_{inh172}$ (asterisks). Histograms of the corresponding current densities (pA/pF) determined at +40 mV. Data are expressed in mean ± SEM, n = 3–5 cells/condition **(E)** Basal: wild-type CFTR expressing cells (left panel) or F508del-CFTR expressing cells (all other panels) in the absence of FSK/IBMX stimulation. Basal-LUM/IVA and basal-TEZ/IVA: F508del-CFTR expressing cells treated with the CFTR modulators only (see above), FSK/IBMX: stimulation of basal or LUM/IVA or TEZ/IVA-treated cells by FSK/IBMX (see above); $CFTR_{inh172}$: basal or LUM/IVA or TEZ/IVA-treated cells in the presence of FSK/IBMX and $CFTR_{inh172}$. Unpaired or paired *t*-test was performed for comparisons. $^{*}p < 0.05$, $^{**}p < 0.01$.

two different combinations of CFTR modulators (LUM/IVA or TEZ/IVA) for 24 h and analyzed Cl^- current density using patch-clamp. CFBE 41o⁻ cells expressing wild-type CFTR showed whole-cell Cl^- currents that could be robustly activated by FSK/IBMX and inhibited by the CFTR selective inhibitor $CFTR_{inh172}$. The peak current-voltage relationship indicated (**Figure 1A**, bottom panel) a linear current-voltage relationship, which was most obvious after FSK/IBMX treatment, that reversed around −40 mV, the expected reversal potential of a Cl^- current calculated from the ionic composition of the pipette-filling and extracellular solutions. The same experiments in CFBE $41o^-$ cells expressing F508del-CFTR resulted in miniature currents that were insensitive to either FSK/IBMX activation or inhibition by $CFTR_{inh172}$ (**Figure 1B**). Most importantly, both combinations of CFTR modulators (LUM/IVA, **Figure 1C**, or TEZ/IVA, **Figure 1D**) significantly increased the basal and the FSK/IBMX-stimulated Cl^- current in comparison to F508del-CFTR basal Cl^- current (**Figures 1B–D**). Moreover, the currents activated by FSK/IBMX treatment were sensitive to $CFTR_{inh172}$ (**Figures 1C,D**). The statistical analysis of the current densities at +40 mV in **Figure 1E** confirms that CFTR modulators corrected F508del-CFTR channel function (**Figure 1E**). The current densities recorded in the presence of FSK/IBMX in cells treated with either LUM/IVA or TEZ/IVA were comparable to the wt-CFTR current density in the absence of the activators (~20 pA/pF) and smaller than wt-CFTR current after stimulation (~80 pA/pF). Of note, TEZ/IVA restored F508del-CFTR Cl^- current density at a moderately higher level than LUM/IVA (9.44 ± 1.01 vs. 8.48 ± 1.14 pA/pF; p = 0.560). In summary, LUM/IVA and TEZ/IVA CFTR modulators partially restored CFTR function in CFBE $41o^-$ cells cultures expressing F508del-CFTR.

CFTR Function Modulates HE4 Concentrations in CFBE 41o⁻ cells Culture Supernatants *in vitro*

CFBE 410-cell cultures expressing F508del-CFTR were treated with CFTR modulators LUM/IVA or TEZ/IVA for 24 h to quantify protein levels of HE4 in the cell culture supernatants. Subsequently, CFBE $41o^-$ cells with wt-CFTR were utilized as controls for HE4 supernatant concentrations. We consistently found that baseline HE4 concentration was higher in F508del-CFTR CFBE $41o^-$ cells than normal cells ($p < 0.01$) and was significantly reduced by LUM/IVA ($p < 0.01$) and TEZ/IVA ($p < 0.001$) treatment compared to

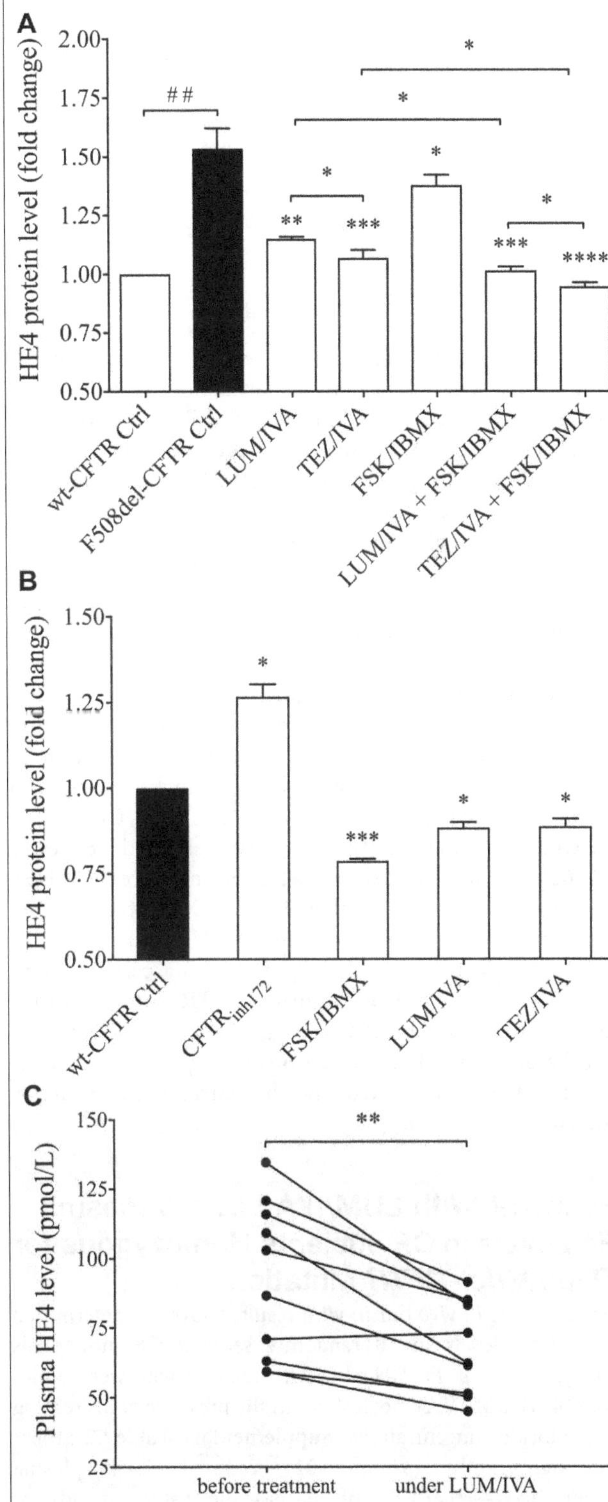

FIGURE 2 | Analysis of HE4 levels in the supernatant of F508del-CFTR or wt-CFTR CFBE 41o⁻ cells with pharmacologically altered CFTR function and in plasma samples of CF subjects under LUM/IVA therapy. Both LUM/IVA (3/10 μM) and TEZ/IVA (5/10 μM) resulted in decreased HE4 in F508del-CFTR CFBE 41o⁻ cells after 24 h approaching the level of normal cells. CFTR activator FSK/IBMX (10/100 μM) alone moderately reduced HE4, while combined treatment of FSK/IBMX with CFTR modulators showed an even

(*Continued*)

FIGURE 2 | larger change in HE4 **(A)** $CFTR_{inh172}$ (20 μM) caused elevated HE4 levels after 24 h while, in turn, improved CFTR function with FSK/IBMX or CFTR modulator reduced HE4 even in wt-CFTR CFBE 41o⁻ cells **(B)** There were lower plasma HE4 values compared to baseline measured in CF subjects (n = 10) after 1 month of Orkambi® in agreement with *in vitro* data with LUM/IVA **(C)** Data are expressed in mean ± SEM (n = 5–6 samples/condition). Unpaired or paired *t*-test or Mann-Whitney *U* test was performed for comparisons. $^{\#\#}p < 0.01$ vs. wt-CFTR cells; $^{*}p < 0.05$, $^{**}p < 0.01$, $^{***}p < 0.001$, and $^{****}p < 0.0001$ vs. F508del-CFTR control (ctrl) cells with DMSO, or baseline plasma samples, respectively.

control samples where the vehicle (i.e., DMSO) was applied. The concentration of HE4 in the supernatant was close to that observed in wt-CFTR CFBE $41o^-$ cells (**Figure 2A**). Interestingly, TEZ/IVA caused a larger decrease of HE4 concentrations compared to LUM/IVA ($p < 0.05$). In parallel, CFTR activator FSK/IBMX was used alone and in combination with aforementioned CFTR modulators in cells with F508del-CFTR. The HE4 protein level was decreased by FSK/IBMX ($p < 0.05$) likely due to the activation of residual CFTR function, while further reduction in HE4 was observed after the combined treatment ($p < 0.05$) vs. using individual CFTR modulator molecules (**Figure 2A**).

To provide further evidence of the inverse association between HE4 expression measured by its concentration in cell culture supernatants and CFTR function, we also applied pharmacological inhibition of CFTR by $CFTR_{inh172}$ in wt-CFTR CFBE $41o^-$ cells, which caused elevated HE4 levels ($p < 0.05$). In contrast, there was a significant decrease in HE4 concentrations ($p < 0.001$) after FSK/IBMX treatment when compared to the controls. Interestingly, LUM/IVA and TEZ/IVA could downregulate HE4 expression to a certain extent even in CFBE $41o^-$ cells with normal CFTR expression ($p < 0.05$) (**Figure 2B**). These data suggest that CFTR function affects basal levels of HE4 expression and impaired function of CFTR could explain elevated HE4 concentration in CF airway epithelial cells *in vitro*.

Treatment With LUM/IVA Lowers Plasma HE4 Levels in CF Subjects Homozygous for *p.Phe508del-CFTR* Mutation

To substantiate *in vivo* our *in vitro* results above, we determined plasma HE4 levels in 10 randomly selected CF individuals homozygous for *p. Phe508del-CFTR* mutation who were under Orkambi® (LUM/IVA) medication. In the presence of decreasing sweat chloride concentrations (**Supplementary Table S2**), there were significantly ($p < 0.01$) reduced HE4 plasma concentrations—regardless of its baseline value—already at 1 month of treatment, this being the earliest follow-up time point of these patients (**Figure 2C**). These clinical data underscore the impact of CFTR modulation therapy on decreasing HE4 plasma concentrations in CF and are in agreement with previous findings in IVA monotherapy in cases with at least one *p. Gly551Asp-CFTR* pathogenic variant (Nagy et al., 2019).

TNF-α Induces Increased *HE4* mRNA Expression in CFBE $41o^-$ cells Cultures *in vitro*

Subsequently, we studied whether *WFDC2/HE4* expression could be further enhanced by an artificial inflammatory stimulus *in vitro*. For this purpose, F508del-CFTR CFBE $41o^-$ cells were stimulated with recombinant TNF-α applied in the range spanning from 1 h up to 1 week. As a result, HE4 mRNA level quantified by RT-qPCR raised already after 1 h of treatment vs. untreated (baseline) sample ($p < 0.05$) and was further elevated within the period of 4 h ($p < 0.001$). Surprisingly, HE4 mRNA levels returned to baseline within 24 h. When TNF-α was administered for longer periods (from 48 h up to 1 week), there was a much higher expression of HE4 mRNA ($p < 0.0001$) in TNF-α stimulated CFBE $41o^-$ cells (**Figure 3A**).

In the same set of samples, mRNA levels of pro-inflammatory cytokines IL-6, IL-8 and IL-1β (**Figures 3B–D**) were also analyzed to ascertain if these mediators were also provoked by TNF-α together with increased expression of HE4. In this regard, IL-6 and IL-8 expression showed similar time-dependent alteration patterns as observed in HE4 mRNA, while elevated IL1B mRNA was sustained from 1 h without a substantial change throughout this time period. Furthermore, the protein concentrations of HE4 and IL-6 were measured in the supernatants of F508del-CFTR CFBE $41o^-$ cells at some selected time points (between 4 and 168 h), whereby HE4 level was significantly elevated after 4 h and gradually increased up to 1 week of treatment, while IL-6 concentration was significantly augmented at all pre-selected time points (**Supplementary Figures S1A,B**). These results imply that expression of HE4 mRNA thus resulting concentrations of HE4 protein are upregulated following TNF-α administration accompanied by different pro-inflammatory cytokines in CFBE cells.

The Pro-inflammatory NF-κB Pathway is Influenced by the Combination of CFTR Modulators in F508del-CFTR CFBE $41o^-$ cells *in vitro*

To establish the relationship between upregulated NF-κB pathway due to CFTR dysfunction and the abnormal HE4 expression in CFBE cells *in vitro*, we applied two experimental approaches. First, the activity of NF-κB pathway was assessed via the p65 nuclear translocation experiments. This protein, also known as RelA (MIM: 164,014), is one of the 5 components that constitute the NF-κB transcription factor family and is used as a marker of NF-κB pathway activation. We applied fluorescence microscopy-based approaches in wt-CFTR and F508del-CFTR CFBE $41o^-$ cells that had been treated with TNF-α vs. untreated controls. Second, the effect of CFTR modulators was studied *in vitro* on basal and induced NF-κB signaling in these CFBE cells after the application of LUM/IVA or TEZ/IVA treatment via p65 nuclear positivity and IL-6 in the cell

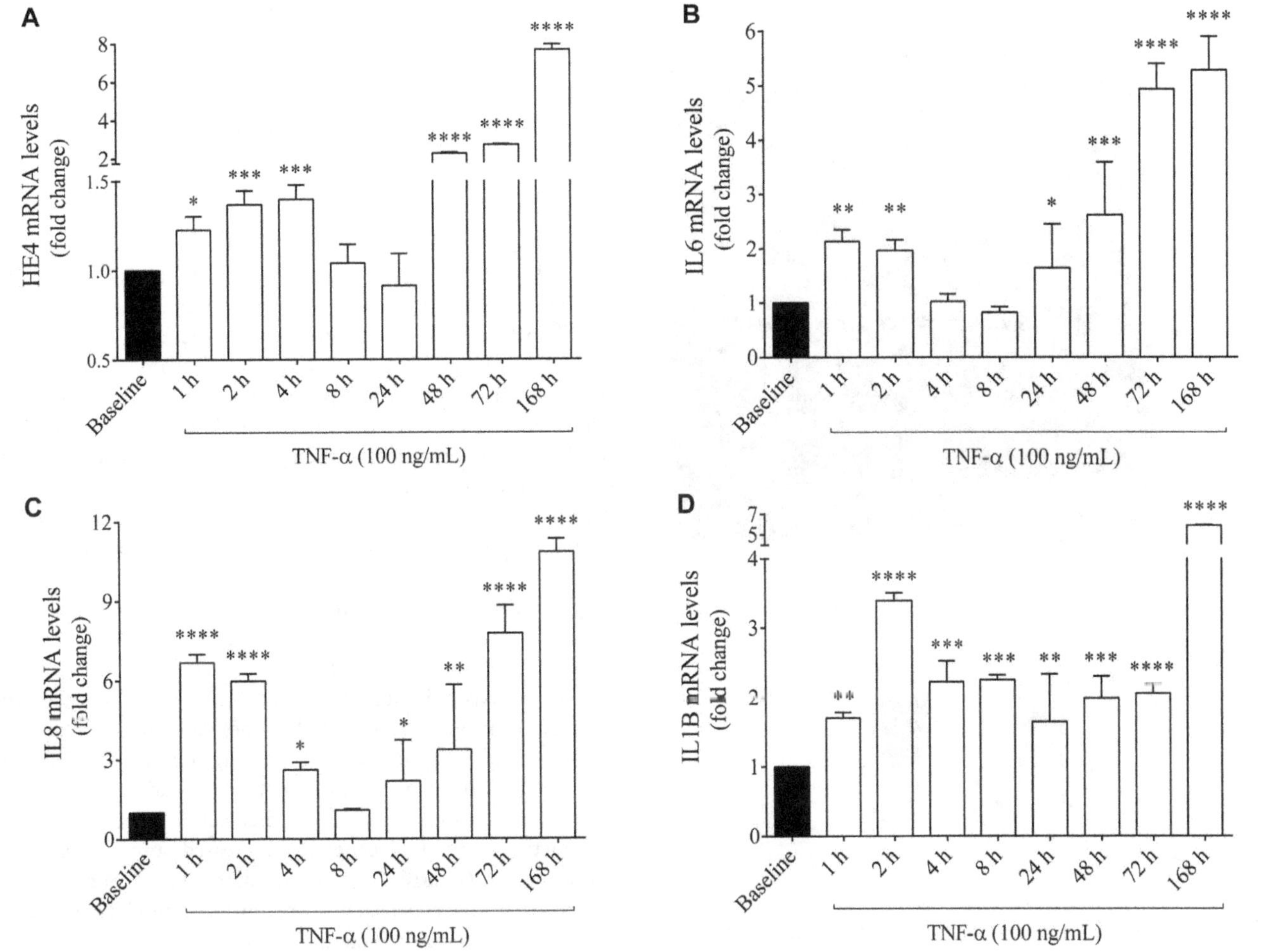

FIGURE 3 | Quantification of HE4, IL6, IL8 and IL1B mRNA levels in F508del-CFTR CFBE 41o⁻ cells after TNF-α stimulation for 1 h up to 1 week *in vitro*. HE4 mRNA level was higher than baseline at 1–4 h that returned to normal range by 24 h and was further induced by TNF-α (100 ng/ml) after 48 h up to 168 h **(A)** IL6 mRNA level was already induced by 1–2 h and was further augmented after 24 h **(B)** In parallel, IL-8 expression showed a similar time-course alteration to HE4 and IL6 **(C)**, while IL1B mRNA level had a sustained elevation without a substantial alteration during this time period **(D)** Mean ± SEM (n = 4–5 samples/condition). $^{*}p < 0.05$, $^{**}p < 0.01$, $^{***}p < 0.001$, and $^{****}p < 0.0001$ vs. baseline, based on ANOVA with Bonferroni's multiple comparison test.

line supernatants. There was a significantly higher baseline level of p65 positivity in the nuclei of F508del-CFTR CFBE 41o$^-$ cells vs. normal cells ($p < 0.01$). When these cell cultures were exposed to TNF-α, significantly higher p65 positivity was seen in both cell types ($p < 0.05$, $p < 0.0001$, respectively), and the difference in p65 translocation between normal and deficient CFBE cells was more pronounced ($p < 0.0001$) (**Figures 4A,B**). These results indicate that there is a higher baseline and induced level of inflammatory status in CF vs. normal CFBE cells. Secondly, CFTR modulators substantially decreased p65 positivity ($p < 0.05$) not only in unstimulated F508del-CFTR CFBE 41o$^-$ cells, but a significant reduction was also observed ($p < 0.001$) after TNF-α treatment compared to baseline (DMSO) sample (**Figures 5A,B**). In parallel, we determined IL-6 protein levels in the supernatants of studied CFBE cell lines which confirmed the anti-inflammatory effect of applied CFTR modulators via downregulation of basal and TNF-α stimulated IL-6 expression (**Figure 5C**). Hence, our data provide evidence that the generally increased levels of NF-κB pathway activation due to CFTR dysfunction could be efficaciously downregulated by the application of LUM/IVA or TEZ/IVA in CFBE cell cultures *in vitro*.

HE4 Concentrations in CFBE 41o$^-$ cells Cultures Are Not Only Upregulated by the NF-κB Pathway and Pro-Inflammatory Signaling but Are Also Directly Influenced by CFTR Activity

Finally, we wanted to examine if TNF-α induced HE4 levels could also be decreased by applying CFTR modulators in F508del-CFTR CFBE 41o$^-$ cells. Administration of either LUM/IVA or TEZ/IVA resulted in a significant reduction in HE4 concentration ($p < 0.001$) when measured in the supernatants of TNF-α activated CFBE 41o$^-$ cells vs. controls with TNF-α and

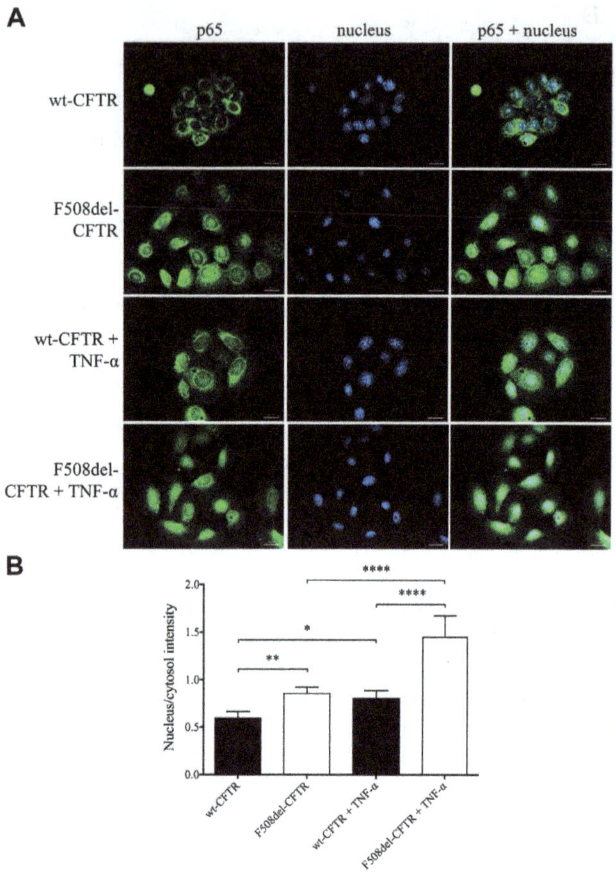

FIGURE 4 | Immunofluorescence staining with the quantification of nuclear/cytosol p65 positivity for detecting NF-κB pathway activation in unstimulated and TNF-α treated CFBE 41o⁻ cells expressing F508del-CFTR or wt-CFTR. The basal level of p65 nuclear translocation was analyzed in respect to CFTR function when normal and F508del-CFTR CFBE 41o⁻ cells were stimulated with 100 ng/ml TNF-α or PBS (baseline) for 4 h. Green: p65 staining; blue: cell nuclei. Scale bar: 20 μm **(A)** Fluorescence intensity of the NF-κB immunostaining was analyzed based on the ratio of the nucleus/cytosol intensity **(B)** Mean ± SEM (n = 6–7 cells/condition). $^{*}p < 0.05$, $^{**}p < 0.01$ and $^{****}p < 0.0001$ based on statistical analyses.

DMSO (**Figure 6A**). Furthermore, FSK/IBMX alone caused a moderate but still significantly reduced HE4 level in the presence of TNF-α ($p < 0.05$), whereas combined administration of LUM/IVA or TEZ/IVA with FSK/IBMX lowered HE4 concentrations by a significantly higher degree ($p < 0.01$; $p < 0.001$, respectively). Similar to the unstimulated samples (**Figure 2A**), TEZ/IVA caused a larger change in HE4 compared to LUM/IVA with or without CFTR activator ($p < 0.05$). (**Figure 6A**). When TNF-α activated wt-CFTR epithelial cells were treated with CFTR activator FSK/IBMX or CFTR modulators, there were similarly reduced HE4 levels ($p < 0.01$) compared to TNF-α activated samples with vehicle (**Figure 6B**). Thus, observed data provide evidence that corrected and/or potentiated CFTR function has a "protective role" against TNF-α-induced upregulation of HE4 expression in CFBE cells *in vitro*.

As we consistently detected enhanced levels of HE4 in the presence of abnormal CFTR function in CFBE 41o⁻ cells bearing F508del-CFTR in contrast to wt-CFTR cells under non-activated and TNF-α activated conditions, we raised the question whether increased HE4 expression in CF is under the regulation of NF-κB mediated pathway directly via impaired CFTR function and related pro-inflammatory stimuli. For this purpose, pretreatment with specific NF-κB pathway inhibitor BAY 11-7082 was used in F508del-CFTR CFBE 41o⁻ cells in the absence or presence of CFTR modulators and TNF-α treatment. In these cell culture samples, supernatant HE4 and IL-6 protein levels were determined. We found that BAY 11-7082 mediated inhibition alone significantly lowered baseline HE4 ($p < 0.05$) and IL-6 levels ($p < 0.01$) after 24 h, while BAY 11-7082 with LUM/IVA or TEZ/IVA resulted in a much stronger reduction in the levels of both proteins ($p < 0.001$; $p < 0.0001$, respectively) (**Figures 7A,B**). TNF-α-induced HE4 expression was also hindered to a large degree via BAY 11-7082-related inhibition of the NF-κB pathway ($p < 0.05$). Moreover, we noted further decrease in HE4 and IL-6 supernatant concentrations when NF-κB pathway inhibitor and CFTR modulators were administered together vs. control samples with TNF-α and DMSO ($p < 0.001$) (**Figures 7A,B**). In turn, CFBE 41o⁻ cells with wt-CFTR were treated with $CFTR_{inh172}$ with or without BAY 11-7082. In contrast to increased HE4 supernatant concentrations, $CFTR_{inh172}$-based inhibition of CFTR was not associated with elevated HE4 concentrations in the supernatant in the presence of the NF-κB pathway inhibitor ($p < 0.05$) (**Figure 7C**). Detected changes in IL-6 supernatant concentrations had similar patterns which underscores the close association between CFTR dysfunction and the generally increased pro-inflammatory status in CF (**Figure 7D**). In summary, HE4 concentrations measured in the supernatants are not only modulated via the NF-κB pathway and pro-inflammatory signaling, but also directly influenced by CFTR in CFBE cell cultures *in vitro*.

DISCUSSION

In this study, we have provided evidence that enhanced *in vitro* expression of HE4 is regulated by CFTR in CFBE cells. Our results add to the increasing line of evidence that CFTR is not only one of the critical regulators of epithelial fluid balance across various apical epithelial membranes, but may also modulate inflammatory signaling (Eidelman et al., 2001). We have recently reported high concentration of HE4 in serum samples accompanied with its elevated expression in airway epithelial biopsy specimens of CF individuals (Nagy et al., 2016). In addition, HE4 level was around two-fold higher in the supernatant of F508del-CFTR vs. wt-CFTR CFBE cells (Nagy et al., 2016). HE4 or WFDC2 protein belongs to the whey acidic protein four-disulfide-core (WFDC) protein family, and its members, such as Secretory Leukocyte Protease Inhibitor (SLPI) and Elafin (PI3) possess anti-protease, anti-bacterial and anti-inflammatory properties (Small et al., 2017). Due to their abundance in the lung, they have been proposed to be involved in lung homeostasis and protection of the lung from proteolytic "attacks" (Bingle et al., 2006; Small et al., 2017). On the other hand, the mechanism of increased production of HE4 in CF airway epithelial cells is yet unknown.

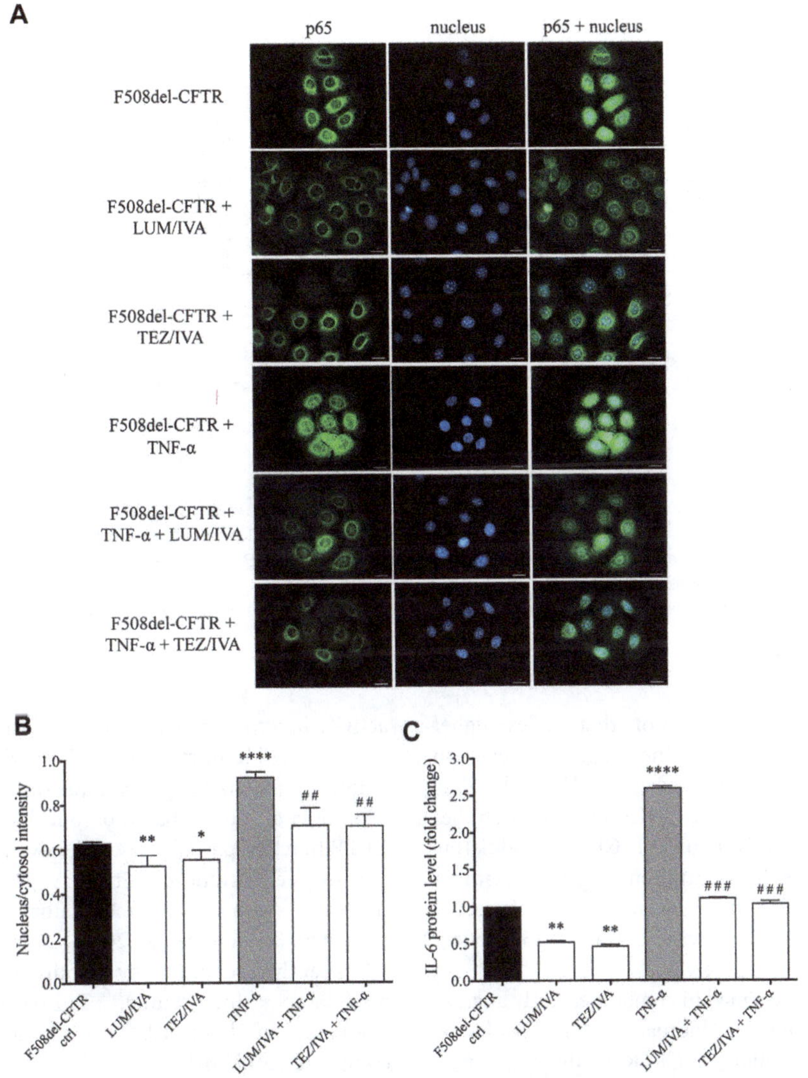

FIGURE 5 | Immunofluorescence staining and quantification of p65 nuclear translocation staining with the analysis of IL-6 protein levels in the presence of CFTR modulators in unstimulated or TNF-α treated CFBE 41o⁻ cells cultures expressing F508del-CFTR. Alteration in p65 nuclear translocation was first analyzed when cells were pretreated with LUM/IVA or TEZ/IVA or DMSO (baseline) for 24 h. CFBE cells were then activated with 100 ng/ml TNF-α or PBS (baseline) for 4 h. Green: p65 staining; blue: cell nuclei. Scale bar: 20 μm **(A)** Fluorescence intensity of the NF-κB immunostaining was analyzed based on the ratio of the nucleus/cytosol intensity **(B)** Downregulated IL-6 protein levels were measured in the supernatants of untreated and TNF-α stimulated CFBE 410-cells to approve the inhibition of NF-κB pathway activation by CFTR modulators by 24 h **(C)** Mean ± SEM, n = 4–5 cells/condition. $^{*}p < 0.05$, $^{**}p < 0.01$, and $^{****}p < 0.0001$ vs. control cells with DMSO; $^{\#\#}p < 0.01$ and $^{\#\#\#}p < 0.001$ vs. CFBE cells with TNF-α and DMSO.

To date, it is still unclear whether CFTR modulators influence airway inflammatory response via moderating abnormal innate immunity or by epithelial cell activation (Hisert et al., 2017). Latest *in vitro* investigations described downregulated IL-1β and IL-18 levels derived from lipopolysaccharide (LPS)-stimulated monocytes after LUM/IVA or TEZ/IVA treatment (Jarosz-Griffith et al., 2020), reduced secretion of pro-inflammatory cytokines with restored macrophage function in response to *P. aeruginosa* after single IVA or combined LUM/IVA therapy (Barnaby et al., 2018), and depressed CXCL8 expression and p38 MAPK phosphorylation in CFBE cells in response to Orkambi® treatment (Ruffin et al., 2018). Accordingly, CFTR corrector and potentiator drugs may have anti-inflammatory capacities through rescued CFTR function and reduced sweat chloride concentration (Ramsey et al., 2011; Hisert et al., 2017). Of note, this is only indirect evidence from clinical trials and post-marketing studies that has not been duly validated *in vitro*. Moreover, these drugs were not always clinically effective in terms of sustained decrease of chronic bronchial inflammation based on studied biomarkers in the sputum (Rowe et al., 2014), and their anti-inflammatory properties could even gradually vanish after 36 h of treatment (Jarosz-Griffith et al., 2020). In this regard, previous studies reported that the general level of inflammation is increased via constitutive activation of the NF-κB

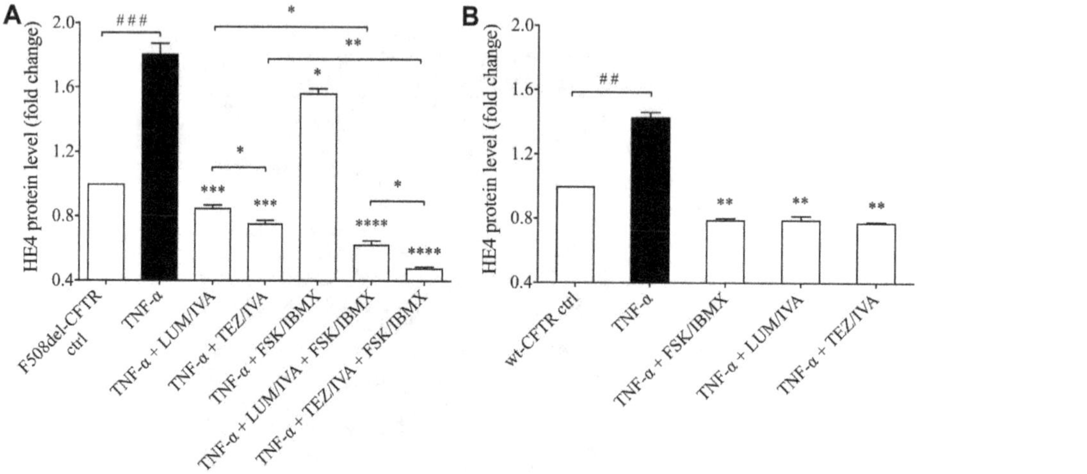

FIGURE 6 | Determination of HE4 level in TNF-α activated F508del-CFTR or wt-CFTR CFBE 41o$^-$ cells with *in vitro* modulated CFTR function. First, TNF-α activated F508del-CFTR CFBE 41o$^-$ cells were analyzed under the treatment with LUM/IVA, TEZ/IVA, FSK/IBMX or their combination for 24 h. TNF-α could not elevate HE4 expression in the presence of improved CFTR function **(A)** In parallel, CFTR function was affected by FSK/IBMX or CFTR modulators in TNF-α-stimulated wt-CFTR CFBE 41o$^-$ cells for 24 h. Similar to the results in F508del-CFTR CFBE 41o$^-$ cells, HE4 expression remained lowered compared to samples with TNF-α but with a smaller extent **(B)** Mean ± SEM, n = 5–6 samples/condition. $^{*}p < 0.05$, $^{**}p < 0.01$, $^{***}p < 0.001$ and $^{****}p < 0.0001$ vs. control samples with TNF-α and DMSO; $^{\#\#}p < 0.01$ and $^{\#\#\#}p < 0.001$ vs. control samples with PBS.

pathway in CF due to CFTR dysfunction that drives higher production of pro-inflammatory cytokines (e.g. IL-8) even in the absence of pathognomonic infectious agents (Vij et al., 2009; Hunter et al., 2010; Wang et al., 2016). Recent clinical studies provide evidence that administration of CFTR modulators normalizes sweat chloride concentration together with a substantial correction of CFTR function in majority of treated subjects (Ramsey et al., 2011; Wainwright et al., 2015; Taylor-Cousar et al., 2017).

Therefore, in this study, we aimed to comprehensively analyze how in our opinion promising biomarker HE4 could be influenced by the administration of CFTR modulators, since the pathogenesis of upregulated HE4 expression in CF is not fully understood. Furthermore, we aimed to provide evidence how treatment with CFTR correctors and potentiators could be monitored using HE4 as a plasma biomarker in routine clinical practice and what the particular diagnostic value of HE4 is in monitoring degree of decreased inflammation in CF patients due to restored function of CFTR. Consequently, we investigated for the first time whether abnormal HE4 expression is directly linked to CFTR dysfunction and is associated with NF-κB pathway in CF. We took aforementioned clinical and laboratory evidence into account when designing our methodological approaches.

For this purpose, we analyzed the change in basal and TNF-α-induced HE4 levels when CFTR function and NF-κB signaling were pharmacologically modulated in CFBE 41o$^-$ cells cultures expressing F508del-CFTR in comparison to cells with wt-CFTR. First, there was about 1.5-fold higher basal HE4 concentration in F508del-CFTR vs. wt-CFTR CFBE 41o$^-$ cells. Both LUM/IVA and TEZ/IVA significantly lowered HE4 in these cells with F508del-CFTR compared to control samples with vehicle. These compounds were formerly tested for the correction of CFTR in CF epithelial cell cultures via the measurement of CFTR activity *in vitro* (Pranke et al., 2017; Kmit et al., 2019). Here, the rescue of CFTR function by CFTR modulators was observed with whole-cell patch-clamp technique similar to a former publication (Boinot et al., 2014). Based on our data, we considered F508del-CFTR function partially rescued, however, Boinot *et al.* suggested that if the current density was greater than 4 pA/pF after treatment with CFTR modulator, the CFTR activity was corrected (Boinot et al., 2014). As a consequence, HE4 was significantly reduced by both combinations of CFTR modulators. Importantly, TEZ/IVA caused a stronger alteration in both Cl$^-$ current and HE4 concentrations compared to LUM/IVA.

Treatment with IVA previously lowered plasma HE4 levels in CF patients bearing a specific Class 3 CFTR pathogenic variant (Nagy et al., 2019), but no data were available on the impact of combined therapy *in vivo* with various CFTR correctors and modulators on plasma HE4 as yet. Hence, we determined plasma HE4 levels in 10 CF individuals homozygous for *p. Phe508del-CFTR* mutation who were taking LUM/IVA regimen. In accordance with *in vitro* data, we provided evidence that this combination of CFTR modulators (Orkambi®) led to significantly decreased HE4 plasma concentrations, regardless of individual baseline HE4 concentrations and already after 1 month since the initiation of treatment. Subsequently, we used pharmacological inhibition of CFTR by $CFTR_{inh172}$ in CFBE 41o$^-$ cells with wt-CFTR that caused elevated HE4 levels *in vitro*. In contrast, there was a significant decrease in HE4 concentrations after CFTR activator FSK/IBMX treatment in wt-CFTR cells compared to controls. These data are in accordance with previous reports on elevated NF-κB activity with higher IL-8 level following $CFTR_{inh172}$ administration and decreased NF-κB activity after FSK/IBMX treatment in another cell culture (Hunter et al., 2010). In addition, FSK/IBMX treatment resulted in a moderate but statistically significant reduction of HE4

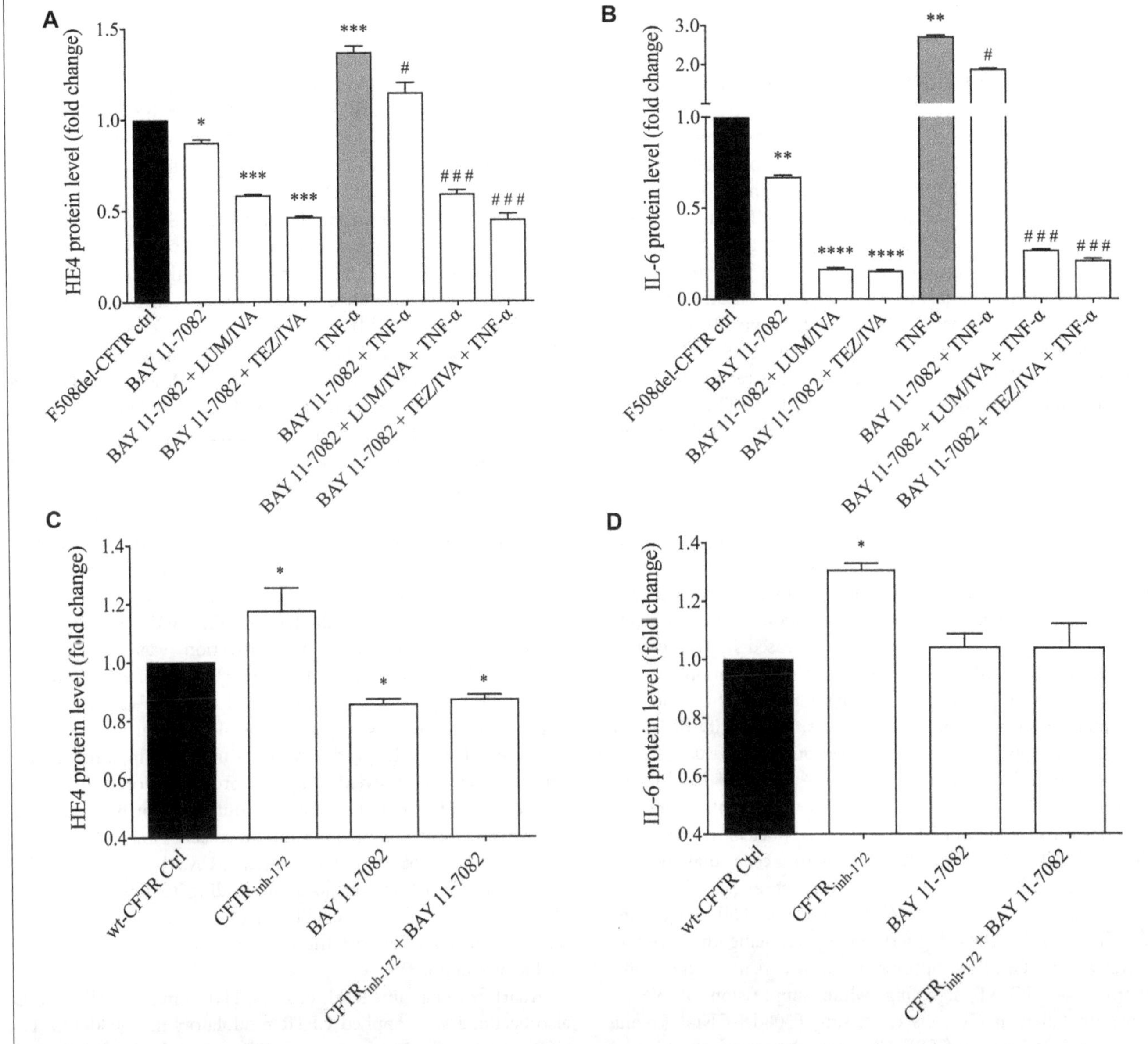

FIGURE 7 | Measurement of HE4 and IL-6 concentrations in non-activated and TNF-α activated F508del-CFTR CFBE 41o⁻ cells in the presence of NF-κB pathway inhibitor and CFTR modulators. BAY 11-7082 (5 μM) was applied to attenuate NF-κB-mediated inflammatory signaling in relation to basal and TNF-α induced HE4 expression in F508del-CFTR CFBE 41o⁻ cells under LUM/IVA or TEZ/IVA or vehicle for 24 h. TNF-α-induced HE4 **(A)** and IL-6 **(B)** expression was prevented by BAY 11–7082, and an even stronger decrease in HE4 and IL-6 was observed when NF-κB inhibitor and CFTR modulators were administered together vs. samples with TNF-α and DMSO. When wt-CFTR CFBE 41o⁻ cells were treated with $CFTR_{inh172}$ with or without BAY 11-7082, $CFTR_{inh172}$ (20 μM) could not elevate HE4 level after incubation with NF-κB inhibitor suggesting the role of NF-κB associated with CFTR **(C)** Changes in IL-6 with the same trend indicates a close relationship between CFTR function and pro-inflammatory conditions in CF **(D)** Mean ± SEM, n = 5–6 samples/condition. $^{*}p < 0.05$, $^{**}p < 0.01$, $^{***}p < 0.001$ and $^{****}p < 0.0001$ vs. control samples with DMSO; $^{\#}p < 0.05$ and $^{\#\#\#}p < 0.001$ vs. control samples with TNF-α and vehicle.

level due to the activation of residual CFTR function of bronchial epithelial cells with F508del-CFTR. However, this particular effect was lower than what we observed in wt-CFTR cells. Finally, when FSK/IBMX was used in combination with CFTR modulators in F508del-CFTR CFBE 41o⁻ cells, HE4 further decreased, especially with TEZ/IVA vs. control samples with DMSO. All these HE4 results are consistent with the change in Cl^- current under different treatments (**Figure 1A**). Based on our results, impaired CFTR function increases baseline HE4 expression in CF airway epithelial cells, which in turn could be efficiently lowered by CFTR modulators.

Next, we wanted to study if *WFDC2/HE4* expression could be upregulated in F508del-CFTR CFBE 41o⁻ cells cultures, so these cells were stimulated *in vitro* with TNF-α for short and long time periods (i.e., for 1 up to 168 h). HE4 mRNA level increased following just 1 h of treatment and remained high for up to 4 h but returned to the baseline by 24 h. Afterward, when HE4 expression was determined up to 168 h, an even higher expression of HE4 was observed in TNF-α stimulated CFBE 41o^{-} cells. To monitor the pro-inflammatory effect of TNF-α on these CFBE cells upon HE4 overexpression, IL6, IL8, and IL1B mRNAs were also analyzed by RT-qPCR in a similar manner. Comparable patterns were found in IL-6 and IL-8 levels as they were upregulated and changed throughout the experiment, while elevated IL1B expression varied only moderately at the different time points. These results indicate that not only pro-inflammatory cytokines are upregulated in CF (Nixon et al., 1998; Cantin et al., 2015), but the expression of HE4 can also be triggered under inflammatory circumstances. As a result, HE4 protein level was significantly elevated after 4 h and gradually increased up to 1 week of treatment, while IL-6 protein concentration was significantly augmented at all time points. Our results are thus reminiscent of a previous report on similar time-dependent regulation of HE4 expression via TLR2 mediated pathway including NF-κB signaling in cancer cells (Janeckova et al., 2015). Similarly, SLPI and Elafin were also induced in response to TNF-α in human alveolar epithelial cells (Sallenave et al., 1994).

Chronic inflammation via upregulated NF-κB signaling leads to gradual progress of structural damage of airways in CF (Cantin et al., 2015). Based on recent findings, ionic imbalance also generated NLRP3-inflammasome activation in CFBE cells exaggerated by LPS/ATP that caused increased IL-18 secretion (Lara-Reyna et al., 2020). To investigate the correlation between enhanced NF-κB pathway caused by CFTR dysfunction and abnormal HE4 expression in CFBE cells, the activity of NF-κB pathway via p65 nuclear translocation was visualized by fluorescence microscopy in wt-CFTR and F508del-CFTR CFBE 41o^{-} cells with or without TNF-α treatment. There was a significantly higher basal level of p65 nuclear positivity in F508del-CFTR vs. wt-CFTR CFBE 41o^{-} cells that was in accordance with former results (Wang et al., 2016). These authors also reported that wt-CFTR regulated TNF-α signaling by enhancing TRADD degradation. By reducing the levels of TRADD, wt-CFTR suppressed downstream the pro-inflammatory NF-κB signaling, while suppression of NF-κB activation failed in CF cells expressing F508del-CFTR (Wang et al., 2016). When our CFBE 41o^{-} cells cultures were activated with TNF-α, the difference in p65 nuclear translocation between normal and deficient CFBE cells was more pronounced. These findings imply that enhanced baseline and triggered NF-κB signaling and abnormal HE4 expression *in vitro* could be related to each other. Therefore, we raised the question of whether application of LUM/IVA or TEZ/IVA treatment could reduce basal and TNF-α induced NF-κB signaling that is responsible for lower HE4 concentrations in the supernatant. We found that CFTR modulators not only attenuated p65 positivity in unstimulated F508del-CFTR CFBE 41o^{-} cells, but a significant reduction was also observed in TNF-α after treatment with CFTR modulators. Decreased baseline and induced IL-6 protein levels in the supernatants of these cells suggest that there are additional anti-inflammatory properties of CFTR modulators apart from decreasing HE4 expression as recently evidenced by others (Ruffin et al., 2018). Overall, these data indicate that the inflammatory status of CF airway epithelial cells could be positively mitigated by CFTR modulators. Our observation is supported by data regarding reduced NLRP3-inflammasome activation in PBMCs observed in CF subjects receiving LUM/IVA or TEZ/IVA via decreased Caspase-1 activity by 3 months of treatment (Jarosz-Griffiths et al., 2020) and by the facts that treatment with Orkambi® restored CFTR dependent chloride efflux (Favia et al., 2020), decreased IL-18 and TNF-α expression in PBMCs (Jarosz-Griffiths et al., 2020), and improved airway epithelial repair (Adam et al., 2018), while Symdeko® downregulated serum IL-1β level in CF subjects (Jarosz-Griffiths et al., 2020). Intriguingly, there were available data, which are contradictory to our results on reduced baseline and TNF-α stimulated IL-6 concentrations in response to LUM/IVA or TEZ/IVA in F508del-CFTR CFBE 41o^{-} cells. Stanton *et al.* reported that PAO1 (MIM:615,854) alone induced a substantial expression of IL-6 and IL-8, while stimulated F508del-CFTR Cl^{-} secretion was reduced despite co-treatment with LUM or LUM/IVA, and IL-6 and IL-8 levels remained unaffected (Stanton et al., 2015). Recently, Laselva *et al.* demonstrated that the levels of IL-6, IL-8 and TNF-α were reduced following Orkambi® and rescued F508del-CFTR HBE cells, which were exposed to PAO1, but only in the presence of antimicrobial peptide or tobramycin (Laselva et al., 2020). In both previous studies, PAO1 resulted in a significant decrease in CFTR expression, but Orkambi® administration was not able to "compensate" for the pro-inflammatory effect of PAO1, which could reflect differences between PAO1 and TNF-α pathway. In our experiments, TNF-α as a pro-inflammatory mediator enhanced IL-6 levels via the NF-κB similar to impaired CFTR function that was prevented by the preincubation with CFTR modulators (**Figure 5C**) with or without inhibitor BAY 11 7082 (**Figure 7B**). Based on the immunofluorescence analysis of CFBE 41o^{-} cells for p65 positivity, either LUM/IVA or TEZ/IVA reduced p65 nuclear translocation leading to lower IL-6 and HE4 levels. Thus, despite this discrepancy, we are convinced that our *in vitro* data support the anti-inflammatory properties of CFTR modulators.

Apart from baseline levels of HE4, TNF-α induced HE4 levels also declined with applied CFTR modulators in F508del-CFTR CFBE 41o^{-} cells. Furthermore, TNF-α stimulated CFBE 41o^{-} cells with wt-CFTR demonstrated lowered HE4 levels in the presence of CFTR activator FSK/IBMX. Since we found enhanced level of NF-κB pathway activity in CFBE cells bearing the F508del-CFTR in contrast to wt-CFTR cells at both basal level and upon TNF-α activation, we finally investigated whether HE4 expression could be altered using specific NF-κB pathway inhibitors. For this purpose, the commercially available BAY 11-7082 inhibitor was applied *in vitro* to attenuate NF-κB mediated signaling in deficient CFBE cells in the absence or presence of TNF-α pretreatment and CFTR modulators. Under these experimental conditions we then determined supernatant HE4 and IL-6 protein levels. We found that both inhibitors significantly lowered the baseline and induced protein level of HE4 and IL-6 (**Figures 7A,B**). Our data implicate that CFTR mediated NF-κB pathway is involved in the regulation of HE4 expression in CFBE cells. The rescue of CFTR function in either unstimulated or TNF-α-activated F508del-

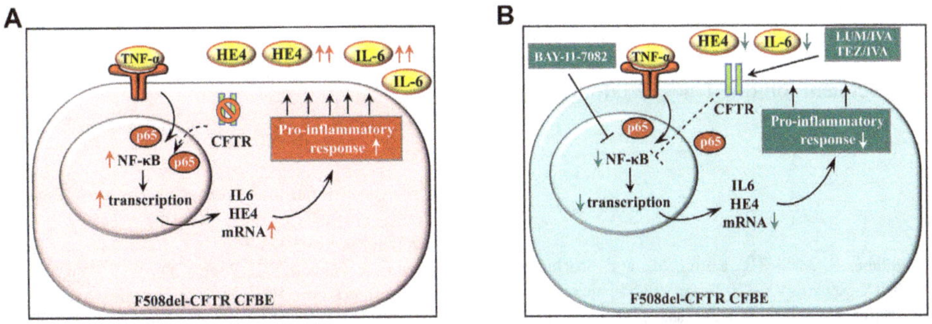

FIGURE 8 | Schematic figure about the model on the regulation of HE4 expression in CF via CFTR and pro-inflammatory signaling. There is an increased basal expression of HE4 with cytokines (e.g., IL-6) in lung epithelial cells of CF that is caused by CFTR dysfunction and external pro-inflammatory stimuli, e.g., TNF-α via the NF-κB pathway **(A)** Blocking the effect of TNF-α by BAY 11-7082 or using CFTR modulators (LUM/IVA or TEZ/IVA) can effectively reduce pro-inflammatory response in CFBE cells by suppressing the NF-κB pathway with a still unknown mechanism (dotted line) that prevents IL-6 and HE4 overexpression **(B)** Abbreviations: CFBE cell: cystic fibrosis bronchial epithelial cell, CFTR: cystic fibrosis transmembrane conductance regulator, TNF-α: tumor necrosis factor alpha, HE4: human epididymis protein 4, IL-6: interleukin-6, NF-κB: nuclear factor-kappa B.

CFTR CFBE 41o$^-$ cells consistently documented reduced HE4 levels not only in the current *in vitro* samples (**Figures 2A, 6A**), but also in CF patients who were on CFTR modulator therapy (**Figure 2C**). These findings were supported with reduced HE4 supernatant levels following BAY 11-7082 CFBE cell culture treatment within the same conditions. In addition, we previously found that in those CF subjects who suffered from more severe inflammation (with acute exacerbation) showing higher CRP values, serum HE4 concentrations were also much higher (Nagy et al., 2016).

Overall, we propose that dual regulation by CFTR and pro-inflammatory signaling via the NF-κB pathway upregulates HE4 expression in CFBE. Bitam and her colleagues formerly reported significantly enhanced CFTR maturation and related chloride currents in F508del-CFTR transfected HeLa cells and primary bronchial epithelial cell cultures after 6 h of treatment with TNF-α, however, CFTR function was only slightly improved within the period of 24 h (Bitam et al., 2015). Therefore, even if TNF-α might rescue CFTR to a certain extent by 24 h under our conditions, HE4 expression was not sufficiently influenced. Earlier, cytokine-mediated induction of Elafin in pulmonary epithelial cells was described to be regulated via an NF-κB site within the proximal promoter of Elafin (Bingle et al., 2001). In addition, a potential NF-κB binding site can be indicated at position -322 relative to the HE4 promoter region (Chen et al., 1998). Hence, we suppose that HE4 is also transcriptionally regulated by the NF-κB, however, further e.g. ChIP-seq-based expression studies are required to support the assertion of any functional relationship.

The manuscript has limitations. Firstly, we have not analyzed whether the absence of CFTR function or the presence of misfolded F508del-CFTR was the cause of increased HE4 expression. Secondly, CF patients on TEZ/IVA medication could not be enrolled for plasma HE4 measurement into this study, because such samples are currently not available, either from CFFT nor from our national studies. Thirdly, the mechanistic relationship between the CF-related inflammation and the expression of HE4 was not fully investigated, thus additional studies are required to reveal further related pathogenetic aspects.

In conclusion, we provide evidence that there is a direct relationship between CFTR function and pro-inflammatory response in F508del-CFTR CFBE cells in terms of increased expression of HE4 measured by its concentrations in the cell culture supernatant *in vitro* (**Figure 8**). CFTR corrector and potentiator administration restores inflammatory balance via correcting CFTR function and reducing NF-κB p65 nuclear translocation in CFBE cells as reflected by lower HE4 concentrations *in vitro* and *in vivo*. Finally, we believe that our study opens novel research avenues in terms of providing evidence for the diagnostic utility of plasma biomarker HE4 in terms of its use in efficient monitoring of anti-inflammatory properties of CFTR modulators.

ETHICS STATEMENT

The studies involving human participants were reviewed and approved by Regional Ethics Committee of the University of Debrecen (permit number: 4813-2017). Written informed consent to participate in this study was provided by the participants' legal guardian/next of kin.

AUTHOR CONTRIBUTIONS

BN designed and performed experiments, analyzed data, provided overall direction and wrote the manuscript. ZB, ZF, TS, FF, and JV performed experiments; LC and GP analyzed data; MM, GP, MA, and IB revised the manuscript and provided critical revisions of the intellectual content of this manuscript. All authors edited, reviewed, and approved the final version of the manuscript.

UNKP-20-4-II-DE-197 New National Excellence Program of The Ministry for Innovation and Technology.

ACKNOWLEDGMENTS

The authors thank Ms Edit Kalina, BSc for excellent technical assistance. BN was a recipient of the Lajos Szodoray Grant (Faculty of Medicine, University of Debrecen). CFFT (Bethesda, MD, United States) is acknowledged to supply the human samples to this study.

REFERENCES

Adam, D., Bilodeau, C., Sognigbé, L., Maillé, É., Ruffin, M., and Brochiero, E. (2018). CFTR Rescue with VX-809 and VX-770 Favors the Repair of Primary Airway Epithelial Cell Cultures from Patients with Class II Mutations in the Presence of *Pseudomonas aeruginosa* Exoproducts. *J. Cystic Fibrosis* 17, 705–714. doi:10.1016/j.jcf.2018.03.010

Barnaby, R., Koeppen, K., Nymon, A., Hampton, T. H., Berwin, B., Ashare, A., et al. (2018). Lumacaftor (VX-809) Restores the Ability of CF Macrophages to Phagocytose and Kill *Pseudomonas aeruginosa*. *Am. J. Physiol.-Lung Cell Mol. Physiol.* 314, L432–L438. doi:10.1152/ajplung.00461.2017

Bene, Z., Fejes, Z., Macek, M., Jr., Amaral, M. D., Balogh, I., and Nagy, B., Jr. (2020). Laboratory Biomarkers for Lung Disease Severity and Progression in Cystic Fibrosis. *Clinica Chim. Acta* 508, 277–286. doi:10.1016/j.cca.2020.05.015

Billet, A., Froux, L., Hanrahan, J. W., and Becq, F. (2017). Development of Automated Patch Clamp Technique to Investigate CFTR Chloride Channel Function. *Front. Pharmacol.* 8, 195. doi:10.3389/fphar.2017.00195

Bingle, L., Cross, S. S., High, A. S., Wallace, W. A., Rassl, D., Yuan, G., et al. (2006). WFDC2 (HE4): a Potential Role in the Innate Immunity of the Oral Cavity and Respiratory Tract and the Development of Adenocarcinomas of the Lung. *Respir. Res.* 7, 61. doi:10.1186/1465-9921-7-61

Bingle, L., Tetley, T. D., and Bingle, C. D. (2001). Cytokine-Mediated Induction of the Human Elafin Gene in Pulmonary Epithelial Cells Is Regulated by Nuclear Factor- κ B. *Am. J. Respir. Cel. Mol. Biol.* 25, 84–91. doi:10.1165/ajrcmb.25.1.4341

Bitam, S., Pranke, I., Hollenhorst, M., Servel, N., Moquereau, C., Tondelier, D., et al. (2015). An Unexpected Effect of TNF-α on F508del-CFTR Maturation and Function. *F1000Res* 4, 218. doi:10.12688/f1000research.6683.1

Boinot, C., Jollivet Souchet, M., Ferru-Clément, R., and Becq, F. (2014). Searching for Combinations of Small-Molecule Correctors to Restore F508del-Cystic Fibrosis Transmembrane Conductance Regulator Function and Processing. *J. Pharmacol. Exp. Ther.* 350, 624–634. doi:10.1124/jpet.114.214890

Bonfield, T. L., Hodges, C. A., Cotton, C. U., and Drumm, M. L. (2012). Absence of the Cystic Fibrosis Transmembrane Regulator (Cftr) from Myeloid-Derived Cells Slows Resolution of Inflammation and Infection. *J. Leukoc. Biol.* 92, 1111–1122. doi:10.1189/jlb.0412188

Cantin, A. M., Hartl, D., Konstan, M. W., and Chmiel, J. F. (2015). Inflammation in Cystic Fibrosis Lung Disease: Pathogenesis and Therapy. *J. Cystic Fibrosis* 14, 419–430. doi:10.1016/j.jcf.2015.03.003

Chen, F. E., Huang, D.-B., Chen, Y.-Q., and Ghosh, G. (1998). Crystal Structure of P50/p65 Heterodimer of Transcription Factor NF-Kb Bound to DNA. *Nature* 391, 410–413. doi:10.1038/34956

Clarke, L. A., Sousa, L., Barreto, C., and Amaral, M. D. (2013). Changes in Transcriptome of Native Nasal Epithelium Expressing F508del-CFTR and Intersecting Data from Comparable Studies. *Respir. Res.* 14, 38. doi:10.1186/1465-9921-14-38

De Boeck, K., and Amaral, M. D. (2016). Progress in Therapies for Cystic Fibrosis. *Lancet Respir. Med.* 4, 662–674. doi:10.1016/s2213-2600(16)00023-0

Eidelman, O., Srivastava, M., Zhang, J., Leighton, X., Murtie, J., Jozwik, C., et al. (2001). Control of the Proinflammatory State in Cystic Fibrosis Lung Epithelial Cells by Genes from the TNF-Ar/nfkb Pathway. *Mol. Med.* 7, 523–534. doi:10.1007/bf03401858

Favia, M., Gallo, C., Guerra, L., De Venuto, D., Diana, A., Polizzi, A. M., et al. (2020). Treatment of Cystic Fibrosis Patients Homozygous for F508del with Lumacaftor-Ivacaftor (Orkambi) Restores Defective CFTR Channel Function in Circulating Mononuclear Cells. *Int. J. Mol. Sci.* 21, 2398. doi:10.3390/ijms21072398

Fejes, Z., Czimmerer, Z., Szük, T., Póliska, S., Horváth, A., Balogh, E., et al. (2018). Endothelial Cell Activation Is Attenuated by Everolimus via Transcriptional and Post-transcriptional Regulatory Mechanisms after Drug-Eluting Coronary Stenting. *PLoS One* 13, e0197890. doi:10.1371/journal.pone.0197890

Hisert, K. B., Heltshe, S. L., Pope, C., Jorth, P., Wu, X., Edwards, R. M., et al. (2017). Restoring Cystic Fibrosis Transmembrane Conductance Regulator Function Reduces Airway Bacteria and Inflammation in People with Cystic Fibrosis and Chronic Lung Infections. *Am. J. Respir. Crit. Care Med.* 195, 1617–1628. doi:10.1164/rccm.201609-1954oc

Hunter, M. J., Treharne, K. J., Winter, A. K., Cassidy, D. M., Land, S., and Mehta, A. (2010). Expression of Wild-type CFTR Suppresses NF-kappaB-Driven Inflammatory Signalling. *PLoS One* 5, e11598. doi:10.1371/journal.pone.0011598

Janeckova, L., Pospichalova, V., Fafilek, B., Vojtechova, M., Tureckova, J., Dobes, J., et al. (2015). HIC1 Tumor Suppressor Loss Potentiates TLR2/NF-Kb Signaling and Promotes Tissue Damage-Associated Tumorigenesis. *Mol. Cancer Res.* 13, 1139–1148. doi:10.1158/1541-7786.mcr-15-0033

Jarosz-Griffiths, H. H., Scambler, T., Wong, C. H., Lara-Reyna, S., Holbrook, J., Martinon, F., et al. (2020). Different CFTR Modulator Combinations Downregulate Inflammation Differently in Cystic Fibrosis. *Elife* 9, e54556. doi:10.7554/elife.54556

Kmit, A., Marson, F. A. L., Pereira, S. V.-N., Vinagre, A. M., Leite, G. S., Servidoni, M. F., et al. (2019). Extent of rescue of F508del-CFTR function by VX-809 and VX-770 in human nasal epithelial cells correlates with SNP rs7512462 in SLC26A9 gene in F508del/F508del Cystic Fibrosis patients. *Biochim. Biophys. Acta (Bba) - Mol. Basis Dis.* 1865, 1323–1331. doi:10.1016/j.bbadis.2019.01.029

Lara-Reyna, S., Holbrook, J., Jarosz-Griffiths, H. H., Peckham, D., and McDermott, M. F. (2020). Dysregulated Signalling Pathways in Innate Immune Cells with Cystic Fibrosis Mutations. *Cell. Mol. Life Sci.* 77, 4485–4503. In press. doi:10.1007/s00018-020-03540-9

Laselva, O., Stone, T. A., Bear, C. E., and Deber, C. M. (2020). Anti-Infectives Restore ORKAMBI Rescue of F508del-CFTR Function in Human Bronchial Epithelial Cells Infected with Clinical Strains of *P. aeruginosa*. *Biomolecules* 10, 334. doi:10.3390/biom10020334

Nagy, B., Jr., Bene, Z., Fejes, Z., Heltshe, S. L., Reid, D., Ronan, N. J., et al. (2019). Human Epididymis Protein 4 (HE4) Levels Inversely Correlate with Lung Function Improvement (Delta FEV1) in Cystic Fibrosis Patients Receiving Ivacaftor Treatment. *J. Cystic Fibrosis* 18, 271–277. doi:10.1016/j.jcf.2018.08.013

Nagy, B., Jr., Nagy, B., Fila, L., Clarke, L. A., Gönczy, F., Bede, O., et al. (2016). Human Epididymis Protein 4: A Novel Serum Inflammatory Biomarker in Cystic Fibrosis. *Chest* 150, 661–672. doi:10.1016/j.chest.2016.04.006

Nixon, L. S., Yung, B., Bell, S. C., Stuart Elborn, J., and Shale, D. J. (1998). Circulating Immunoreactive Interleukin-6 in Cystic Fibrosis. *Am. J. Respir. Crit. Care Med.* 157, 1764–1769. doi:10.1164/ajrccm.157.6.9704086

Pranke, I. M., Hatton, A., Simonin, J., Jais, J. P., Le Pimpec-Barthes, F., Carsin, A., et al. (2017). Correction of CFTR Function in Nasal Epithelial Cells from Cystic Fibrosis Patients Predicts Improvement of Respiratory Function by CFTR Modulators. *Sci. Rep.* 7, 7375. doi:10.1038/s41598-017-07504-1

Ramsey, B. W., Davies, J., McElvaney, N. G., Tullis, E., Bell, S. C., Dřevínek, P., et al. (2011). A CFTR Potentiator in Patients with Cystic Fibrosis and theG551DMutation. *N. Engl. J. Med.* 365, 1663–1672. doi:10.1056/nejmoa1105185

Rowe, S. M., Heltshe, S. L., Gonska, T., Donaldson, S. H., Borowitz, D., Gelfond, D., et al. (2014). GOAL Investigators of the Cystic Fibrosis Foundation Therapeutics Development Network. (Clinical Mechanism of the Cystic Fibrosis Transmembrane Conductance Regulator Potentiator Ivacaftor in G551D-Mediated Cystic Fibrosis. *Am. J. Respir. Crit. Care Med.* 190, 175–184. doi:10.1164/rccm.201404-0703oc

Rowe, S. M., Miller, S., and Sorscher, E. J. (2005). Cystic Fibrosis. *N. Engl. J. Med.* 352, 1992–2001. doi:10.1056/nejmra043184

Ruffin, M., Roussel, L., Maillé, É., Rousseau, S., and Brochiero, E. (2018). Vx-809/Vx-770 Treatment Reduces Inflammatory Response to *Pseudomonas aeruginosa* in Primary Differentiated Cystic Fibrosis Bronchial Epithelial Cells. *Am. J. Physiol.-Lung Cell Mol. Physiol.* 314, L635–L641. doi:10.1152/ajplung.00198.2017

Sallenave, J. M., Shulmann, J., Crossley, J., Jordana, M., and Gauldie, J. (1994). Regulation of Secretory Leukocyte Proteinase Inhibitor (SLPI) and Elastase-specific Inhibitor (ESI/elafin) in Human Airway Epithelial Cells by Cytokines and Neutrophilic Enzymes. *Am. J. Respir. Cell Mol. Biol.* 11, 733–741. doi:10.1165/ajrcmb.11.6.7946401

Small, D. M., Doherty, D. F., Dougan, C. M., Weldon, S., and Taggart, C. C. (2017). The Role of Whey Acidic Protein Four-Disulfide-Core Proteins in Respiratory Health and Disease. *Biol. Chem.* 398, 425–440. doi:10.1515/hsz-2016-0262

Stanton, B. A., Coutermarsh, B., Barnaby, R., and Hogan, D. (2015). *Pseudomonas aeruginosa* Reduces VX-809 Stimulated F508del-CFTR Chloride Secretion by Airway Epithelial Cells. *PLoS One* 10, e0127742. doi:10.1371/journal.pone.0127742

Taylor-Cousar, J. L., Munck, A., McKone, E. F., van der Ent, C. K., Moeller, A., Simard, C., et al. (2017). Tezacaftor-Ivacaftor in Patients with Cystic Fibrosis Homozygous for Phe508del. *N. Engl. J. Med.* 377, 2013–2023. doi:10.1056/nejmoa1709846

Vij, N., Mazur, S., and Zeitlin, P. L. (2009). CFTR Is a Negative Regulator of NFkappaB Mediated Innate Immune Response. *PLoS One* 4, e4664. doi:10.1371/journal.pone.0004664

Wainwright, C. E., Elborn, J. S., Ramsey, B. W., Marigowda, G., Huang, X., Cipolli, M., et al. (2015). TRAFFIC Study Group; TRANSPORT Study GroupLumacaftor-Ivacaftor in Patients with Cystic Fibrosis Homozygous for Phe508del CFTR. *N. Engl. J. Med.* 373, 220–231. doi:10.1056/nejmoa1409547

Wang, H., Cebotaru, L., Lee, H. W., Yang, Q., Pollard, B. S., Pollard, H. B., et al. (2016). CFTR Controls the Activity of NF-Kb by Enhancing the Degradation of TRADD. *Cell. Physiol. Biochem.* 40, 1063–1078. doi:10.1159/000453162

11

CFTR Modulator Therapy Enhances Peripheral Blood Monocyte Contributions to Immune Responses in People with Cystic Fibrosis

Katherine B. Hisert[1,2], Timothy P. Birkland[2], Kelly Q. Schoenfelt[3], Matthew E. Long[2], Brenda Grogan[4], Suzanne Carter[4], W. Conrad Liles[2], Edward F. McKone[4], Lev Becker[3†], Anne M. Manicone[2†] and Sina A. Gharib[2†]*

[1] Division of Pulmonary, Critical Care, and Sleep Medicine, Department of Medicine, National Jewish Health, Denver, CO, United States, [2] Center for Lung Biology, Division of Pulmonary, Critical Care, and Sleep Medicine, Department of Medicine, University of Washington, Seattle, WA, United States, [3] Ben May Department for Cancer Research, University of Chicago, Chicago, IL, United States, [4] Department of Medicine, St. Vincent's University Hospital, Dublin, Ireland

***Correspondence:**
Katherine B. Hisert
hisertk@njhealth.org

[†]These authors have contributed equally to this work

Background: CFTR modulators decrease some etiologies of CF airway inflammation; however, data indicate that non-resolving airway infection and inflammation persist in individuals with CF and chronic bacterial infections. Thus, identification of therapies that diminish airway inflammation without allowing unrestrained bacterial growth remains a critical research goal. Novel strategies for combatting deleterious airway inflammation in the CFTR modulator era require better understanding of cellular contributions to chronic CF airway disease, and how inflammatory cells change after initiation of CFTR modulator therapy. Peripheral blood monocytes, which traffic to the CF airway, can develop both pro-inflammatory and inflammation-resolving phenotypes, represent intriguing cellular targets for focused therapies. This therapeutic approach, however, requires a more detailed knowledge of CF monocyte cellular programming and phenotypes.

Material and Methods: In order to characterize the inflammatory phenotype of CF monocytes, and how these cells change after initiation of CFTR modulator therapy, we studied adults (n=10) with CF, chronic airway infections, and the *CFTR-R117H* mutations before and 7 days after initiation of ivacaftor. Transcriptomes of freshly isolated blood monocytes were interrogated by RNA-sequencing (RNA-seq) followed by pathway-based analyses. Plasma concentrations of cytokines and chemokines were evaluated by multiplex ELISA.

Results: RNAseq identified approximately 50 monocyte genes for which basal expression was significantly changed in all 10 subjects after 7 days of ivacaftor. Of these, the majority were increased in expression post ivacaftor, including many genes traditionally associated with enhanced inflammation and immune responses. Pathway analyses confirmed that transcriptional programs were overwhelmingly up-regulated in monocytes after 7 days of ivacaftor, including biological modules associated with immunity, cell cycle, oxidative phosphorylation, and the unfolded protein response.

Ivacaftor increased plasma concentrations of CXCL2, a neutrophil chemokine secreted by monocytes and macrophages, and CCL2, a monocyte chemokine.

Conclusions: Our results demonstrate that ivacaftor causes acute changes in blood monocyte transcriptional profiles and plasma chemokines, and suggest that increased monocyte inflammatory signals and changes in myeloid cell trafficking may contribute to changes in airway inflammation in people taking CFTR modulators. To our knowledge, this is the first report investigating the transcriptomic response of circulating blood monocytes in CF subjects treated with a CFTR modulator.

Keywords: cystic fibrosis, monocytes, ivacaftor, inflammation, transcriptome

INTRODUCTION

Although chronic airways diseases are a leading cause of morbidity and mortality in the world, therapies that dampen airway inflammation without inducing broad systemic immunosuppression or exerting clinically significant side effects are still lacking for many of these diseases. In cystic fibrosis (CF), a disease of chronic airway infection and chronic inflammation, NSAIDs and steroids improve lung function and decrease symptoms (Cheng et al., 2013); however, adverse side effects limit their use (Mogayzel, Jr. et al., 2013; Cantin et al., 2015). Development of effective inflammation-dampening therapies for people with CF is further complicated by the fact that some components of the immune response are necessary for controlling airway infections, while others may only enhance tissue damage (Doring et al., 2014; Konstan et al., 2014), thus therapies ideally would target specific arms of the inflammatory response (Lin and Kazmierczak, 2017). However, the contributions of specific cell populations and inflammatory mediators to persistence of non-resolving inflammation remain incompletely understood in CF, like in many chronic lung diseases, largely due to a lack of animal models that recapitulate chronic airway inflammation,

Research in human subjects indicates that peripheral blood monocytes participate in inflammation in many chronic diseases by trafficking to sites of damage and infection where they develop into macrophages (Byers and Holtzman, 2011; Dewhurst et al., 2017; Kapellos et al., 2019). Because macrophages are long-lived cells that can initiate, modulate, and resolve inflammation (Johnston et al., 2012; Wynn and Vannella, 2016; Puttur et al., 2019), pharmacologic manipulation of monocytes and macrophages to shift these cells toward disease-resolving phenotypes has been suggested as a therapeutic strategy in a number of chronic inflammatory diseases including pulmonary fibrosis and cardiac disease (Cheng and Rong, 2018; Liu et al., 2019). In CF, neutrophils and macrophages make up the majority of cells in the airway lumen (Henig et al., 2001; Hisert et al., 2019), and many CF airway macrophages appear to be derived from blood monocytes (Wright et al., 2009; Garratt et al., 2012), thus medications that target peripheral blood monocytes could be an effective anti-inflammatory strategy in CF as well.

Cell-focused therapies require knowledge of both how the cell population participates in disease pathophysiology as well as how the disease state alters immune cell programming and function. Multiple studies have shown that CF monocytes and macrophages mount aberrant immune responses (Bruscia and Bonfield, 2016). Monocytes from people with CF demonstrate tolerance to LPS (del Fresno et al., 2008) and impaired adhesion and trafficking (Sorio et al., 2015) compared to cells from healthy donors, and some monocyte defects seen in CF can be induced in healthy donor cells by exposure to CF plasma (Zhang et al., 2019). In contrast, studies using cells from CFTR deficient animals (that have not developed chronic lung infections and inflammation) and human CF macrophages cultured *in vitro* indicate that lack of CFTR activity causes macrophages to mount overly robust inflammatory responses (Bruscia et al., 2009; Bonfield et al., 2012). Thus, monocytes that migrate to the CF airway and become macrophages could have abnormal immune responses for at least two distinct, but intertwined, reasons: a direct effect of lack of sufficient CFTR activity, and the secondary effects of exposure to plasma containing products of non-resolving infection and chronic disease. Understanding the *in vivo* phenotypes of CF monocytes and macrophages is an essential first step towards devising methods to manipulate the cellular programs of these key regulatory cells to help dampen or resolve inflammation.

As we enter the era of highly effective CFTR modulator therapy, drivers of inflammation in CF will change for patients receiving these medications. Inflammation resulting directly from a lack of CFTR activity will become less pronounced, if not eliminated, by CFTR modulators (Sorio et al., 2015; Barnaby et al., 2018; Rosen et al., 2018). However, studies indicate that chronic airway infection and inflammation, particularly in subjects with advanced lung disease, will continue to cause symptoms and progressive lung damage (Rowe et al., 2014; Heltshe et al., 2015; Hisert et al., 2017). Based on prior studies of CF monocytes and macrophages exposed *ex vivo* to CFTR modulators, restoration of CFTR activity could either enhance or dampen cellular responses (Barnaby et al., 2018; Zhang et al., 2018). In order to characterize the inflammatory phenotype of *in vivo* blood monocytes in people with CF, and to determine how cellular phenotypes change in response to CFTR modulator therapy, we have used unbiased "omics" methods to identify changes in freshly isolated peripheral blood monocytes following initiation of ivacaftor in people with susceptible *CFTR* mutations. Previously we identified changes in the monocyte plasma-membrane associated proteome in subjects with *CFTR-G551D* mutations that suggested that CFTR modulator therapy causes a decrease in monocyte IFNγ responses (Hisert et al., 2016), a hypothesis that we have since confirmed (Hisert et al., 2020). Here we describe how restoration of CFTR activity by ivacaftor acutely changes the peripheral blood monocyte transcriptome and plasma chemokines in a cohort of adults with CF and the *CFTR* mutation *R117H.*

MATERIALS AND METHODS

Patient Cohort and Study Design

Ten patients (6 male and 4 female) from the Adult Cystic Fibrosis Clinic at St. Vincent's University Hospital in Dublin, Ireland were enrolled in this study. Human subject recruitment was approved by the Research Ethics Committee, and all study participants provided written informed consent. Subjects were excluded if they had participated in the VX-770 (ivacaftor) Extended Access Program or had used ivacaftor within 6 months prior to the day 0 visit, or if they had required treatment with oral, inhaled or IV antibiotics within the 2 weeks prior to the day 0 visit. Subjects were,thus, considered at their clinical baseline at the day 0 visit. Subjects were allowed to continue other standard CF therapies. The day 0 visit for all subjects occurred during a two-week period in fall of 2016, and all subjects were started on ivacaftor treatment during the same week. At each study visit subjects provided sputum and blood specimens and underwent assessment of vital signs, weight, sweat chloride, and spirometry. Ivacaftor treatment was initiated following the day 0 study visit. Subjects were grouped into cohorts of three to four subjects on each day, and specimens from each cohort were processed in parallel on the same day.

Processing of Blood and Isolation of Monocytes

Whole blood was collected into K-EDTA tubes from subjects before (day 0) and seven days after initiation of ivacaftor (**Figure 1**). One aliquot was used for separation of plasma from blood cells. The remaining blood was separated using

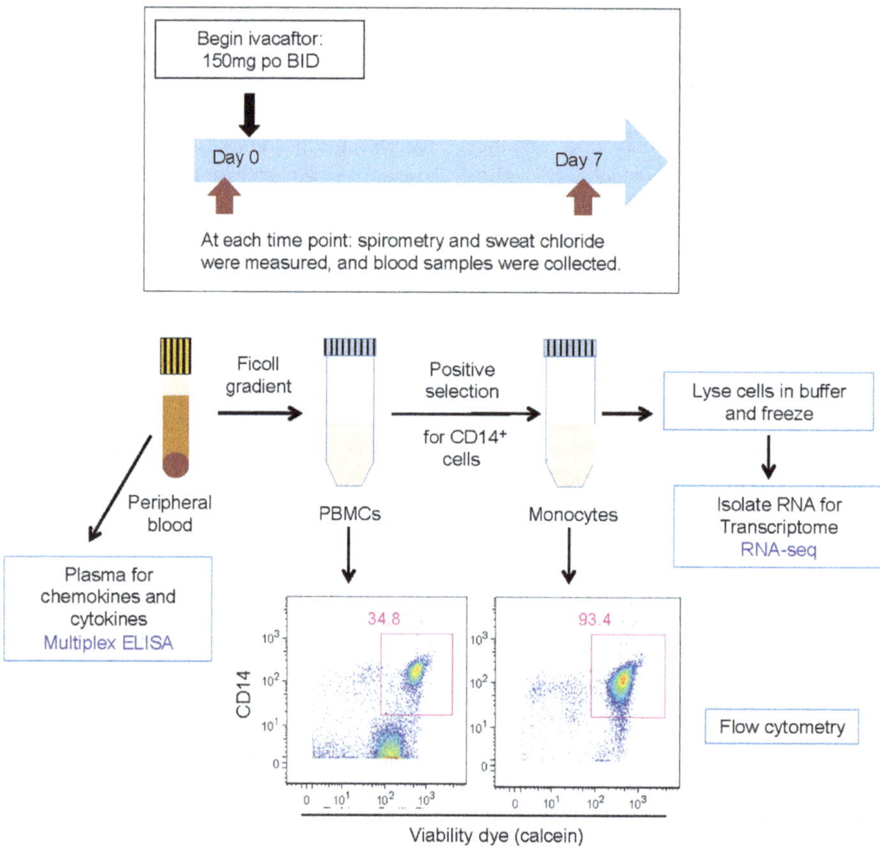

FIGURE 1 | Schematic for study design. Subjects were evaluated on day 0 and day 7. Subjects initiated ivacaftor treatment following the day 0 study visit. During each visit, subjects underwent a physical examination and sweat chloride evaluation, performed spirometry, and had blood drawn. Blood samples, acquired into K-EDTA tubes, were brought to the laboratory on ice. One tube of blood was centrifuged to obtain plasma. The remaining blood was processed to isolate PBMCs and then monocytes. Aliquots of PBMCs and monocytes were removed for quantification of cells and flow cytometric analysis to determine abundance of leukocyte sub-populations and purity of isolated monocytes. Cells recovered from CD14 positive selection column were immediately lysed in RLT buffer (Qiagen) and frozen.

gradient centrifugation over Ficoll-paque (GE) to separate peripheral blood mononuclear cells (PBMCs) from neutrophils and red blood cells. The Miltenyi Monocyte Isolation Kit (a positive selection kit that uses magnetic beads conjugated to CD14 antibody) was used to isolate monocytes. Numbers of PBMCs and cells recovered by magnetic beads were quantified using a Neubauer hemocytometer, and values pre- and post-ivacaftor were compared using Student's *t*-test. Efficacy of monocyte isolation was confirmed by assessing proportions of T cells (CD3+ cells), B-cells (CD19+ cells), and monocytes (CD14+ cells) before and after cells were subjected to the Monocyte Isolation Kit.

Quantification of Plasma Cytokines and Chemokines

Plasma cytokines and chemokines were measured using a custom Human Magnetic Luminex pre-mixed multiplex assay (R&D Systems). Plasma levels of IL-8, IL-10, G-CSF, IL-6, CCL4, CXCL1, Il-1β, TNF, GM-CSF, and IL-12p40 were all below the limit of detection in most subjects at both time points. For those analytes that were detected, statistically significant differences between day 0 and day 7 were determined by using the Wilcoxon Signed-Rank test.

RNA Isolation

RNA was isolated from human peripheral blood monocytes using Qiagen's RNeasy Plus kit per manufacturer's instructions. Briefly, freshly isolate monocytes were homogenized in Qiagen RLT buffer, snap frozen, and stored at –80°C until further processing *via* the Qiagen kit. Purified RNA from samples was eluted in Ambion's RNA storage solution and stored frozen at –80°C until use.

RNA Sequencing

RNA-seq was performed by the Genomics Core at the Benaroya Research Institute. For each sample, libraries were constructed from 100 ng of total RNA using the TruSeq Stranded mRNA kit (Illumina) with poly(A) selection. Libraries were pooled and quantified using a Qubit® Fluorometer (Life Technologies). Single-read sequencing of pooled libraries was carried out on a HiSeq2500 sequencer (Illumina) with 58-base reads, using HiSeq v4 Cluster and SBS kits (Illumina) with a target depth of 10 million reads per sample. Basecalls were processed to FASTQs on BaseSpace (Illumina), and a base call quality trimming step was applied to remove low-confidence base calls from the ends of reads. The FASTQs were aligned to the human reference genome (GRCh38.91), using STAR v.2.4.2a (Dobin et al., 2013) and gene counts were generated using htseq-count (Anders et al., 2015). QC and metrics analysis were performed using the Picard family of tools (v1.134) (https://broadinstitute.github.io/picard/). All RNA-seq data meeting MINSEQE (Minimum Information About a Next-generation Sequencing Experiment) have been deposited at Gene Expression Omnibus repository (https://www.ncbi.nlm.nih.gov/geo/, GSE148076).

RNA-Sequencing Data Analysis

To explore the overall changes in monocyte transcriptome in response to ivacaftor, we applied multidimensional scaling using Principal Components Analysis (PCA) to the entire RNA-seq profiles. Since each subject was assessed twice (day 0, day 7), we used a multilevel decomposition for repeated measures as implemented by the "mixOmics" package in R statistical environment (Rohart et al., 2017).

Differentially expressed genes between day 0 (untreated baseline) and day 7 (after ivacaftor therapy) were identified using paired statistical analysis for each subject (pre vs. post treatment) with "DESeq2" package in R (Love et al., 2014). Adjustment for multiple hypothesis testing was implemented using Benjamini-Hochberg's false discovery rate (FDR) analysis, with an FDR < 0.05 designating significant differential gene expression. Two-dimensional hierarchical clustering of $\log_2$ [Day 7/Day 0] gene expression ratios was performed using a Euclidian distance metric.

Gene product interaction network analysis was applied to the differentially expressed genes (FDR < 0.05) based on experimentally verified relationships derived from Ingenuity (Calvano et al., 2005) and STRING (v.11, https://string-db.org/) (Szklarczyk et al., 2019).

Pathway enrichment was performed using the Gene Set Enrichment Analysis (GSEA) program (Subramanian et al., 2005), where all unique transcripts were rank-ordered based on their DESeq2 statistic and over 7,000 gene sets derived from canonical pathways (Hallmark, KEGG, Reactome, Biocarta) and Gene Ontology (GO) annotations were assessed. An FDR < 0.05 was used to identify significant enrichment based on 1000 random gene set permutations. Enrichment Map (Isserlin et al., 2014), an application within the Cytoscape software platform (Cline et al., 2007), was used to create a network-based visualization of the GSEA results. To simplify the pathway enrichment network, only the most significantly enriched gene sets (FDR=0) were used as nodes. Edges were drawn between gene sets if at least 50% of their gene members overlapped. The emerging topology of the network allowed identification of aggregates of highly connected nodes that defined distinct biological modules. To compare our study with the GOAL cohort, we performed Gene Ontology enrichment analysis on differentially up and down-regulated genes between the subset of subjects that had clinical response to one month of ivacaftor therapy ("responders") vs. those that did not ("non-responders") using Webgestalt program (Liao et al., 2019). An enrichment FDR < 0.05 was used to designate significantly enriched processes.

RESULTS

Cohort Characteristics

All subjects were heterozygous for the *R117H-CFTR* gene allele (5T Poly T tract), and seven subjects' second mutation was *ΔF508;* none of the subjects had 2 ivacaftor-sensitive CFTR mutations (**Table 1**). Subjects were all adults with an age range of 25 – 52 years old (median, 40.5 years), baseline sweat ranged from 61 to 98 mM (median 79 mM), and body mass index (BMI) ranged from 18.5 to 32.5 (median 25.1). The cohort subjects demonstrated a wide range of baseline forced expiratory volume in one second (FEV_1), from 35% to 109% (median, 72%); 3 subjects had a baseline FEV_1 > 75% predicted, 5 subjects had a baseline FEV_1 of 60% to 75% predicted, and 2 subjects had a

TABLE 1 | Subject Demographics.

Non-R117H CFTR mutation	**7: ΔF508** **2: M156R** **1: 2622+1G→A**
Age	40.5 years (25 – 52)
Gender	6 male; 4 female
BMI	25.1 (18.5 – 32.5)
Baseline sweat chloride (mM)	79 (61 – 98)
Baseline FEV_1, % predicted	72% (35 – 109%)
Clinical laboratory sputum culture data	• 5 recent +*S. aureus* (± *Haemophilus*, *Pseudomonas* or *Acinetobacter* species) • 2 recent + *P. aeruginosa* • 3 prior + *P. aeruginosa* • 1 with no recent sputum production

Data presented as median (ranges) unless stated otherwise.

baseline FEV_1 < 50% predicted. None of the subjects had CF-related diabetes (CFRD); seven of the subjects were pancreatic sufficient, and three subjects were being evaluated for pancreatic insufficiency, but had recent normal fecal elastase values. Five subject had recent clinical sputum cultures positive for *Staphylococcus aureus* (± *Haemophilus, Pseudomonas* or *Acinetobacter* species), two subjects had recent *Pseudomonas aeruginosa* positive sputum cultures, three subjects had a history of *P. aeruginosa* positive sputum cultures, and one subject had not recently produced sputum. All subjects experienced a pronounced decrease in sweat chloride, and the cohort also experienced a statistically significant increase in FEV_1, within 48 h of ivacaftor treatment, and both changes were maintained at day 7 (Hisert et al., 2020).

Ivacaftor-Induced Changes in Plasma Chemokines Suggest Inflammatory Pathways Altered by CFTR Restoration Differ From Pathways Involved in CF Pulmonary Exacerbations

For this study, we chose to evaluate specimens at day 7 after subjects started ivacaftor because we hoped to identify changes that may be direct consequences of CFTR restoration by ivacaftor, rather than secondary effects of improved mucociliary clearance in the lung and decreased airway inflammation and bacterial burden. In our prior studies of subjects with *CFTR-G551D* mutations starting ivacaftor, GSEA analysis determined that proteomic changes that were significant at day 7 could be detected at day 2; however, most were not significant at day 2 (Hisert et al., 2016). Thus, although sweat chloride is changed by day 2 of treatment (Hisert et al., 2017), we deemed this timepoint likely too early to identify significant changes in plasma proteins and monocyte transcriptomes.

Identification of biomarkers that reflect systemic changes in inflammation in people with CF has been an area of intense interest, especially changes that predict CF pulmonary exacerbations and response to antibiotic therapy. Serum CRP level, calprotectin concentrations, and white blood cell counts decline following antibiotic treatment of exacerbations, and changes in some of these markers may predict response to therapy (Horsley et al., 2013; Sagel et al., 2015; Waters et al., 2015). We predicted that plasma biomarkers associated with decreases in bacterial burden in the airway would not be changed during the first week of ivacaftor therapy. In our prior cohort of subjects with *CFTR-G551D* mutations who started ivacaftor, we did not detect changes in plasma CRP levels or in numbers of PBMCs or monocytes, T cells or B cells in blood following 7 days of ivacaftor treatment (Hisert et al., 2016), consistent with our hypothesis that ivacaftor-induced changes in the airways during the first week of treatment likely had not yet translated to secondary effects in the systemic circulation. In the current cohort, we likewise observed that one week of ivacaftor treatment did not lead to detectable differences in numbers PBMCs and cells subsets (**Figure 2A**).

We then investigated whether ivacaftor changed levels of other plasma biomarkers that have been associated with inflammation in CF. Calprotectin, or S100A8/9, decreases in both sputum and serum following treatment of CF pulmonary exacerbations with antibiotics (Gray et al., 2010). In our study, we did not detect differences in levels of plasma S100A9 following initiation of ivacaftor (**Figure 2B**). We also found no changes in levels of plasma IL-1Ra (**Figure 2C**), a suppressor of inflammation that decreases in CF plasma during treatment of pulmonary exacerbations with intravenous antibiotics, and remains at lower levels during clinical stability as compared to during the exacerbation state (Sagel et al., 2015). CD163, a monocyte and macrophage surface protein that is shed when cells become activated (Davis and Zarev, 2005; Moller, 2012), has also been associated with CF disease state. Expression of CD163 mRNA is elevated in monocytes isolated from people with CF compared to cells from healthy controls, and was identified as part of a peripheral blood monocyte gene expression signature associated with successful treatment of CF pulmonary exacerbations (Saavedra et al., 2008; Nick et al., 2013). However in our study, there were no detectable changes in plasma levels of soluble CD163 (sCD163) at day 7 after initiation of ivacaftor (**Figure 2D**).

Although ivacaftor treatment did not change plasma levels of biomarkers associated with treatment of CF pulmonary exacerbations, we detected statistically significant increased plasma concentrations of two myeloid chemokines that are likely relevant to CF disease. CCL2 and CXCL2 were both increased at day 7 as compared to both pre-ivacaftor levels (**Figures 2E, F**). CCL2, also known as monocyte chemoattractant protein 1, or MCP-1, is elevated in both sputum and plasma of people with CF as compared to healthy controls (Brennan et al., 2009; Rao et al., 2009). CXCL2, also known as macrophage inflammatory protein-2, or MIP-2, is a key chemokine for activation and recruitment of neutrophils to sites of inflammation, and is produced by monocytes, macrophages, epithelial cells, and other cells in response to injury (Huang et al., 2001; De Filippo et al., 2013). Free DNA content in human CF sputum correlates with both airway levels of CXCL2 and airflow obstruction, with increased airway free DNA and CXCL2 associating with lower FEV_1, and similar findings were demonstrated in a CF mouse model (Marcos et al., 2015).

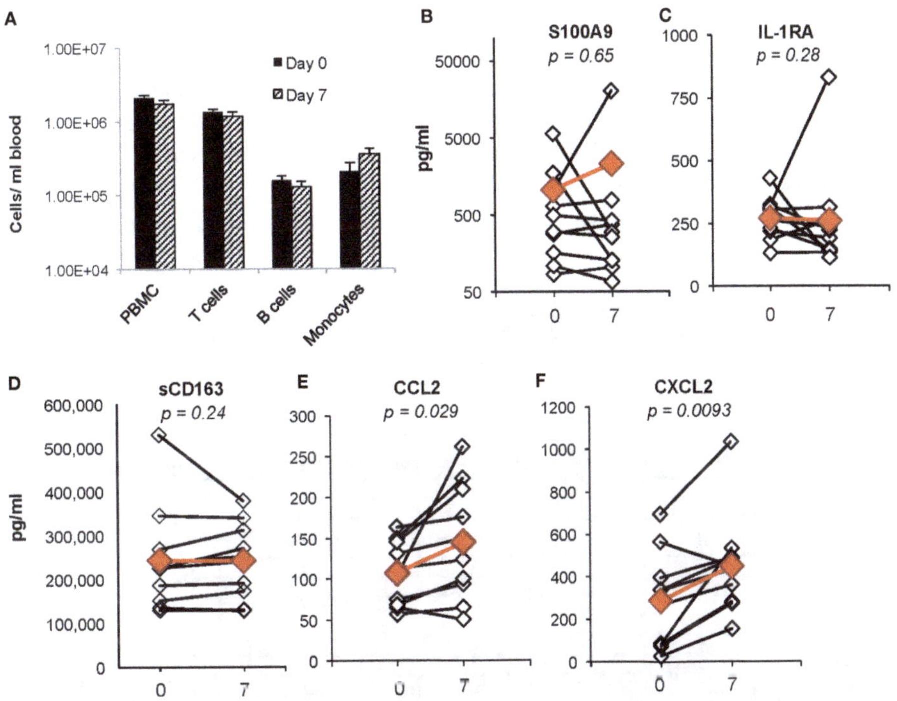

FIGURE 2 | Changes in blood cells, proposed CF biomarkers, and chemokines following 1 week of ivacaftor therapy. **(A)** Total numbers of PBMCs/ml blood as determined by (i) quantitation of PBMCs using a hemocytometer and (ii) flow cytometric analysis of PBMCs (pre-selection for CD14+ cells) using antibodies for CD3 (T cells), CD19 (B cells), and CD14 (monocytes). **(B–F)** Plasma cytokine concentrations were determined in sample obtained before (day 0) and after (day 7) initiation of ivacaftor treatment using multiplex ELISA. Students' *t*-test was used to compare data in panel **(A)**. Open simples with black lines are individual subjects. Red symbols indicate the mean value. Wilcoxon signed-rank test used to generate p-values for comparison of day 0 vs day 7 in **(B–F)**.

Transcriptomic Analyses Reveal That Ivacaftor Treatment Activates Monocytes and Up-Regulates Inflammatory Pathways

Although there have been several published reports on gene expression profiling of PBMCs or whole blood from people with CF, we sought specifically to characterize the monocyte transcriptome, and determine how restoration of CFTR activity by initiation of ivacaftor acutely changes monocyte transcriptional signals. We thus performed RNA-seq on monocytes isolated from subjects before and 7 days after initiation of ivacaftor therapy. We initially performed exploratory analysis using Principal Components Analysis (PCA), a statistical method for reducing high dimensional data while retaining the drivers of expression variability, on the entire RNA-seq dataset. To capture the repeated measure structure of the study, we applied a multi-level implementation of PCA. We observed that most of the samples segregated based on pre- and post-ivacaftor time points (**Figure 3**), indicating that despite inter-individual variability, ivacaftor treatment led to global transcriptional changes in circulating monocytes.

Next, we applied a subject-specific (paired) gene-based statistical method and identified 49 differentially expressed genes after adjustment for multiple comparisons (FDR < 0.05) with significant differences between pre-ivacaftor and day 7 post

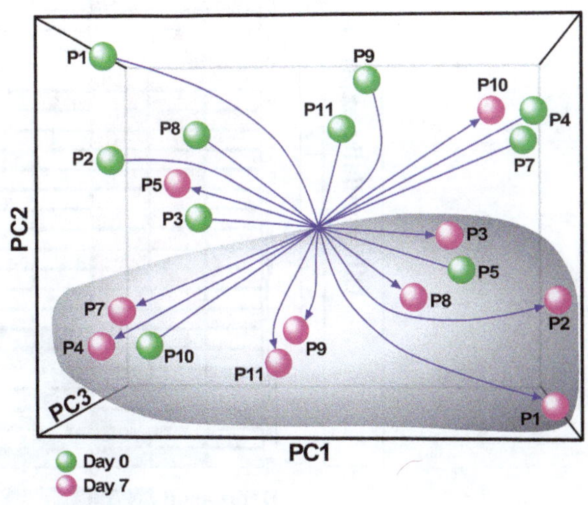

FIGURE 3 | Principal components analysis (PCA) of monocyte transcriptome data. Multivariate decomposition PCA was applied to gene expression data from individual subjects pre-ivacaftor (day 0, green spheres) and post ivacaftor (day 7, magenta spheres) and plotted using the first three principal components (PC). Arrows are used to highlight the pre and post states. Despite variability across subjects, there is separation between day 0 and day 7 indicating that ivacaftor elicits a global transcriptional signal in monocytes.

ivacaftor conditions (**Figure 4**, **Table S1**). Of these differentially expressed genes, 42 were up-regulated following ivacaftor treatment and 7 were down-regulated. The predominance of up-regulated genes was surprising because monocytes are key innate immune activators of inflammation, and ivacaftor has been shown to reduce markers of inflammation in people with CF (Hisert et al., 2017; Ronan et al., 2018), as well as cellular responses and markers of inflammation (Bratcher et al., 2016; Barnaby et al., 2018; Zhang et al., 2018). Also remarkable were the identities of the significantly up-regulated transcripts: many of these genes code for canonical pro-inflammatory factors, including cytokines (TNF, IL-1β) and chemokines (CCL4, CXCL2). To better elucidate the relationship among these differentially expressed genes, we performed gene product interaction network analysis. As depicted in **Figure 5** (with additional details in **Figure S1**), the resulting interactome

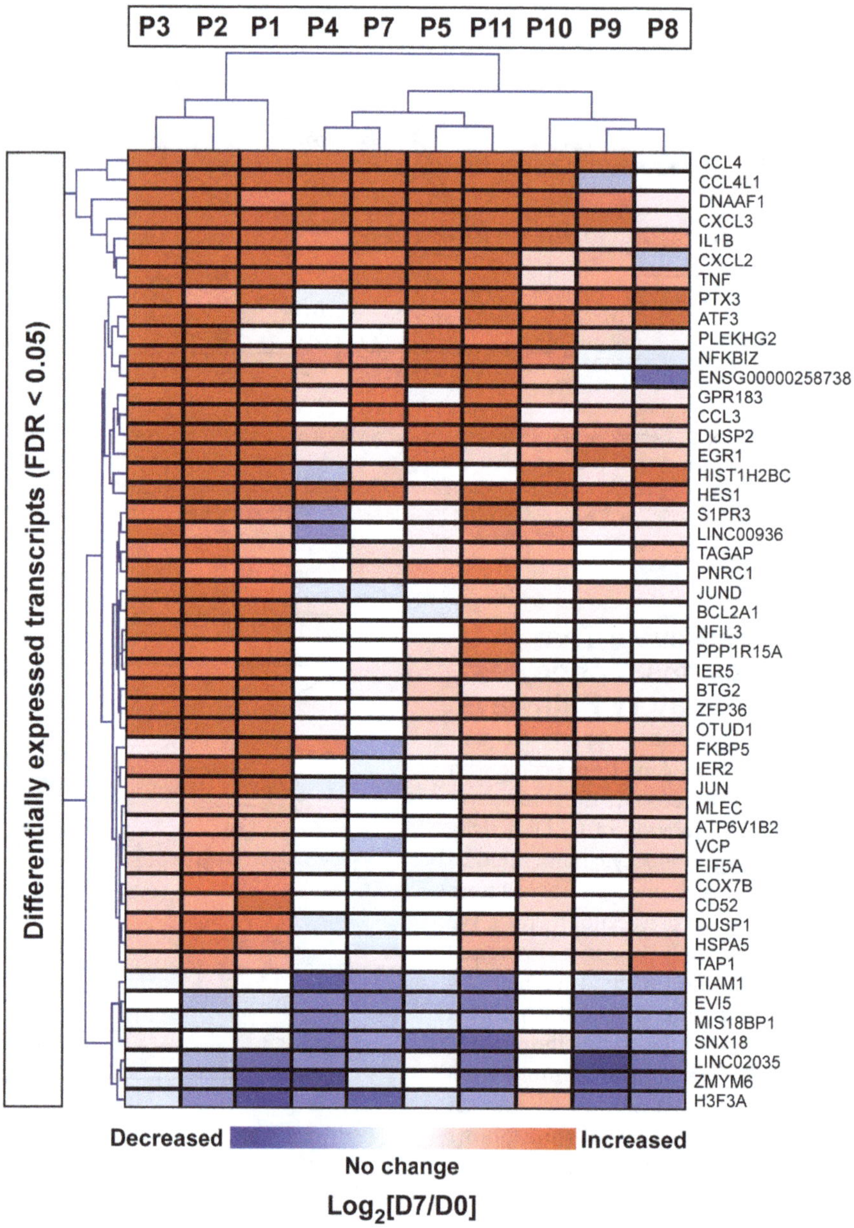

FIGURE 4 | Two-dimensional hierarchical cluster analysis of statistically significantly differentially expressed monocyte genes in response to ivacaftor. The Heatmap depicts differentially expressed genes with FDR < 0.05 in rows and subjects in columns. The relative expression of each gene on day 7 vs. day 0 is shown with red indicating that the gene was increased in expression at day 7 compared to day 0, and blue indicating decreased expression at day 7 compared to day 0. Complete list with details is provided in **Supplementary Table S1**.

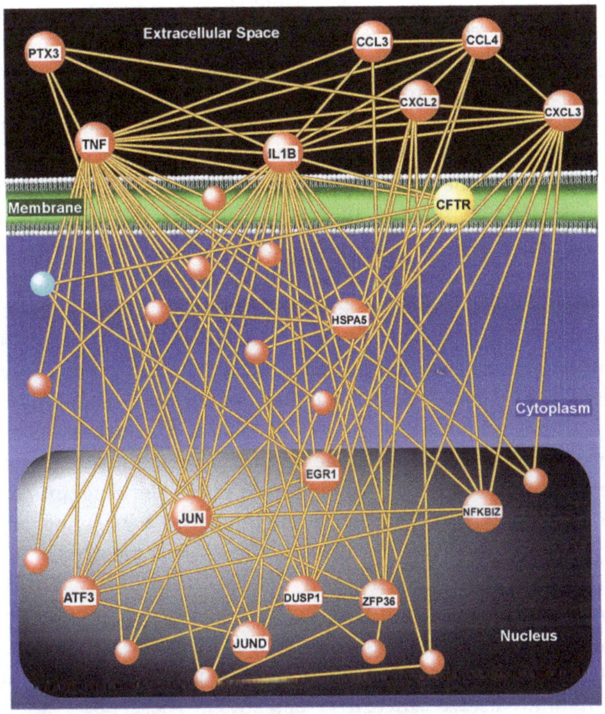

FIGURE 5 | Gene product interaction network analysis of differentially expressed monocyte genes after 1 week of ivacaftor therapy. This "interactome" was constructed based on known relationships among the differentially expressed genes. To depict interaction of these nodes with the target of ivacaftor, we also added CFTR as a seed to the network. Note the presence of several highly connected nodes (or hubs), such as IL1B, TNF, CXCL3, CXCL2, that are up-regulated (red spheres) and are key modulators of immune signaling.

revealed complex relationships among the network nodes and identified several densely connected "hubs," such as TNF, IL1B, CXCL3, CXCL2, ZPF36, JUN, and DUSP1 that may be important drivers of the monocyte transcriptional response to ivacaftor treatment. Furthermore, by adding CFTR as a network node, we observed that several of these hubs (e.g., TNF, IL1B, CXCL3, JUN) also interact with the functional target of ivacaftor.

Since genes do not exert their biological influence in isolation (Hartwell et al., 1999), we applied pathway enrichment analyses based on the entire transcriptome using GSEA to further understand the ivacaftor-induced changes in monocyte functional state. We found that treatment with ivacaftor induced an overwhelming up-regulation of cellular pathways in monocytes, with over 1,000 being enriched at FDR < 0.05 (**Table S2**). In contrast, only three gene sets were down-regulated at day 7 (FDR < 0.05) (**Table S3**). This finding indicates that restoring CF function elicits activation of a diverse set of transcriptional programs in peripheral blood monocytes. To visualize the enrichment pattern following ivacaftor therapy, we applied a network-based method to the most significantly up-regulated gene sets (N = 177, FDR = 0). The topology of the resultant network revealed several clusters of highly connected pathways defined as "modules" with distinct biological themes including "immunity and cell cycle," "oxidative phosphorylation," "transcription/translation," "unfolded protein response," and "Oxidative stress" (**Figure 6**). The largest module was comprised of many immune-related pathways including TNF signaling *via* NF-κB, IFNγ response, inflammatory response, IFNα response, cytokine signaling, and response to bacterium. Collectively, these results indicate that 7 days of ivacaftor treatment in CF subjects alters the functional state of their circulating monocytes by promoting the widespread activation of immuno-inflammatory programs.

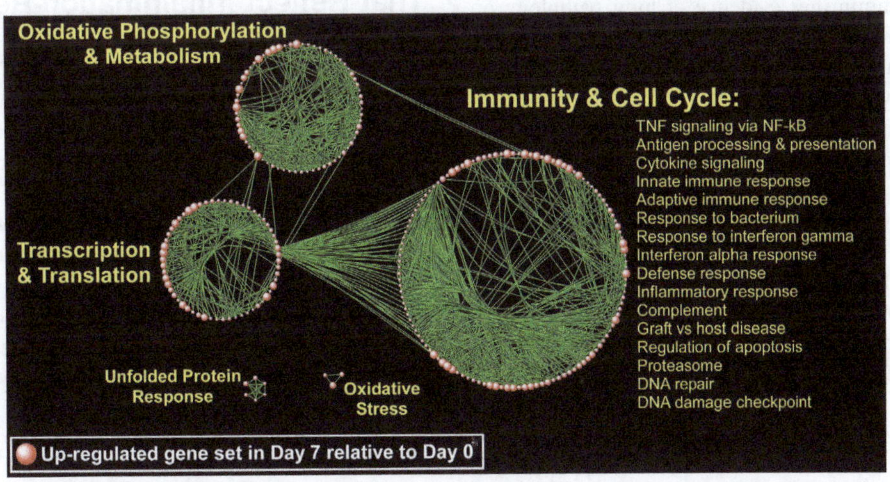

FIGURE 6 | A network-based illustration of enriched monocyte gene sets 1 week after ivacaftor treatment. Each sphere represents an up-regulated gene set and in order to simplify the figure, only the most significantly enriched gene sets are depicted (N = 177, FDR = 0). Connectivity between the pathways is based on 50% or greater overlap among their member genes. The topology of the network is characterized by the emergence of biological modules comprised of highly interconnected gene sets that possess similar functional themes; notable modules include "immunity and cell cycle," "oxidative phosphorylation and metabolism," "transcription and translation," "unfolded protein response," and "oxidative stress." representative processes mapping to the most prominent module, "Immunity and Cell Cycle" are shown, and a complete list of all enriched gene sets (FDR < 0.05) is included in **Supplementary Table S2**.

DISCUSSION

Despite many recent advances in CF care, therapies are still needed to dampen baseline chronic CF airway inflammation and to treat enhanced inflammation during CF pulmonary exacerbations. An improved understanding of the molecular and cellular basis of CF inflammation is critical to developing focused anti-inflammatory strategies that will not compromise host defenses or cause significant long-term side effects. Blood monocytes are intriguing therapeutic targets because they can traffic to the inflamed CF airway (Wright et al., 2009; Garratt et al., 2012; Hisert et al., 2019), and they mount aberrant responses in people with CF (del Fresno et al., 2008; Sorio et al., 2015; Hisert et al., 2016), which may contribute to CF disease pathology. Here we use transcriptomics to characterize the phenotypes of peripheral blood monocytes in people with CF before and 7 days after initiation of highly effective modulator therapy with ivacaftor. Our data demonstrate that ivacaftor therapy leads to an rapid change in the transcriptional programming of blood monocytes, predominantly activating genes and transcriptional modules in several broad functional categories, although may are associated with innate immunity and inflammation (**Figure 6**). Ivacaftor also rapidly increased plasma levels of CXCL2 and CCL2, chemokines that summon neutrophils and monocytes respectively. We did not, however, detect changes in several plasma biomarkers that had previously been associated with changes in CF airway inflammation following antibiotic treatment of pulmonary exacerbations.

Are CFTR Modulators Pro- or Anti-Inflammatory?

From a clinical perspective, ivacaftor appears to decrease inflammation in people with CF: ivacaftor acutely improves lung function and lessens symptoms (Ramsey et al., 2011; Rowe et al., 2014; Hisert et al., 2017), and over time reduces frequency of pulmonary exacerbations (Ramsey et al., 2011; Rowe et al., 2014), diminishes evidence of lung pathology on CT scans (Chassagnon et al., 2016; Hisert et al., 2017; Ronan et al., 2018), and may decrease inflammatory biomarkers in sputum and blood over time (Hisert et al., 2017; Ronan et al., 2018). In addition, macrophages lacking CFTR activity mount hyperinflammatory responses compared to cells with functional CFTR (Bruscia et al., 2009; Bruscia and Bonfield, 2016), and some of these overly exuberant responses are reversed by CFTR modulators (Barnaby et al., 2018; Zhang et al., 2018). It therefore may seem counter-intuitive for restoration of CFTR activity by ivacaftor to enhance multiple monocyte transcriptional pathways associated with inflammation, monocyte expression of canonical inflammatory cytokines, such as TNF and IL-αβ, and plasma levels of chemokines for neutrophils and monocytes. However, studies have shown that *ex vivo* peripheral blood immune cells isolated from people with CF actually exist in an immune-suppressed (or tolerant) state compared to cells from healthy donors. Blood monocytes from people with CF have decreased responses to LPS (del Fresno et al., 2008), and this is thought to be due to exposure of CF monocytes to low levels of LPS that translocate form the CF airway into the plasma (del Campo et al., 2011). Similarly, cells in CF whole blood exposed to multiple toll-like receptor (TLR) agonists mounted less robust inflammatory responses than cells from healthy donors (Kosamo et al., 2019), including decreased secretion of TNF and other NF-κB-induced cytokines.

Is this relative immune-suppressed state of CF peripheral immune cells adaptive and protective, or does it contribute to CF disease pathogenesis? CF subjects with the most robust TLR responses had the most preserved lung function (FEV_1) and the slowest decline in lung function over time (Kosamo et al., 2019); in other words, impaired peripheral immune cell inflammatory responses in CF are associated with worse lung disease. One explanation for these findings is that impaired immune cell responses in people with CF contribute to airway pathology, and stronger immune responses protect the lung, possibly by fighting bacterial pathogens. Another possibility is that more advanced lung disease results in a leakier barrier between the lungs and the bloodstream, thus exposing peripheral immune cells to higher doses of tolerizing antigens compared to people with less severe lung disease. In support for this second possibility, healthy donor PMBCs cultured in CF plasma experienced marked decreases in transcription compared to cells cultured in healthy donor plasma, and plasma from subjects with severe CF lung disease caused a greater suppression of transcription than plasma from subjects with mild disease (Ideozu et al., 2019). These observations suggest that the *in vivo* plasma milieu in CF can override the hyper-inflammatory influences of intrinsic CFTR dysfunction on innate immune cells' phenotypes (Murphy and Ribeiro, 2019), and that CFTR modulators therefore potentially exert both pro- and anti-inflammatory effects on immune cells in people with CF.

Biomarkers That Measure Changes in Inflammation Following Restoration of CFTR Activity May Differ From Biomarkers That Reflect Inflammation Related to Airway Infection

In our prior study of patients with *CFTR-G551D* mutations initiating ivacaftor, we detected no difference in plasma C-reactive protein (CRP) after 1 week of therapy (Hisert et al., 2016). We measured CRP because it is used broadly as a clinical marker of systemic inflammation, and has also been evaluated in a number of studies as a biomarker to detect onset of CF pulmonary exacerbation, efficacy of treatment of CF exacerbations, or severity of CF lung disease (with one parameter for disease severity being whether or not subjects have chronic *P. aeruginosa* infection) (Sharma et al., 2017; Loh et al., 2018; Sagel et al., 2019). In the current study, we evaluated other plasma mediators that have been proposed as biomarkers of inflammation in people with CF. However, many of the analytes tested were below the limit of detection in our assay. We were able to detect high levels of S100A9, IL-1Ra, CXCL2, CCL2, and sCD163 in subject's plasma pre-ivacaftor. Changes in plasma S100A9, IL-1Ra, and sCD163 have been observed in people with CF who are being treated with antibiotics for pulmonary exacerbations; however, as with CRP, we detected no change in these analytes after 7 days of ivacaftor.

These results could reflect that our small cohort was under-powered to detect changes. Alternately, it may be that inflammation caused by an exacerbation/bacteria may be a different phenomenon than inflammation resulting from insufficient CFTR activity. The CF community may need different biomarkers to assess efficacy of CFTR modulators than what are used for measuring onset of exacerbation or efficacy of antibiotics to treat exacerbations.

CXCL2 and CCL2 were both elevated in people with CF compared to healthy controls, and thus the increase in plasma levels of both of these myeloid chemokines after ivacaftor treatment was unexpected. These increases, though, are consistent with our transcriptomic data indicating activation of immuno-inflammatory programs and chemokines in circulating monocytes. Future longitudinal studies of plasma mediators will be important to understand whether there are immediate and delayed changes in plasma inflammatory mediators following restoration of CFTR, and the roles CXCL2 and CCL2 may play in modulating CF airway inflammation.

Comparisons With Prior CF Immune Cell Transcriptomics Studies

A number of previous studies have characterized the transcriptomes of CF immune cells, and a few have evaluated changes in gene expression following CFTR modulator therapy. To our knowledge, our study is the first report to focus specifically on the transcriptomes of CF monocytes. The most comparable previous study was performed by Sun et al., who characterized the transcriptome of PBMCs collected from subjects enrolled in the GOAL study, a multi-center, prospective characterization of ivacaftor-induced changes in people with *CFTR-G551D* mutations in the USA (Sun et al., 2019). They identified 239 differentially expressed genes (DEGs) when comparing PBMCs pre-ivacaftor and 1 month post-ivacaftor, using a false discovery rate < 0.1; the majority of these genes were decreased in expression after 1 month of ivacaftor treatment. There were no DEGs in common between the GOAL cohort data set, and our data from monocytes isolated pre- and post-ivacaftor. It should be noted that there were many differences between our study and that by Sun et al. In addition to differences in the cell types (PBMCs vs. monocytes) and time points analyzed (1 month vs. 1 week post-ivacaftor), Sun et al. applied a different statistical analysis to their data. We performed a paired analysis, in which all subjects that provided a pre-ivacaftor specimen also provided a post-ivacaftor specimen. Sun et al. included 56 subjects, of which 37 provided both pre- and post-ivacaftor samples, and 19 provided only one sample.

Additionally, the cohort used in the Sun et al. paper differed from our cohort in several important ways. Their cohort (a subset of the total GOAL cohort) (1) had a lower median age than our cohort, (2) was made up of people with *CFTR-G551D* mutations (whereas our cohort all had *CFTR-R117H* mutations), and (3) did not experience a statistically significant increase in FEV_1 by one month after ivacaftor treatment, when their post-ivacaftor samples were collected. In our cohort, we detected a statistically significant improvement in FEV_1 by 2 days post ivacaftor that was maintained at day 7, when our post-ivacaftor specimens were collected. The difference in clinical response to ivacaftor may be the key distinction between the two studies. Although the total cohort in the Sun et al. study did not demonstrate a statistically significant improvement in FEV_1 following ivacaftor treatment, a subset of subjects did experience a clinical response to ivacaftor. Sun et al. distinguished subjects as either "responders" or "non-responders" to ivacaftor based on FEV_1, body mass index (BMI), and Cystic Fibrosis Questionnaire-Revised (CFQR) respiratory scores (Sun et al., 2019). When we performed functional enrichment analysis on the DEGs with increased expression in the subset of subjects who were "responders" relative to "non-responders" in the Sun et al. cohort, we identified multiple pathways associated with immune function that were significantly up-regulated (**Table S4**). This result suggests that, consistent with our CF cohort findings, peripheral blood immune/inflammatory program activation following initiation of ivacaftor therapy is associated with significant clinical improvements in the GOAL study.

Kopp et al. also characterized immune cell transcriptomes in subjects starting CFTR modulator therapy, and performed both a paired comparison of subjects pre- and post-modulator, and also compared both datasets to transcriptomes from cells from non-CF control subject. Their study examined whole blood from a cohort of delta F508 homozygous subjects, starting lumacaftor/ivacaftor, and they examined a later time point (comparison of pre- and 6 months post-lumacaftor/ivacaftor) (Kopp et al., 2019). In addition to this difference in study design, the clinical response of subjects in this study to lumacaftor/ivacaftor was not as robust, based on change in FEV_1, as that seen in subjects from studies in which the subjects had ivacaftor-sensitive mutations. Overall, these authors found that blood cells from people with CF both before and after modulator therapy had higher expression of inflammation and apoptosis related genes than cells from healthy donors, and lumacaftor/ivacaftor modestly decreased expression of some inflammatory genes.

In both the studies by Kopp et al. and Sun et al., CFTR modulator treatment was associated with a general dampening of peripheral immune cell inflammatory phenotypes, whereas we found up-regulation of immune and inflammatory transcripts and pathways in blood monocytes one week after initiation of ivacaftor. This difference in trend could be due to the differences in cell populations studied or demographics of the study populations. The choice of time point for assessing changes post initiation of modulator therapy might also be the critical distinction between these studies, indicating that there may be phases of responses to CFTR modulators. CFTR modulators may initially enhance immune cells transcriptional pathways, and then later, when there are decreased airway bacteria and mucous plugging (Hisert et al., 2017), and different or less stimuli in the blood, peripheral blood cell phenotypes may reflect a less inflamed state. As with plasma biomarkers, there are likely both acute and direct effects, as well as the secondary and later effects, of CFTR modulators on immune cells and thus inflammation.

Interpretation of transcriptomics data, particularly when determining whether changes are pro- or anti-inflammatory, is also complicated by the fact that some genes with increased expression may be inhibitors of inflammatory pathways. In fact, several of the most significantly up-regulated genes following ivacaftor treatment in our study are known inhibitors of inflammation. OTUD1 (Ovarian Tumor Family Deubiquitinase 1, FDR = 3.74×10^{-13}) can inhibit nuclear translocation and transcriptional activity of the IFNγ-activated transcription factor IRF3 (Lu et al., 2018), and loss of function of OTUD1 is associated with auto-immune diseases mediated by interferons (Lu et al., 2018). DUSP2 (Dual Specificity Protein Phosphatase 2, FDR = 1.07×10^{-10}) belongs to a family of phosphatases that can de-phosphorylate STAT proteins (involved in interferon signaling, in addition to other intracellular signaling cascades), and ERK proteins (involved in toll-like receptor intracellular signaling (Lang et al., 2006; Lu et al., 2015). ATF3 (Activating Transcription Factor 3, FDR = 3.11×10^{-10}) binds CRE elements in DNA and represses transcription, and has been shown to negatively regulate pro-inflammatory cytokine expression in macrophages (Rosenberger et al., 2008; Labzin et al., 2015). We recently showed that monocytes from the same cohort described here exhibit a decrease in *ex vivo* responsiveness to IFNγ after subjects have received ivacaftor for 7 days (Hisert et al., 2020). An increased expression of genes that deactivate or dampen inflammatory signaling could partly explain why transcriptome data predicted that these monocytes have a more inflammatory phenotype while the same cells, when stimulated *ex vivo*, exhibited decreased IFNγ responses.

Study Limitations and Strengths

Our study has several limitations. First, our cohort was small, which may have limited our ability to detect important changes in monocyte activation states or plasma biomarkers. Second, we performed our analysis at a single time point after treatment, and thus our data capture an early snapshot of acute changes in monocytes after initiation of ivacaftor, which may not reflect chronic therapy. Most studies evaluating changes in cells and biomarkers following initiation of CFTR modulators have sampled subjects at only one time point, with few longitudinal studies (Rowe et al., 2014; Hisert et al., 2017; Ronan et al., 2018; Kopp et al., 2019; Sun et al., 2019; Harris et al., 2020); however, the synthesis of individual time points with the longitudinal studies suggest that there may be phases of changes in inflammation following restoration of CFTR activity with modulators. The changes reported here occurred within the first week of ivacaftor treatment, and thus reflect acute responses to ivacaftor, and may not reflect a longer term steady-state that incorporates both primary and secondary changes induced by ivacaftor. In future studies of subjects initiating highly active modulator therapy, analyses of changes in inflammatory endpoints at multiple time points should be performed. Third, we did not assess transcriptional profiles of monocytes from healthy control subjects in this study, and therefore we cannot draw conclusions about the relative inflammatory state of CF monocytes compared to those from healthy donors. However, building on the prior literature, we hypothesize that the overall increase in activation of transcriptional programs in CF monocytes post ivacaftor reflects a change from the tolerant state of monocytes pre-ivacaftor, and a return towards the activation state of healthy "wildtype" monocytes following restoration of CFTR activity. Finally, although we investigated an early timepoint to try to detect direct consequences of CFTR restoration by ivacaftor, our data cannot ultimately discriminate whether the changes in monocyte transcriptomes post-ivacaftor are due to direct effects of ivacaftor on monocyte CFTR activity, indirect effects of ivacaftor increasing CFTR activity on other cells in the body (such as airway epithelial cells), or off target effects of ivacaftor on monocytes. The literature suggests that some CF PBMC impairments are likely an indirect consequence of CFTR activity, resulting from exposure of the cells to an altered milieu of CF plasma (Zhang et al., 2019).

Nevertheless, our cohort's unique design provided several strengths. Our ability to compare cells from the same individuals pre- and post-ivacaftor minimized confounding and maximized statistical power, allowing for detection of statistically significant changes despite the small cohort size. The fact that all subjects were from one institution allowed for processing of specimens on site, and the application of multiple studies to the same specimens, resulting in a deeply phenotyped cohort. Third, we detected a clinically meaningful response to ivacaftor within 48 hours, which provides additional confidence that the changes in immune cells and mediators were related to restoration of CFTR activity and could contribute to changes in airway inflammation. Finally, our data here and in our previous publications describe changes in one immune cell population (monocytes) before and after CFTR modulator therapy, thus providing a detailed functional description of a target cell for potential therapeutic manipulation.

SUMMARY

Peripheral blood monocytes travel to sites of inflammation, including the CF airway, and are attractive therapeutic targets for dampening the deleterious inflammation in CF lungs. Leveraging an unbiased transcriptomics approach, we systematically characterized changes in the inflammatory phenotypes of these cells following restoration of CFTR activity with ivacaftor. Unexpectedly, our findings revealed that multiple transcriptional programs, including pathways associated with immunity and inflammation, are up-regulated in circulating CF monocytes after one week of ivacaftor treatment. Coincident with this early enhancement of monocyte immuno-inflammatory signals, we identified significant increases in plasma levels of the myeloid chemokines CCL2 and CXCL2 and an overall improvement in FEV_1. Collectively, our results demonstrate that ivacaftor causes acute alterations in the inflammatory state of blood monocytes in people with CF, which in turn, may modulate airway inflammation and influence lung function. Future studies are necessary to determine if this enhancement of monocyte transcriptional pathways associated with inflammation and immunity is a transient phenomenon, or reflects the new steady state of people with CF receiving highly effective CFTR modulator therapy.

ETHICS STATEMENT

The studies involving human participants were reviewed and approved by Research Ethics Committee at St. Vincent's Hospital, Dublin, Ireland. The patients/participants provided their written informed consent to participate in this study.

AUTHOR CONTRIBUTIONS

KH, LB, and EM conceived of the hypothesis and designed the study. KH, TB, KS, BG, SC, and EM acquired and processed specimens. KH, TB, ML, WL, EM, LB, AM, and SG analyzed the data. KH, WL, LB, AM, and SG prepared the manuscript.

(ISS-2016-105055) from Vertex Pharmaceuticals, Inc. Funding was also provided by a K08 award (1 K08 HL136786-01A1) and two R01 awards (R01 AI137111 and R01 HL152724) from the National Institutes of Health.

ACKNOWLEDGMENTS

We thank Vivian Gersuk (Benaroya Research Institute, Seattle, WA) for her help with RNA-sequencing. We thank Pradeep Singh (U of Washington) for inviting us to join the research team in Dublin. We thank Michael Welsh (U of Iowa), David Stoltz (U of Iowa), Jan Launspach (U of Iowa), Mavra Nasir (Dartmouth University), Anina Ratjen (U of Washington), Robert Gray (U of Edinburgh), and Gareth Hardisty (U of Edinburgh) for collegial interactions and strategic support during specimen collection and initial specimen processing in Dublin. We are also grateful to Drs. Kong Chen and Tao Sun for sharing GOAL cohort transcriptomics data.

REFERENCES

Anders, S., Pyl, P. T., and Huber, W. (2015). HTSeq–a Python framework to work with high-throughput sequencing data. *Bioinformatics* 31, 166–169. doi: 10.1093/bioinformatics/btu638

Barnaby, R., Koeppen, K., Nymon, A., Hampton, T. H., Berwin, B., Ashare, A., et al. (2018). Lumacaftor (VX-809) restores the ability of CF macrophages to phagocytose and kill Pseudomonas aeruginosa. *Am. J. Physiol. Lung Cell. Mol. Physiol.* 314, L432–L438. doi: 10.1152/ajplung.00461.2017

Bonfield, T. L., Hodges, C. A., Cotton, C. U., and Drumm, M. L. (2012). Absence of the cystic fibrosis transmembrane regulator (Cftr) from myeloid-derived cells slows resolution of inflammation and infection. *J. Leukocyte Biol.* 92, 1111–1122. doi: 10.1189/jlb.0412188

Bratcher, P. E., Rowe, S. M., Reeves, G., Roberts, T., Szul, T., Harris, W. T., et al. (2016). Alterations in blood leukocytes of G551D-bearing cystic fibrosis patients undergoing treatment with ivacaftor. *J. Cystic Fibrosis* 15, 67–73. doi: 10.1016/j.jcf.2015.02.010

Brennan, S., Sly, P. D., Gangell, C. L., Sturges, N., Winfield, K., Wikstrom, M., et al. (2009). Alveolar macrophages and CC chemokines are increased in children with cystic fibrosis. *Eur. Respiratory J.* 34, 655–661. doi: 10.1183/09031936.00178508

Bruscia, E. M., and Bonfield, T. L. (2016). Cystic fibrosis lung immunity: the role of the Macrophage. *J. Innate Immun.* 8, 550–563. doi: 10.1159/000446825

Bruscia, E. M., Zhang, P. X., Ferreira, E., Caputo, C., Emerson, J. W., Tuck, D., et al. (2009). Macrophages directly contribute to the exaggerated inflammatory response in cystic fibrosis transmembrane conductance regulator-/- mice. *Am. J. Respiratory Cell Mol. Biol.* 40, 295–304. doi: 10.1165/rcmb.2008-0170OC

Byers, D. E., and Holtzman, M. J. (2011). Alternatively activated macrophages and airway disease. *Chest* 140, 768–774. doi: 10.1378/chest.10-2132

Calvano, S. E., Xiao, W., Richards, D. R., Felciano, R. M., Baker, H. V., Cho, R. J., et al. (2005). Host Response to Injury Large Scale Collab. Res, a network-based analysis of systemic inflammation in humans. *Nature* 437, 1032–1037. doi: 10.1038/nature03985

Cantin, A. M., Hartl, D., Konstan, M. W., and Chmiel, J. F. (2015). Inflammation in cystic fibrosis lung disease: Pathogenesis and therapy. *J. Cystic Fibrosis* 14, 419–430. doi: 10.1016/j.jcf.2015.03.003

Chassagnon, G., Hubert, D., Fajac, I., Burgel, P. R., and Revel, M. P. (2016). and investigators, Long-term computed tomographic changes in cystic fibrosis patients treated with ivacaftor. *Eur. Respiratory J.* 48, 249–252. doi: 10.1183/13993003.01918-2015

Cheng, Y., and Rong, J. (2018). Macrophage polarization as a therapeutic target in Myocardial infarction. *Curr. Drug Targets* 19, 651–662. doi: 10.2174/1389450118666171031115025

Cheng, K., Ashby, D., and Smyth, R. L. (2013). Oral steroids for long-term use in cystic fibrosis. *Cochrane Database System. Rev.* 6, CD000407. doi: 10.1002/14651858.CD000407.pub3

Cline, M. S., Smoot, M., Cerami, E., Kuchinsky, A., Landys, N., Workman, C., et al. (2007). Integration of biological networks and gene expression data using Cytoscape. *Nat. Protoc.* 2, 2366–2382. doi: 10.1038/nprot.2007.324

Davis, B. H., and Zarev, P. V. (2005). Human monocyte CD163 expression inversely correlates with soluble CD163 plasma levels. Cytometry. Part B. *Clin. Cytometry* 63, 16–22. doi: 10.1002/cyto.b.20031

De Filippo, K., Dudeck, A., Hasenberg, M., Nye, E., van Rooijen, N., Hartmann, K., et al. (2013). Mast cell and macrophage chemokines CXCL1/CXCL2 control the early stage of neutrophil recruitment during tissue inflammation. *Blood* 121, 4930–4937. doi: 10.1182/blood-2013-02-486217

del Campo, R., Martinez, E., del Fresno, C., Alenda, R., Gomez-Pina, V., Fernandez-Ruiz, I., et al. (2011). Translocated LPS might cause endotoxin tolerance in circulating monocytes of cystic fibrosis patients. *PloS One* 6, e29577. doi: 10.1371/journal.pone.0029577

del Fresno, C., Gomez-Pina, V., Lores, V., Soares-Schanoski, A., Fernandez-Ruiz, I., Rojo, B., et al. (2008). Monocytes from cystic fibrosis patients are locked in an LPS tolerance state: down-regulation of TREM-1 as putative underlying mechanism. *PloS One* 3, e2667. doi: 10.1371/journal.pone.0002667

Dewhurst, J. A., Lea, S., Hardaker, E., Dungwa, J. V., Ravi, A. K., and Singh, D. (2017). Characterisation of lung macrophage subpopulations in COPD patients and controls. *Sci. Rep.* 7, 7143. doi: 10.1038/s41598-017-07101-2

Dobin, A., Davis, C. A., Schlesinger, F., Drenkow, J., Zaleski, C., Jha, S., et al. (2013). STAR: ultrafast universal RNA-seq aligner. *Bioinformatics* 29, 15–21. doi: 10.1093/bioinformatics/bts635

Doring, G., Bragonzi, A., Paroni, M., Akturk, F. F., Cigana, C., Schmidt, A., et al. (2014). BIIL 284 reduces neutrophil numbers but increases P. aeruginosa bacteremia and inflammation in mouse lungs. *J. Cystic Fibrosis* 13, 156–163. doi: 10.1016/j.jcf.2013.10.007

Garratt, L. W., Wright, A. K., Ranganathan, S. C., Grigg, J., Sly, P. D.A.C. behalf of (2012). Small macrophages are present in early childhood respiratory disease. *J. Cystic Fibrosis* 11, 201–208. doi: 10.1016/j.jcf.2011.11.008

Gray, R. D., Imrie, M., Boyd, A. C., Porteous, D., Innes, J. A., and Greening, A. P. (2010). Sputum and serum calprotectin are useful biomarkers during CF exacerbation. *J. Cystic Fibrosis* 9, 193–198. doi: 10.1016/j.jcf.2010.01.005

Harris, J. K., Wagner, B. D., Zemanick, E. T., Robertson, C. E., Stevens, M. J., Heltshe, S. L., et al. (2020). Changes in airway microbiome and inflammation with Ivacaftor treatment in patients with cystic fibrosis and the G551D mutation. *Ann. Am. Thoracic Soc.* 17, 212–220. doi: 10.1513/AnnalsATS.201907-493OC

Hartwell, L. H., Hopfield, J. J., Leibler, S., and Murray, A. W. (1999). From molecular to modular cell biology. *Nature* 402, C47–C52. doi: 10.1038/35011540

Heltshe, S. L., Mayer-Hamblett, N., Burns, J. L., Khan, U., Baines, A., Ramsey, B. W., et al. (2015). Network, Pseudomonas aeruginosa in cystic fibrosis patients with

G551D-CFTR treated with ivacaftor. *Clin. Infect. Dis.* 60, 703–712. doi: 10.1093/cid/ciu944

Henig, N. R., Tonelli, M. R., Pier, M. V., Burns, J. L., and Aitken, M. L. (2001). Sputum induction as a research tool for sampling the airways of subjects with cystic fibrosis. *Thorax* 56, 306–311. doi: 10.1136/thorax.56.4.306

Hisert, K. B., Schoenfelt, K. Q., Cooke, G., Grogan, B., Launspach, J. L., Gallagher, C. G., et al. (2016). Ivacaftor-induced proteomic changes suggest monocyte defects may contribute to the pathogenesis of Cystic Fibrosis. *Am. J. Respiratory Cell Mol. Biol.* 54, 594–597. doi: 10.1165/rcmb.2015-0322LE

Hisert, K. B., Heltshe, S. L., Pope, C., Jorth, P., Wu, X., Edwards, R. M., et al. (2017). Restoring CFTR function reduces airway bacteria and inflammation in people with Cystic fibrosis and chronic lung infections. *Am. J. Respiratory Crit. Care Med.* 195 (12), 1617–1628. doi: 10.1164/rccm.201609-1954OC

Hisert, K. B., Liles, W. C., and Manicone, A. M. (2019). A flow cytometric method for isolating Cystic fibrosis airway Macrophages from expectorated sputum. *Am. J. Respiratory Cell Mol. Biol.* 61, 42–50. doi: 10.1165/rcmb.2018-0236MA

Hisert, K. B., Birkland, T. P., Schoenfelt, K. Q., Long, M. E., Grogan, B., Carter, S., et al. (2020). Ivacaftor decreases monocyte sensitivity to interferon-gamma in people with cystic fibrosis. *ERJ Open Res.* 6 (2), 00318–2019. doi: 10.1183/23120541.00318-2019

Horsley, A. R., Davies, J. C., Gray, R. D., Macleod, K. A., Donovan, J., Aziz, Z. A., et al. (2013). Changes in physiological, functional and structural markers of cystic fibrosis lung disease with treatment of a pulmonary exacerbation. *Thorax* 68, 532–539. doi: 10.1136/thoraxjnl-2012-202538

Huang, X. R., Chun Hui, C. W., Chen, Y. X., Wong, B. C., Fung, P. C., Metz, C., et al. (2001). Macrophage migration inhibitory factor is an important mediator in the pathogenesis of gastric inflammation in rats. *Gastroenterology* 121, 619–630. doi: 10.1053/gast.2001.27205

Ideozu, J. E., Rangaraj, V., Abdala-Valencia, H., Zhang, X., Kandpal, M., Sala, M. A., et al. (2019). Transcriptional consequences of impaired immune cell responses induced by cystic fibrosis plasma characterized via dual RNA sequencing. *BMC Med. Genomics* 12, 66. doi: 10.1186/s12920-019-0529-0

Isserlin, R., Merico, D., Voisin, V., and Bader, G. D. (2014). Enrichment Map - a Cytoscape app to visualize and explore OMICs pathway enrichment results. *F1000Research* 3, 141. doi: 10.12688/f1000research.4536.1

Johnston, L. K., Rims, C. R., Gill, S. E., McGuire, J. K., and Manicone, A. M. (2012). Pulmonary macrophage subpopulations in the induction and resolution of acute lung injury. *Am. J. Respiratory Cell Mol. Biol.* 47, 417–426. doi: 10.1165/rcmb.2012-0090OC

Kapellos, T. S., Bonaguro, L., Gemund, I., Reusch, N., Saglam, A., Hinkley, E. R., et al. (2019). Human monocyte subsets and phenotypes in major chronic inflammatory diseases. *Front. Immunol.* 10, 2035. doi: 10.3389/fimmu.2019.02035

Konstan, M. W., Doring, G., Heltshe, S. L., Lands, L. C., Hilliard, K. A., Koker, P., et al. (2014). A randomized double blind, placebo controlled phase 2 trial of BIIL 284 BS (an LTB4 receptor antagonist) for the treatment of lung disease in children and adults with cystic fibrosis. *J. Cystic Fibrosis* 13, 148–155. doi: 10.1016/j.jcf.2013.12.009

Kopp, B. T., Fitch, J., Jaramillo, L., Shrestha, C. L., Robledo-Avila, F., Zhang, S., et al. (2019). Whole-blood transcriptomic responses to lumacaftor/ivacaftor therapy in cystic fibrosis. *J. Cystic Fibrosis.* 19 (2), 245–254. doi: 10.1016/j.jcf.2019.08.021

Kosamo, S., Hisert, K. B., Dmyterko, V., Nguyen, C., Black, R. A., Holden, T. D., et al. (2019). Strong toll-like receptor responses in cystic fibrosis patients are associated with higher lung function. *J. Cystic Fibrosis.* 19 (4), 608–613. doi: 10.1016/j.jcf.2019.11.009

Labzin, L. I., Schmidt, S. V., Masters, S. L., Beyer, M., Krebs, W., Klee, K., et al. (2015). ATF3 is a key regulator of Macrophage IFN responses. *J. Immunol.* 195, 4446–4455. doi: 10.4049/jimmunol.1500204

Lang, R., Hammer, M., and Mages, J. (2006). DUSP meet immunology: dual specificity MAPK phosphatases in control of the inflammatory response. *J. Immunol.* 177, 7497–7504. doi: 10.4049/jimmunol.177.11.7497

Liao, Y., Wang, J., Jaehnig, E. J., Shi, Z., and Zhang, B. (2019). WebGestalt 2019: gene set analysis toolkit with revamped UIs and APIs. *Nucleic Acids Res.* 47, W199–W205. doi: 10.1093/nar/gkz401

Lin, C. K., and Kazmierczak, B. I. (2017). Inflammation: a double-edged sword in the response to Pseudomonas aeruginosa infection. *J. Innate Immun.* 9, 250–261. doi: 10.1159/000455857

Liu, G., Zhai, H., Zhang, T., Li, S., Li, N., Chen, J., et al. (2019). New therapeutic strategies for IPF: based on the "phagocytosis-secretion-immunization" network regulation mechanism of pulmonary macrophages. *BioMed. Pharmacother.* 118, 109230. doi: 10.1016/j.biopha.2019.109230

Loh, G., Ryaboy, I., Skabelund, A., and French, A. (2018). Procalcitonin, erythrocyte sedimentation rate and C-reactive protein in acute pulmonary exacerbations of cystic fibrosis. *Clin. Respir. J.* 12, 1545–1549. doi: 10.1111/crj.12703

Love, M. I., Huber, W., and Anders, S. (2014). Moderated estimation of fold change and dispersion for RNA-seq data with DESeq2. *Genome Biol.* 15, 550. doi: 10.1186/s13059-014-0550-8

Lu, D., Liu, L., Ji, X., Gao, Y., Chen, X., Liu, Y., et al. (2015). The phosphatase DUSP2 controls the activity of the transcription activator STAT3 and regulates TH17 differentiation. *Nat. Immunol.* 16, 1263–1273. doi: 10.1038/ni.3278

Lu, D., Song, J., Sun, Y., Qi, F., Liu, L., Jin, Y., et al. (2018). Mutations of deubiquitinase OTUD1 are associated with autoimmune disorders. *J. Autoimmun* 94, 156–165. doi: 10.1016/j.jaut.2018.07.019

Marcos, V., Zhou-Suckow, Z., Onder Yildirim, A., Bohla, A., Hector, A., Vitkov, L., et al. (2015). Free DNA in cystic fibrosis airway fluids correlates with airflow obstruction. *Mediators Inflammation* 2015, 408935. doi: 10.1155/2015/408935

Mogayzel, P. J. Jr., Naureckas, E. T., Robinson, K. A., Mueller, G., Hadjiliadis, D., Hoag, J. B., et al. (2013). Cystic fibrosis pulmonary guidelines. Chronic medications for maintenance of lung health. *Am. J. Respiratory Crit. Care Med.* 187, 680–689. doi: 10.1164/rccm.201207-1160OE

Moller, H. J. (2012). Soluble CD163. *Scand. J. Clin. Lab. Invest.* 72, 1–13. doi: 10.3109/00365513.2011.626868

Murphy, S. V., and Ribeiro, C. M. P. (2019). Cystic fibrosis inflammation: hyperinflammatory, hypoinflammatory, or both? *Am. J. Respiratory Cell Mol. Biol.* 61, 273–274. doi: 10.1165/rcmb.2019-0107ED

Nick, J. A., Sanders, L. A., Ickes, B., Briones, N. J., Caceres, S. M., Malcolm, K. C., et al. (2013). Blood mRNA biomarkers for detection of treatment response in acute pulmonary exacerbations of cystic fibrosis. *Thorax* 68, 929–937. doi: 10.1136/thoraxjnl-2012-202278

Puttur, F., Gregory, L. G., and Lloyd, C. M. (2019). Airway macrophages as the guardians of tissue repair in the lung. *Immunol. Cell Biol.* 97, 246–257. doi: 10.1111/imcb.12235

Ramsey, B. W., Davies, J., McElvaney, N. G., Tullis, E., Bell, S. C., Drevinek, P., et al. (2011). A CFTR potentiator in patients with cystic fibrosis and the G551D mutation. *New Engl. J. Med.* 365, 1663–1672. doi: 10.1056/NEJMoa1105185

Rao, S., Wright, A. K., Montiero, W., Ziegler-Heitbrock, L., and Grigg, J. (2009). Monocyte chemoattractant chemokines in cystic fibrosis. *J. Cystic Fibrosis* 8, 97–103. doi: 10.1016/j.jcf.2008.09.009

Rohart, F., Gautier, B., Singh, A., and Le Cao, K. A. (2017). mixOmics: an R package for 'omics feature selection and multiple data integration. *PloS Comput. Biol.* 13, e1005752. doi: 10.1371/journal.pcbi.1005752

Ronan, N. J., Einarsson, G. G., Twomey, M., Mooney, D., Mullane, D., NiChroinin, M., et al. (2018). CORK Study in Cystic Fibrosis: sustained improvements in ultra-low-dose chest CT scores after CFTR modulation with Ivacaftor. *Chest* 153, 395–403. doi: 10.1016/j.chest.2017.10.005

Rosen, B. H., Evans, T. I. A., Moll, S. R., Gray, J. S., Liang, B., Sun, X., et al. (2018). Infection is not required for mucoinflammatory lung disease in CFTR-knockout ferrets. *Am. J. Respiratory Crit. Care Med.* 197, 1308–1318. doi: 10.1164/rccm.201708-1616OC

Rosenberger, C. M., Clark, A. E., Treuting, P. M., Johnson, C. D., and Aderem, A. (2008). ATF3 regulates MCMV infection in mice by modulating IFN-gamma expression in natural killer cells. *Proc. Natl. Acad. Sci. U. States America* 105, 2544–2549. doi: 10.1073/pnas.0712182105

Rowe, S. M., Heltshe, S. L., Gonska, T., Donaldson, S. H., Borowitz, D., Gelfond, D., et al. (2014). Network, clinical mechanism of the cystic fibrosis transmembrane conductance regulator potentiator ivacaftor in G551D-mediated cystic fibrosis. *Am. J. Respiratory Crit. Care Med.* 190, 175–184. doi: 10.1164/rccm.201404-0703OC

Saavedra, M. T., Hughes, G. J., Sanders, L. A., Carr, M., Rodman, D. M., Coldren, C. D., et al. (2008). Circulating RNA transcripts identify therapeutic response in cystic fibrosis lung disease. *Am. J. Respiratory Crit. Care Med.* 178, 929–938. doi: 10.1164/rccm.200803-387OC

Sagel, S. D., Thompson, V., Chmiel, J. F., Montgomery, G. S., Nasr, S. Z., Perkett, E., et al. (2015). Effect of treatment of cystic fibrosis pulmonary exacerbations on systemic inflammation. *Ann. Am. Thoracic Soc.* 12, 708–717. doi: 10.1513/AnnalsATS.201410-493OC

Sagel, S. D., Wagner, B. D., Ziady, A., Kelley, T., Clancy, J. P., Narvaez-Rivas, M., et al. (2019). Utilizing centralized biorepository samples for biomarkers of cystic fibrosis lung disease severity. *J. Cystic Fibrosis.* 19 (4), 632–640. doi: 10.1016/j.jcf.2019.12.007

Sharma, A., Kirkpatrick, G., Chen, V., Skolnik, K., Hollander, Z., Wilcox, P., et al. (2017). Clinical utility of C-reactive protein to predict treatment response during cystic fibrosis pulmonary exacerbations. *PloS One* 12, e0171229. doi: 10.1371/journal.pone.0171229

Sorio, C., Montresor, A., Bolomini-Vittori, M., Caldrer, S., Rossi, B., Dusi, S., et al. (2015). Mutations of Cystic Fibrosis Transmembrane Conductance Regulator (CFTR) gene cause a monocyte-selective adhesion deficiency. *Am. J. Respiratory Crit. Care Med.* 193 (10), 1123–1133. doi: 10.1164/rccm.201510-1922OC

Subramanian, A., Tamayo, P., Mootha, V. K., Mukherjee, S., Ebert, B. L., Gillette, M. A., et al. (2005). Gene set enrichment analysis: a knowledge-based approach for interpreting genome-wide expression profiles. *Proc. Natl. Acad. Sci. U. S. A.* 102, 15545–15550. doi: 10.1073/pnas.0506580102

Sun, T., Sun, Z., Jiang, Y., Ferguson, A. A., Pilewski, J. M., Kolls, J. K., et al. (2019). Transcriptomic responses to Ivacaftor and prediction of Ivacaftor clinical responsiveness. *Am. J. Respiratory Cell Mol. Biol.* 61, 643–652. doi: 10.1165/rcmb.2019-0032OC

Szklarczyk, D., Gable, A. L., Lyon, D., Junge, A., Wyder, S., Huerta-Cepas, J., et al. (2019). STRING v11: protein-protein association networks with increased coverage, supporting functional discovery in genome-wide experimental datasets. *Nucleic Acids Res.* 47, D607–D613. doi: 10.1093/nar/gky1131

Waters, V. J., Stanojevic, S., Sonneveld, N., Klingel, M., Grasemann, H., Yau, Y. C., et al. (2015). Factors associated with response to treatment of pulmonary exacerbations in cystic fibrosis patients. *J. Cystic Fibrosis* 14, 755–762. doi: 10.1016/j.jcf.2015.01.007

Wright, A. K., Rao, S., Range, S., Eder, C., Hofer, T. P., Frankenberger, M., et al. (2009). Pivotal advance: expansion of small sputum macrophages in CF: failure to express MARCO and mannose receptors. *J. Leukocyte Biol.* 86, 479–489. doi: 10.1189/jlb.1108699

Wynn, T. A., and Vannella, K. M. (2016). Macrophages in tissue repair, regeneration, and fibrosis. *Immunity* 44, 450–462. doi: 10.1016/j.immuni.2016.02.015

Zhang, S., Shrestha, C. L., and Kopp, B. T. (2018). Cystic fibrosis transmembrane conductance regulator (CFTR) modulators have differential effects on cystic fibrosis macrophage function. *Sci. Rep.* 8, 17066. doi: 10.1038/s41598-018-35151-7

Zhang, X., Pan, A., Jia, S., Ideozu, J. E., Woods, K., Murkowski, K., et al. (2019). Cystic fibrosis plasma blunts the immune response to bacterial infection. *Am. J. Respiratory Cell Mol. Biol.* 61, 301–311. doi: 10.1165/rcmb.2018-0114OC

12

Mitochondrial Stress Responses and "Mito-Inflammation" in Cystic Fibrosis

Simone Patergnani[1], *Veronica A.M. Vitto*[1], *Paolo Pinton*[1,2] *and Alessandro Rimessi*[1,2*]

[1] *Department of Medical Sciences and Laboratory for Technologies of Advanced Therapies (LTTA), University of Ferrara, Ferrara, Italy,* [2] *Center of Research for Innovative Therapies in Cystic Fibrosis, University of Ferrara, Ferrara, Italy*

Correspondence:
Alessandro Rimessi
alessandro.rimessi@unife.it

Cystic fibrosis (CF) is a genetic disease associated to mutations in the cystic fibrosis transmembrane conductance regulator gene, which results in the alteration of biological fluid and electrolyte homeostasis. The characteristic pathological manifestation is represented by exaggerated proinflammatory response in lung of CF patients, driven by recurrent infections and worsen by hypersecretion of proinflammatory mediators and progressive tissue destruction. Treating inflammation remains a priority in CF. However, current anti-inflammatory treatments, including non-steroidal agents, are poorly effective and present dramatic side effects in CF patients. Different studies suggest an intimate relationship between mitochondria and CF lung disease, supporting the hypothesis that a decline in mitochondrial function endorses the development of the hyperinflammatory phenotype observed in CF lung. This allowed the implementation of a new concept: the "mito-inflammation," a compartmentalization of inflammatory process, related to the role of mitochondria in engage and sustain the inflammatory responses, resulting a druggable target to counteract the amplification of inflammatory signals in CF. Here, we will offer an overview of the contribution of mitochondria in the pathogenesis of CF lung disease, delving into mitochondrial quality control responses, which concur significantly to exacerbation of CF lung inflammatory responses. Finally, we will discuss the new therapeutic avenues that aim to target the mito-inflammation, an alternative therapeutic advantage for mitochondrial quality control that improves CF patient's inflammatory state.

Keywords: mitochondria, inflammation, cystic fibrosis, mitochondrial stress response, lung

INTRODUCTION

Cystic fibrosis (CF) is a genetic and multi-organ disease, caused by mutations in the cystic fibrosis transmembrane conductance regulator (CFTR) gene, resulting in lacked or reduced expression and function of protein (Elborn, 2016). ΔF508 is the most common mutation that displays a frequency of ~66% worldwide, which determine the inadequate processing of protein with consequent trapping in the endoplasmic reticulum (ER) (Marson et al., 2016). CFTR protein functions as cyclic adenosine monophosphate-regulated chloride channel and regulator of epithelial transport proteins, including epithelial sodium channel (Csanady et al., 2019). Defective CFTR alters fluid and electrolyte homeostasis, resulting in abnormally viscous and sticky secretions that at pulmonary level facilitates the adhesion and proliferation of pathogens, especially by *Pseudomonas aeruginosa* (*P. aeruginosa*), triggering exaggerated pro-inflammatory responses characterized by elevated secretion of pro-inflammatory mediators (such as the interleukin (IL)-8, IL-1β, and IL-18) (Malhotra et al., 2019). The intrinsic defects associated with CFTR deficiency and the repeated pulmonary infections induce hyperinflammation, leading to reduced bacterial clearance capacity and tissue damage in airways, compromising the respiration (Rafeeq and Murad, 2017).

While the underlying mechanisms that promote CF lung disease progression are not fully delineated, more studies highlighted the connection between mitochondrial health and CF pathogenesis, shading light on this organelle's role in regulating host response and inflammation.

Mitochondria are central signaling hub that communicate with the cell to regulate several functions, such as metabolism, regulation of calcium (Ca^{2+}) homeostasis, inflammation, stress responses, and cell death. Differently from other organelles, mitochondria present two membranes constituted by low levels of sphingolipids and cholesterol with exclusively components, such as posphosphatidylglycerol and cardiolipin (CL). The outer mitochondrial membrane (OMM) fully surrounds the inner mitochondrial membrane, separating the intermembrane space (IMS) from the matrix (Mejia and Hatch, 2016). They create a dynamic tubular and organized network, where the shape is continuously controlled by opposing fission and fusion events. These dynamic events are relevant during cell cycle in mitochondrial movement and in the interaction with other intracellular organelles (Nunnari and Suomalainen, 2012).

The interorganelle communication plays a key role in the mitochondrial functions, in particular with ER. Approximately, 5–20% of mitochondria surface is juxtaposed to specialized ER regions, linked by specific physical tethers at distance of 10–30 nm distance. Functional ER-mitochondria tethering is due by inositol 1,4,5-trisphosphate (IP3) receptors (IP3Rs), glucose-regulated protein 75, and voltage-dependent anion channels (VDAC) to transfer Ca^{2+} from ER to mitochondria (Giorgi et al., 2018a). While among structural tethering: the ER-located mitofusin 2 (MFN2) that builds a bridge with a heterodimer complex with MFN1/2 on OMM, and the integral ER protein vesicle-associated membrane protein-associated protein B (VAPB), which interacts with protein tyrosine phosphatase-interacting protein-51 (PTPIP51) (Lee and Min, 2018). Disruption or remodeling of ER-mitochondria tethering lead to a mismatch between the two organelles, causing dysregulation of lipid trafficking, Ca^{2+} signaling, autophagosome formation and apoptosis progression (Rowland and Voeltz, 2012; Rimessi et al., 2020a).

The mitochondria's innermost compartment is the matrix, where resides the mitochondrial DNA (mtDNA) that contains genetic coding information for 13 proteins, core constituents of the mitochondrial respiratory complexes I-IV. The matrix is also site of replication and transcription of mtDNA, protein biosynthesis, and ATP synthesis. During this last process, electrons move along the respiratory complexes of the mitochondrial electron transport chain (mETC). This flow is coupled to the pumping of protons from matrix into IMS, creating an electromotive force used to produce ATP (Turrens, 2003). During this process, some electrons leak out of ETC, interact with oxygen to produce reactive oxygen species (ROS), in particular the superoxide anion (O_2^-). Complex-I (NADH dehydrogenase) and complex-III (CoQH2-cytochrome c reductase) result the primary sites where electron leak occurs and ROS are produced.

The mitochondrial membrane potential ($\Delta\psi$) is the driving force necessary for protein import *via* translocase of outer membrane/translocase of inner membrane complex and for mitochondrial Ca^{2+}-uptake into the matrix through the mitochondrial Ca^{2+} uniporter (MCU). The Ca^{2+}-released from ER, *via* IP3Rs, may enter into matrix through VDAC and MCU (Giorgi et al., 2018b). Mitochondrial Ca^{2+} may stimulate OXPHOS, but upon cell stress, excessive mitochondrial Ca^{2+} accumulation induces ROS production, autophagic flux reduction, and mitochondrial permeability transition pore (mPTP) opening, which lead to an irreversible collapse of $\Delta\psi$, swelling of mitochondria, and release of pro-apoptotic factors, such as cytochrome c (Pedriali et al., 2017).

In this review, we highlight the role of mitochondria in the pathogenesis of CF lung disease. In particular, we will discuss of role of mitochondrial quality control responses, which are modulated by defective CFTR and persistent infections, contributing significantly to CF lung hyperinflammation. The complete understanding of these alterations, their molecular mechanisms, and the importance of each compensatory pathways engaged will help us to find new CF therapy strategies.

MITOCHONDRIAL DYSFUNCTION IN CYSTIC FIBROSIS

Endogenous and/or environmental stresses may perturb the mitochondrial homeostasis and interfere with the steady-state activity of mitochondrial functions, promoting a state of mitochondrial stress characterized by the inability to maintain basal $\Delta\psi$ and mitochondrial ROS production, with repercussions on mitochondrial protein import, mitochondrial Ca^{2+} signaling, and oxidation state. All this could harm airway epithelial and immune cells, contributing to the development and exacerbation of CF lung disease. Studies revealed that the mitochondrial impairments in the CF lung and the mitochondrial quality control responses are associated with CFTR deficiency and inflammatory environment.

MITOCHONDRIAL DEFECTS ASSOCIATED TO CFTR DEFICIENCY

The first evidence of mitochondrial defects related to CFTR deficiency was obtained in the 80s, showing that the oxygen consumption rate of isolated mitochondria from CF patients was affected due to complex-I and Na^+/K^+ ATPase alterations (Feigal and Shapiro, 1979; Shapiro et al., 1979). Consistently, the gene MT-ND4 and CISD1, fundamentals for a proper functioning of mETC, resulted downregulated in CF patient-derived tracheal cells (Valdivieso et al., 2007). Indeed, case reports of CF patients reported impairments in cytochrome c oxidase and in 6-phosphate dehydrogenase (Congdon et al., 1981; Battino et al., 1986). Oxygen consumption, complex-I activity, $\Delta\psi$, and OXPHOS were also found dysregulated in CFTR-silencing intestinal epithelial and in F508del-CFTR airway cells (Kleme et al., 2018). However, treatment with "CFTR correctors," including VX809 and 4,6,4'-trimethylangelicin, improved all the mitochondrial parameters, indicating that the CFTR rescue is linked to recovery of mitochondrial function (Atlante et al., 2016).

Other mitochondrial defects, such as the mitochondrial protein pattern, the intracellular pH and mitochondrial Ca^{2+} signaling have been described in CF to be sufficient to promote ROS production and membrane lipid peroxidation (Turrens et al., 1982; Picci et al., 1991; de Meer et al., 1995; Rimessi et al., 2015). Mitochondrial alteration due to oxidative stress has been also reported in CFTR-knockout mice, where oxidative mtDNA damage and reduced aconitase activity were described (Velsor et al., 2006). Also the ROS detoxification capacity in CF appears compromised. Low levels of mitochondrial reduced glutathione (mtGSH) and defects in GSH transport have been found in CF patient-derived airway cells and in CFTR-knockout, resulting in an altered extracellular ratio between reduced and oxidized GSH (Gao et al., 1999; Velsor et al., 2006; Kelly-Aubert et al., 2011). Accordingly, functional CFTR reintroduction restored mtGSH levels, attenuating the $\Delta\psi$ depolarization and IL-8 secretion[28].

MITOCHONDRIAL DEFECTS ASSOCIATED TO PERSISTENCE INFECTIONS

Pathogens affect mitochondria, generally causing $\Delta\psi$ loss and mitochondrial fragmentation, to influence their intracellular survival or to evade host immunity (Tiku et al., 2020). Airway epithelial and immune cells are sensitive to pathogen upon infection, activating mitochondrial stress responses to preserve the mitochondrial homeostasis.

In uninfected conditions, no significant differences in mitochondrial physiology and in inflammatory profile were detected between human CF and non-CF airway cells. Both mitochondrial networks exhibited the classical ultrastructure integrity of a well-defined OMM with numerous pleomorphic cristae. Contrariwise, the exposition to *P. aeruginosa* strains displayed extensive mitochondrial swollen and fragmentation with derangement of cristae in CF airway epithelial cells, resulting in $\Delta\psi$ loss, excessive O_2^- production, and nod-like receptor 3 (NLRP3) inflammasome activation (Rimessi et al., 2015). Using non-motile *P. aeruginosa* mutants, it has been demonstrated that the mitochondrial dysfunction in CF airway epithelial cells is triggered by the bacterial constituent flagellin through a Toll-like receptor 5 (TLR5)-dependent pathway (Rimessi et al., 2015). The recovery of mitochondrial integrity in CF airway epithelial cells during infection was obtained silencing or pharmacologically inhibiting MCU, with KB-R7943, indicating that mitochondrial Ca^{2+} signaling has a role in *P. aeruginosa*-dependent mitochondrial impairments in CF (Rimessi et al., 2015; Rimessi et al., 2020b).

These data show that a functional CFTR channel may prevent the *P. aeruginosa*-triggered mitochondrial dysfunction, regulating the susceptibility of airway cells to infection and thus conditioning the degree of innate immune response.

MITOCHONDRIAL STRESS RESPONSES IN CYSTIC FIBROSIS

It is not yet entirely clear whether mitochondrial dysfunction is a trigger for, a consequence, or both for CF lung disease. In resting conditions, compensatory mitochondrial stress responses are transiently activated to restore the mitochondrial homeostasis, while during the recurrent infections, the chronic mitochondrial stress condition leads to amplification and persistence of these responses. Functional fusion complementation, mitophagy, mitochondrial unfolded protein response (UPR^{mt}), and apoptosis are recruited to recover and preserve the mitochondrial homeostasis to regulate metabolism and innate immune response and cell viability. In CF, the persistent infections and the defects associated with CFTR deficiency alter the mitochondria quality control machinery, acquiring potential relevance to the disease state.

FUNCTIONAL FUSION COMPLEMENTATION AND MITOPHAGY

The morphology of mitochondrial network is regulated by fusion/fission events and mitophagy to sustain an adequate supply of healthy mitochondria. Mitochondrial fusion compensation optimize the functional efficiency of organelle under stressful conditions, allowing the exchange of materials among partially damaged mitochondria (Campello and Scorrano, 2010). The MFN1/2 are pivotal mediators of this process (Song et al., 2009). A sustained stress condition favors the segregation of damaged/depolarized parts of mitochondria in autophagosomes that then will be eliminated through lysosomal degradation by mitophagy. This catabolic process minimizes the quote of dysfunctional mitochondria, removing excess of ROS, oxidized mtDNA, and other mitochondrial dangerous factors relevant to disease state (Eisner et al., 2018) (**Figure 1**, mitophagy). Mitochondrial-targeted kinase PINK1 and E3 ubiquitin ligase Parkin have a central role for mitophagy. Parkin is recruited to OMM by perturbed mitochondrial import of PINK1 in stressed mitochondria, where catalyzes the ubiquitination of MFNs and other OMM proteins to sequester the organelle in autophagosome. At the same time, PINK1 contributes to strengthen the mitophagic response, phosphorylating

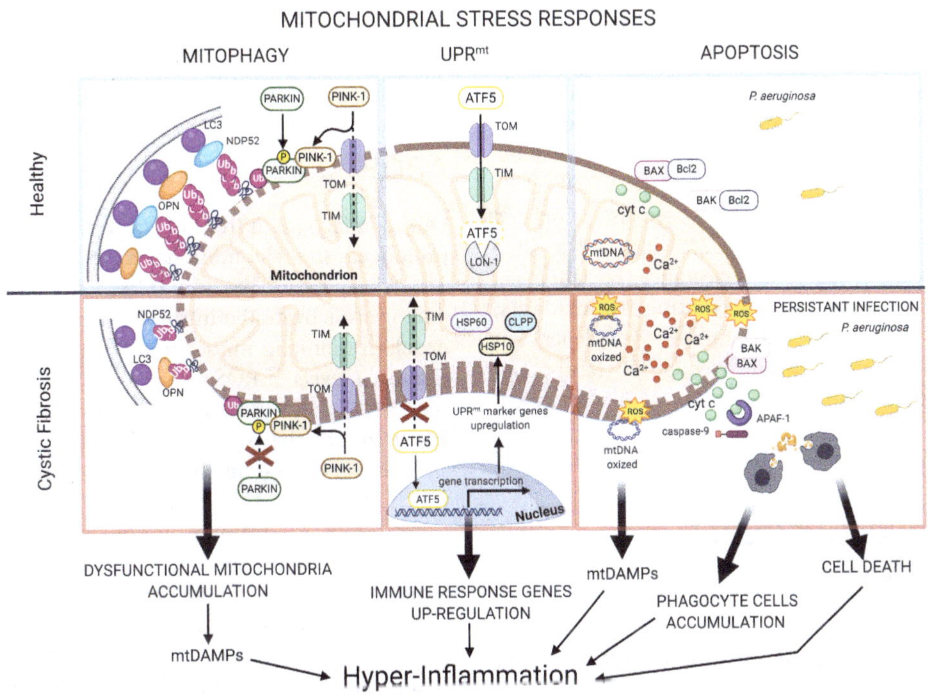

FIGURE 1 | Mitochondrial stress responses in cystic fibrosis. Schematic representation of mitochondrial stress response pathways in healthy and in CF. In healthy condition, compensatory mitochondrial stress responses are transiently triggered to restore the mitochondrial homeostasis during *P. aeruginosa* infection. Damaged mitochondrial portions are removed by mitophagy, where the PINK1-Parkin signaling pathway promotes ubiquitination of OMM proteins while the mitophagic receptors, optineurin (OPN) and NDP52, act as adaptors to recruit autophagosomal membranes to mitochondria, interacting with LC3. In CF, defective mitophagy leads to dysfunctional mitochondria accumulation with consequent release of mitochondrial DAMPs, which contribute to hyper-inflammatory responses in CF airway cells during the persistent *P. aeruginosa* infection. The mammalian UPR^{mt} is regulated by the transcription factors ATF5, which in healthy condition is imported into mitochondria to be degraded. In CF, the persistent mitochondrial stress in airway cells induces abnormal UPR^{mt} activation with consequent nuclear translocation of ATF5, which supports the regulation of innate immunity response during pathogen infection. At front of the mitochondrial Ca^{2+}-overload, a higher susceptibility to irreversible damages in response to pathogen infection occur in CF airway cells, contributing to promote organelle dysfunction and cell death. In CF, the exacerbation of inflammatory environment is due also by mtDAMPs release and by accumulation of phagocyte cells that intervene to scavenge the dying cells and pathogens. PTEN induced kinase 1 (PINK-1); Microtubule-associated proteins 1A/1B light chain 3B (LC3); Nuclear domain 10 protein 52 (NDP52); Optineurin (OPN); Translocase of the outer membrane (TOM); Translocase of the inner membrane (TIM); Activating Transcription Factor 5 (ATF5); Lon protease homolog 1 (LON-1); heat shock protein 60 (HSP60); heat shock protein 10 (HSP10); Caseinolytic Mitochondrial Matrix Peptidase Proteolytic Subunit (CLPP); mitochondrial deoxyribonucleic acid (mtDNA); cytochrome c (cyt c); B-cell lymphoma 2 protein (Bcl2); BCL2 Associated X protein (BAX); Bcl-2 homologous antagonist/killer protein (BAK); reactive oxygen species (ROS); calcium (Ca^{2+}); *Pseudomonas aeruginosa* (*P. aeruginosa*); apoptotic protease activating factor-1 (APAF-1). This figure has been created with "BioRender.com".

both parkin and ubiquitin and recruiting the mitophagic receptors NDP-52 and optineurin to mitochondria (Koyano et al., 2014; Lazarou et al., 2015).

In airway epithelial cells the accumulation of NDP-52, optineurin and autophagic form of microtubule-associated protein light chain 3 (LC3-II) to mitochondria triggers mitophagy during *P. aeruginosa* infection. The minor mitochondrial redistribution of LC3-II indicated a slower kinetic of mitochondrial sequestration into autophagosome in CF cells respect to non-CF cells, confirmed also by a reduced recruitment of Parkin to stressed mitochondria (Rimessi et al., 2020b) (**Figure 1**, mitophagy). Defective mitophagy led to excessive O_2^- production and NLRP3 inflammasome activation in CF airway cells during *P. aeruginosa* infection (Rimessi et al., 2015; Rimessi et al., 2020b). Similar defect was emerged also in xenophagy, the selective autophagic response involved to sequester into the cell invading pathogens (Gatica et al., 2018). The higher number of colony-forming unit/ml and of interactions between xenophagic receptors and invading *P. aeruginosa* in CF airway cells compared with non-CF cells, indicated a reduced bacterial clearance capacity of CF airway cells, resulting in further cell stress and pyroptosis induction (Rimessi et al., 2020b). The worsening of mitophagy and xenophagy in CF cells during infection is consequence of an enhanced ER-mitochondria juxtaposition, which making the organelles more prone to interorganelle Ca^{2+}-exchange. CF airway cells exposed to *P. aeruginosa* showed increased expression and interaction between ER protein VAPB and OMM protein PTPIP51, which induced tightening of tethers and concomitant impairment of selective autophagic responses (Rimessi et al., 2020b). Pharmacologically control of mitochondria Ca^{2+}-uptake, by MCU inhibitor KB-R7943, abrogated the inhibitory effects of VAPB and PTPIP51 on the selective autophagic responses, promoting cellular and mitochondrial resistance to infection and inflammatory reduction (Rimessi et al., 2020b). This highlights a central role for mitochondrial stress in progression of CF lung inflammatory state, with detrimental repercussions on the autophagic responses, which may further affect the expression, trafficking, and function of CFTR channel (Luciani et al., 2010; Villella et al., 2013). Defective macroautophagy in CF has been also associated to upregulation of transglutaminase (TG2), which led to ROS production and decrease of aggresomes clearance (Luciani et al., 2010). The rescue of autophagy, mediating antioxidants, cystamine (TG2 inhibitor), or modulators of Ca^{2+}-dependent signaling (KB-R7943), resulted in improved CFTR transport to PM, reduced oxidative stress, and cytokines release in CF airway cells[30,37].

MITOCHONDRIAL UNFOLDED PROTEIN RESPONSE

Perturbed mitochondrial protein import and the accumulation misfolded proteins within of organelle induces UPR^{mt} activation, a transcriptional program that results in a number of cellular- and mito-protective outcomes (Melber and Haynes, 2018). In *C. elegans*, the *P. aeruginosa* exposure induced mitochondrial stress and recruitment of stress-activated transcription factor 1, which induced the transcription of mitochondrial chaperones [such as heat shock protein (HSP) 10 and HSP 60], proteases (including the caseinolytic mitochondrial matrix peptidase proteolytic subunit), ROS detoxification, and innate immune genes, resulting a key regulator of UPR^{mt} (Nargund et al., 2012; Pellegrino et al., 2014). A similar transcriptional response has been described in mammals, identifying ATF5, which upon mitochondrial stress, fails to be imported into mitochondria for its degradation by mitochondrial protease lon protease homolog 1 but moves to the nucleus inducing gene transcription (**Figure 1**, UPR^{mt}) (Fiorese et al., 2016).

Rimessi et al. demonstrated that CFTR deficiency reduced the mitophagic clearance during infection with detrimental repercussion on mitochondrial homeostasis, triggering an abnormal UPR^{mt} activation in CF airway epithelial cells (Rimessi et al., 2020b). An extensive nuclear ATF5 redistribution, associated to an increased expression levels of UPR^{mt} reporters, was measured in CF airway cells during *P. aeruginosa* infection. The persistent UPR^{mt} activation also increased the inflammatory-sensitivity of CF cells to pathogen, as shown by higher levels of NLRP3 inflammasome-dependent IL-1β and IL-18 released during infection (Rimessi et al., 2020b). The amplitude of inflammasome responses were correlated to amount of dysfunctional mitochondria accumulated and by the levels of nuclear ATF5. UPR^{mt} and NLRP3 inflammasome activation in turn led to worsening of mitophagic and xenophagic defects in CF cells, favoring a vicious cycle that contributed to exacerbate the *P. aeruginosa*-dependent cellular and mitochondrial stress (Rimessi et al., 2020b). These findings showed as the impairments in selective autophagy in CF are sustained by abnormal UPR^{mt} and NLRP3 activation, contributing to persistent damaged mitochondria and invading bacteria accumulation in CF cells.

APOPTOSIS

During infection, in front of irreversible damages in response to prolonged stress conditions, mitochondria may activate the intrinsic apoptotic pathway (Green and Kroemer, 2004). Many pathogens activate the intrinsic apoptotic pathway, causing $\Delta\psi$ depolarization and mitochondrial permeabilization followed by enhanced levels of ROS and pro-apoptotic Bcl2 family proteins, such as Bax and Bid (Green and Kroemer, 2004; Wood et al., 2015). In turn, the excessive oxidative stress may oxidize mtDNA and active redox-sensitive kinases and transcription factors, which exacerbates the inflammatory environment contributing significantly to promote apoptosis in CF cells (**Figure 1**, apoptosis) (Jendrossek et al., 2001; Rottner et al., 2007; Kamdar et al., 2008; Galli et al., 2012; Rimessi et al., 2016).

Other studies suggest that the increased apoptotic susceptibility in CF cells is dependent by CFTR deficiency; e.g., I) due by abnormal intracellular Ca^{2+} signaling, which upon stress sensitizes the cell to organelle dysfunction and death (Antigny et al., 2011; Rimessi et al., 2020b); II) due to a reduced antioxidant activity, CFTR deficiency induced dysregulation of GSH concentration and transport, while reducing the expression of superoxide dismutase in F508del-CFTR mutant pancreatic cells (Gao et al., 1999; L'hoste et al., 2010; Kelly-Aubert et al., 2011; Rottner et al., 2011); III) due to a reduced expression of anti-apoptotic proteins, such as Bcl2 in CFTR-silencing intestinal cells[20]; IV) due to altered intracellular pH (de Meer et al., 1995; Barriere et al., 2001).

In any case, the enhanced apoptosis in CF cells contributes to hasten the tissue damage and functional loss in CF, worsening the disease state.

MITO-INFLAMMATION IN CYSTIC FIBROSIS

The extensive studies of these years revealed a supplementary role of mitochondria as drivers of inflammatory responses, leading us to reflect on new concept: the mito-inflammation. A compartmentalization of inflammatory process related to the role of mitochondria in engage and sustain the inflammatory responses and thus a druggable target to counteract the exacerbations of responses. In CF, mitochondria function as central regulator of danger signals, arbitrators with a double role in the pathogenesis of hyperinflammatory state.

Firstly, they act as checkpoints of intracellular downstream signal cascades to pathogen recognition receptor responses, induced by exogenous pathogen-associated molecular patterns. Bacterial ligands induce macrophage bactericidal-activity binding TLR 1, 2 and 4, which modulate the mitochondrial respiratory chain assembly factor, ECSIT, to increase mitochondrial ROS production (West et al., 2011). Again, the mitochondrial antiviral signaling protein (MAVS), located on the OMM regulates the transduction of interferon-dependent signaling pathway to amplify antiviral innate immune responses (Banoth and Cassel, 2018).

Second, mitochondria act as a key source of mitochondrial danger-associated molecular patterns (DAMPs), where ROS, mtDNA, ATP, CL and Ca^{2+} are released as danger signals into the cytosol or in the extracellular milieu, which recognized by TLRs and/or the cytosolic nucleotide-binding oligomerization domain-like receptors (NLRs) trigger the inflammatory responses inducing the expression and secretion of numerous pro-inflammatory mediators (**Figure 2**) (Lavelle et al., 2010).

Upon stress, the mitochondrial ROS production results excessive in CF cells, determining (**Figure 2**, ROS): I) oxidative damage to intracellular macromolecules, including mtDNA; II) activation of redox-sensitive transcription factors, inducing the up-regulation of cytokines and inflammasomes. The transcription factors NF-kB, AP-1 and HIF-1 result hyperactivated in murine and human CF airway cells, due to also by intrinsic defects associated to defective CFTR (like abnormal intracellular Ca^{2+} signaling), causing production of chemokine IL-8 and priming of NLRP3 and pro-IL-1β expression (McNamara et al., 2006; Tabary et al., 2006; Levy et al., 2009; Legendre et al., 2011; Saadane et al., 2011; Nichols and Chmiel, 2015); III) NLRP3 inflammasome activation; and IV) additional mitochondrial impairments in a feed-back stimulatory manner that exacerbates the inflammatory response (Brookes et al., 2004; Rimessi et al., 2016).

mtDNA may be oxidized by ROS and its damages may alter the OXPHOS activity, producing additional ROS (**Figure 2**, mtDNA). mtDNA may escape from matrix, due to impaired mitophagy or Ca^{2+}- and oxidative stress-dependent mPTP opening, and binds directly the NLR component of inflammasomes to trigger theirs activation (Escames et al., 2012). CL is accidentally released from damaged mitochondria and acts as direct activator of NLRP3 inflammasome in the cytosol (Iyer et al., 2013).

ATP released from mitochondria acts in the extracellular milieu as ligand of purinergic receptors, resulting in increased ROS production and cytokines release, influencing also NLRP3 activation (Bonora et al., 2012). Finally, dysfunctional mitochondria present altered mitochondrial Ca^{2+} signals, critical for inflammation, which influence the mitochondrial stress responses with consequent repercussions on inflammasome activation and on up-regulation and release of cytokines (Rimessi et al., 2015).

The mitochondrial DAMPs are preferentially bound by different NLRs to modulate the amplitude of immune responses activating the inflammasomes, multiprotein complexes that lead to caspase-1 activation and subsequent maturation of the pro-inflammatory cytokines IL-1β, IL-18, and IL-33 (**Figure 2**) (Broz and Dixit, 2016). Elevated concentrations of IL-1β and IL-18 were detected in human airway epithelial cells, monocytes and serum of CF patients (Levy et al., 2009; Rimessi et al., 2015; Iannitti et al., 2016; Scambler et al., 2019). Mitochondrial DAMPs are the principal initiator of NLRP3 inflammasome activation. NLRP3 is a cytosolic receptor that, once activated, interacts with mitochondria where oligomerizes recruiting the adaptor protein apoptosis-associated speck-like protein containing a caspase recruitment domain (ASC) and the procaspase-1 (Zhou et al., 2011). Its mitochondrial localization and association depends by MAVS, which promotes also its activation, and by mitochondrial-anchored protein ligase (Park et al., 2013; Subramanian et al., 2013). Rimessi et al. showed the NLRP3 mitochondrial recruitment and activation in CF airway cells during *P. aeruginosa* infection, since defective CFTR induced mitochondrial Ca^{2+}-overload and ROS production, which in turn driven the NLRP3 inflammasome activation and release of IL-1β and IL-18 (Rimessi et al., 2015). The increased susceptibility to pathogen-dependent mitochondrial dysfunction and the mitochondrial Ca^{2+}-overload in human CF airway cells resulted in the recruitment of both NLRP3 and NLRC4 inflammasome with consequent worsen of inflammation (Rimessi et al., 2015). NLRC4/IPAF inflammasome activation has been associated to mitochondrial DAMPs during *P. aeruginosa* infection also in macrophages, due to ROS and direct binding with oxidized mtDNA (Jabir et al., 2015). Typically, it activated by TLR5-recognition on PM *via* bacterial flagellin and in the cytosol *via* the microbial type III secretion system (Sutterwala et al., 2007; Tolle et al., 2015). The interplay between NLRP3 and NLRC4 inflammasome has been also reported in CFTR-null mouse model and in alveolar CF macrophages and neutrophils, where NLRP3 greatly contributed (Iannitti et al., 2016). In CF airway cells, NLRP3 inflammasome activation induces also the downregulation of mitophagy and xenophagy, promoting the accumulation of damaged mitochondria and invading bacteria into the cells (Rimessi et al., 2020b). In turn, released IL-1β induces mitochondrial ROS production, down-regulating the complex-I activity and $\Delta\psi$, and NF-kB activation, generating a loop that sustain and exacerbate the inflammatory response (Lopez-Armada et al., 2006; Escames et al., 2012).

The hyperinflammation observed in CF lung is in part conditioned by altered phenotype of airway immune cells associated to defective CFTR. CF neutrophils exhibit altered chlorination of phagocytosed bacteria while the macrophages showed reduced selective autophagic activity, becoming a replicative niche for bacteria (Painter et al., 2006; Lamothe and Valvano, 2008; Ratner and Mueller, 2012; Assani et al., 2014). Mitochondrial metabolism and the metabolic state of the cell drive the pro- or anti-inflammatory responses, regulating the polarization and activation of different immune cells, including neutrophils and macrophages (Michalek et al., 2011; Tarique et al., 2015). Accordingly, a compromised metabolism was found in CF neutrophils in response to LPS, shifting to a state of increased aerobic glycolysis with consequent exacerbation of IL-1β production (McElvaney et al., 2019). CF macrophages did not respond to IL-13/IL-4 and failed to polarize into M2, contributing to excessive production of cytokines

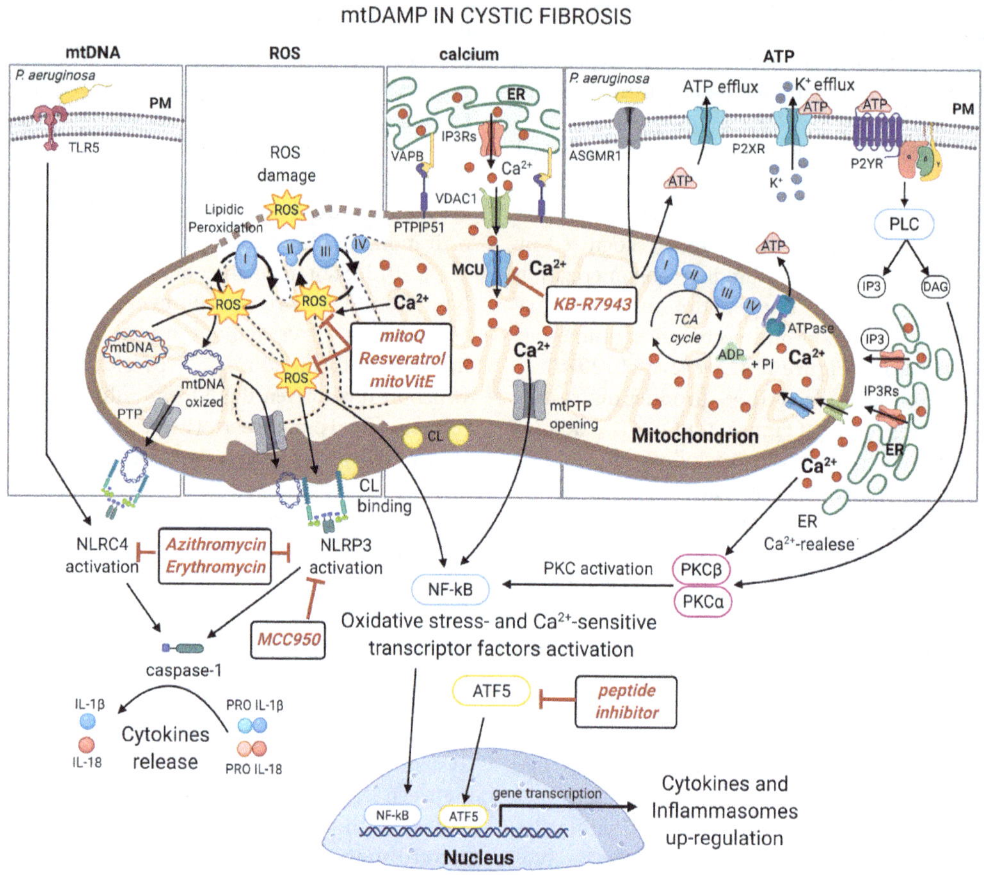

FIGURE 2 | mtDAMPs in cystic fibrosis Under stress, mitochondria generate and/or release immunogenic molecules, named mitochondrial damage associated molecular patters (mtDAMPs), that influence significantly the inflammatory response in CF lung disease. The accumulation of dysfunctional mitochondria leads to excessive ROS production in CF airway cells with detrimental effects on mitochondrial constituents, inducing oxidative damages on mtDNA and mitochondrial respiratory complexes or the lipidic peroxidation of mitochondrial membranes. The ROS may also active: I) oxidative-stress sensitive transcriptor factors, which after nuclear translocation, up-regulate the expression of cytokines and inflammasomes; II) or the NLRP3 inflammasome to promote the release of interleukine-1β (IL-1β) and IL-18. NLRP3 and NLRC4 inflammasomes are also activated by direct interaction with mtDNA and cardiolipin (CL), released following mitochondrial damage or PTP opening, with consequent activation of caspase-1. The abnormal ER-mitochondria Ca^{2+} transfer, due by increased interorganelle crosstalk mediated by VAPB-PTPIP51 tethering during pathogen infection in CF, contributes to mitochondrial stress inducing ROS production, PTP opening and UPR^{mt} activation, which facilitate the activation of NF-kB and NLRP3 inflammasome. Increased levels of extracellular ATP, induced by *P. aeruginosa*-ASGMR1 signaling pathway, mediate ionic flux and intracellular potassium (K^+) depletion through the ATP-binding to ligand-gated ion channels P2X receptors, sensitizing the CF airway cells to NLRP3 inflammasome activation. Indeed, mediating P2Y receptors, the extracellular ATP induces the Ca^{2+}-dependent activation of classical Protein Kinase C (PKC) isoforms through the IP3-triggering ER Ca^{2+}-release, resulting in NF-kB activation (Pinton et al., 2004). Several classes of molecules may exert anti-inflammatory activity targeting mitochondria at different levels. In this figure are shown the discussed drugs that may counteract the mito-inflammation in CF lung disease. Plasma membrane (PM); Toll-like receptor 5 (TLR5); NLR Family CARD Domain Containing 4 (NLRC4); permeability transition pore (PTP); NLR Family Pyrin Domain Containing 3 (NLRP3); Mitochondrial Calcium Uniporter (MCU); Voltage-dependent anion-selective channel 1 (VDAC1); Vesicle-associated membrane protein-associated protein B (VAPB); Protein tyrosine phosphatase interacting protein 51 (PTPIP51); Inositol 1,4,5-Triphosphate (IP3); diacylglycerol (DAG); Inositol trisphosphate receptors (IP3Rs); Endoplasmic Reticulum (ER); nuclear factor-κB (NF-kB); adenosine triphosphate (ATP); adenosine diphosphate (ADP); Asialo GM1 receptor (ASGMR1); P2X purinoceptor (P2XR); Purinergic Receptor (P2YR); Phospholipase C (PLC). This figure has been created with "BioRender.com".

(Tarique et al., 2017). The pro-inflammatory Th17 cells are highly glycolytic; meanwhile the immunosuppressive Treg cells present an elevated rate of lipid oxidation. In CF patients, the differentiation of T lymphocytes to Th17 phenotype was increased (Kushwah et al., 2013), indicating that the maintenance of mitochondrial homeostasis and of a functional metabolic reprogramming are critical conditions to regulate the immune responses also in CF.

TARGETING MITO-INFLAMMATION AS THERAPEUTIC APPROACH IN CYSTIC FIBROSIS

In CF, the ideal drug should be one that interrupts the vicious CF cycle that sustains lung hyperinflammation, but also generates favorable conditions to rescue or potentiate the residue functionality of defective CFTR. In this regard, several modulators of mitochondrial behaviors have shown anti-inflammatory activity, such as mitochondrial antioxidants, modulators of mitochondrial Ca^{2+}-exchange, selective autophagic-inducing compounds and inflammasome and IL-1β inhibitors.

Strategies that limit mitochondrial ROS production may be useful to control the hyperactivation of redox-sensitive inflammatory transcription factors and inflammasomes (**Figure 2**, ROS). An example may be found in the natural phenolic antioxidant resveratrol (3,4′,5-trihydroxystilbene), which efficiently reduces oxidative stress and subsequent inflammation, preserving mitochondrial $\Delta\psi$ and mtDNA *in vitro* and *in vivo* (Manna et al., 2000; Xu et al., 2012). At high concentration, in preclinical studies resveratrol rescues the expression of F508del-CFTR, the chloride secretion and the intracellular transport in human primary airway epithelial cells and CF mouse models (Hamdaoui et al., 2011; Dhooghe et al., 2015; Lu et al., 2020). Indeed, in presence of the modulator, ivacaftor, resveratrol augmented the G155D-CFTR activation in human primary sinonasal cells (Cho et al., 2019). Unfortunately, resveratrol exhibits poor bioavailability with maximal achievable plasma concentration of about 2 μM (a concentration no effective to improve CFTR function), that could limit its clinical usefulness (Walle, 2011; Jai et al., 2015). However, different therapies in CF involve topical application of drugs to lung mediating aerosol, a strategy that may overcome the limit of bioavailability.

Other antioxidants, such NAC, have been locally administrated to CF adults and children in different clinical trials. Acute administration of NAC was found to be well tolerated and free of adverse effects. Despite this, it was only found beneficial variations in sputum rheology and hydration, two factors that may be predictive of improved airway mucus clearance. Any significant change in pulmonary function and in clinical indicator were registered (App et al., 2002). Of more interest were the results obtained in a phase II randomized placebo-controlled trial, where it was performed long-term treatment with oral NAC (Conrad et al., 2015). Indeed, authors found improvements in lung functions, reduction in the incidence of pulmonary exacerbations. Unfortunately, they found no change in sputum human neutrophil elastase activity and other biomarkers of inflammation, suggesting to consider more specialized antioxidants as therapeutic strategy in CF (Cantin, 2004). Antioxidants that have shown promising results in oxidative stress-related diseases are mitovitamin E (MitoVit-E) and mitoquinone (Mito-Q), mitochondrial antioxidants that contain the triphenylphosphonium cation moiety that facilitates theirs accumulation into the organelle (Smith et al., 2003). MitoVit-E suppressed the sepsi-induced peripheral and myocardial production of cytokines, including IL-1β, improving mitochondrial function and heart activity, while Mito-Q restored mitochondrial function in chronic obstructive pulmonary disease (COPD) patients, reducing inflammation and IL-8 release in preclinical studies (Zang et al., 2012; Wiegman et al., 2015). In CF patients, the low level of vitamin-E in serum is normally correct with a dietary supplement, this implementation should be enriched also with MitoVit-E to safeguard the mitochondrial function (Sokol et al., 1989).

The hyperinflammation in CF lung is due also by altered mitochondrial Ca^{2+} exchange, in which MCU is involved (Rimessi et al., 2015; Rimessi et al., 2020b). Pharmacological MCU inhibition, mediating KB-R7943, attenuated *in vitro* and *in vivo* the *P. aeruginosa*-dependent mitochondrial dysfunction and hyperinflammation in CF lung, controlling UPR^{mt} and NLRP3 inflammasome activation (**Figure 2**, calcium) (Rimessi et al., 2020b). KB-R7943 is the first freely PM permeable and only one available dose-selective MCU inhibitor, in opposing to more used MCU inhibitors, Ruthenium Red and Ru360 that are cell impermeable (Santo-Domingo et al., 2007). A new class of cell-permeable selective MCU inhibitors are now available, and Ru265 and DS16570511 are minimally toxic *in vitro* and could have important implications in CF in the future (Kon et al., 2017; Woods et al., 2019). KB-R7943 also restored mitophagy and xenophagy in CF, removing stressed mitochondria and pathogens able to induce mtDAMPs release, it attenuated the inflammatory state (Rimessi et al., 2020b). Thus, selective autophagic inducers may mitigate the hyperinflammation in CF. Rapamycin and MK-2206, both inhibitors of PI3K/Akt/mTOR pathway, reduced the severity of CF inflammation and improved the CFTR stability in airway epithelial cells in preclinical studies (Abdulrahman et al., 2011; Reilly et al., 2017). In a perspective of mitochondrial quality control based therapy, the synthetic cell-penetrating dominant negative ATF5 peptide (Cs Bio®) should be useful to dampen the persistent UPR^{mt} activation in CF, restoring the autophagy process (**Figure 2**) (Sheng et al., 2011).

Inflammasome and IL-1β inhibitors may rescue selective autophagy and attenuate the hyperinflammation in CF. MCC950 inhibits NLRP3 and AIM2 inflammasome, but not NLRC4, blocking the formation of ASC complexes (Coll et al., 2011). *In vivo*, MCC950 improved the clearance of *P. aeruginosa* and reduced IL-1β release in the lung (McElvaney et al., 2019). The pathogenic NLRP3 activity in CF may be reduced using the IL-1 antagonist receptor Anakinra, that by blocking the biological IL-1α and IL-1β activity ameliorated tissue damage and inflammation against *P. aeruginosa* in CF, with positive repercussion also on autophagy and neutrophils infiltration (Iannitti et al., 2016). The questionable limit of this approach is the indiscriminate block of IL-1 activity, which may compromise the global inflammatory responses important in fighting the persistent infections, in particular in those body areas where the microbe-host interactions are strategic. Despite this consideration, a phase 2 study (ClinicalTrials.gov Identifier: NCT03925194) to evaluate safety and efficacy on lung function of Anakinra subcutaneous administration in CF patients is ongoing. Recently, it has been demonstrated that also azithromycin and erythromycin (macrolides used in antibiotic CF therapies) inhibit the activation of inflammasome NLRP3 and NLRC4, which attenuated lung injury and inflammation enhancing the *P. aeruginosa* clearance in mice and in bronchiectasis patients (**Figure 2**) (Fan et al., 2017). Considering that the beneficial effects of these antibiotics is difficult to maintain over the years, treatments engaging specific inflammasome inhibitors may be used to improve the effects of these drugs in long-term treatment (Samson et al., 2016).

In conclusion, all these studies reveal the pathogenic role of mito-inflammation in CF and support mitochondria as new pharmacological targets. Emerging concepts of mitochondrial quality control provide opportunities to develop mitochondrial therapies, which aim to preserve the mitochondrial function as an alternative anti-inflammatory approach. The therapeutically restoring of mitochondrial homeostasis will be useful to improve the clinical state of CF lung disease, avoiding the overstimulation of inflammatory signals.

AUTHOR CONTRIBUTIONS

All authors contributed to the article and approved the submitted version.

FUNDING

The research was funded by grants from Italian Cystic Fibrosis Research Foundation FFC#12/2010 and #19/2014, Italian Association for Cancer Research (AIRC, IG-23670), Telethon (GGP11139B), local funds from the University of Ferrara, and the Italian Ministry of Education, University and Research (PRIN grant 2017E5L5P3) to PP. SP is supported by Fondazione Umberto Veronesi. AR is supported by Italian Cystic Fibrosis Research Foundation grant FFC #20/2015, local funds from University of Ferrara, FIR-2017, the Italian Ministry of Health (GR-2016-02364602), and the Italian Ministry of Education, University and Research (PRIN grant 2017XA5J5N). PP is grateful to Camilla degli Scrovegni for continuous support.

REFERENCES

Abdulrahman, B. A., Khweek, A. A., Akhter, A., Caution, K., Kotrange, S., Abdelaziz, D. H., et al. (2011). Autophagy stimulation by rapamycin suppresses lung inflammation and infection by Burkholderia cenocepacia in a model of cystic fibrosis. *Autophagy* 7, 1359–1370. doi: 10.4161/auto.7.11.17660

Antigny, F., Norez, C., Becq, F., and Vandebrouck, C. (2011). CFTR and Ca Signaling in Cystic Fibrosis. *Front. Pharmacol.* 2, 67. doi: 10.3389/fphar.2011.00067

App, E. M., Baran, D., Dab, I., Malfroot, A., Coffiner, M., Vanderbist, F., et al. (2002). Dose-finding and 24-h monitoring for efficacy and safety of aerosolized Nacystelyn in cystic fibrosis. *Eur. Respir. J.* 19, 294–302. doi: 10.1183/09031936.02.00025802

Assani, K., Tazi, M. F., Amer, A. O., and Kopp, B. T. (2014). IFN-gamma stimulates autophagy-mediated clearance of Burkholderia cenocepacia in human cystic fibrosis macrophages. *PloS One* 9, e96681. doi: 10.1371/journal.pone.0096681

Atlante, A., Favia, M., Bobba, A., Guerra, L., Casavola, V., and Reshkin, SJ. (2016). Characterization of mitochondrial function in cells with impaired cystic fibrosis transmembrane conductance regulator (CFTR) function. *J. Bioenerg. Biomembr.* 48, 197–210. doi: 10.1007/s10863-016-9663-y

Banoth, B., and Cassel, S. L. (2018). Mitochondria in innate immune signaling. *Transl. Res.* 202, 52–68. doi: 10.1016/j.trsl.2018.07.014

Barriere, H., Poujeol, C., Tauc, M., Blasi, J. M., Counillon, L., and Poujeol, P. (2001). CFTR modulates programmed cell death by decreasing intracellular pH in Chinese hamster lung fibroblasts. *Am. J. Physiol. Cell Physiol.* 281, C810–C824. doi: 10.1152/ajpcell.2001.281.3.C810

Battino, M., Rugolo, M., Romeo, G., and Lenaz, G. (1986). Kinetic alterations of cytochrome-c oxidase in cystic fibrosis. *FEBS Lett.* 199, 155–158. doi: 10.1016/0014-5793(86)80470-7

Bonora, M., Patergnani, S., Rimessi, A., De Marchi, E., Suski, J. M., Bononi, A., et al. (2012). ATP synthesis and storage. *Purinergic Signal* 8, 343–357. doi: 10.1007/s11302-012-9305-8

Brookes, P. S., Yoon, Y., Robotham, J. L., Anders, M. W., and Sheu, S. S. (2004). Calcium, ATP, and ROS: a mitochondrial love-hate triangle. *Am. J. Physiol. Cell Physiol.* 287, C817–C833. doi: 10.1152/ajpcell.00139.2004

Broz, P., and Dixit, V. M. (2016). Inflammasomes: mechanism of assembly, regulation and signalling. *Nat. Rev. Immunol.* 16, 407–420. doi: 10.1038/nri.2016.58

Campello, S., and Scorrano, L. (2010). Mitochondrial shape changes: orchestrating cell pathophysiology. *EMBO Rep.* 11, 678–684. doi: 10.1038/embor.2010.115

Cantin, A. M. (2004). Potential for antioxidant therapy of cystic fibrosis. *Curr. Opin. Pulm. Med.* 10, 531–536. doi: 10.1097/01.mcp.0000138997.29276.a1

Cho, D. Y., Zhang, S., Lazrak, A., Grayson, J. W., Pena Garcia, J. A., Skinner, D. F., et al. (2019). Resveratrol and ivacaftor are additive G551D CFTR-channel potentiators: therapeutic implications for cystic fibrosis sinus disease. *Int. Forum Allergy Rhinol.* 9, 100–105. doi: 10.1002/alr.22202

Coll, R. C., Robertson, A., Butler, M., Cooper, M., and O'Neill, L. A. (2011). The cytokine release inhibitory drug CRID3 targets ASC oligomerisation in the NLRP3 and AIM2 inflammasomes. *PloS One* 6, e29539. doi: 10.1371/journal.pone.0029539

Congdon, P. J., Littlewood, J. M., Aggarwal, R. K., and Shapiro, H. (1981). Glucose 6-phosphate dehydrogenase deficiency and cystic fibrosis. *Postgrad. Med. J.* 57, 453–454. doi: 10.1136/pgmj.57.669.453

Conrad, C., Lymp, J., Thompson, V., Dunn, C., Davies, Z., Chatfield, B., et al. (2015). Long-term treatment with oral N-acetylcysteine: affects lung function but not sputum inflammation in cystic fibrosis subjects. A phase II randomized placebo-controlled trial. *J. Cyst. Fibros* 14, 219–227. doi: 10.1016/j.jcf.2014.08.008

Csanady, L., Vergani, P., and Gadsby, D. C. (2019). Structure, Gating, and Regulation of the Cftr Anion Channel. *Physiol. Rev.* 99, 707–738. doi: 10.1152/physrev.00007.2018

De Meer, K., Jeneson, J. A., Gulmans, V. A., van der Laag, J., and Berger, R. (1995). Efficiency of oxidative work performance of skeletal muscle in patients with cystic fibrosis. *Thorax* 50, 980–983. doi: 10.1136/thx.50.9.980

Dhooghe, B., Bouckaert, C., Capron, A., Wallemacq, P., Leal, T., Noel, S., et al. (2015). Resveratrol increases F508del-CFTR dependent salivary secretion in cystic fibrosis mice. *Biol. Open* 4, 929–936. doi: 10.1242/bio.010967

Eisner, V., Picard, M., and Hajnoczky, G. (2018). Mitochondrial dynamics in adaptive and maladaptive cellular stress responses. *Nat. Cell Biol.* 20, 755–765. doi: 10.1038/s41556-018-0133-0

Elborn, J. S. (2016). Cystic fibrosis. *Lancet* 388, 2519–2531. doi: 10.1016/S0140-6736(16)00576-6

Escames, G., Lopez, L. C., Garcia, J. A., Garcia-Corzo, L., Ortiz, F., and Acuna-Castroviejo, D. (2012). Mitochondrial DNA and inflammatory diseases. *Hum. Genet.* 131, 161–173. doi: 10.1007/s00439-011-1057-y

Fan, L. C., Lin, J. L., Yang, J. W., Mao, B., Lu, H. W., Ge, B. X., et al. (2017). Macrolides protect against Pseudomonas aeruginosa infection via inhibition of inflammasomes. *Am. J. Physiol. Lung Cell Mol. Physiol.* 313, L677–L686. doi: 10.1152/ajplung.00123.2017

Feigal, R. J., and Shapiro, B. L. (1979). Mitochondrial calcium uptake and oxygen consumption in cystic fibrosis. *Nature* 278, 276–277. doi: 10.1038/278276a0

Fiorese, C. J., Schulz, A. M., Lin, Y. F., Rosin, N., Pellegrino, M. W., and Haynes, C. M. (2016). The Transcription Factor ATF5 Mediates a Mammalian Mitochondrial UPR. *Curr. Biol.* 26, 2037–2043. doi: 10.1016/j.cub.2016.06.002

Galli, F., Battistoni, A., Gambari, R., Pompella, A., Bragonzi, A., Pilolli, F., et al. (2012). Oxidative stress and antioxidant therapy in cystic fibrosis. *Biochim. Biophys. Acta* 1822, 690–713. doi: 10.1016/j.bbadis.2011.12.012

Gao, L., Kim, K. J., Yankaskas, J. R., and Forman, H. J. (1999). Abnormal glutathione transport in cystic fibrosis airway epithelia. *Am. J. Physiol.* 277, L113–L118. doi: 10.1152/ajplung.1999.277.1.L113

Gatica, D., Lahiri, V., and Klionsky, D. J. (2018). Cargo recognition and degradation by selective autophagy. *Nat. Cell Biol.* 20, 233–242. doi: 10.1038/s41556-018-0037-z

Giorgi, C., Danese, A., Missiroli, S., Patergnani, S., and Pinton, P. (2018a). Calcium Dynamics as a Machine for Decoding Signals. *Trends Cell Biol.* 28, 258–273. doi: 10.1016/j.tcb.2018.01.002

Giorgi, C., Marchi, S., and Pinton, P. (2018b). The machineries, regulation and cellular functions of mitochondrial calcium. *Nat. Rev. Mol. Cell Biol.* 19, 713–730. doi: 10.1038/s41580-018-0052-8

Green, D. R., and Kroemer, G. (2004). The pathophysiology of mitochondrial cell death. *Science* 305, 626–629. doi: 10.1126/science.1099320

Hamdaoui, N., Baudoin-Legros, M., Kelly, M., Aissat, A., Moriceau, S., Vieu, D. L., et al. (2011). Resveratrol rescues cAMP-dependent anionic transport in the cystic fibrosis pancreatic cell line CFPAC1. *Br. J. Pharmacol.* 163, 876–886. doi: 10.1111/j.1476-5381.2011.01289.x

Iannitti, R. G., Napolioni, V., Oikonomou, V., De Luca, A., Galosi, C., Pariano, M., et al. (2016). IL-1 receptor antagonist ameliorates inflammasome-dependent inflammation in murine and human cystic fibrosis. *Nat. Commun.* 7, 10791. doi: 10.1038/ncomms10791

Iyer, S. S., He, Q., Janczy, J. R., Elliott, E. I., Zhong, Z., Olivier, A. K., et al. (2013). Mitochondrial cardiolipin is required for Nlrp3 inflammasome activation. *Immunity* 39, 311–323. doi: 10.1016/j.immuni.2013.08.001

Jabir, M. S., Hopkins, L., Ritchie, N. D., Ullah, I., Bayes, H. K., Li, D., et al. (2015). Mitochondrial damage contributes to Pseudomonas aeruginosa activation of the inflammasome and is downregulated by autophagy. *Autophagy* 11, 166–182. doi: 10.4161/15548627.2014.981915

Jai, Y., Shah, K., Bridges, R. J., and Bradbury, N. A. (2015). Evidence against resveratrol as a viable therapy for the rescue of defective DeltaF508 CFTR. *Biochim. Biophys. Acta* 1850, 2377–2384. doi: 10.1016/j.bbagen.2015.08.020

Jendrossek, V., Grassme, H., Mueller, I., Lang, F., and Gulbins, E. (2001). Pseudomonas aeruginosa-induced apoptosis involves mitochondria and stress-activated protein kinases. *Infect. Immun.* 69, 2675–2683. doi: 10.1128/IAI.69.4.2675-2683.2001

Kamdar, O., Le, W., Zhang, J., Ghio, A. J., Rosen, G. D., and Upadhyay, D. (2008). Air pollution induces enhanced mitochondrial oxidative stress in cystic fibrosis airway epithelium. *FEBS Lett.* 582, 3601–3606. doi: 10.1016/j.febslet.2008.09.030

Kelly-Aubert, M., Trudel, S., Fritsch, J., Nguyen-Khoa, T., Baudouin-Legros, M., Moriceau, S. , et al. (2011). GSH monoethyl ester rescues mitochondrial defects in cystic fibrosis models. *Hum. Mol. Genet.* 20, 2745–2759. doi: 10.1093/hmg/ddr173

Kleme, M. L., Sane, A., Garofalo, C., Seidman, E., Brochiero, E., Berthiaume, Y., et al. (2018). CFTR Deletion Confers Mitochondrial Dysfunction and Disrupts Lipid Homeostasis in Intestinal Epithelial Cells. *Nutrients* 10. doi: 10.3390/nu10070836

Kon, N., Murakoshi, M., Isobe, A., Kagechika, K., Miyoshi, N., and Nagayama, T. (2017). DS16570511 is a small-molecule inhibitor of the mitochondrial calcium uniporter. *Cell Death Discovery* 3, 17045. doi: 10.1038/cddiscovery.2017.45

Koyano, F., Okatsu, K., Kosako, H., Tamura, Y., Go, E., Kimura, M., et al. (2014). Ubiquitin is phosphorylated by PINK1 to activate parkin. *Nature* 510, 162–166. doi: 10.1038/nature13392

Kushwah, R., Gagnon, S., and Sweezey, N. B. (2013). Intrinsic predisposition of naive cystic fibrosis T cells to differentiate towards a Th17 phenotype. *Respir. Res.* 14, 138. doi: 10.1186/1465-9921-14-138

Lamothe, J., and Valvano, M. A. (2008). Burkholderia cenocepacia-induced delay of acidification and phagolysosomal fusion in cystic fibrosis transmembrane conductance regulator (CFTR)-defective macrophages. *Microbiology* 154, 3825–3834. doi: 10.1099/mic.0.2008/023200-0

Lavelle, E. C., Murphy, C., O'Neill, L. A., and Creagh, E. M. (2010). The role of TLRs, NLRs, and RLRs in mucosal innate immunity and homeostasis. *Mucosal Immunol.* 3, 17–28. doi: 10.1038/mi.2009.124

Lazarou, M., Sliter, D. A., Kane, L. A., Sarraf, S. A., Wang, C., Burman, J. L., et al. (2015). The ubiquitin kinase PINK1 recruits autophagy receptors to induce mitophagy. *Nature* 524, 309–314. doi: 10.1038/nature14893

Lee, S., and Min, K. T. (2018). The Interface Between ER and Mitochondria: Molecular Compositions and Functions. *Mol. Cells* 41, 1000–1007. doi: 10.14348/molcells.2018.0438

Legendre, C., Mooij, M. J., Adams, C., and O'gara, F. (2011). Impaired expression of hypoxia-inducible factor-1alpha in cystic fibrosis airway epithelial cells - a role for HIF-1 in the pathophysiology of CF? *J. Cyst. Fibros* 10, 286–290. doi: 10.1016/j.jcf.2011.02.005

Levy, H., Murphy, A., Zou, F., Gerard, C., Klanderman, B., Schuemann, B., et al. (2009). IL1B polymorphisms modulate cystic fibrosis lung disease. *Pediatr. Pulmonol.* 44, 580–593. doi: 10.1002/ppul.21026

Lopez-Armada, M. J., Carames, B., Martin, M. A., Cillero-Pastor, B., Lires-Dean, M., Fuentes- Boquete, I., et al. (2006). Mitochondrial activity is modulated by TNFalpha and IL-1beta in normal human chondrocyte cells. *Osteoarthritis Cartilage* 14, 1011–1022. doi: 10.1016/j.joca.2006.03.008

L'hoste, S., Chargui, A., Belfodil, R., Corcelle, E., Duranton, C., Rubera, I., et al. (2010). CFTR mediates apoptotic volume decrease and cell death by controlling glutathione efflux and ROS production in cultured mice proximal tubules. *Am. J. Physiol. Renal Physiol.* 298, F435–F453. doi: 10.1152/ajprenal.00286.2009

Lu, B., Corey, D. A., and Kelley, T. J. (2020). Resveratrol restores intracellular transport in cystic fibrosis epithelial cells. *Am. J. Physiol. Lung Cell Mol. Physiol.* 318, L1145–L1157. doi: 10.1152/ajplung.00006.2020

Luciani, A., Villella, V. R., Esposito, S., Brunetti-Pierri, N., Medina, D., Settembre, C., et al. (2010). Defective CFTR induces aggresome formation and lung inflammation in cystic fibrosis through ROS-mediated autophagy inhibition. *Nat. Cell Biol.* 12, 863–875. doi: 10.1038/ncb2090

Malhotra, S., Hayes, D.Jr., and Wozniak, D. J. (2019). Cystic Fibrosis and Pseudomonas aeruginosa: the Host-Microbe Interface. *Clin. Microbiol. Rev.* 32, e00138-18. doi: 10.1128/CMR.00138-18

Manna, S. K., Mukhopadhyay, A., and Aggarwal, B. B. (2000). Resveratrol suppresses TNF-induced activation of nuclear transcription factors NF-kappa B, activator protein-1, and apoptosis: potential role of reactive oxygen intermediates and lipid peroxidation. *J. Immunol.* 164, 6509–6519. doi: 10.4049/jimmunol.164.12.6509

Marson, F. A. L., Bertuzzo, C. S., and Ribeiro, J. D. (2016). Classification of CFTR mutation classes. *Lancet Respir. Med.* 4, e37–e38. doi: 10.1016/S2213-2600(16)30188-6

McElvaney, O. J., Zaslona, Z., Becker-Flegler, K., Palsson-Mcdermott, E. M., Boland, F., Gunaratnam, C., et al. (2019). Specific Inhibition of the NLRP3 Inflammasome as an Antiinflammatory Strategy in Cystic Fibrosis. *Am. J. Respir. Crit. Care Med.* 200, 1381–1391. doi: 10.1164/rccm.201905-1013OC

McNamara, N., Gallup, M., Sucher, A., Maltseva, I., Mckemy, D., and Basbaum, C. (2006). AsialoGM1 and TLR5 cooperate in flagellin-induced nucleotide signaling to activate Erk1/2. *Am. J. Respir. Cell Mol. Biol.* 34, 653–660. doi: 10.1165/rcmb.2005-0441OC

Mejia, E. M., and Hatch, G. M. (2016). Mitochondrial phospholipids: role in mitochondrial function. *J. Bioenerg. Biomembr.* 48, 99–112. doi: 10.1007/s10863-015-9601-4

Melber, A., and Haynes, C. M. (2018). UPR(mt) regulation and output: a stress response mediated by mitochondrial-nuclear communication. *Cell Res.* 28, 281–295. doi: 10.1038/cr.2018.16

Michalek, R. D., Gerriets, V. A., Jacobs, S. R., Macintyre, A. N., Maciver, N. J., Mason, E. F., et al. (2011). Cutting edge: distinct glycolytic and lipid oxidative metabolic programs are essential for effector and regulatory CD4+ T cell subsets. *J. Immunol.* 186, 3299–3303. doi: 10.4049/jimmunol.1003613

Nargund, A. M., Pellegrino, M. W., Fiorese, C. J., Baker, B. M., and Haynes, C. M. (2012). Mitochondrial import efficiency of ATFS-1 regulates mitochondrial UPR activation. *Science* 337, 587–590. doi: 10.1126/science.1223560

Nichols, D. P., and Chmiel, J. F. (2015). Inflammation and its genesis in cystic fibrosis. *Pediatr. Pulmonol.* 50 Suppl 40, S39–S56. doi: 10.1002/ppul.23242

Nunnari, J., and Suomalainen, A. (2012). Mitochondria: in sickness and in health. *Cell* 148, 1145–1159. doi: 10.1016/j.cell.2012.02.035

Painter, R. G., Valentine, V. G., Lanson, N. A. Jr., Leidal, K., Zhang, Q., Lombard, G., et al. (2006). CFTR Expression in human neutrophils and the phagolysosomal chlorination defect in cystic fibrosis. *Biochemistry* 45, 10260–10269. doi: 10.1021/bi060490t

Park, S., Juliana, C., Hong, S., Datta, P., Hwang, I., Fernandes-Alnemri, T., et al. (2013). The mitochondrial antiviral protein MAVS associates with NLRP3 and regulates its inflammasome activity. *J. Immunol.* 191, 4358–4366. doi: 10.4049/jimmunol.1301170

Pedriali, G., Rimessi, A., Sbano, L., Giorgi, C., Wieckowski, M. R., Previati, M., et al. (2017). Regulation of Endoplasmic Reticulum-Mitochondria Ca(2+) Transfer and Its Importance for Anti-Cancer Therapies. *Front. Oncol.* 7, 180. doi: 10.3389/fonc.2017.00180

Pellegrino, M. W., Nargund, A. M., Kirienko, N. V., Gillis, R., Fiorese, C. J., and Haynes, C. M. (2014). Mitochondrial UPR-regulated innate immunity provides resistance to pathogen infection. *Nature* 516, 414–417. doi: 10.1038/nature13818

Picci, L., Brentagni, L., Mastella, G., Scarso, E., Pizzochero, P., Mattiazzo, P., et al. (1991). 2D-electrophoresis of mitochondrial proteins from cystic fibrosis patients. *Adv. Exp. Med. Biol.* 290, 379–381. doi: 10.1007/978-1-4684-5934-0_44

Pinton, P., Leo, S., Wieckowski, M. R., Di Benedetto, G., and Rizzuto, R. (2004). Long-term modulation of mitochondrial Ca2+ signals by protein kinase C isozymes. *J. Cell Biol.* 165, 223–232. doi: 10.1083/jcb.200311061

Rafeeq, M. M., and Murad, H. A. S. (2017). Cystic fibrosis: current therapeutic targets and future approaches. *J. Transl. Med.* 15, 84. doi: 10.1186/s12967-017-1193-9

Ratner, D., and Mueller, C. (2012). Immune responses in cystic fibrosis: are they intrinsically defective? *Am. J. Respir. Cell Mol. Biol.* 46, 715–722. doi: 10.1165/rcmb.2011-0399RT

Reilly, R., Mroz, M. S., Dempsey, E., Wynne, K., Keely, S. J., Mckone, E. F., et al. (2017). Targeting the PI3K/Akt/mTOR signalling pathway in Cystic Fibrosis. *Sci. Rep.* 7, 7642. doi: 10.1038/s41598-017-06588-z

Rimessi, A., Bezzerri, V., Patergnani, S., Marchi, S., Cabrini, G., and Pinton, P. (2015). Mitochondrial Ca2+-dependent NLRP3 activation exacerbates the Pseudomonas aeruginosa-driven inflammatory response in cystic fibrosis. *Nat. Commun.* 6 (19), eaax9093. doi: 10.1038/ncomms7201

Rimessi, A., Previati, M., Nigro, F., Wieckowski, M. R., and Pinton, P. (2016). Mitochondrial reactive oxygen species and inflammation: Molecular mechanisms, diseases and promising therapies. *Int. J. Biochem. Cell Biol.* 81, 281–293. doi: 10.1016/j.biocel.2016.06.015

Rimessi, A., Pedriali, G., Vezzani, B., Tarocco, A., Marchi, S., Wieckowski, M. R., et al. (2020a). Interorganellar calcium signaling in the regulation of cell metabolism: A cancer perspective. *Semin. Cell Dev. Biol.* 98, 167–180. doi: 10.1016/j.semcdb.2019.05.015

Rimessi, A., Pozzato, C., Carparelli, L., Rossi, A., Ranucci, S., De Fino, I., et al. (2020b). Pharmacological modulation of Mitochondrial Calcium Uniporter controls lung inflammation in cystic fibrosis. *Sci. Adv.* 6 (19), eaax9093. doi: 10.1126/sciadv.aax9093

Rottner, M., Kunzelmann, C., Mergey, M., Freyssinet, J. M., and Martinez, M. C. (2007). Exaggerated apoptosis and NF-kappaB activation in pancreatic and tracheal cystic fibrosis cells. *FASEB J.* 21, 2939–2948. doi: 10.1096/fj.06-7614com

Rottner, M., Tual-Chalot, S., Mostefai, H. A., Andriantsitohaina, R., Freyssinet, J. M., and Martinez, M. C. (2011). Increased oxidative stress induces apoptosis in human cystic fibrosis cells. *PloS One* 6, e24880. doi: 10.1371/journal.pone.0024880

Rowland, A. A., and Voeltz, G. K. (2012). Endoplasmic reticulum-mitochondria contacts: function of the junction. *Nat. Rev. Mol. Cell Biol.* 13, 607–625. doi: 10.1038/nrm3440

Saadane, A., Eastman, J., Berger, M., and Bonfield, T. L. (2011). Parthenolide inhibits ERK and AP-1 which are dysregulated and contribute to excessive IL-8 expression and secretion in cystic fibrosis cells. *J. Inflammation (Lond).* 8, 26. doi: 10.1186/1476-9255-8-26

Samson, C., Tamalet, A., Thien, H. V., Taytard, J., Perisson, C., Nathan, N., et al. (2016). Long-term effects of azithromycin in patients with cystic fibrosis. *Respir. Med.* 117, 1–6. doi: 10.1016/j.rmed.2016.05.025

Santo-Domingo, J., Vay, L., Hernandez-Sanmiguel, E., Lobaton, C. D., Moreno, A., Montero, M., et al. (2007). The plasma membrane Na+/Ca2+ exchange inhibitor KB-R7943 is also a potent inhibitor of the mitochondrial Ca2+ uniporter. *Br. J. Pharmacol.* 151, 647–654. doi: 10.1038/sj.bjp.0707260

Scambler, T., Jarosz-Griffiths, H. H., Lara-Reyna, S., Pathak, S., Wong, C., Holbrook, J., et al. (2019). ENaC-mediated sodium influx exacerbates NLRP3-dependent inflammation in cystic fibrosis. *Elife* 8. doi: 10.7554/eLife.49248

Shapiro, B. L., Feigal, R. J., and Lam, L. F. (1979). Mitrochondrial NADH dehydrogenase in cystic fibrosis. *Proc. Natl. Acad. Sci. U. S. A.* 76, 2979–2983. doi: 10.1073/pnas.76.6.2979

Sheng, Z., Ma, L., Sun, J. E., Zhu, L. J., and Green, M. R. (2011). BCR-ABL suppresses autophagy through ATF5-mediated regulation of mTOR transcription. *Blood* 118, 2840–2848. doi: 10.1182/blood-2010-12-322537

Smith, R. A., Porteous, C. M., Gane, A. M., and Murphy, M. P. (2003). Delivery of bioactive molecules to mitochondria in vivo. *Proc. Natl. Acad. Sci. U. S. A.* 100, 5407–5412. doi: 10.1073/pnas.0931245100

Sokol, R. J., Reardon, M. C., Accurso, F. J., Stall, C., Narkewicz, M., Abman, S. H., et al. (1989). Fat-soluble-vitamin status during the first year of life in infants with cystic fibrosis identified by screening of newborns. *Am. J. Clin. Nutr.* 50, 1064–1071. doi: 10.1093/ajcn/50.5.1064

Song, Z., Ghochani, M., McCaffery, J. M., Frey, T. G., and Chan, D. C. (2009). Mitofusins and OPA1 mediate sequential steps in mitochondrial membrane fusion. *Mol. Biol. Cell* 20, 3525–3532. doi: 10.1091/mbc.e09-03-0252

Subramanian, N., Natarajan, K., Clatworthy, M. R., Wang, Z., and Germain, R. N. (2013). The adaptor MAVS promotes NLRP3 mitochondrial localization and inflammasome activation. *Cell* 153, 348–361. doi: 10.1016/j.cell.2013.02.054

Sutterwala, F. S., Mijares, L. A., Li, L., Ogura, Y., Kazmierczak, B. I., and Flavell, R. A. (2007). Immune recognition of Pseudomonas aeruginosa mediated by the IPAF/NLRC4 inflammasome. *J. Exp. Med.* 204, 3235–3245. doi: 10.1084/jem.20071239

Tabary, O., Boncoeur, E., De Martin, R., Pepperkok, R., Clement, A., Schultz, C., et al. (2006). Calcium-dependent regulation of NF-(kappa)B activation in cystic fibrosis airway epithelial cells. *Cell Signal* 18, 652–660. doi: 10.1016/j.cellsig.2005.06.004

Tarique, A. A., Logan, J., Thomas, E., Holt, P. G., Sly, P. D., and Fantino, E. (2015). Phenotypic, functional, and plasticity features of classical and alternatively activated human macrophages. *Am. J. Respir. Cell Mol. Biol.* 53, 676–688. doi: 10.1165/rcmb.2015-0012OC

Tarique, A. A., Sly, P. D., Holt, P. G., Bosco, A., Ware, R. S., Logan, J., et al. (2017). CFTR-dependent defect in alternatively-activated macrophages in cystic fibrosis. *J. Cyst. Fibros* 16, 475–482. doi: 10.1016/j.jcf.2017.03.011

Tiku, V., Tan, M. W., and Dikic, I. (2020). Mitochondrial Functions in Infection and Immunity. *Trends Cell Biol.* 30, 263–275. doi: 10.1016/j.tcb.2020.01.006

Tolle, L., Yu, F. S., Kovach, M. A., Ballinger, M. N., Newstead, M. W., Zeng, X., et al. (2015). Redundant and cooperative interactions between TLR5 and NLRC4 in protective lung mucosal immunity against Pseudomonas aeruginosa. *J. Innate Immun.* 7, 177–186. doi: 10.1159/000367790

Turrens, J. F., Freeman, B. A., Levitt, J. G., and Crapo, J. D. (1982). The effect of hyperoxia on superoxide production by lung submitochondrial particles. *Arch. Biochem. Biophys.* 217, 401–410. doi: 10.1016/0003-9861(82)90518-5

Turrens, J. F. (2003). Mitochondrial formation of reactive oxygen species. *J. Physiol.* 552, 335–344. doi: 10.1113/jphysiol.2003.049478

Valdivieso, A. G., Marcucci, F., Taminelli, G., Guerrico, A. G., Alvarez, S., Teiber, M. L., et al. (2007). The expression of the mitochondrial gene MT-ND4 is downregulated in cystic fibrosis. *Biochem. Biophys. Res. Commun.* 356, 805–809. doi: 10.1016/j.bbrc.2007.03.057

Velsor, L. W., Kariya, C., Kachadourian, R., and Day, B. J. (2006). Mitochondrial oxidative stress in the lungs of cystic fibrosis transmembrane conductance regulator protein mutant mice. *Am. J. Respir. Cell Mol. Biol.* 35, 579–586. doi: 10.1165/rcmb.2005-0473OC

Villella, V. R., Esposito, S., Bruscia, E. M., Vicinanza, M., Cenci, S., Guido, S., et al. (2013). Disease-relevant proteostasis regulation of cystic fibrosis transmembrane conductance regulator. *Cell Death Differ.* 20, 1101–1115. doi: 10.1038/cdd.2013.46

Walle, T. (2011). Bioavailability of resveratrol. *Ann. N. Y. Acad. Sci.* 1215, 9–15. doi: 10.1111/j.1749-6632.2010.05842.x

West, A. P., Brodsky, I. E., Rahner, C., Woo, D. K., Erdjument-Bromage, H., Tempst, P., et al. (2011). TLR signalling augments macrophage bactericidal activity through mitochondrial ROS. *Nature* 472, 476–480. doi: 10.1038/nature09973

Wiegman, C. H., Michaeloudes, C., Haji, G., Narang, P., Clarke, C. J., Russell, K. E., et al. (2015). Oxidative stress-induced mitochondrial dysfunction drives inflammation and airway smooth muscle remodeling in patients with chronic obstructive pulmonary disease. *J. Allergy Clin. Immunol.* 136, 769–780. doi: 10.1016/j.jaci.2015.01.046

Wood, S. J., Goldufsky, J. W., Bello, D., Masood, S., and Shafikhani, S. H. (2015). Pseudomonas aeruginosa ExoT Induces Mitochondrial Apoptosis in Target Host Cells in a Manner That Depends on Its GTPase-activating Protein (GAP) Domain Activity. *J. Biol. Chem.* 290, 29063–29073. doi: 10.1074/jbc.M115.689950

Woods, J. J., Nemani, N., Shanmughapriya, S., Kumar, A., Zhang, M., Nathan, S. R., et al. (2019). A Selective and Cell-Permeable Mitochondrial Calcium Uniporter (MCU) Inhibitor Preserves Mitochondrial Bioenergetics after Hypoxia/Reoxygenation Injury. *ACS Cent. Sci.* 5, 153–166. doi: 10.1021/acscentsci.8b00773

Xu, Y., Nie, L., Yin, Y. G., Tang, J. L., Zhou, J. Y., Li, D. D., et al. (2012). Resveratrol protects against hyperglycemia-induced oxidative damage to mitochondria by activating SIRT1 in rat mesangial cells. *Toxicol. Appl. Pharmacol.* 259, 395–401. doi: 10.1016/j.taap.2011.09.028

Zang, Q. S., Sadek, H., Maass, D. L., Martinez, B., Ma, L., Kilgore, J. A., et al. (2012). Specific inhibition of mitochondrial oxidative stress suppresses inflammation and improves cardiac function in a rat pneumonia-related sepsis model. *Am. J. Physiol. Heart Circ. Physiol.* 302, H1847–H1859. doi: 10.1152/ajpheart.00203.2011

Zhou, R., Yazdi, A. S., Menu, P., and Tschopp, J. (2011). A role for mitochondria in NLRP3 inflammasome activation. *Nature* 469, 221–225. doi: 10.1038/nature09663

13

Update on Calcium Signaling in Cystic Fibrosis Lung Disease

Alessandro Rimessi[1,2†], *Veronica A. M. Vitto*[1†], *Simone Patergnani*[1] *and Paolo Pinton*[1,2*]

[1]Department of Medical Sciences and Laboratory for Technologies of Advanced Therapies (LTTA), University of Ferrara, Ferrara, Italy, [2]Center of Research for Innovative Therapies in Cystic Fibrosis, University of Ferrara, Ferrara, Italy

***Correspondence:**
Paolo Pinton
paolo.pinton@unife.it

†These authors have contributed equally to this work

Cystic fibrosis (CF) is an autosomal recessive disorder characterized by mutations in the cystic fibrosis transmembrane conductance regulator gene, which causes multifunctional defects that preferentially affect the airways. Abnormal viscosity of mucus secretions, persistent pathogen infections, hyperinflammation, and lung tissue damage compose the classical pathological manifestation referred to as CF lung disease. Among the multifunctional defects associated with defective CFTR, increasing evidence supports the relevant role of perturbed calcium (Ca^{2+}) signaling in the pathophysiology of CF lung disease. The Ca^{2+} ion is a critical player in cell functioning and survival. Its intracellular homeostasis is maintained by a fine balance between channels, transporters, and exchangers, mediating the influx and efflux of the ion across the plasma membrane and the intracellular organelles. An abnormal Ca^{2+} profile has been observed in CF cells, including airway epithelial and immune cells, with heavy repercussions on cell function, viability, and susceptibility to pathogens, contributing to proinflammatory overstimulation, organelle dysfunction, oxidative stress, and excessive cytokines release in CF lung. This review discusses the role of Ca^{2+} signaling in CF and how its dysregulation in airway epithelial and immune cells contributes to hyperinflammation in the CF lung. Finally, we provide an outlook on the therapeutic options that target the Ca^{2+} signaling to treat the CF lung disease.

Keywords: inflammatory disease, calcium signaling, lung disease, inflammation, cystic fibrosis, calcium

INTRODUCTION

Cystic fibrosis (CF) is a multiorgan genetic disease associated with mutations in the cystic fibrosis transmembrane conductance regulator (CFTR) gene, which preferentially affects the airways causing abnormal infiltration of polymorphonucleated cells, hyperinflammation, and severe lung damage (Riordan, 1993). According to the CF foundation patient registries, more than 70,000 people are living with CF worldwide and about one thousand new cases of CF are diagnosed only in United States each year. The CF is a complex disease, in which the type and severity of symptoms may differ from patient to patient, influencing the individual's health and the course of disease in a different manner.

The gene's product is a plasma membrane (PM) ion channel protein located on the apical surface of epithelial cells. Its activation is due by ATP and cAMP-dependent protein kinase A phosphorylations, which extrudes chloride (Cl-) and bicarbonate ions from airway cells (Jacquot et al., 2008). Although CF has long been recognized as an epithelial disease, the channel is expressed also in immune cells (Di et al., 2006; Ng et al., 2016). The most common mutation is the deletion of phenylalanine at position 508 (F508del-CFTR) and the substitution of the amino acid glycine by aspartate at position 551 (G551D-CFTR). The first mutation results in a misfolded protein retained in the endoplasmic reticulum (ER) to be prematurely degraded through the ubiquitin-proteasome pathway. The second is the most prevalent gating mutation, which abolishing the ATP-dependent gating led to a pronounced reduction of channel activity (Pedemonte et al., 2005; Farinha et al., 2013).

Moreover, defective CFTR induces an increased absorption of sodium (Na^+) coupled with the absence of Cl- secretion. This electrolytic disorder causes the dehydration of periciliary and mucus layers, leading to mucociliary dysfunction and airway mucus plugging (Boucher et al., 1988). An increased susceptibility to pathogen infections, including *Pseudomonas aeruginosa* (*P. aeruginosa*), is associated with defective CFTR, which leads to exaggerated lung inflammatory responses (Bruscia and Bonfield, 2016). In addition, CF patients airways are characterized by abnormal infiltration of neutrophils, which synthesize and release abundant proinflammatory mediators such as interleukin-8 (IL-8) and IL-1β, that contribute to overstimulating the inflammatory responses and worsening the pulmonary injury (Bruscia and Bonfield, 2016).

To improve the lung function, airway clearance techniques and administration of mucus thinner, such as mucolytics, contribute to maintaining the lung clear. Meanwhile, antibiotics and anti-inflammatory drugs fight the infection and consequent hyperinflammation, conditioning the days of CF patients. Recently, a new class of CFTR modulators has been introduced in CF therapy to correct and potentiate the defective CFTR channel. "Correctors" and "potentiators" have garnered much attention in the CF community, although their impact on downstream consequences, such as inflammation, remains debated. The new advances in CF care have drastically ameliorated the quality and duration of life of CF patients.

The calcium ion (Ca^{2+}) is a second messenger, which fulfills a plethora of intracellular functions (Giorgi et al., 2018). In addition to its prominent but ambiguous role in energy metabolism and cell death, Ca^{2+} is intimately involved in various cellular processes, such as autophagy and inflammation (Carafoli and Krebs, 2016; Marchi et al., 2018; Patergnani et al., 2020a). Therefore, it is not surprising that altered Ca^{2+} signaling represents a key factor in several inflammatory diseases, including CF. Airway epithelial and immune cells are critically dependent on Ca^{2+} signaling function and integrity. Consequently, perturbations in Ca^{2+} signaling have been observed in CF and are caused by intrinsic defects associated with CFTR deficiency and environmental stress related to recurrent bacterial infections, resulting in an exacerbated inflammatory response that favors lung injury (Ribeiro and Boucher, 2010; Antigny et al., 2011a; Rimessi et al., 2015a).

This review analyzes Ca^{2+} signaling in CF and how its dysregulation contributes to CF lung disease. We summarize the current knowledge and provide an outlook on the therapeutic options to treat the CF lung disease. In particular, we will focus on compounds that target the Ca^{2+} signaling and potentially would lead to adjusting the inflammatory response, thus suggesting new therapeutic strategies for this pulmonary disease.

CA^{2+} SIGNALING IN AIRWAY EPITHELIAL AND IMMUNE CELLS

The free cytosolic Ca^{2+} concentration $[Ca^{2+}]_{cyt}$ is very low with concentrations in the order of hundreds of nM. This characteristic is guaranteed by a regulated activity of pumps, exchangers, and channels that reside on the PM and by intracellular organelles, such as ER and Golgi, that act as intracellular Ca^{2+} store by accumulating ions in the order of hundreds of μM (**Figure 1**) (Bootman and Bultynck, 2020).

The advancements in the definition of Ca^{2+} signaling have evidenced the high spatiotemporal complexity and asynchronicity of Ca^{2+} responses. These responses are represented by localized $[Ca^{2+}]_{cyt}$ spikes that gradually propagate into the cell as Ca^{2+} waves (Berridge et al., 2003). In nonexcitable cells, such as airway epithelial and immune cells, the $[Ca^{2+}]_{cyt}$ spikes are caused by extracellular stimuli, which result in a Ca^{2+}-influx from the extracellular space. Agonists, including some proinflammatory and infectious stimuli (e.g., cytokines, bradykinin, prostaglandins, lipopolysaccharides, bacterial flagellin, and pili), are translated in intracellular Ca^{2+} signals through their interaction and subsequent activation of membrane receptors, such as Toll-Like Receptors (TLR) and G protein coupled receptors (GPCRs) linked to phospholipase C (PLC) (Wootten et al., 2018). Activating PLC types, such as PLCβ or γ, catalyzes the hydrolysis of phosphatidylinositol 4,5-bisphosphate (PIP2), giving rise to two second messengers: diacylglycerol (DAG) and 1,4,5-inositol trisphosphate (IP3) (**Figure 1i**) (Bill and Vines, 2020). DAG may activate transient receptor potential (TRP) canonic (TRPC) channels and classical and novel protein kinase C (PKC) isoforms (Rimessi et al., 2007; Curcic et al., 2019) (**Figure 1ii**). The DAG-triggering $[Ca^{2+}]_i$ spikes occur through the direct binding with TRPC channels in PM, in a PKC-independent manner (Curcic et al., 2019). The subfamily of TRPC channels is composed of seven members (TRPC1-7). They are nonselective ion channels permeable to Na^+ and Ca^{2+}. TRPC3, TRPC6, and TRPC7 are the principal contributors of DAG-dependent Ca^{2+}-entry in nonexcitable and excitable cells (**Figure 1ii**).

IP3 induces a transient increase in $[Ca^{2+}]_{cyt}$ through the binding with IP3 receptors (IP3Rs), which in turn trigger ER Ca^{2+}-release (Foskett et al., 2007) (**Figure 1v**). The temporal kinetics, the amplitude, and localization of generated Ca^{2+} spikes are strictly dependent on the nature of stimuli. All three IP3Rs induce local Ca^{2+} spikes with similar mean amplitudes, temporal characteristics, and spatial extents (Lock et al., 2018). Normally, IP3Rs are localized in cluster positioned near ER-mitochondria and ER-PM junctions, where the stromal interaction molecule (STIM)/Orai (Ca^{2+}-release activated Ca^{2+} modulator 1) complex accumulates Ca^{2+} after the ER store depletion (Thillaiappan et al., 2017; Marchi et al., 2018; Taylor and Machaca, 2019). Intraluminal $[Ca^{2+}]$ depletion induces a conformational change in STIM1 and STIM2 isoforms, which translocate in ER-PM interface to bind the PM Orai channel (**Figure 1iii**). The STIM/Orai complex stimulates the Orai channel opening, giving rise to the store operated Ca^{2+}-entry (SOCE) process from the extracellular space. This Ca^{2+}-influx mechanism replenishes

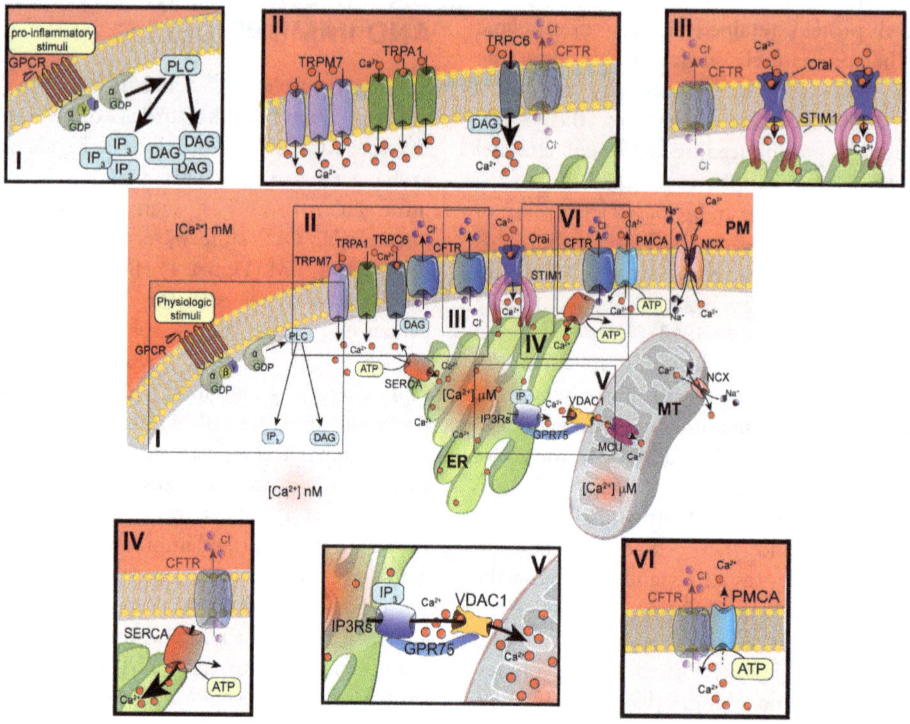

FIGURE 1 | Principal defects in Ca^{2+} signaling associated with defective CFTR channel. Schematic representation of intracellular Ca^{2+} signaling in airway cells. The cellular Ca^{2+} homeostasis is regulated by systems of Ca^{2+}-entry and Ca^{2+}-efflux located in plasma membrane and organelles. In the inset are reported the principal molecular systems involved in the abnormal intracellular Ca^{2+} signaling associated with defective CFTR channel, where the their dysfunction contributes to physiopathology of CF lung disease: I) increased PLC activity, due to GPCR-dependent overstimulation; II) increased TRP-dependent Ca^{2+}-entry, due to enhanced functional activity and/or expression; III) increased Orai insertion with consequent augments in Ca^{2+}-influx; IV) increased SERCA activity; V) increased MCU activity; and VI) reduced Ca^{2+}-efflux, due to altered PMCA activity. ATP, adenosine triphosphate; Ca^{2+}, calcium; CFTR, cystic fibrosis transmembrane conductance regulator; Cl-, chloride; DAG, diacylglycerol; ER, endoplasmic reticulum; GPCR, G protein coupled receptor; GPD, guanosine diphosphate; GRP75, glucose-related protein 75; IP3, inositol 1,4,5-triphosphate; IP3Rs; inositol trisphosphate receptors; MCU, mitochondrial calcium uniporter; NCX, sodium-calcium exchanger; Orai, calcium release activated calcium channel; PLC, phospholipase C; PM, plasma membrane; PMCA, PM-resident Ca^{2+}-ATPase; SERCA, ER-resident Ca^{2+}-ATPase; STIM1; stromal interaction molecule 1; TRPC, transient receptor potential (TRP) channels; VDAC1, voltage-dependent anion-selective channel 1.

the ER Ca^{2+} stores and sustains the IP3Rs-dependent phase of increased $[Ca^{2+}]_{cyt}$ (Bodnar et al., 2017). A preferential platform for clustering SOCE channels is the caveolae, PM lipid raft microdomains, where Ca^{2+} channels and their regulators are grouped to provide the Ca^{2+}-entry also in an IP3R-dependent manner upon the intracellular administration of IP_3 (Pani et al., 2008; Pulli et al., 2015).

Most of this free intracellular Ca^{2+} is bound by cytosolic proteins or organelles, such as mitochondria and lysosomes, which act as Ca^{2+} buffers (Schwaller, 2020). Another cytosolic Ca^{2+}-binding protein involved in the regulation of intracellular Ca^{2+} signaling is Calmodulin. It binds Ca^{2+} through four high affinity binding sites, promoting a direct association and opening of CFTR channel (Bozoky et al., 2017) and regulation of the activity of protein kinases and Ca^{2+}-pumps (Villalobo et al., 2018).

Mitochondria influence the $[Ca^{2+}]_{cyt}$ by inducing a transient sequestering of the Ca^{2+} released at the ER-mitochondria interfaces (Marchi et al., 2018). In these intimate and dynamic regions between ER and mitochondrial outer membranes (OMMs), called also mitochondria-associated ER membranes (MAMs), a series of specialized molecular bridges control the frequency of interactions, the size and the spacing between the organelles, and changing at front of cellular and functional requests (Simmen and Herrera-Cruz, 2018; Bootman and Bultynck, 2020). Thus, the mitochondrial Ca^{2+}-transfer is firstly favored by the distance from ER and number of mitochondria involved in these interorganelle couplings and secondly by the negative membrane potential in mitochondrial matrix generated by the respiratory chain (Csordas et al., 2010; Rimessi et al., 2015b). The Ca^{2+} is then transmitted into the matrix by the mitochondrial Ca^{2+} uniporter (MCU) (**Figure 1v**) (Baughman et al., 2011; De Stefani et al., 2011). MCU is a transmembrane protein of inner mitochondrial membrane (IMM), assembled as tetramer, which forms a high selective Ca^{2+}-channel with low affinity for the ion. Its activity is regulated by the EF-hand-containing Ca^{2+}-binding proteins mitochondrial calcium uptake 1 (MICU1) and MICU2, which together with other forming-channel elements, such as MCUb and essential MCU regulator (EMRE), constitute the MCU complex (**Figure 2**) (Marchi and Pinton, 2014). However, before reaching the IMM, Ca^{2+} must cross the OMM

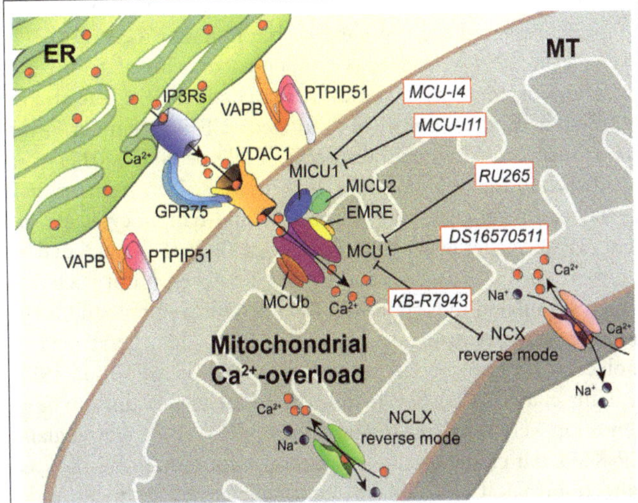

FIGURE 2 | Dampening the mitochondrial Ca^{2+}-overload in cystic fibrosis. The dysregulation of Ca^{2+} signaling in CF causes mitochondrial Ca^{2+}-overload in airway cells during the recurrent pathogen infections, which leads to organelle dysfunction with repercussion on ROS production and inflammatory responses. The mitochondrial Ca^{2+}-overload is mediated by an increased ER-mitochondria Ca^{2+} transfer through the IP3Rs-VDAC-MCU axis due to the stabilization of VAPB-PTPIP51 tethers. Indeed, the increased ENaC-dependent Na^+ absorption due to defective CFTR in CF could stimulate NCX and NCLX exchangers to work in reverse mode triggering intracellular and mitochondrial Ca^{2+}-influx, which may worsen the excessive mitochondrial Ca^{2+}-uptake. To dampen the detrimental Ca^{2+} accumulation in matrix, a new class of Ca^{2+} modulator drugs are under investigation; the mitochondrial Ca^{2+}-overload inhibitors act on MCU complex and mitochondrial Ca^{2+} exchangers in reverse mode to control the amount of Ca^{2+} imported into the matrix to avoid mitochondrial injury and oxidative stress in CF. Ca^{2+}, calcium; EMRE, essential MCU regulator; ER, endoplasmic reticulum; GRP75, glucose-related protein 75; IP3Rs, inositol trisphosphate receptors; MCU, mitochondrial Ca^{2+} uniporter; MICU1, mitochondrial calcium uptake protein 1; MICU2, mitochondrial calcium uptake protein 2; MT, mitochondrion; Na^+, sodium; NCX, sodium-calcium exchanger; NCLX, mitochondrial Na/Ca exchanger; PTPIP51, protein tyrosine phosphatase interacting protein 51; VAPB, vesicle-associated membrane protein-associated protein B; VDAC1, voltage-dependent anion-selective channel 1.

mediating the voltage-dependent anion channels (VDACs), involved also in the transport of adenosines (ATP, ADP) and metabolites, including pyruvate and malate (Shoshan-Barmatz et al., 2010). Three different isoforms of VDAC have been identified: VDAC1-3. Among them, VDAC1 has Ca^{2+} binding sites and is highly Ca^{2+} permeable and modulates the accessibility of ion to the mitochondrial intermembrane space (IMS) (Gincel et al., 2001). The mitochondrial Ca^{2+} is released more slowly back into the cytosol by Na^+-dependent exchange mechanisms in excitable and nonexcitable cells via Na^+/Ca^{2+} exchanger (NCX) and $Na^+/Ca^{2+}/Li^+$ exchanger (NCLX) (Khananshvili, 2014; Kostic and Sekler, 2019). NCX, located on the OMM, may operate either in forward mode, extruding one Ca^{2+} ion from mitochondrial intermembrane space *vs* three Na^+ ions in influx from cytosol, or in reverse mode, exchanging Ca^{2+}-influx/Na^+-efflux. NCLX, located on the IMM, transports Ca^{2+} outside the matrix in exchange of either Na^+ or Li^+ at similar rates (**Figures 1, 2**). In nonexcitable cells, the mitochondrial Ca^{2+} is also extruded by H^+/Ca^{2+} exchanger (Nishizawa et al., 2013).

However, after removing the stimulus, the $[Ca^{2+}]_{cyt}$ is rapidly lowered through the activation of Ca^{2+}-ATPase pumps located on the PM and ER, respectively (**Figure 1iv–vi**). PM Ca^{2+}-ATPase (PMCA) push out Ca^{2+} from cell while sarco/endoplasmic reticulum Ca^{2+}-ATPase (SERCA) pumps Ca^{2+} back into the ER (Domi et al., 2007). These pumps are P-type ATPase, which exchange one (PMCA) or two (SERCA) Ca^{2+} ions for hydrolyzed ATP (Strehler and Treiman, 2004; Chen et al., 2020a). PMCA presents a high Ca^{2+}-affinity but low Ca^{2+}-transporting rate. In support of the PM Na^+/Ca^{2+} exchangers, a second Ca^{2+}-efflux system with low Ca^{2+}-affinity but high Ca^{2+}-transporting rate contributes to clamping the $[Ca^{2+}]_{cyt}$ at homeostatic levels.

ABNORMAL CA^{2+} SIGNALING IN CYSTIC FIBROSIS AND PHYSIOPATHOLOGICAL CONSEQUENCES

To date, increasing evidence highlights the importance of perturbed Ca^{2+} signaling in CF lung disease's physiopathology. The abnormal Ca^{2+} profile observed in CF airway epithelial and immune cells is initially due to intrinsic defects associated with mutated CFTR. It is sustained successively by recurrent pathogen infections and by overstimulation of released proinflammatory mediators, resulting in detrimental lung inflammation (Ribeiro, 2006; Antigny et al., 2011a).

Defective CFTR and Ca^{2+} Signaling

Ca^{2+} signals have key roles in the CFTR channel function and in airway immune responses, which are perturbed in CF. Ca^{2+} signaling controls the CFTR protein expression levels and internalization (Bargon et al., 1992; Patel et al., 2019), while at level of airways, it regulates ciliary beating and secretion of fluid and antimicrobial agents (Salathe, 2007; Waterer, 2012; Lee and Foskett, 2014).

In CF, Ca^{2+} exacerbates the airway inflammatory responses (**Figure 1i**). Its dysregulation has been observed in several human CF patient-derived primary cells: airway epithelial cells (Rimessi et al., 2015a), bronchial goblet cells (Roomans, 1986), skin fibroblasts (Shapiro et al., 1978), kidney cells (Katz et al., 1988), and immune cells such as leukocytes, neutrophils, and lymphocytes (Banschbach et al., 1978; Waller et al., 1984; Robledo-Avila et al., 2018). In all of them, the $[Ca^{2+}]_{cyt}$ was increased compared to non-CF cells, demonstrating that functional CFTR regulates the Ca^{2+} homeostasis conditioning and in turn the interorganelle Ca^{2+}-transfer evoked by stimuli (Rimessi et al., 2015a).

The increased $[Ca^{2+}]_{cyt}$ in CF airways results from an enhanced Ca^{2+}-entry mediated by PM Ca^{2+}-channels and reduced Ca^{2+}-efflux operated by PMCA, influencing the Ca^{2+} accumulation into the stores (**Figures 1i,ii,vi**) (Philippe et al., 2015). In particular, the TRP channel family is involved in abnormal Ca^{2+}-entry in CF airway cells (reviewed in (Grebert et al., 2019)) (**Figure 1ii**). TRPC6-mediated Ca^{2+}-influx was increased in F508del-CFTR and G551D-CFTR airway cells with respect to non-CF cells when exposed to 1-oleoyl-sn-glycerol, a synthetic, cell-permeable compound analogous to DAG, used as an activator of PKC (Antigny et al., 2011b). No difference in TRPC6 expression justified the discrepancy, but it has been observed that the physical interaction between WT-CFTR and TRPC6 channel downregulated the Ca^{2+}-influx in airway epithelial cells, suggesting that the lacked or reduced CFTR expression in PM in CF cells perturbs the functional coupling between the two channels favoring the abnormal Ca^{2+}-entry (Antigny et al., 2011b). However, specific TRPC6-silencing or the CFTR-corrector agent's administration, VX-770, reduced the abnormal $[Ca^{2+}]_{cyt}$ increment and IL-8 release, indicating that defective CFTR worsens the inflammatory response affecting the TRPC6 activity (Vachel et al., 2013). Similar effects were also observed for TRP vanilloid 4 and 6 channels (TRPV4 and TRPV6), respectively. The intracellular Ca^{2+} elevation by TRPV4 stimulation led to CFTR channel activation in bronchial epithelial cells in physiological condition (Genovese et al., 2019). The increased Ca^{2+}-influx and the inflammatory response in CF were attenuated by genetic manipulation of TRPV channels and by low temperature-mediated F508del-CFTR rescue in CFTR-deficient cells, mediating reduction of $[Ca^{2+}]_{cyt}$ mitigated release of IL-8, prostaglandin E2 and keratinocyte chemo-attractant (Vachel et al., 2015; Henry et al., 2016).

In addition, an increased expression in PM of nonselective Ca^{2+} channel TRP subfamily M member 7 (TRPM7) has been observed in both F508del-CFTR- and G551D-CFTR-expressing cells, resulting in higher Ca^{2+}-influx than WT-CFTR-expressing cells (Huguet et al., 2016). A similar increase in expression of TRP ankyrin subtype 1 channel (TRPA1) was observed in human CF respiratory epithelium and in CF airway cells. Here, TRPA1 pharmacological modulation controls the transcription and release of several proinflammatory mediators, including IL-8 and IL-1β, in a Ca^{2+}-dependent manner (Prandini et al., 2016). Orai expression resulted in enhanced CF airway cells with a consequent increase in Ca^{2+}-entry and release of IL-8 (**Figure 1iii**) (Balghi et al., 2011). The STIM1 migration and Orai activity do not occur only during ER depletion but may also occur upon mitochondrial Ca^{2+}-efflux, as demonstrated in basophilic leukemia, embryonic fibroblast, and kidney cells, with dangerous repercussions on inflammation (Singaravelu et al., 2011; Delmotte et al., 2012).

Abnormal Ca^{2+}-entry is a primary signal associated with defective CFTR that conditions the ER Ca^{2+}-accumulation and mitochondrial Ca^{2+}-overload elicited in CF cells, already due also to increased SERCA activity (**Figure 1vi**) (Philippe et al., 2015). The functional interaction between WT-CFTR with SERCA2b and PMCA observed in non-CF cells is partially lost in CF cells, due to ER retention of F508del-CFTR mutant, with several implications on the ER and PM Ca^{2+} channel activities, which potentiate the intraluminal Ca^{2+} accumulation (Norez et al., 2006). A study identified Calumenin as interactor of CFTR channel, a Ca^{2+}-binding protein located primarily in the ER able to regulate ER Ca^{2+} homeostasis, interacting with SERCA and the ER Ca^{2+} channel ryanodine receptors (RyRs) (Vorum et al., 1999; Jung et al., 2006; Sahoo et al., 2009; Teng et al., 2012). The binding between Calumenin and CFTR increased when the channel presented the prevalent gating mutation G551D-CFTR (Teng et al., 2012). Indeed, Calumenin contributed to the ER retention of mutated F508del-CFTR channel, if silenced PM expression and activity of mutated CFTR channel were restored in bronchial epithelial cells (Philippe et al., 2017).

Mitochondrial Ca^{2+}-uptake was increased in primary CF airway epithelial cells, skin fibroblasts, and lymphocytes (Feigal et al., 1982; Waller et al., 1984; Rimessi et al., 2015a), mediated by a greater ER Ca^{2+}-transfer and by perturbed respiratory activity, which stimulated mitochondrial ROS production, mitochondrial injury, and release of mitochondrial damage-associated molecular patterns in CF lung (**Figure 1v**) (Feigal et al., 1982; Antigny et al., 2011a). Severe mitochondrial dysfunctions in basal condition were restricted to human F508del-CFTR tracheal gland CF-KM4 cell clone. In this cell clone, authors found a reduced mitochondrial Ca^{2+} uptake consequence of mitochondrial membrane depolarization and perturbed network, resulting from an altered mitochondrial physiology (Antigny et al., 2009).

At demonstration of the presence of an abnormal mitochondrial Ca^{2+} accumulation, different studies unveiled that, by using corrector agents, such as VX-770 and VX-809, or by rescuing functional F508del-CFTR, it is possible to normalize the mitochondrial $[Ca^{2+}]$ levels with beneficial repercussions on oxidative stress and the levels of proinflammatory mediators released, such as IL-8 and the inflammasome-dependent cytokine IL-1β (Vachel et al., 2013; Rimessi et al., 2015a; Philippe et al., 2015).

Ca^{2+} Signaling in CF Infection and Inflammation

Airway epithelial cells respond to pathogens, such as *P. aeruginosa*, through Ca^{2+}-dependent mechanisms to produce proinflammatory mediators to initiate the inflammatory response (Ratner et al., 2001; Fu et al., 2007). Different bacterial constituents, including LPS, promote TRP-dependent Ca^{2+}-entry and ER Ca^{2+}-release via IP3Rs (Buyck et al., 2013). Pili and flagellin interact with TLR2, TLR4, TLR5, and Asialo ganglio-N-tetraosylceramide (Asialo GM1) receptor and induce the expression of IL-8 mediating the activation of NF-kB, which is also phosphorylated by Ca^{2+}-dependent PKC isoforms α and β that respond to intracellular Ca^{2+} flux following IP3R-dependent ER Ca^{2+}-release (Pinton et al., 2004; Asehnoune et al., 2005; Chun and Prince, 2006). This Ca^{2+}-dependent activation of NF-kB is also sustained by Asialo GM1-dependent nucleotides released from airway epithelial cells that interact with flagellin, which binds the purinergic P2Y receptors active intracellular Ca^{2+}-signaling (Mcnamara et al., 2006; Billet and Hanrahan, 2013).

In CF, the airway epithelial cells respond to the recurrent infection generating abnormal Ca^{2+} mobilization to produce many cytokines and chemokines, useful to recruit leukocytes to contrast the accumulated bacteria in the airways. This overstimulation determines a Ca^{2+}-dependent hyperinflammation phenotype. CF airway epithelial cells result in hyperresponsiveness to pathogens due to the increased $[Ca^{2+}]_{cyt}$, which contributes to 1) ER expansion and increased intraluminal [Ca^{2+}]; 2) mitochondrial Ca^{2+}-overload and consequent organelle dysfunction; and 3) an exuberant and more prolonged NF-kB activation, priming the cells to excessive expression and release of proinflammatory mediators (Ribeiro et al., 2005; Tabary et al., 2006; Rimessi et al., 2015a; Rimessi et al., 2020).

The ER Ca^{2+} store expansion in CF airway cells is due to activation of the inositol-requiring enzyme 1 (IRE1)/X-box binding 1 (XBP-1) pathway, which is not the consequence of misfolded CFTR. Reductions in ER Ca^{2+}-release in CF samples were also obtained by correcting F508del-CFTR trafficking by miglustat (N-butyldeoxynojirimycin) or low temperature (27°C) (Antigny et al., 2008a; Antigny et al., 2008b). Antigny et al. demonstrated that the abnormal ER Ca^{2+}-release in CF gland CF-KM4 clone was due to a dysfunctional IP3Rs, consequence of ER retention of mutant CFTR channel (Antigny et al., 2008b). The importance of IP3Rs in CF was then confirmed by Martins et al. in nasal epithelial cells, where it was demonstrated that the ER retention of F508del-CFTR determined a functional interference with IP3-receptor binding protein IRBIT, which suppresses the activation of IP3Rs by competing with IP3 for binding to the ligand-binding domain (Ando et al., 2006; Martins et al., 2011).

However, the increased flux of newly synthesized proinflammatory mediators into the ER in response to recurrent infections contributes to ER expansion (Ribeiro and Lubamba, 2017). Besides, changes in the intracellular redistribution of ER have been observed in response to pathogens. In this case, the ER moved to the apical level of polarized CF airway epithelial cells to facilitate the GPCR-induced Ca^{2+} responses (Ribeiro et al., 2005).

Recently, Rimessi et al. demonstrated that *P. aeruginosa* infection increases ER-mitochondria juxtapositions in CF airway epithelial cells by stabilizing the ER protein vesicle-associated membrane protein-associated protein B (VAPB) and the outer mitochondrial membrane protein tyrosine phosphatase interacting protein 51 (PTPIP51) tethers, favoring the mitochondrial Ca^{2+} transfer via MCU (**Figure 2**) (Rimessi et al., 2020). This led to mitochondrial membrane potential loss, ROS production, and organelle dysfunction, inducing persistent mitochondrial Unfolding Protein Response (UPR^{mt}) and NLRP3 inflammasome activation. In turn, these processes downregulated the selective autophagic responses, mitophagy, and xenophagy, resulting in augmented pathogen survival and worsening of inflammatory response (Rimessi et al., 2015a; Rimessi et al., 2020). Thus, the mitochondrial Ca^{2+}-overload in CF airway cells plays a crucial role in the evolution of CF pulmonary inflammation. Preventing the mitochondrial Ca^{2+}-overload, via MCU inhibition, the *P. aeruginosa*-dependent mitochondrial dysfunction was abrogated in CF airway cells, while the selective autophagic responses were rectified (Rimessi et al., 2020).

A higher predisposition of CF airway cells to NLRP3 inflammasome activation is also due to the dysregulation of ENaC-dependent Na^+-influx associated with defective CFTR, which predisposes the cells to K^+-efflux, a further activating signal to NLRP3 inflammasome (Scambler et al., 2019).

Excessive Ca^{2+}-dependent IL-8 secretion is critical for CF lung disease development and is responsible for abundant neutrophil recruitment into the lung. IL-8 production is 13-fold higher in CF bronchial cells than non-CF cells and occurs through persistent and prolonged NF-kB activation (Tabary et al., 2000). A Single Nucleotide Polymorphisms (SNP) genetic study from a panel of 135 genes implicated in the signal transduction for neutrophil recruitment, identifying PLC beta-3 (PLCB3) gene on top of the rank, involved in the excessive expression and release of IL-8 during *P. aeruginosa* infection in F508del-CFTR patients (Bezzerri et al., 2011). The c.2534C > T (p.S845L) PLCB3 is a loss-of-function variant associated with a mild progression of CF lung disease, where its inability to trigger intracellular Ca^{2+} transient limited the activation of Ca^{2+}-dependent PKCs and NF-kB, reducing the *P. aeruginosa*-dependent induction of IL-8 transcription and protein release in primary CF patient-derived airway epithelial cells (Rimessi et al., 2018). Similar effects have been observed by inhibiting the Ca^{2+}-dependent PKCα isoform with β-sitosterol, which blocked the *P. aeruginosa*-triggering IL-8 induction and release in CF airway cells (Lampronti et al., 2017).

The abnormal intracellular Ca^{2+} signaling associated with defective CFTR also implies the abundant neutrophils recruited into CF lung during the recurrent bacterial infections. An increased $[Ca^{2+}]_{cyt}$ has been measured in human CF neutrophils compared to non-CF, which correlates with a reduced antimicrobial killing capacity due to diminished NADPH oxidase response and impaired secretion of neutrophil extracellular traps (Robledo-Avila et al., 2018). The higher $[Ca^{2+}]_{cyt}$ in CF neutrophils is sustained by increased Ca^{2+}-entry via TRP channels, especially TRPM2 and TRPM7 channels, which when inhibited with 2-aminoethoxydiphenylborane restored the antimicrobial response of CF neutrophils during infection, preventing the intracellular Ca^{2+}-overloading (Heiner et al., 2005; Park et al., 2014; Robledo-Avila et al., 2018).

TARGETING CA^{2+} SIGNALING AS ALTERNATIVE ANTI-INFLAMMATORY APPROACH

Understanding the molecular mechanisms that induce hyperinflammation in CF lung through the Ca^{2+} signaling impairment helps to identify new and alternative therapeutic targets to treat the CF lung disease. Thus, pharmacological Ca^{2+} signaling-targeting agents aim to control the increased $[Ca^{2+}]_{cyt}$, ER, and mitochondrial Ca^{2+}-overload in CF airway epithelial and immune cells, which may be considered a new class of anti-inflammatory drugs to prevent the hyperinflammatory response in CF.

TRP Channel Inhibitors

TRPA1 results in a druggable target to control the excessive inflammation in CF. The selective inhibition of TRPA1, by HC03 or A96 antagonist, reduced the induction and release of IL-8, IL-1β, and TNFα in CF patient-derived airway cells during *P. aeruginosa* infection (Prandini et al., 2016). Recently, the new antagonists of TRPA1 ODM-108, CB-625, CB-189625, and HX-100, which were under investigation in different phases of clinical trials to treat asthma and chronic obstructive pulmonary disease, have been discontinued for pharmacokinetics reasons (Chen and Terrett, 2020). In addition, GRC-17536, which had obtained promising results in preclinical studies on inflammatory animal models, has been suspended from clinical trials (Preti et al., 2012; Mukhopadhyay et al., 2014; Chen and Terrett, 2020). Also, TRPV4 plays a role in the excessive Ca^{2+}-entry in CF. A new inhibitor derived from the TRPV4-inhibitor GSK205, called compound 16-8, has been developed to target simultaneously TRPV4 and TRPA1 channel to block the Ca^{2+}-influx, showing the potentially advantageous property to apply to CF hyperinflammation (Kanju et al., 2016).

TRPC6 is another druggable target to counteract the increased $[Ca^{2+}]_{cyt}$ in CF. BI-749327 is an orally selective TRPC6-inhibitor used to suppress renal inflammatory cell infiltration and fibrosis, ameliorating renal stress-induced disease (Lin et al., 2019). SAR7334 was initially identified as a potent TRPC6-inhibitor, but this agent may inhibit the Ca^{2+}-influx mediated by TRPC3 and TRPC7. SAR7334 attenuated the IL-6 and IL-8 release in human bronchial epithelial cells exposed to ozone (O_3), protecting from the O_3-induced airway inflammatory response *in vivo* (Chen et al., 2020b). The nonselectivity of TRPC antagonist SKF-96365 limits the clinical usefulness of this drug although it reduced the LPS-dependent secretion of TNFα and IL-6 in microglia. In contrast, carvacrol, a phenolic monoterpene, through the selective inhibition of TRPM7, reduced the oversecretion of proinflammatory cytokines such as IL-1β, TNFα, and IL-6 in endotoxemic rats (Heo et al., 2015; Gatica et al., 2019).

PLC Inhibitors

PLC activity concurs to abnormal Ca^{2+} signaling in CF inducing the TRP channels activation and ER Ca^{2+}-release through the recurrent generation of DAG and IP3. Thus, the inhibition of PLC may contribute to attenuating the hyperinflammatory response in CF, reducing the Ca^{2+}-entry and the mitochondrial Ca^{2+}-overload limiting TRP channels activation and ER-mitochondria Ca^{2+}-transfer, respectively. Edelfosine was the first PLC inhibitor identified, decreasing the ER Ca^{2+}-release in tumor cells, but its cytotoxicity limits the clinical usefulness (Berkovic, 1998). U73122 is another PLC inhibitor and is used as an anti-inflammatory agent in different pathological contexts. U73122 may inhibit the LPS- or influenza A virus-induced expression of cytokines IL-1β and TNFα in human promonocyte U937 cells and in mouse primary peritoneal macrophages (Zhu et al., 2015; Zhu et al., 2016). Unfortunately, accumulating reports highlight off-target effects of U73122, including SERCA, Kir3, and Ca^{2+}-activated K^+ channels, calling into question its selectivity (Klose et al., 2008; Hollywood et al., 2010). A high-throughput analysis has been performed on 6,280 compounds, identifying three putative PLC activity inhibitors. Unfortunately, these compounds are not optimal to inhibit cellular PLC activity because they present a reduced cell permeability and a limited potency. Nevertheless, these compounds may be useful for development of new drugs to interrupt the abnormal signaling cascades controlled by PLCs, for the treatment of human diseases, including cancer (Huang et al., 2013).

Mitochondrial Ca^{2+}-Overload Inhibitors

The mitochondrial Ca^{2+}-overload inhibitors are pharmacological agents that by preventing the detrimental Ca^{2+} accumulation in the matrix reduce mitochondrial injury and oxidative stress, which are necessary to amplify the proinflammatory signals and activate NLRP3 inflammasome in CF lung disease (**Figure 2**) (Rimessi et al., 2015a; Rimessi et al., 2020). Limiting the excessive Ca^{2+} transport into mitochondria, via MCU, represents the first therapeutic approach with promising results both *in vitro* and *in vivo* in CF (Rimessi et al., 2015a; Rimessi et al., 2020). The MCU inhibitor, KB-R7943, reduced lung inflammation in *P. aeruginosa*-inoculated CF mice. The treated mice showed a reduction of interstitial inflammatory infiltrate with a general reduction in the congestion of lung parenchyma and restoration at the level of interalveolar septa of inflammatory infiltrate clearing conditions (Rimessi et al., 2020). Indeed, KB-R7943 rectified the unbalanced selective autophagic activities, thus restoring mitochondrial quality control and bacterial clearance capacity in CF airway cells. KB-R7943, designed to inhibit NCX in reverse mode, is the first cell-permeable MCU inhibitor available (Iwamoto et al., 1996; Santo-Domingo et al., 2007). Its nonspecificity and toxicity at high concentrations have limited its clinical usefulness, but its multitasking activity in CF on inflammation, mitochondrial stress response, and autophagy could represent an important starting point to develop new drugs to treat CF (**Figure 2**). A new class of selective and cell-permeable MCU inhibitors is now commercially available, namely, Ru265 and DS16570511, until now used only *in vitro*, but could have therapeutic implications in CF in the future (Kon et al., 2017; Woods et al., 2019).

The abnormal mitochondrial Ca^{2+}-uptake in CF may be controlled through MCU and mitochondrial NCX reverse targeting. The increased ENaC-dependent Na^+ absorption in CF could stimulate NCX and NCLX exchanger to work in reverse mode, triggering intracellular and mitochondrial Ca^{2+}-influx (Berdiev et al., 2009; Verkhratsky et al., 2018).

As an alternative, mitochondrial Ca^{2+}-overload may be prevented by inhibiting MICU1 activity (**Figure 2**). MCU complex comprises the pore-forming MCU protein, EMRE, and the gatekeepers MICU1 and MICU2, which regulate the MCU activity sensing the changes in $[Ca^{2+}]_{cyt}$. Recently, two new pharmacological MICU1 inhibitors have been developed, MCU-i4 and MCU-i11, both blocking the IP3-dependent mitochondrial Ca^{2+}-uptake, maintaining the gatekeeping role of their target (Di Marco et al., 2020). Hence, the MICU1 inhibitors should allow a greater fine-tuning modulation of mitochondrial Ca^{2+}-uptake than the known MCU inhibitors. This aspect could be relevant to treat the hyperinflammation in CF lung disease. The last strategy feasible should be to activate the mitochondrial Ca^{2+}-efflux mechanisms, but selective activators or inducer have not been identified.

Some potential pitfalls could emerge about mitochondrial Ca^{2+}-overload inhibitors, concerning the safety and biochemical stability of new molecules *in vivo*, the limitations in current knowledge (being recently discovered), and the long-term efficacy of mitochondrial Ca^{2+} signaling modulation that would be expected to alter the cell metabolism. However, no differences in basal oxygen consumption have been observed between WT and MCU-KO mice, suggesting that basal metabolism was not markedly altered in absence of mitochondrial Ca^{2+} signal (Pan et al., 2013; Murphy et al., 2014).

The enhancement of mitochondrial quality control through the pharmacological modulation of mitochondrial Ca^{2+} signaling is emerging as alternative anti-inflammatory strategy for the prevention or treatment of mitochondrial-associated disorders, such as CF (Patergnani et al., 2020b). Drugs that directly affect mitochondria, and thus mitochondrial Ca^{2+} signaling, have been recently used as a main mode of action to treat diseases, such as type 2 diabetes and cancer, as well as upregulating the immune system to clear infection with promising success (Stoker et al., 2019).

CONCLUSION

Substantial evidence supports the theory that the dysregulation in Ca^{2+} signaling associated with defective CFTR is essential for the development of the hyperinflammatory phenotype observed in CF lungs. This dysregulation involves different cells leading to multifunctional defects in CF patients. Both airway epithelial and immune cells are affected, with heavy repercussions on cell function, viability, and susceptibility to pathogens, which contribute significantly to the degeneration of pathological conditions of CF lung disease. Targeting the abnormal Ca^{2+} signaling in CF represents a new and attractive therapeutic strategy useful for reducing the proinflammatory overstimulation, organelle dysfunction, oxidative stress, and cytokines release in the CF lung.

"Correctors" and "potentiators" that are the new frontier in CF therapy, despite their positive impact in the CF community, are debated about their downstream consequences, in particular on inflammation. Evidence shows that *P. aeruginosa* burden decreased in the first six months of modulator therapy but rebounded thereafter, increasing the inflammatory response (Hisert et al., 2017). In addition, *P. aeruginosa* has been shown to directly reduce the apical membrane expression of rescued ΔF508CFTR and the following chloride secretion (Rubino et al., 2014). These facts are relevant since the presence of *P. aeruginosa* infection could *per se* render the recent CF therapies less effective. Therefore, alternative approaches aimed at activating early anti-inflammatory pathways to prevent organ damage before patients become symptomatic are needed. To date, new class of alternative anti-inflammatory drugs is emerging to prevent the inflammatory signal amplification and tissue degeneration related to chronic inflammation in CF. The cure of the lung pathology of CF patients will rely on the association of drugs acting as "correctors" and "potentiators" on the mutated CFTR protein together with novel anti-inflammatory drugs, such as the Ca^{2+}-modulators, and more active antibacterial drugs against *P. aeruginosa*.

AUTHOR CONTRIBUTIONS

All authors listed have made a substantial, direct, and intellectual contribution to the work and approved it for publication.

FUNDING

AR is supported by the Italian Cystic Fibrosis Research Foundation, grant FFC #20/2015, local funds from the University of Ferrara, FIR-2017, the Italian Ministry of Health (GR-2016-02364602), and the Italian Ministry of Education, University and Research (PRIN Grant 2017XA5J5N). The research was funded by grants from the Italian Cystic Fibrosis Research Foundation, FFC#12/2010 and #19/2014, Italian Association for Cancer Research (AIRC, IG-23670), Telethon (GGP11139B), local funds from the University of Ferrara, and the Italian Ministry of Education, University and Research (PRIN Grant 2017E5L5P3) to PP. PP is grateful to Camilla degli Scrovegni for continuous support. SP is supported by Fondazione Umberto Veronesi.

REFERENCES

Ando, H., Mizutani, A., Kiefer, H., Tsuzurugi, D., Michikawa, T., and Mikoshiba, K. (2006). IRBIT suppresses IP3 receptor activity by competing with IP3 for the common binding site on the IP3 receptor. *Mol. Cel.* 22, 795–806. doi:10.1016/j.molcel.2006.05.017

Antigny, F., Girardin, N., Raveau, D., Frieden, M., Becq, F., and Vandebrouck, C. (2009). Dysfunction of mitochondria Ca^{2+} uptake in cystic fibrosis airway epithelial cells. *Mitochondrion* 9, 232–241. doi:10.1016/j.mito.2009.02.003

Antigny, F., Norez, C., Becq, F., and Vandebrouck, C. (2008a). Calcium homeostasis is abnormal in cystic fibrosis airway epithelial cells but is normalized after rescue of F508del-CFTR. *Cell Calcium* 43, 175–183. doi:10.1016/j.ceca.2007.05.002

Antigny, F., Norez, C., Becq, F., and Vandebrouck, C. (2011a). CFTR and Ca signaling in cystic fibrosis. *Front. Pharmacol.* 2, 67. doi:10.3389/fphar.2011.00067

Antigny, F., Norez, C., Cantereau, A., Becq, F., and Vandebrouck, C. (2008b). Abnormal spatial diffusion of Ca^{2+} in F508del-CFTR airway epithelial cells. *Respir. Res.* 9, 70. doi:10.1186/1465-9921-9-70

Antigny, F., Norez, C., Dannhoffer, L., Bertrand, J., Raveau, D., Corbi, P., et al. (2011b). Transient receptor potential canonical channel 6 links Ca^{2+} mishandling to cystic fibrosis transmembrane conductance regulator channel dysfunction in cystic fibrosis. *Am. J. Respir. Cel Mol. Biol.* 44, 83–90. doi:10.1165/rcmb.2009-0347OC

Asehnoune, K., Strassheim, D., Mitra, S., Yeol Kim, J., and Abraham, E. (2005). Involvement of PKCalpha/beta in TLR4 and TLR2 dependent activation of NF-kappaB. *Cell Signal* 17, 385–394. doi:10.1016/j.cellsig.2004.08.005

Balghi, H., Robert, R., Rappaz, B., Zhang, X., Wohlhuter-Haddad, A., Evagelidis, A., et al. (2011). Enhanced Ca^{2+} entry due to Orai1 plasma membrane insertion increases IL-8 secretion by cystic fibrosis airways. *FASEB J.* 25, 4274–4291. doi:10.1096/fj.11-187682

Banschbach, M. W., Karam, A. G., Love, P. K., and Hilman, B. C. (1978). Cystic fibrosis serum promotes [45Ca] uptake by normal human leukocytes. *Biochem. Biophys. Res. Commun.* 84, 922–927. doi:10.1016/0006-291x(78)91671-6

Bargon, J., Trapnell, B. C., Chu, C. S., Rosenthal, E. R., Yoshimura, K., Guggino, W. B., et al. (1992). Down-regulation of cystic fibrosis transmembrane conductance regulator gene expression by agents that modulate intracellular divalent cations. *Mol. Cel Biol.* 12, 1872–1878. doi:10.1128/mcb.12.4.1872

Baughman, J. M., Perocchi, F., Girgis, H. S., Plovanich, M., Belcher-Timme, C. A., Sancak, Y., et al. (2011). Integrative genomics identifies MCU as an essential component of the mitochondrial calcium uniporter. *Nature* 476, 341–345. doi:10.1038/nature10234

Berdiev, B. K., Qadri, Y. J., and Benos, D. J. (2009). Assessment of the CFTR and ENaC association. *Mol. Biosyst.* 5, 123–127. doi:10.1039/b810471a

Berkovic, D. (1998). Cytotoxic etherphospholipid analogues. *Gen. Pharmacol.* 31, 511–517. doi:10.1016/s0306-3623(98)00081-0

Berridge, M. J., Bootman, M. D., and Roderick, H. L. (2003). Calcium signalling: dynamics, homeostasis and remodelling. *Nat. Rev. Mol. Cel Biol.* 4, 517–529. doi:10.1038/nrm1155

Bezzerri, V., D'adamo, P., Rimessi, A., Lanzara, C., Crovella, S., Nicolis, E., et al. (2011). Phospholipase C-beta3 is a key modulator of IL-8 expression in cystic fibrosis bronchial epithelial cells. *J. Immunol.* 186, 4946–4958. doi:10.4049/jimmunol.1003535

Bill, C. A., and Vines, C. M. (2020). Phospholipase C. *Adv. Exp. Med. Biol.* 1131, 215–242. doi:10.1007/978-3-030-12457-1_9

Billet, A., and Hanrahan, J. W. (2013). The secret life of CFTR as a calcium-activated chloride channel. *J. Physiol. (Lond)* 591, 5273–5278. doi:10.1113/jphysiol.2013.261909

Bodnar, D., Chung, W. Y., Yang, D., Hong, J. H., Jha, A., and Muallem, S. (2017). STIM-TRP pathways and microdomain organization: Ca^{2+} influx channels: the orai-STIM1-TRPC complexes. *Adv. Exp. Med. Biol.* 993, 139–157. doi:10.1007/978-3-319-57732-6_8

Bootman, M. D., and Bultynck, G. (2020). Fundamentals of cellular calcium signaling: a primer. *Cold Spring Harb Perspect. Biol.* 12, a038802. doi:10.1101/cshperspect.a038802

Boucher, R. C., Cotton, C. U., Gatzy, J. T., Knowles, M. R., and Yankaskas, J. R. (1988). Evidence for reduced Cl- and increased Na^{+} permeability in cystic fibrosis human primary cell cultures. *J. Physiol. (Lond)* 405, 77–103. doi:10.1113/jphysiol.1988.sp017322

Bozoky, Z., Ahmadi, S., Milman, T., Kim, T. H., Du, K., Di Paola, M., et al. (2017). Synergy of cAMP and calcium signaling pathways in CFTR regulation. *Proc. Natl. Acad. Sci. USA* 114, E2086–E2095. doi:10.1073/pnas.1613546114

Bruscia, E. M., and Bonfield, T. L. (2016). Innate and adaptive immunity in cystic fibrosis. *Clin. Chest Med.* 37, 17–29. doi:10.1016/j.ccm.2015.11.010

Buyck, J. M., Verriere, V., Benmahdi, R., Higgins, G., Guery, B., Matran, R., et al. (2013). P. aeruginosa LPS stimulates calcium signaling and chloride secretion via CFTR in human bronchial epithelial cells. *J. Cyst Fibros* 12, 60–67. doi:10.1016/j.jcf.2012.06.007

Carafoli, E., and Krebs, J. (2016). Why calcium? How calcium became the best communicator. *J. Biol. Chem.* 291, 20849–20857. doi:10.1074/jbc.R116.735894

Chen, H., and Terrett, J. A. (2020). Transient receptor potential ankyrin 1 (TRPA1) antagonists: a patent review (2015–2019). *Expert Opin. Ther. Pat.* 30, 643–657. doi:10.1080/13543776.2020.1797679

Chen, J., Sitsel, A., Benoy, V., Sepúlveda, M. R., and Vangheluwe, P. (2020a). Primary active Ca^{2+} transport systems in health and disease. *Cold Spring Harb Perspect. Biol.* 12, a035113. doi:10.1101/cshperspect.a035113

Chen, Q., Zhou, Y., Zhou, L., Fu, Z., Yang, C., Zhao, L., et al. (2020b). TRPC6-dependent Ca^{2+} signaling mediates airway inflammation in response to oxidative stress via ERK pathway. *Cell Death Dis.* 11, 170. doi:10.1038/s41419-020-2360-0

Chun, J., and Prince, A. (2006). Activation of Ca^{2+}-dependent signaling by TLR2. *J. Immunol.* 177, 1330–1337. 177/2/133010.4049/jimmunol.177.2.1330.

Csordas, G., Várnai, P., Golenár, T., Roy, S., Purkins, G., Schneider, T. G., et al. (2010). Imaging interorganelle contacts and local calcium dynamics at the ER-mitochondrial interface. *Mol. Cel.* 39, 121–132. doi:10.1016/j.molcel.2010.06.029

Curcic, S., Schober, R., Schindl, R., and Groschner, K. (2019). TRPC-mediated Ca^{2+} signaling and control of cellular functions. *Semin. Cel Dev. Biol.* 94, 28–39. doi:10.1016/j.semcdb.2019.02.001

De Stefani, D., Raffaello, A., Teardo, E., Szabò, I., and Rizzuto, R. (2011). A forty-kilodalton protein of the inner membrane is the mitochondrial calcium uniporter. *Nature* 476, 336–340. doi:10.1038/nature10230

Delmotte, P., Yang, B., Thompson, M. A., Pabelick, C. M., Prakash, Y. S., and Sieck, G. C. (2012). Inflammation alters regional mitochondrial Ca^{2+} in human airway smooth muscle cells. *Am. J. Physiol. Cel Physiol.* 303, C244–C256. doi:10.1152/ajpcell.00414.2011

Di, A., Brown, M. E., Deriy, L. V., Li, C., Szeto, F. L., Chen, Y., et al. (2006). CFTR regulates phagosome acidification in macrophages and alters bactericidal activity. *Nat. Cel Biol.* 8, 933–944. doi:10.1038/ncb1456

Di Marco, G., Vallese, F., Jourde, B., Bergsdorf, C., Sturlese, M., De Mario, A., et al. (2020). A high-throughput screening identifies MICU1 targeting compounds. *Cell Rep.* 30, 2321–2331.e6. doi:10.1016/j.celrep.2020.01.081

Domi, T., Di Leva, F., Fedrizzi, L., Rimessi, A., and Brini, M. (2007). Functional specificity of PMCA isoforms? *Ann. N. Y Acad. Sci.* 1099, 237–246. doi:10.1196/annals.1387.043

Farinha, C. M., King-Underwood, J., Sousa, M., Correia, A. R., Henriques, B. J., Roxo-Rosa, M., et al. (2013). Revertants, low temperature, and correctors reveal the mechanism of F508del-CFTR rescue by VX-809 and suggest multiple agents for full correction. *Chem. Biol.* 20, 943–955. doi:10.1016/j.chembiol.2013.06.004

Feigal, R. J., Tomczyk, M. S., and Shapiro, B. L. (1982). The calcium abnormality in cystic fibrosis mitochondria: relative role of respiration and ATP hydrolysis. *Life Sci.* 30, 93–98. doi:10.1016/0024-3205(82)90640-3

Foskett, J. K., White, C., Cheung, K. H., and Mak, D. O. (2007). Inositol trisphosphate receptor Ca^{2+} release channels. *Physiol. Rev.* 87, 593–658. doi:10.1152/physrev.00035.2006

Fu, Z., Bettega, K., Carroll, S., Buchholz, K. R., and Machen, T. E. (2007). Role of Ca^{2+} in responses of airway epithelia to *Pseudomonas aeruginosa*, flagellin, ATP, and thapsigargin. *Am. J. Physiol. Lung Cel. Mol. Physiol.* 292, L353–L364. doi:10.1152/ajplung.00042.2006

Gatica, S., Eltit, F., Santibanez, J. F., Varela, D., Cabello-Verrugio, C., and Simon, F. (2019). Expression suppression and activity inhibition of TRPM7 regulate cytokine production and multiple organ dysfunction syndrome during endotoxemia: a new target for sepsis. *Curr. Mol. Med.* 19, 547–559. doi:10.2174/1566524019666190709181726

Genovese, M., Borrelli, A., Venturini, A., Guidone, D., Caci, E., Viscido, G., et al. (2019). TRPV4 and purinergic receptor signalling pathways are separately linked in airway epithelia to CFTR and TMEM16A chloride channels. *J. Physiol.* 597, 5859–5878. doi:10.1113/JP278784

Gincel, D., Zaid, H., and Shoshan-Barmatz, V. (2001). Calcium binding and translocation by the voltage-dependent anion channel: a possible regulatory mechanism in mitochondrial function. *Biochem. J.* 358, 147–155. doi:10.1042/0264-6021:3580147

Giorgi, C., Danese, A., Missiroli, S., Patergnani, S., and Pinton, P. (2018). Calcium dynamics as a machine for decoding signals. *Trends Cel Biol.* 28, 258–273. doi:10.1016/j.tcb.2018.01.002

Grebert, C., Becq, F., and Vandebrouck, C. (2019). Focus on TRP channels in cystic fibrosis. *Cell Calcium* 81, 29–37. doi:10.1016/j.ceca.2019.05.007

Heiner, I., Radukina, N., Eisfeld, J., Kühn, F., and Lückhoff, A. (2005). Regulation of TRPM2 channels in neutrophil granulocytes by ADP-ribose: a promising pharmacological target. *Naunyn Schmiedebergs Arch. Pharmacol.* 371, 325–333. doi:10.1007/s00210-005-1033-y

Henry, C. O., Dalloneau, E., Pérez-Berezo, M. T., Plata, C., Wu, Y., Guillon, A., et al. (2016). *In vitro* and *in vivo* evidence for an inflammatory role of the calcium channel TRPV4 in lung epithelium: potential involvement in cystic fibrosis. *Am. J. Physiol. Lung Cel. Mol. Physiol.* 311, L664–L675. doi:10.1152/ajplung.00442.2015

Heo, D. K., Lim, H. M., Nam, J. H., Lee, M. G., and Kim, J. Y. (2015). Regulation of phagocytosis and cytokine secretion by store-operated calcium entry in primary isolated murine microglia. *Cel Signal* 27, 177–186. doi:10.1016/j.cellsig.2014.11.003

Hisert, K. B., Heltshe, S. L., Pope, C., Jorth, P., Wu, X., Edwards, R. M., et al. (2017). Restoring cystic fibrosis transmembrane conductance regulator function reduces airway bacteria and inflammation in people with cystic fibrosis and chronic lung infections. *Am. J. Respir. Crit. Care Med.* 195, 1617–1628. doi:10.1164/rccm.201609-1954OC

Hollywood, M. A., Sergeant, G. P., Thornbury, K. D., and Mchale, N. G. (2010). The PI-PLC inhibitor U-73122 is a potent inhibitor of the SERCA pump in smooth muscle. *Br. J. Pharmacol.* 160, 1293–1294. doi:10.1111/j.1476-5381.2010.00795.x

Huang, W., Barrett, M., Hajicek, N., Hicks, S., Harden, T. K., Sondek, J., et al. (2013). Small molecule inhibitors of phospholipase C from a novel high-throughput screen. *J. Biol. Chem.* 288, 5840–5848. doi:10.1074/jbc.M112.422501

Huguet, F., Calvez, M. L., Benz, N., Le Hir, S., Mignen, O., Buscaglia, P., et al. (2016). Function and regulation of TRPM7, as well as intracellular magnesium content, are altered in cells expressing DeltaF508-CFTR and G551D-CFTR. *Cell Mol. Life Sci.* 73, 3351–3373. doi:10.1007/s00018-016-2149-6

Iwamoto, T., Watano, T., and Shigekawa, M. (1996). A novel isothiourea derivative selectively inhibits the reverse mode of Na^+/Ca^{2+} exchange in cells expressing NCX1. *J. Biol. Chem.* 271, 22391–22397. doi:10.1074/jbc.271.37.22391

Jacquot, J., Tabary, O., Le Rouzic, P., and Clement, A. (2008). Airway epithelial cell inflammatory signalling in cystic fibrosis. *Int. J. Biochem. Cel Biol* 40, 1703–1715. doi:10.1016/j.biocel.2008.02.002

Jung, D. H., Mo, S. H., and Kim, D. H. (2006). Calumenin, a multiple EF-hands Ca^{2+}-binding protein, interacts with ryanodine receptor-1 in rabbit skeletal sarcoplasmic reticulum. *Biochem. Biophys. Res. Commun.* 343, 34–42. doi:10.1016/j.bbrc.2006.02.115

Kanju, P., Chen, Y., Lee, W., Yeo, M., Lee, S. H., Romac, J., et al. (2016). Small molecule dual-inhibitors of TRPV4 and TRPA1 for attenuation of inflammation and pain. *Sci. Rep.* 6, 26894. doi:10.1038/srep26894

Katz, S. M., Krueger, L. J., and Falkner, B. (1988). Microscopic nephrocalcinosis in cystic fibrosis. *N. Engl. J. Med.* 319, 263–266. doi:10.1056/NEJM198808043190502

Khananshvili, D. (2014). Sodium-calcium exchangers (NCX): molecular hallmarks underlying the tissue-specific and systemic functions. *Pflugers Arch.* 466, 43–60. doi:10.1007/s00424-013-1405-y

Klose, A., Huth, T., and Alzheimer, C. (2008). 1-[6-[[(17beta)-3-methoxyestra-1,3,5(10)-trien-17-yl]amino]hexyl]-1H-pyrrole-2,5-dione (U73122) selectively inhibits Kir3 and BK channels in a phospholipase C-independent fashion. *Mol. Pharmacol.* 74, 1203–1214. doi:10.1124/mol.108.047837

Kon, N., Murakoshi, M., Isobe, A., Kagechika, K., Miyoshi, N., and Nagayama, T. (2017). DS16570511 is a small-molecule inhibitor of the mitochondrial calcium uniporter. *Cell Death Discov.* 3, 17045. doi:10.1038/cddiscovery.2017.45

Kostic, M., and Sekler, I. (2019). Functional properties and mode of regulation of the mitochondrial Na^+/Ca^{2+} exchanger, NCLX. *Semin. Cel Dev. Biol.* 94, 59–65. doi:10.1016/j.semcdb.2019.01.009

Lampronti, I., Dechecchi, M. C., Rimessi, A., Bezzerri, V., Nicolis, E., Guerrini, A., et al. (2017). Beta-sitosterol reduces the expression of chemotactic cytokine genes in cystic fibrosis bronchial epithelial cells. *Front. Pharmacol.* 8, 236. doi:10.3389/fphar.2017.00236

Lee, R. J., and Foskett, J. K. (2014). Ca^{2+} signaling and fluid secretion by secretory cells of the airway epithelium. *Cell Calcium* 55, 325–336. doi:10.1016/j.ceca.2014.02.001

Lin, B. L., Matera, D., Doerner, J. F., Zheng, N., Del Camino, D., Mishra, S., et al. (2019). *In vivo* selective inhibition of TRPC6 by antagonist BI 749327 ameliorates fibrosis and dysfunction in cardiac and renal disease. *Proc. Natl. Acad. Sci. U S A.* 116, 10156–10161. doi:10.1073/pnas.1815354116

Lock, J. T., Alzayady, K. J., Yule, D. I., and Parker, I. (2018). All three IP3 receptor isoforms generate Ca^{2+} puffs that display similar characteristics. *Sci. Signal.* 11, 11. doi:10.1126/scisignal.aau0344

Marchi, S., Patergnani, S., Missiroli, S., Morciano, G., Rimessi, A., Wieckowski, M. R., et al. (2018). Mitochondrial and endoplasmic reticulum calcium homeostasis and cell death. *Cell Calcium* 69, 62–72. doi:10.1016/j.ceca.2017.05.003

Marchi, S., and Pinton, P. (2014). The mitochondrial calcium uniporter complex: molecular components, structure and physiopathological implications. *J. Physiol. (Lond)* 592, 829–839. doi:10.1113/jphysiol.2013.268235

Martins, J. R., Kongsuphol, P., Sammels, E., Dahimène, S., Aldehni, F., Clarke, L. A., et al. (2011). F508del-CFTR increases intracellular Ca^{2+} signaling that causes enhanced calcium-dependent Cl(−) conductance in cystic fibrosis. *Biochim. Biophys. Acta* 1812, 1385–1392. doi:10.1016/j.bbadis.2011.08.008

Mcnamara, N., Gallup, M., Sucher, A., Maltseva, I., Mckemy, D., and Basbaum, C. (2006). AsialoGM1 and TLR5 cooperate in flagellin-induced nucleotide signaling to activate Erk1/2. *Am. J. Respir. Cel. Mol. Biol.* 34, 653–660. doi:10.1165/rcmb.2005-0441OC

Mukhopadhyay, I., Kulkarni, A., Aranake, S., Karnik, P., Shetty, M., Thorat, S., et al. (2014). Transient receptor potential ankyrin 1 receptor activation *in vitro* and *in vivo* by pro-tussive agents: GRC 17536 as a promising anti-tussive therapeutic. *PLoS One* 9, e97005. doi:10.1371/journal.pone.0097005

Murphy, E., Pan, X., Nguyen, T., Liu, J., Holmström, K. M., and Finkel, T. (2014). Unresolved questions from the analysis of mice lacking MCU expression. *Biochem. Biophys. Res. Commun.* 449, 384–385. doi:10.1016/j.bbrc.2014.04.144

Ng, H. P., Valentine, V. G., and Wang, G. (2016). CFTR targeting during activation of human neutrophils. *J. Leukoc. Biol.* 100, 1413–1424. doi:10.1189/jlb.4A0316-130RR

Nishizawa, T., Kita, S., Maturana, A. D., Furuya, N., Hirata, K., Kasuya, G., et al. (2013). Structural basis for the counter-transport mechanism of a H^+/Ca^{2+} exchanger. *Science* 341, 168–172. doi:10.1126/science.1239002

Norez, C., Antigny, F., Becq, F., and Vandebrouck, C. (2006). Maintaining low Ca^{2+} level in the endoplasmic reticulum restores abnormal endogenous F508del-CFTR trafficking in airway epithelial cells. *Traffic* 7, 562–573. doi:10.1111/j.1600-0854.2006.00409.x

Pan, X., Liu, J., Nguyen, T., Liu, C., Sun, J., Teng, Y., et al. (2013). The physiological role of mitochondrial calcium revealed by mice lacking the mitochondrial calcium uniporter. *Nat. Cel Biol.* 15, 1464–1472. doi:10.1038/ncb2868

Pani, B., Ong, H. L., Liu, X., Rauser, K., Ambudkar, I. S., and Singh, B. B. (2008). Lipid rafts determine clustering of STIM1 in endoplasmic reticulum-plasma membrane junctions and regulation of store-operated Ca^{2+} entry (SOCE). *J. Biol. Chem.* 283, 17333–17340. doi:10.1074/jbc.M800107200

Park, H. S., Hong, C., Kim, B. J., and So, I. (2014). The pathophysiologic roles of TRPM7 channel. *Korean J. Physiol. Pharmacol.* 18, 15–23. doi:10.4196/kjpp.2014.18.1.15

Patel, W., Moore, P. J., Sassano, M. F., Lopes-Pacheco, M., Aleksandrov, A. A., Amaral, M. D., et al. (2019). Increases in cytosolic Ca^{2+} induce dynamin- and calcineurin-dependent internalisation of CFTR. *Cel. Mol. Life Sci.* 76, 977–994. doi:10.1007/s00018-018-2989-3

Patergnani, S., Danese, A., Bouhamida, E., Aguiari, G., Previati, M., Pinton, P., et al. (2020a). Various aspects of calcium signaling in the regulation of apoptosis, autophagy, cell proliferation, and cancer. *Int. J. Mol. Sci.* 21, 8323. doi:10.3390/ijms21218323

Patergnani, S., Vitto, V. A. M., Pinton, P., and Rimessi, A. (2020b). Mitochondrial stress responses and "Mito-Inflammation" in cystic fibrosis. *Front. Pharmacol.* 11, 581114. doi:10.3389/fphar.2020.581114

Pedemonte, N., Sonawane, N. D., Taddei, A., Hu, J., Zegarra-Moran, O., Suen, Y. F., et al. (2005). Phenylglycine and sulfonamide correctors of defective delta F508 and G551D cystic fibrosis transmembrane conductance regulator chloride-channel gating. *Mol. Pharmacol.* 67, 1797–1807. doi:10.1124/mol.105.010959

Philippe, R., Antigny, F., Buscaglia, P., Norez, C., Becq, F., Frieden, M., et al. (2015). SERCA and PMCA pumps contribute to the deregulation of Ca^{2+} homeostasis in human CF epithelial cells. *Biochim. Biophys. Acta* 1853, 892–903. doi:10.1016/j.bbamcr.2015.01.010

Philippe, R., Antigny, F., Buscaglia, P., Norez, C., Huguet, F., Castelbou, C., et al. (2017). Calumenin contributes to ER-Ca^{2+} homeostasis in bronchial epithelial cells expressing WT and F508del mutated CFTR and to F508del-CFTR retention. *Cell Calcium* 62, 47–59. doi:10.1016/j.ceca.2017.01.011

Pinton, P., Leo, S., Wieckowski, M. R., Di Benedetto, G., and Rizzuto, R. (2004). Long-term modulation of mitochondrial Ca^{2+} signals by protein kinase C isozymes. *J. Cel Biol.* 165, 223–232. doi:10.1083/jcb.200311061

Prandini, P., De Logu, F., Fusi, C., Provezza, L., Nassini, R., Montagner, G., et al. (2016). Transient receptor potential ankyrin 1 channels modulate inflammatory response in respiratory cells from patients with cystic fibrosis. *Am. J. Respir. Cel Mol Biol* 55, 645–656. doi:10.1165/rcmb.2016-0089OC

Preti, D., Szallasi, A., and Patacchini, R. (2012). TRP channels as therapeutic targets in airway disorders: a patent review. *Expert Opin. Ther. Pat* 22, 663–695. doi:10.1517/13543776.2012.696099

Pulli, I., Blom, T., Löf, C., Magnusson, M., Rimessi, A., Pinton, P., et al. (2015). A novel chimeric aequorin fused with caveolin-1 reveals a sphingosine kinase 1-regulated Ca^{2+} microdomain in the caveolar compartment. *Biochim. Biophys. Acta* 1853, 2173–2182. doi:10.1016/j.bbamcr.2015.04.005

Ratner, A. J., Bryan, R., Weber, A., Nguyen, S., Barnes, D., Pitt, A., et al. (2001). Cystic fibrosis pathogens activate Ca^{2+}-dependent mitogen-activated protein kinase signaling pathways in airway epithelial cells. *J. Biol. Chem.* 276, 19267–19275. doi:10.1074/jbc.M007703200

Ribeiro, C. M., and Boucher, R. C. (2010). Role of endoplasmic reticulum stress in cystic fibrosis-related airway inflammatory responses. *Proc. Am. Thorac. Soc.* 7, 387–394. doi:10.1513/pats.201001-017AW

Ribeiro, C. M., and Lubamba, B. A. (2017). Role of IRE1alpha/XBP-1 in cystic fibrosis airway inflammation. *Int. J. Mol. Sci.* 18, ijms18010118. doi:10.3390/ijms18010118

Ribeiro, C. M., Paradiso, A. M., Carew, M. A., Shears, S. B., and Boucher, R. C. (2005). Cystic fibrosis airway epithelial Ca^{2+} i signaling: the mechanism for the larger agonist-mediated Ca^{2+} i signals in human cystic fibrosis airway epithelia. *J. Biol. Chem.* 280, 10202–10209. doi:10.1074/jbc.M410617200

Ribeiro, C. M. (2006). The role of intracellular calcium signals in inflammatory responses of polarised cystic fibrosis human airway epithelia. *Drugs R. D* 7, 17–31. doi:10.2165/00126839-200607010-00002

Rimessi, A., Bezzerri, V., Patergnani, S., Marchi, S., Cabrini, G., and Pinton, P. (2015a). Mitochondrial Ca^{2+}-dependent NLRP3 activation exacerbates the *Pseudomonas* aeruginosa-driven inflammatory response in cystic fibrosis. *Nat. Commun.* 6, 6201. doi:10.1038/ncomms7201

Rimessi, A., Bezzerri, V., Salvatori, F., Tamanini, A., Nigro, F., Dechecchi, M. C., et al. (2018). PLCB3 loss of function reduces *Pseudomonas* aeruginosa-dependent IL-8 release in cystic fibrosis. *Am. J. Respir. Cel Mol Biol* 59, 428–436. doi:10.1165/rcmb.2017-0267OC

Rimessi, A., Patergnani, S., Bonora, M., Wieckowski, M. R., and Pinton, P. (2015b). Mitochondrial Ca^{2+} remodeling is a prime factor in oncogenic behavior. *Front. Oncol.* 5, 143. doi:10.3389/fonc.2015.00143

Rimessi, A., Pozzato, C., Carparelli, L., Rossi, A., Ranucci, S., De Fino, I., et al. (2020). Pharmacological modulation of mitochondrial calcium uniporter controls lung inflammation in cystic fibrosis. *Sci. Adv.* 6, eaax9093. doi:10.1126/sciadv.aax9093

Rimessi, A., Rizzuto, R., and Pinton, P. (2007). Differential recruitment of PKC isoforms in HeLa cells during redox stress. *Cell Stress Chaperones* 12, 291–298. doi:10.1379/csc-211.1

Riordan, J. R. (1993). The cystic fibrosis transmembrane conductance regulator. *Annu. Rev. Physiol.* 55, 609–630. doi:10.1146/annurev.ph.55.030193.003141

Robledo-Avila, F. H., Ruiz-Rosado, J. D., Brockman, K. L., Kopp, B. T., Amer, A. O., Mccoy, K., et al. (2018). Dysregulated calcium homeostasis in cystic fibrosis neutrophils leads to deficient antimicrobial responses. *J. Immunol.* 201, 2016–2027. doi:10.4049/jimmunol.1800076

Roomans, G. M. (1986). Calcium and cystic fibrosis. *Scan Electron. Microsc.* 165–178.

Rubino, R., Bezzerri, V., Favia, M., Facchini, M., Tebon, M., Singh, A. K., et al. (2014). Pseudomonas aeruginosa reduces the expression of CFTR via post-translational modification of NHERF1. *Pflugers Arch.* 466, 2269–2278. doi:10.1007/s00424-014-1474-6

Sahoo, S. K., Kim, T., Kang, G. B., Lee, J. G., Eom, S. H., and Kim, D. H. (2009). Characterization of calumenin-SERCA2 interaction in mouse cardiac sarcoplasmic reticulum. *J. Biol. Chem.* 284, 31109–31121. doi:10.1074/jbc.M109.031989

Salathe, M. (2007). Regulation of mammalian ciliary beating. *Annu. Rev. Physiol.* 69, 401–422. doi:10.1146/annurev.physiol.69.040705.141253

Santo-Domingo, J., Vay, L., Hernández-Sanmiguel, E., Lobatón, C. D., Moreno, A., Montero, M., et al. (2007). The plasma membrane Na^{+}/Ca^{2+} exchange inhibitor KB-R7943 is also a potent inhibitor of the mitochondrial Ca^{2+} uniporter. *Br. J. Pharmacol.* 151, 647–654. doi:10.1038/sj.bjp.0707260

Scambler, T., Jarosz-Griffiths, H. H., Lara-Reyna, S., Pathak, S., Wong, C., Holbrook, J., et al. (2019). ENaC-mediated sodium influx exacerbates NLRP3-dependent inflammation in cystic fibrosis. *Elife* 8. doi:10.7554/eLife.49248

Schwaller, B. (2020). Cytosolic Ca^{2+} buffers are inherently Ca^{2+} signal modulators. *Cold Spring Harb Perspect. Biol.* 12, a035543. doi:10.1101/cshperspect.a035543

Shapiro, B. L., Feigal, R. J., Laible, N. J., Biros, M. H., and Warwick, W. J. (1978). Doubling time alpha-aminoisobutyrate transport and calcium exchange in cultured fibroblasts from cystic fibrosis and control subjects. *Clin. Chim. Acta* 82, 125–131. doi:10.1016/0009-8981(78)90035-9

Shoshan-Barmatz, V., De Pinto, V., Zweckstetter, M., Raviv, Z., Keinan, N., and Arbel, N. (2010). VDAC, a multi-functional mitochondrial protein regulating cell life and death. *Mol. Aspects Med.* 31, 227–285. doi:10.1016/j.mam.2010.03.002

Simmen, T., and Herrera-Cruz, M. S. (2018). Plastic mitochondria-endoplasmic reticulum (ER) contacts use chaperones and tethers to mould their structure and signaling. *Curr. Opin. Cel Biol.* 53, 61–69. doi:10.1016/j.ceb.2018.04.014

Singaravelu, K., Nelson, C., Bakowski, D., De Brito, O. M., Ng, S. W., Di Capite, J., et al. (2011). Mitofusin 2 regulates STIM1 migration from the Ca^{2+} store to the plasma membrane in cells with depolarized mitochondria. *J. Biol. Chem.* 286, 12189–12201. doi:10.17402910.1074/jbc.M110.174029

Stoker, M. L., Newport, E., Hulit, J. C., West, A. P., and Morten, K. J. (2019). Impact of pharmacological agents on mitochondrial function: a growing opportunity? *Biochem. Soc. Trans.* 47, 1757–1772. doi:10.1042/BST20190280

Strehler, E. E., and Treiman, M. (2004). Calcium pumps of plasma membrane and cell interior. *Curr. Mol. Med.* 4, 323–335. doi:10.2174/1566524043360735

Tabary, O., Boncoeur, E., De Martin, R., Pepperkok, R., Clément, A., Schultz, C., et al. (2006). Calcium-dependent regulation of NF-(kappa)B activation in cystic fibrosis airway epithelial cells. *Cel Signal* 18, 652–660. doi:10.1016/j.cellsig.2005.06.004

Tabary, O., Escotte, S., Couetil, J. P., Hubert, D., Dusser, D., Puchelle, E., et al. (2000). High susceptibility for cystic fibrosis human airway gland cells to produce IL-8 through the I kappa B kinase alpha pathway in response to extracellular NaCl content. *J. Immunol.* 164, 3377–3384. doi:10.4049/jimmunol.164.6.3377

Taylor, C. W., and Machaca, K. (2019). IP3 receptors and store-operated Ca^{2+} entry: a license to fill. *Curr. Opin. Cel. Biol.* 57, 1–7. doi:10.1016/j.ceb.2018.10.001

Teng, L., Kerbiriou, M., Taiya, M., Le Hir, S., Mignen, O., Benz, N., et al. (2012). Proteomic identification of calumenin as a G551D-CFTR associated protein. *PLoS One* 7, e40173. doi:10.1371/journal.pone.0040173

Thillaiappan, N. B., Chavda, A. P., Tovey, S. C., Prole, D. L., and Taylor, C. W. (2017). Ca^{2+} signals initiate at immobile IP3 receptors adjacent to ER-plasma membrane junctions. *Nat. Commun.* 8, 1505. doi:10.1038/s41467-017-01644-8

Vachel, L., Norez, C., Becq, F., and Vandebrouck, C. (2013). Effect of VX-770 (ivacaftor) and OAG on Ca^{2+} influx and CFTR activity in G551D and F508del-CFTR expressing cells. *J. Cyst Fibros* 12, 584–591. doi:10.1016/j.jcf.2013.05.008

Vachel, L., Norez, C., Jayle, C., Becq, F., and Vandebrouck, C. (2015). The low PLC-delta1 expression in cystic fibrosis bronchial epithelial cells induces upregulation of TRPV6 channel activity. *Cell Calcium* 57, 38–48. doi:10.1016/j.ceca.2014.11.005

Verkhratsky, A., Trebak, M., Perocchi, F., Khananshvili, D., and Sekler, I. (2018). Crosslink between calcium and sodium signalling. *Exp. Physiol.* 103, 157–169. doi:10.1113/EP086534

Villalobo, A., Ishida, H., Vogel, H. J., and Berchtold, M. W. (2018). Calmodulin as a protein linker and a regulator of adaptor/scaffold proteins. *Biochim. Biophys. Acta Mol. Cel. Res.* 1865, 507–521. doi:10.1016/j.bbamcr.2017.12.004

Vorum, H., Hager, H., Christensen, B. M., Nielsen, S., and Honoré, B. (1999). Human calumenin localizes to the secretory pathway and is secreted to the medium. *Exp. Cel. Res.* 248, 473–481. doi:10.1006/excr.1999.4431

Waller, R. L., Brattin, W. J., and Dearborn, D. G. (1984). Cytosolic free calcium concentration and intracellular calcium distribution in lymphocytes from cystic fibrosis patients. *Life Sci.* 35, 775–781. doi:10.1016/0024-3205(84)90347-3

Waterer, G. W. (2012). Airway defense mechanisms. *Clin. Chest Med.* 33, 199–209. doi:10.1016/j.ccm.2012.03.003

Woods, J. J., Nemani, N., Shanmughapriya, S., Kumar, A., Zhang, M., Nathan, S. R., et al. (2019). A selective and cell-permeable mitochondrial calcium uniporter (MCU) inhibitor preserves mitochondrial bioenergetics after hypoxia/

reoxygenation injury. *ACS Cent. Sci.* 5, 153–166. doi:10.1021/acscentsci.8b00773

Wootten, D., Christopoulos, A., Marti-Solano, M., Babu, M. M., and Sexton, P. M. (2018). Mechanisms of signalling and biased agonism in G protein-coupled receptors. *Nat. Rev. Mol. Cel Biol.* 19, 638–653. doi:10.1038/s41580-018-0049-3

Zhu, L., Yuan, C., Ding, X., Xu, S., Yang, J., Liang, Y., et al. (2016). PLC-gamma1 is involved in the inflammatory response induced by influenza A virus H1N1 infection. *Virology* 496, 131–137. doi:10.1016/j.virol.2016.06.003

Zhu, L., Yuan, C., Ma, Y., Ding, X., Zhu, G., and Zhu, Q. (2015). Anti-inflammatory activities of phospholipase C inhibitor U73122: inhibition of monocyte-to-macrophage transformation and LPS-induced pro-inflammatory cytokine expression. *Int. Immunopharmacol.* 29, 622–627. doi:10.1016/j.intimp.2015.09.019

14

Glycosaminoglycans as Multifunctional Anti-Elastase and Anti-Inflammatory Drugs in Cystic Fibrosis Lung Disease

Judith A. Voynow, Shuo Zheng and Apparao B. Kummarapurugu*

Department of Pediatric Pulmonology, Children's Hospital of Richmond at VCU, Richmond, VA, United States

***Correspondence:**
Judith A. Voynow
judith.voynow@vcuhealth.org

Neutrophil elastase (NE) is a major protease in the airways of patients with cystic fibrosis (CF) that activates airway inflammation by several mechanisms. NE stimulates epithelial toll like receptors (TLR) resulting in cytokine upregulation and release, upregulates MUC5AC, a major airway mucin, degrades both phagocytic receptors and opsonins resulting in both neutrophil and macrophage phagocytic failure, generates oxidative stress *via* extracellular generation and uptake of heme free iron, and activates other proteases. Altogether, these mechanisms create a significant inflammatory challenge that impairs innate immune function and results in airway remodeling. Currently, a major gap in our therapeutic approach to CF lung disease is the lack of an effective therapeutic strategy targeting active NE and its downstream pro-inflammatory sequelae. Polysulfated glycosaminoglycans (GAGs) are potent anti-elastase drugs that have additional anti-inflammatory properties. Heparin is a prototype of a glycosaminoglycan with both anti-elastase and anti-inflammatory properties. Heparin inhibits NE in an allosteric manner with high potency. Heparin also inhibits cathepsin G, blocks P-selectin and L-selectin, hinders ligand binding to the receptor for advanced glycation endproducts, and impedes histone acetyltransferase activity which dampens cytokine transcription and High Mobility Group Box 1 release. Furthermore, nebulized heparin treatment improves outcomes for patients with chronic obstructive pulmonary disease (COPD), asthma, acute lung injury and smoke inhalation. However, the anticoagulant activity of heparin is a potential contraindication for this therapy to be developed for CF lung disease. Therefore, modified heparins and other GAGs are being developed that retain the anti-elastase and anti-inflammatory qualities of heparin with minimal to no anticoagulant activity. The modified heparin, 2-O, 3-O desulfated heparin (ODSH), maintains anti-elastase and anti-inflammatory activities *in vitro* and *in vivo*, and has little residual anticoagulant activity. Heparan sulfate with O-sulfate residues but not N-sulfate residues blocks allergic asthmatic inflammation in a murine model. Polysulfated hyaluronic acid abrogates allergen- triggered rhinosinusitis in a murine model. Finally, nonsaccharide glycosaminoglycan mimetics with specific sulfate modifications can be designed to inhibit NE activity. Altogether, these novel GAGs or GAG mimetics hold significant promise to address the unmet need for inhaled anti-elastase and anti-inflammatory therapy for patients with CF.

Keywords: neutrophil elastase, cystic fibrosis, glycosaminoglycans, heparin, hyaluronic acid, High Mobility Group Box 1

INTRODUCTION

Cystic fibrosis (CF) lung disease is marked by recurrent exacerbations of acute bronchitis with an overexuberant inflammatory response and markedly high airway concentrations of neutrophil elastase (NE). A major gap in current therapy for patients with CF is the lack of anti-protease and anti-inflammatory therapies to inhibit NE and NE-activated sequelae. In this review, we will discuss the impact of NE on CF lung biology, review the current landscape of anti-protease and anti-inflammatory therapies for CF lung disease, and then discuss the biology and pharmacology of glycosaminoglycans (GAGs) as potential anti-protease and anti-inflammatory therapies for CF.

Neutrophil Elastase and Cystic Fibrosis Lung Disease

The primary defect in CF, an autosomal recessive disorder, is the loss of function of the Cystic Fibrosis Transmembrane Conductance Regulator protein, which results in abnormal airway mucus (Stoltz et al., 2015; Boucher, 2019). CF airway mucus is tethered to submucosal ducts and airway epithelia (Ostedgaard et al., 2017; Ermund et al., 2018) with subsequent mucus stasis and failure to clear infections. Thus, recurrent cycles of infection and inflammation are established and neutrophils are recruited to the airway. In addition, mucus stasis alone may be sufficient to increase neutrophilic inflammation (Rosen et al., 2018), possibly by generating airway hypoxemic stress which triggers IL-1β and IL-1α cytokine release (Chen et al., 2019). The CF airway milieu, characterized by viscous sputum containing microbes and pro-inflammatory cytokines, further impairs neutrophil function and clearance (Voynow et al., 2008). Ultimately, in the CF airways, neutrophils release extracellular traps (Gray et al., 2018) or undergo necrosis (Vandivier et al., 2002), and release DNA and granule contents including proteases. The most abundant protease released into the CF airway is neutrophil elastase (NE).

NE is present in the bronchoalveolar lavage (BAL) fluid in infants with CF, and BAL NE concentrations are directly associated with lung disease progression starting in infancy (Sagel et al., 2012; Sly et al., 2013; Rosenow et al., 2019). NE accelerates the progression of CF lung disease by several mechanisms (Voynow et al., 2008; McKelvey et al., 2019). First, NE contributes to altered ion flux in the CF airway by activating the epithelial sodium channel (Caldwell et al., 2005) and degrading CFTR *via* an endogenous proteinase, calpain (Le Gars et al., 2013). These NE actions further aggravate altered ion and water flux across the CF airway. Second, NE activates signaling pathways that promote abnormal epithelial structure and repair. NE upregulates mucin expression and goblet cell metaplasia (Voynow et al., 2004; Park et al., 2013); and triggers epithelial apoptosis (Suzuki et al., 2009) and/or premature senescence (Fischer et al., 2013), which impair epithelial proliferation and restoration following injury. Third, NE employs several mechanisms to promote airway inflammation (Voynow et al., 2008; Bruscia and Bonfield, 2016; Roesch et al., 2018). NE amplifies inflammation by upregulating neutrophil chemokines, e.g. IL-8 (Cosgrove et al., 2011), proteolytically activating chemokines such as IL-1α or IL-33 (Clancy et al., 2018), and releasing damage associated molecular pattern proteins such as High Mobility Group Box 1 (HMGB1) (Griffin et al., 2014) which binds to the Receptor for Advanced Glycation End-products (RAGE) or facilitates ligand binding to TLR2 and TLR4 (Lotze and Tracey, 2005). NE further contributes to airway inflammation by increasing the expression of pro-inflammatory long chain ceramides (Karandashova et al., 2018; Horati et al., 2020); these lipids impact plasma membrane structure and receptor clustering. NE degrades innate immune proteins including lactoferrin and surfactant proteins A and D, and cleaves both complement and complement receptors causing impaired neutrophil and macrophage phagocytic activity (Voynow et al., 2008). NE increases the activity of other proteases; NE activates matrix metalloproteinase 9 (MMP 9) by cleavage of its prodomain and by degradation of its inhibitor, Tissue inhibitor of metalloprotease-1 (Jackson et al., 2010). In addition, the protease load is further exaggerated by the loss of endogenous anti-proteases. Anti-NE capacity is depleted in the CF airway due to NE degradation of elafin (Guyot et al., 2008), secretory leucoprotease inhibitor (Weldon et al., 2009; Twigg et al., 2015) and both oxidation and protease degradation of alpha-1- protease inhibitor (A1-PI) (Twigg et al., 2015). Finally, NE generates oxidative stress in epithelial cells and macrophages by degrading heme-containing proteins and releasing heme-free iron which is taken up by cells (Fischer et al., 2009); this process occurs in the airways of patients with CF (Ghio et al., 2013) and with COPD (Fischer et al., 2009). NE has a broad repertoire of activities that increase inflammation, impair host immunity and result in airway remodeling. Although NE appears to be a central regulator of inflammation in CF lung disease, NE actions are amplified by ligand-receptor interactions, oxidative stress, and the presence of other active proteases that contribute to a complex pro-inflammatory milieu. This may be one reason why the strategy of therapy for a single target, NE activity, in the CF airway, has not yet been successful.

Status of Current Anti-Proteases and Anti-Inflammatory Therapies for Cystic Fibrosis

Currently, there are two anti-inflammatory therapies approved for CF: azithromycin for patients with *Pseudomonas aeruginosa* infections (Nichols et al., 2020) and ibuprofen high dose oral therapy (Konstan et al., 1995). These therapies blunt the rate of decline of lung function over time; however, they do not resolve the high airway protease load that is associated with progression of bronchiectasis and lung injury. Many anti-protease candidate drugs have been tested in the CF airway (reviewed in (Voynow et al., 2008) and (Twigg et al., 2015)). An oral neutrophil elastase inhibitor, AZD9668, was tested in a Phase II randomized, double-blind, placebo-controlled trial in patients with CF (Elborn et al., 2012). Although AZD9668 treatment was associated with decreased urine desmosine, a marker of NE activity, and decreased sputum IL-6 and Regulated on Activation, Normal T Expressed and Secreted (RANTES), there was no improvement in sputum NE activity, sputum neutrophil counts, or measures of quality of life. A recent Phase IIa randomized, placebo-controlled clinical trial of inhaled alpha1 proteinase inhibitor (A1-HC) (Gaggar et al., 2016) revealed that the treatment group had increased sputum concentrations of A1-HC, but there was no significant change in lung function, quality of life measures, or sputum NE activity or sputum cytokine levels. Recently, an inhaled anti-NE therapy, POL6014, was studied in a Phase I trial using an ascending dose schedule in both healthy volunteers and participants with CF (Barth et al., 2019). A single inhaled dose was safe in both healthy volunteers and subjects with CF. Sputum active NE levels were reduced by greater than 1-log at 3 h after treatment at all doses. Therapy with POL6014 for subjects with CF is currently being evaluated in a Phase IIa/IIb randomized, placebo-controlled, double-blind study (NCT03748199). This initial report of POL6014 activity is promising; however, there is still a compelling need to develop drugs with multifunctional anti-protease and anti-inflammatory activities that are resistant to protease degradation or oxidation.

GAGs: Structure and Function

GAGs are polymers composed primarily of disaccharides which consist of a D-glucosamine bound to either uronic acid (D-glucuronic acid or L-iduronic acid) or galactose (Morla, 2019). The composition and linkage of monosaccharides and addition of modifications define the four major classes of GAGs: heparin/heparan sulfate (HS), chondroitin sulfate, dermatan sulfate, and hyaluronan. The uronic acid has a carboxylic acid unit and both monosaccharides are decorated with N- and O-linked sulfate residues that together confer a negative charge to the polymers. Native hyaluronan is not sulfated. In the CF lung, there are high levels of chondroitin sulfate and hyaluronan. Chondroitin sulfate proteoglycans contribute to turbidity and the mass of insoluble pellet in CF sputum; these qualities are relieved by depolymerization with chondroitinase ABC (Khatri et al., 2003). Low molecular weight hyaluronan may contribute to inflammation in the CF lung *via* TLR2 and TLR4 signaling and downstream NK-κB signaling (reviewed in (Reeves et al., 2011)). However, GAG structures can be modified to alter sulfation which plays a critical role in mediating biological effects. Moreover, GAG mimetics are being generated to achieve optimal drug characteristics while minimizing adverse properties. Heparin and HS proteoglycans bind to predicted basic amino acid-rich domains (Cardin and Weintraub, 1989; Hileman et al., 1998). GAGs have many biological effects that impact coagulation, infection, inflammation, cell adhesion, metastasis, cell matrix structure, and tissue differentiation and repair (Lima et al., 2017; Morla, 2019). Importantly, heparin can be taken up by cells and localized to cytoplasm and nucleus (Richardson et al., 2001; Raman et al., 2013) (**Figure 1A**). The localization of administered heparin to both extracellular and intracellular domains permits a wide array of anticipated functions including enzyme inhibition and interference with cell- cell receptor interactions, microbe- cell interactions, and HS proteoglycan pro-inflammatory activities. In this review, we will focus on GAG properties that impact CF and other chronic lung diseases.

Modified Non-Anticoagulant Heparins and Anti-Inflammatory Activity

Heparin is well known for its anticoagulant activity, but in addition, heparin has a broad repertoire of anti-inflammatory functions including anti-NE and anti-cathepsin G activity, inhibition of NF-kB, blockade of L- and P-selectin binding, and interference with HMGB1 release and interaction with its receptor, RAGE (Morla, 2019; Mulloy, 2019). At least three modified heparins have been developed to reduce anti-coagulant activity but retain anti-inflammatory activity: glycol-split heparin, sulfated-non-anticoagulant Low Molecular Weight Heparin (S- NACH) and 2-O, 3-O desulfated heparin (ODSH). Glycol-split heparin, generated by periodate oxidation of porcine mucosal heparin, is characterized by a cleavage between C2 and C3 of the nonsulfated uronic acid residue (Naggi et al., 2005). Glycol split heparin, administered subcutaneously to mice daily starting 10 days after establishment of chronic *P. aeruginosa*-agar bead pneumonia, decreases inflammatory cytokines, BAL neutrophil counts, and bacterial lung burden at 28 days (Lore et al., 2018). S-NACH is a purified fraction of low molecular weight heparin isolated to select drug with minimal anti-coagulant activity (Shastri et al., 2015). In a murine asthma model generated by ovalbumin (OVA)-sensitization and challenge, S-NACH intraperitoneal administration following OVA challenge blunted BAL inflammation by eosinophils, macrophages, and neutrophils, blocked goblet cell metaplasia, and blocked T2 cytokine expression in serum and BAL (Ghonim et al., 2018).

Of the modified non-anticoagulant heparins tested for anti-inflammatory efficacy, there is the most experience with 2-O, 3-O, desulfated heparin (ODSH). Fryer et al. (1997) lyophilized heparin under alkaline condition to produce ODSH. ODSH has substantially reduced anticoagulant activity compared to heparin as determined by activated partial thromboplastin time (APTT) and anti-Xa clotting assays. But the anti-neutrophil protease activities, including anti-NE and anti-cathepsin G activities, are largely unchanged in ODSH compared to heparin. ODSH also retains the pharmacological properties of heparin *in vivo*, including inhibition of bronchial hyperreactivity after antigen challenge, and prevention of airway smooth muscle cell proliferation (Fryer et al., 1997). Importantly, ODSH does not bind to platelet factor 4 and thus doesn't trigger heparin-induced thrombocytopenia (Rao et al., 2010). ODSH interrupts ligand-receptor interactions, blunting pro-inflammatory signaling

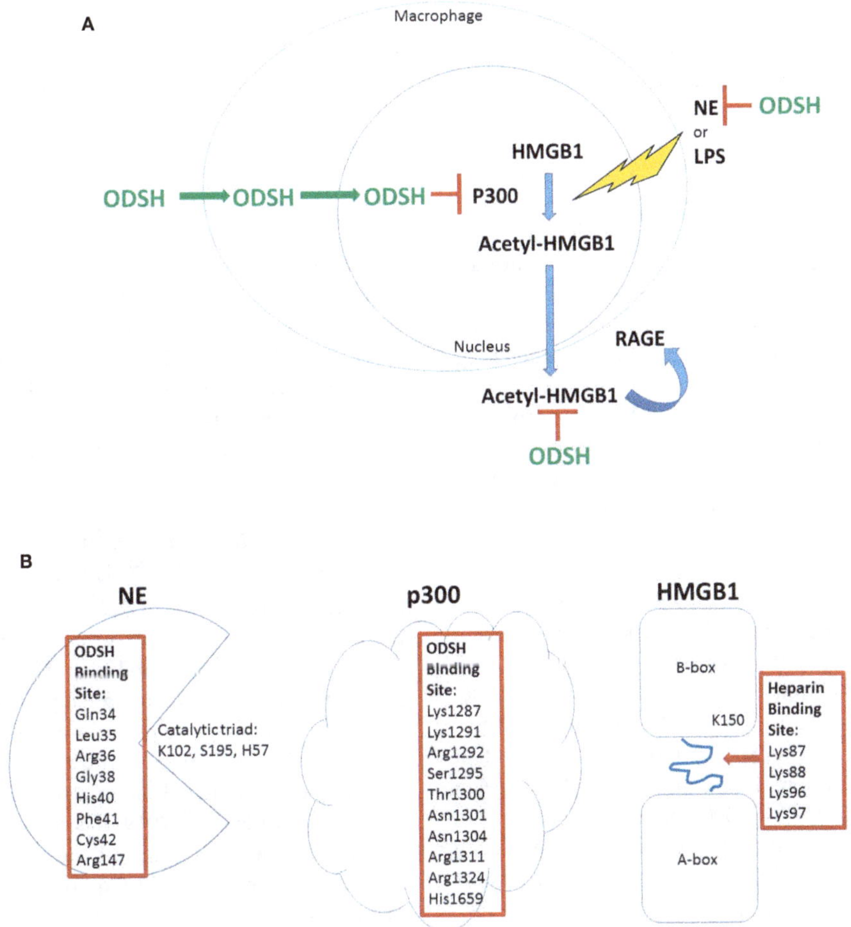

FIGURE 1 | ODSH localization and function in a macrophage cell line. ODSH is taken up by a mouse macrophage cell line (RAW264.7) into the cytoplasm within 2 h and into the nucleus by 24 h (Zheng et al., 2017) **(A)**. ODSH has anti-NE activity and blocks HMGB1-RAGE interaction in the extracellular domain, and inhibits p300 lysine acetyltransferase activity in the nucleus **(A)**. ODSH inhibits NE activity by binding to an allosteric inhibitory site (Kummarapurugu et al., 2018), and ODSH inhibits p300 enzyme activity by binding to the acetyl-CoA binding site in the catalytic domain (Zheng et al., 2017) **(B)**. In contrast, ODSH binds to the loop connecting the A-box and B-box of HMGB1, blocking interaction with heparan sulfate proteoglycans required for HMGB1 ligation of the RAGE receptor (Xu et al., 2011) **(B)**. Amino acid residues required for ODSH or heparin inhibitory activity are shown (Red Box).

cascades. Both heparin and ODSH inhibit RAGE- HMGB1 interaction and RAGE-S100A9/calgranulin interaction *in vitro* (Rao et al., 2010). The ODSH concentrations (IC_{50}) to inhibit NE activity (0.14 µg/ml), and to block HMGB1-RAGE binding (0.23 µg/ml) are similar, supporting the concept that ODSH (MW approximately 10 kD) achieves both anti-protease and anti-inflammatory activities within a nanomolar concentration range.

Heparin and ODSH Anti-HMGB1 Activity

HMGB1 is recognized as a major inflammatory mediator in CF plasma and sputum that is strongly associated with lung disease progression (Liou et al., 2012; Chirico et al., 2015). Therefore, HMGB1 is likely to be an important target for CF anti-inflammatory therapy. HMGB1 has two major functions; it is a nuclear non-histone chromatin binding protein that facilitates transcriptional regulation, and it is an extracellular damage associated molecule pattern or alarmin that is secreted by activated macrophages as a delayed mediator of inflammation (Lotze and Tracey, 2005). HMGB1 release is triggered by HMGB1 lysine acetylation which is activated following exposure to microbial products (LPS), cytokines (TNFα) (Lotze and Tracey, 2005), or NE (Griffin et al., 2014). HMGB1 can also be released from necrotic cells. HMGB1 has been reported to transduce cellular signals by interacting with at least three receptors: RAGE, TLR2 and TLR4 (Park et al., 2004; Sharma et al., 2014). Binding of HMGB1 to RAGE activates NF-κB and the ERK/p38 pathway which promotes cytokine production (TNF, IL-6, and IFN-γ). Binding of HMGB1 to TLR2/TLR4 leads to NF-κB activation through a MyD88 (myeloid differentiation primary-response protein 88)-dependent mechanism. Importantly, ODSH blocks both HMGB1 release and HMGB1 ligation of receptors both *in vitro* and *in vivo*. Intratracheal HMGB1 in a mouse model induces significant pulmonary inflammation with increased BAL total cells, neutrophils, and TNF-α levels at 24 hr. Simultaneous intratracheal ODSH administered with HMGB1 decreased all of these BAL measures, indicating that ODSH can inhibit HMGB1-RAGE- induced inflammatory responses *in vivo* (Rao et al., 2010). A summary of glycol split heparin, S-NACH, and ODSH activities *in vivo* in preclinical models relevant to CF is summarized in **Table 1**.

ODSH is effective in preclinical models of infection and inflammation to blunt these pathologic processes. In a *P. aeruginosa* (PA)-induced murine pneumonia model, intranasal ODSH decreases BAL HMGB1 levels, reduces pulmonary bacterial burden, ameliorates PA-induced lung injury, and improves survival (Sharma et al., 2014). In a murine model of intratracheal NE-induced lung inflammation and remodeling, ODSH pretreatment blocks NE-induced neutrophil influx, upregulation of KC, and release of HMGB1 into BAL (Griffin et al., 2014). To investigate the mechanism of ODSH inhibition of HMGB1 release, the impact of fluorescein-labeled (FITC)-ODSH on NE- or LPS-treated mouse macrophage cells (RAW264.7) was investigated. ODSH is taken up by RAW264.7 cells, and is localized to the cytoplasm and nucleus (Zheng et al., 2017). The sulfation pattern of modified heparins influence intracellular uptake and localization that is specific for different cell types (Raman et al., 2013). In RAW264.7 cells treated with NE or LPS, ODSH blocks HMGB1 lysine-acetylation in a dose-dependent manner, by inhibiting P300 histone (lysine) acetyltransferase (HAT) activity. Spectrofluorometry reveals that ODSH binding to p300 results in a conformational change in p300, and further tightens ODSH-p300 binding; this mechanism is supported by a complementary approach of in silico modeling with combinatorial virtual library screening of interactions between p300 and ODSH (Zheng et al., 2017) (**Figure 1B**). Importantly, heparin also interacts directly with HMGB1, changing its conformation and reducing its affinity for RAGE which interrupts the HMGB1-RAGE signaling cascade (Ling et al., 2011). Furthermore, heparin and ODSH bind to NE and inhibit its activity.

Heparin and ODSH Anti-NE Activity in *Ex Vivo* CF Sputum

High concentrations of NE released by neutrophils are found in CF sputum. Importantly NE, a cationic serine protease, binds to the copious polyanionic polymers in sputum including DNA (Gray et al., 2015); mucins (Nadziejko and Finkelstein, 1994) and actin filaments (Broughton-Head et al., 2007; Kater et al., 2007). Dornase alfa (Fuchs et al., 1994) and 7% hypertonic saline (HTS) (Elkins et al., 2006), the mainstay mucoactive therapies for patients with CF, improve pulmonary function, and decrease the frequency of pulmonary exacerbations. However, both therapies have been reported to increase NE activity in CF sputum (Cantin, 1998; Chen et al., 2006). ODSH is a robust inhibitor of NE activity *in vitro* with a low IC_{50} (Griffin et al., 2014; Kummarapurugu et al., 2018), but in CF sputum, both ODSH and heparin inhibition of NE activity requires DNA depolymerization by DNase-1 (Kummarapurugu et al., 2018). This observation suggests that anionic DNA polymers compete with anionic ODSH for binding to NE. When these interactions were investigated, it was discovered by both pharmacokinetic studies and by combinatorial virtual library screening, that both DNA and ODSH bind to the same allosteric domain on NE that is required for inhibition (Kummarapurugu et al., 2018) (**Figure 1B**). Furthermore, inhibition of NE activity in sputum by heparin or DNA is chain length dependent, with a requirement for a larger size than approximately 15 monosaccharides for heparins (Spencer et al., 2006; Kummarapurugu et al., 2018) or 12-mer for DNA oligomers (Kummarapurugu et al., 2018). Neither fondiparinux, a heparin pentasaccharide (1.8 kDa) nor a DNA hexamer have anti-NE activity, confirming that a threshold length is necessary for heparin and DNA to bind to NE and exert anti-elastase activity (Kummarapurugu et al., 2018). Interestingly, unfractionated heparin releases soluble DNA from sputum that is available for dornase alfa cleavage (Broughton-Head et al., 2007). Thus, heparin enhances DNase activity.

Novel Glycosaminoglycan Therapeutics as Anti-Protease, Anti-Microbial, and/or Anti-Inflammatory Therapies

Glycosaminoglycans have a broad array of functions both in native tissues and when modified to be used as competitors for endogenous heparan sulfate proteoglycans or for their properties to bind to cationic proteins and modify activities. Development of small synthetic non-saccharide glycosaminoglycan mimetics (NSGMs) offer modifiable alternatives for polysaccharide GAGs. NSGM 32 (Morla et al., 2019) has robust anti-elastase activity *in vitro* and has a mixed allosteric and orthosteric mechanism of action. However, NSGM 32 requires DNA depolymerization for anti-elastase activity in CF sputum, and is less potent than ODSH (Kummarapurugu et al., 2018). It was speculated that NSGM 32 binds to other positively charged moieties in CF sputum and therefore higher concentrations of drug are required for inhibition of NE activity (Morla et al., 2019). A sulfated synthetic lignin, sulfated dehydropolymer caffeic acid (CDSO3), inhibits the development of emphysema in a VEGFR-inhibitor-induced rat model *via* multiple functions including anti-oxidant activity, and prevention of epithelial and endothelial cell death *via* iron-chelation- induced stabilization of HIF-1α and VEGF signaling (Truong et al., 2017). These two compounds illustrate the exquisite target specificity due to sulfation patterns incorporated into small synthetically produced GAG mimetics. Another advantage of synthetic sulfated lignins is that they are homogeneous compounds that do not require porcine or bovine bioproducts for production.

Polysulfated hyaluronan is a modified hyaluronic acid which has potent anti-inflammatory properties (Zhang et al., 2011). Low molecular weight polysulfated hyaluronan blocks LPS-stimulated macrophage release of cytokines including TNFα, IL-6, IL-12, MCP-1, and increases expression of antioxidants, superoxide 2 and 3 (Jouy et al., 2017). In a murine model of second hand smoke induced lung disease, a polysulfated hyaluronan administered by intraperitoneal (i.p.) injection inhibits release of

TABLE 1 | *In vivo* models of chronic lung diseases treated with modified or non-saccharide GAGs.

Animal Model	Treatment (Dose and Administration)	Outcome Measures	Reference
Balb/c mice: NE airway inflammation model NE (o.a.) ± **ODSH** (o.a.)	Days 1, 4, 7: NE (44 μM) or NS **ODSH** (635 μM) or NS o.a. Day 8: BAL/lung harvest	NE induces BAL cells & PMN, KC, HMGB1 **ODSH**+NE: decreases total cells and PMN; decreases KC and HMGB1	Griffin et al. (2014)
C57BL/6 mice: *P. aeruginosa* (PA01) pneumonia model PA01 (i.n.) PA01 (i.t.) ± **ODSH** (s.c.)	Day 1: PA01 i.n. **ODSH** (8.3- 75 mg/kg) or NS s.c. q 12 h x 2 Day 2: BAL/lung harvest Day 1: PA01 i.t. **ODSH** (75 mg/kg) or NS s.c. 12 h x 4 Day 3: survival	**ODSH** decreases PA01 CFU; decreases lung protein content and edema; decreases total and PMN cell count; decreases BAL HMGB1; inhibits TLR2 and TLR4 binding **ODSH** improves mouse survival	Sharma et al. (2014)
C57Bl/6N *P.aeruginosa* pneumonia model (PA) CF isolate AA43- embedded in agar beads (i.t.) ± **glycol split LMWH, C3gs20 vs. N-acetyl LMWH, C23** s.c.	Day 1: PA- agar beads (1-2 x 10^6) vs. sterile beads i.t. Day 1-14: **C3gs20 or C23** (30 mg/kg/d) or vehicle s.c. Day 14: BAL and lung harvest Day 1: PA- agar beads (1-2 x 10^6) vs. sterile beads i.t. Day 10-28: **C3gs20 or C23** (30 mg/kg/d) or vehicle s.c. Day 28: BAL and lung harvest	**C23** decreased BAL total cells and PMN; No significant change in PA CFU. **C3gs and C23** decreased BAL total cells and PMN, decreased total PA CFU, and decreased IL-17A **C3gs20** decreased IL-1β, IL-12pp40, G-CSF, and KC	Lore et al. (2018)
C57BL/6J mice Allergic Asthma model OVA i.p. sensitization and challenge with Ova ± **sulfated non-anticoagulant LMWH (S-NACH) i.p.**	Wk 1: Alum/Ova i.p.once per wk x 2 Wk 2-4: Ova 3% inhaled 3x per week **S-NACH** (10 mg/kg) or NS i.p. Week 5: BAL and lung harvest	**S-NACH** decreased Ova-triggered eosinophils, macrophages, lymphocytes in BAL, decreased goblet cell metaplasia, decreased lung tissue hydroxyproline, decreased BAL and serum T2 cytokines, decreased Ova-IgE.	Ghonim et al. (2018)
C57BL/6 mice: LL-37- induced rhinosinusitis model LL37 i.n.± **polysulfated HA (GM-0111)** or HA i.n.	Day 1: LL-37 (115 μg) **GM-0111** or HA (800μg) Day 2: sinus harvest	LL-37 increases Mast cells, MPO, lamina propria (LP) thickening and cell death **GM-0111**+LL-37: Decreased Mast cells, MPO, LP thickening and cell death **GM-0111** more effective than HA	Pulsipher et al. (2017)
BALB/c mice: Aspergillus chronic rhinosinusitis (CRS) model A.fumigatus extract ± **polysulfated HA (GM-1111) or PBS** i.n. 3 Groups: 1. 1. PBS 2. 2. A fumigatus+ PBS 3. 3. A. fumigatus+ GM-1111	Week 0: All groups sensitized with Alum + PBS or *A.fumigatus* i.p. Weeks 1-8: PBS or *A.fumigatus* extract (20,000 PNU i.n.) 3 x per wk. Weeks 5-8: PBS or GM-1111 (600 μg) i.n.5x per wk Week 9: Collect blood and sinonasal tissue	**GM-1111**+ *A.fumigatus* (Af) extract decreased Af-induced CRS symptoms, mucosal edema and injury, goblet cells, TLR2 and TLR4, T2 cytokines, and IgE	Alt et al. (2018)
C57BL/6 mice Second hand smoke model of lung disease ± **sulfated semisynthetic HA GAG ethers (SAGEs)**	SHS vs. Rm air nasal inhalation 10 min/day x 5 d/wk 4 weeks exposure **SAGE** (30 mg/kg) i.p. for 3 d/wk Collect BAL and lung RNA and protein	**SAGEs** effect on SHS exposure: Blocked lung RAGE expression Blocked BAL protein, total cells, and cytokines: IL-α, IL-2, TNFα	Tsai et al. (2019)
Sprague Dawley rats Rat Emphysema Model with SU51416 (VEGFR inhibitor)±	Day 1: SU5416 (20 mg/kg) s.c. ± Day 1–Day 21:	**CDSO3** prevented SU5416-induced emphysema, improved rat exercise endurance, decreased oxidative stress,	Truong et al. (2017)

(Continued)

TABLE 1 | Continued

Animal Model	Treatment (Dose and Administration)	Outcome Measures	Reference
polysulfated dehydropolymer of caffeic acid (CDSO3) 3 Groups: Untreated healthy SU5416 + NS SU5416 + **CDSO3**	**CDSO3** (60 μg/kg) or NS inhaled 3x per week	and increased VEGF and HIF-1α, and decreased cleaved caspase-3	

BAL, bronchoalveolar lavage; HIF-1α, hypoxia inducible factor- 1α; i.n., intranasal; i.p., intraperitoneal; i.t., intratracheal; KC, keratinocyte chemoattractant; LMWH, low molecular weight heparin; MPO, myeloperoxidase; PMN, neutrophil; PNU, protein neoantigen units; o.a., oropharyngeal aspiration; RAGE, receptor for advanced glycation end products; s.c., subcutaneous; SHS, second hand smoke; TNFα, tumor necrosis factor α; VEGF, vascular endothelial growth factor.
The bolded text are to emphasize the stimuli for the model type and the drugs used to treat this model.

BAL TNFα, IL-1α, and IL-2, and decreases BAL inflammation and lung permeability (Tsai et al., 2019). A sulfated semisynthetic low molecular weight hyaluronan, GM-1111, (molecular weight 5.5 kD), has been tested for anti-inflammatory properties. In a mouse model of rhinosinusitis generated by intranasal administration of a cathelicidin fragment, LL37, GM-1111 blocks neutrophil and mast cell mucosal infiltration and significantly decreases epithelial apoptosis (Pulsipher et al., 2017). In vitro, in nasal epithelial cells, LL37 stimulates inflammation and cell death; another GM compound, GM-0111, inhibits IL-6 and IL-8 release and blocks Caspase-1- and Caspase-8 -induced cell death (Thomas et al., 2017). In an *A.fumigatus*- intranasal allergen-sensitization mouse model of chronic rhinosinusitis, intranasal GM-1111 introduced 3 weeks after *A. fumigatus* sensitization, significantly inhibits goblet cell metaplasia and mucosal T2 inflammation, and decreases TLR2 and TLR4 expression (Alt et al., 2018). In addition, in a periodontitis model, GM-0111 suppresses the growth of *P. gingivalis* and *A. actinomycetemcomitans* and biofilm formation, demonstrating antimicrobial activity (Savage et al., 2016). A summary of polysulfated hyaluronan activities *in vivo* in preclinical models of chronic lung disease is summarized in **Table 1**.

Heparan sulfate (HS) is expressed widely on many cell types as a proteoglycan. HS proteoglycans regulate inflammation by binding to ELR (Glu Leu Arg)- CXC chemokines at conserved His, Lys, Arg residues, controlling chemotactic gradients in the extracellular and pericellular matrices (Rajarathnam KaD, 2020). However, in the CF lung, endogenous HS proteoglycans have pro-inflammatory properties (Reeves et al., 2011); HS stabilizes cytokine and chemokine ligands, preventing protease digestion, thus increasing CXCL ligation to CXCR1 and 2 to upregulate inflammation (Rajarathnam KaD, 2020). HS enables RAGE hexamer formation for more efficient intracellular signaling (Xu et al., 2013), and binds L-selectin to promote neutrophil slowing and diapedesis across endothelial cells into tissues (Farrugia et al., 2018). HS also serves as a cell receptor for microbe adhesion and invasion (Rostand and Esko, 1997) (**Figure 2**). Bacteria, *P. aeruginosa* (Paulsson et al., 2019) and *nontypable H. influenza* (NTHi) (Su et al., 2019), and viruses, adenovirus (Dechecchi et al., 2001) and Severe Acute Respiratory Syndrome-Coronavirus (SARS-CoV) (Lang et al., 2011) and SARS-CoV-2 spike protein (So Young Kim et al., 2020) all bind to HS proteoglycans. Importantly, exposure to heparin competes with and inhibits binding to HS proteoglycans (**Figure 2**) resulting in inhibition of binding of *P. aeruginosa* (Paulsson et al., 2019) and NTHi (Su et al., 2019) to laminin, a major component of the basal lamina in the airway, and inhibition of binding of adenovirus (Dechecchi et al., 2001) and SARS-CoV (Lang et al., 2011) to epithelia, and inhibition of SARS-CoV-2 (So Young Kim et al., 2020) spike protein to HS as detected by surface plasmon resonance. Treatment with synthetic HS or heparin inhibits cytokine/chemokine binding to G-protein coupled receptors and blocks neutrophil interaction with endothelial selectins resulting in decreased neutrophil influx (Lore et al., 2018) (**Figure 2**). Altered sulfation of HS affects pro- vs anti-inflammatory behavior; increased N- and 6-O-sulfation increase cytokine ligation and neutrophil recruitment while increased 2-O-sulfation blunts neutrophilic inflammation (Axelsson et al., 2012). HS is also required for HMGB1-RAGE receptor binding; heparin can compete with HS and interrupt RAGE ligation by binding to HMGB1 (Xu et al., 2011).

Clinical Trials Using GAGs for Respiratory Diseases

Unfractionated heparin is the only GAG used in clinical trials to date. Inhaled heparin was tested in healthy volunteers and is safe and well tolerated. When delivered by nebulization, approximately 8% of the nebulized dose of heparin is delivered to the lower respiratory tract (Bendstrup et al., 1999). Importantly, inhaled doses up to 400,000 IU, did not affect lung function, but did increase circulating anti-Factor Xa activity and activated partial thromboplastin time (APTT) (Bendstrup et al., 2002). BAL fluid was tested for anti-coagulant activity in the presence of control plasma and by this method, the half-life of inhaled heparin was determined to be 28 h (Markart et al., 2010).

Inhalation of unfractionated heparin has been tested as a therapeutic for severe COPD (Shute et al., 2018), asthma (Yildiz-Pekoz and Ozsoy, 2017), smoke inhalation (Miller et al., 2014), and acute lung injury (ALI) (Dixon et al., 2010; Tuinman et al., 2012; Juschten et al., 2017), but the number of randomized, double-blind, placebo-controlled studies for these indications is limited (**Table 2**). There is one randomized, double- blind, placebo-controlled, crossover trial of twice daily inhaled heparin (50,000 IU per dose) for 2 weeks in adults with CF, which demonstrates a good safety profile, but does not show any significant improvement in lung function, sputum inflammatory markers or mucus clearance (Serisier et al., 2006). In contrast, a

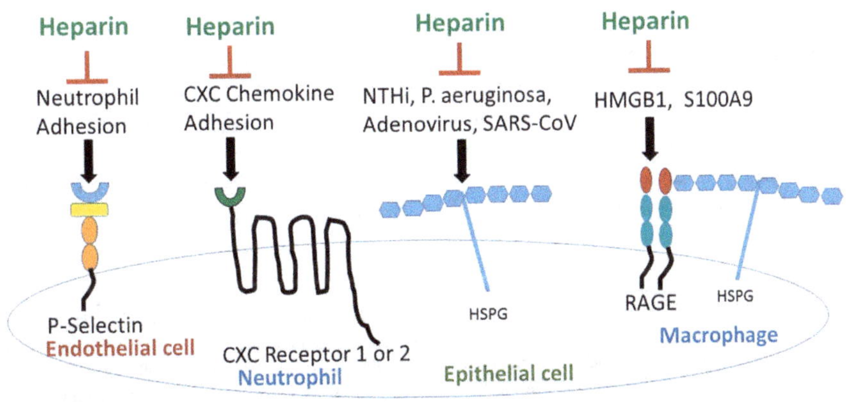

FIGURE 2 | Heparin/ODSH interrupts cell- cell interactions and ligand-receptor binding to block pro-inflammatory pathways. Heparin/ODSH oligosaccharides bind to P- and L-selectins and block neutrophil adhesion and chemotaxis (Nelson et al., 1993; Rao et al., 2010). Heparin inhibits CXCL8/IL-8 and other ELR (Glu Leu Arg)-CXC chemokines from binding to G-protein coupled receptors CXCR1 and CXCR2 (Rajarathnam KaD, 2020). Heparin competes with HSPG for binding to microbial proteins which prevents bacterial or viral-epithelial adhesion and invasion (Rostand and Esko, 1997). Heparin/ODSH bind to HMGB1 and S100A9 and interrupt RAGE ligation (Rao et al., 2010). HSPG, heparan sulfate proteoglycan; NTHi, non-typeable H. influenza; S100A9, calgranulin; SARS-CoV, Severe acute respiratory syndrome- corona virus.

randomized, double-blind, placebo-controlled single site study for COPD using twice daily inhaled heparin (150,000 IU per dose) in addition to inhaled twice daily salbutamol & beclomethasone and airway clearance for 21 days reveals that heparin improves lung function including FEV_1, 6 minute walk distance, and Borg dyspnea score (Shute et al., 2018). The contrast between the COPD study (Shute et al., 2018) and the previously cited CF study (Serisier et al., 2006) suggests that possible reasons for the failure of heparin to improve lung function in patients with CF were an insufficient dose of heparin and/or a limited trial duration to observe clinically significant changes in pulmonary function.

SUMMARY

There are many challenges for developing anti-protease and anti-inflammatory drugs for patients with CF. The innate immune

TABLE 2 | Clinical trials using heparin for chronic lung diseases*.

Disease	Trial design	Drug: dose and administration mode	Outcomes compared to placebo	Reference
Cystic Fibrosis	R, PC, DB- 2 weeks; CF adults; moderate to severe lung disease;N=18	Heparin (50,000 U) inhaled every 12 h	No change in FEV_1 serum CRP sputum IL-8, MPO, NE, TCC, sputum volume	Serisier et al. (2006)
COPD	R, PC, DB- 3 weeks; COPD- GOLD II- IV; N=40	Heparin (75,000 or 150,000 IU) Inhaled twice per day	Adherence 56% Improved FEV_1 Improved 6MWD Increased SpO2	Shute et al. (2018)
Asthma	R, PC, DB crossover; Allergic to dust mite; N=10	Heparin (20,000 U) inhaled 10 min before inhaled dust mite extract bronchoprovocation challenge	Heparin increased the Log_2 provocation dose of dust mite protein nitrogen units causing 20% fall in FEV_1	Bowler et al. (1993)
Asthma	R, PC, DB crossover; Allergic to dust mite; N=8	Heparin (1000 U/kg/dose) inhaled: 90 min and 30 min pre-dust mite inhaled challenge, and 2, 4, 6 h post-dust mite inhaled challenge	Heparin blunted the severity of FEV_1% decrease in late asthmatic responses compared to placebo	Diamant et al. (1996)
Asthma EIB	R, PC, SB, cross-over—5 days; Asymptomatic; N = 12	Day 1: baseline PFT and exercise challenge; Day 3-5: Heparin (1000 U/kg) or cromolyn (20 mg) or placebo inhaled followed by exercise challenge	Heparin blocks post-exercise decrease in SGaw	Ahmed et al. (1993)
Asthma EIB	R, PC, DB, cross-over -7 days; Asymptomatic; N=13	Day 1: baseline PFT and exercise challenge; days 3–7: inhaled Heparin (80,0000 U) or Enoxaparin (0.5, 1, 2 mg/kg) or placebo 45 min before baseline PFTs and then serially post-exercise	Decrease in FEV_1 was blocked by heparin and enoxaparin	Ahmed et al. (1999)

**Only trials with randomized, double or single blind, placebo controlled design were included. 6MWD, 6 minute walk distance test; CRP, C-reactive protein; DB, double-blind; EIB, exercise-induced bronchospasm; FEV_1, Forced expiratory volume at 1 sec; MPO, myeloperoxidase; NE, neutrophil elastase; PC, placebo controlled; R, randomized; SB, single-blind; SGaw, Specific conductance of the airways; SpO2, oxyhemoglobin saturation; TCC, terminal complement complex.*

response is impaired for both viral (Zheng et al., 2003; Berkebile et al., 2020) and bacterial infections. The CF airway milieu is typified by high concentrations of several proteases including neutrophil serine proteases: NE, proteinase 3, Cathepsin G; lysosomal proteases: Cathepsins B, L, and S; and matrix metalloproteases: MMP-9, MMP-8 and MMP-12 (McKelvey et al., 2019) which stimulate downstream signaling cascades that perpetuate oxidative stress and inflammation. The strategy of directing therapy to one target is unlikely to be successful to control inflammation and prevent lung injury. Instead, we propose that GAGs can be developed and harnessed as multi-functional anti-elastase and anti-inflammatory therapies and serve an important function as part of the armamentarium for CF lung disease.

AUTHOR CONTRIBUTIONS

All authors wrote the text and edited the text. JV designed the figures.

REFERENCES

Ahmed, T., Garrigo, J., and Danta, I. (1993). Preventing bronchoconstriction in exercise-induced asthma with inhaled heparin. *N Engl. J. Med.* 329, 90–95. doi: 10.1056/NEJM199307083290204

Ahmed, T., Gonzalez, B. J., and Danta, I. (1999). Prevention of exercise-induced bronchoconstriction by inhaled low-molecular-weight heparin. *Am. J. Respir. Crit. Care Med.* 160, 576–581. doi: 10.1164/ajrccm.160.2.9812076

Alt, J. A., Lee, W. Y., Davis, B. M., Savage, J. R., Kennedy, T. P., Prestwich, G. D., et al. (2018). A synthetic glycosaminoglycan reduces sinonasal inflammation in a murine model of chronic rhinosinusitis. *PloS One* 13, e0204709. doi: 10.1371/journal.pone.0204709

Axelsson, J., Xu, D., Kang, B. N., Nussbacher, J. K., Handel, T. M., Ley, K., et al. (2012). Inactivation of heparan sulfate 2-O-sulfotransferase accentuates neutrophil infiltration during acute inflammation in mice. *Blood* 120, 1742–1751. doi: 10.1182/blood-2012-03-417139

Barth, P., Bruijnzeel, P., Wach, A., Sellier Kessler, O., Hooftman, L., Zimmermann, J., et al. (2019). Single dose escalation studies with inhaled POL6014, a potent novel selective reversible inhibitor of human neutrophil elastase, in healthy volunteers and subjects with cystic fibrosis. *J. Cyst. Fibros.* 19, 299–304. doi: 10.1016/j.jcf.2019.08.020

Bendstrup, K. E., Chambers, C. B., Jensen, J. I., and Newhouse, M. T. (1999). Lung deposition and clearance of inhaled (99m)Tc-heparin in healthy volunteers. *Am. J. Respir. Crit. Care Med.* 160, 1653–1658. doi: 10.1164/ajrccm.160.5.9809123

Bendstrup, K. E., Gram, J., and Jensen, J. I. (2002). Effect of inhaled heparin on lung function and coagulation in healthy volunteers. *Eur. Respir. J.* 19, 606–610. doi: 10.1183/09031936.02.00105202

Berkebile, A. R., Bartlett, J. A., Abou Alaiwa, M., Varga, S. M., Power, U. F., and McCray, P. B.Jr. (2020). Airway Surface Liquid Has Innate Antiviral Activity That Is Reduced in Cystic Fibrosis. *Am. J. Respir. Cell Mol. Biol.* 62, 104–111. doi: 10.1165/rcmb.2018-0304OC

Boucher, R. C. (2019). Muco-Obstructive Lung Diseases. *N Engl. J. Med.* 380, 1941–1953. doi: 10.1056/NEJMra1813799

Bowler, S. D., Smith, S. M., and Lavercombe, P. S. (1993). Heparin inhibits the immediate response to antigen in the skin and lungs of allergic subjects. *Am. Rev. Respir. Dis.* 147, 160–163. doi: 10.1164/ajrccm/147.1.160

Broughton-Head, V. J., Shur, J., Carroll, M. P., Smith, J. R., and Shute, J. K. (2007). Unfractionated heparin reduces the elasticity of sputum from patients with cystic fibrosis. *Am. J. Physiol. Lung Cell Mol. Physiol.* 293, L1240–L1249. doi: 10.1152/ajplung.00206.2007

Bruscia, E. M., and Bonfield, T. L. (2016). Innate and Adaptive Immunity in Cystic Fibrosis. *Clin. Chest Med.* 37, 17–29. doi: 10.1016/j.ccm.2015.11.010

Caldwell, R. A., Boucher, R. C., and Stutts, M. J. (2005). Neutrophil elastase activates near-silent epithelial Na+ channels and increases airway epithelial Na + transport. *Am. J. Physiol. Lung Cell Mol. Physiol.* 288, L813–L819. doi: 10.1152/ajplung.00435.2004

Cantin, A. M. (1998). DNase I acutely increases cystic fibrosis sputum elastase activity and its potential to induce lung hemorrhage in mice. *Am. J. Respir. Crit. Care Med.* 157, 464–469. doi: 10.1164/ajrccm.157.2.9608033

Cardin, A. D., and Weintraub, H. J. (1989). Molecular modeling of protein-glycosaminoglycan interactions. *Arteriosclerosis* 9, 21–32. doi: 10.1161/01.ATV.9.1.21

Chen, Y., Hashiguchi, N., Yip, L., and Junger, W. G. (2006). Hypertonic saline enhances neutrophil elastase release through activation of P2 and A3 receptors. *Am. J. Physiol. Cell Physiol.* 290, C1051 C1059. doi: 10.1152/ajpcell.00216.2005

Chen, G., Sun, L., Kato, T., Okuda, K., Martino, M. B., Abzhanova, A., et al. (2019). IL-1beta dominates the promucin secretory cytokine profile in cystic fibrosis. *J. Clin. Invest.* 129, 4433–4450. doi: 10.1172/JCI125669

Chirico, V., Lacquaniti, A., Leonardi, S., Grasso, L., Rotolo, N., Romano, C., et al. (2015). Acute pulmonary exacerbation and lung function decline in patients with cystic fibrosis: high-mobility group box 1 (HMGB1) between inflammation and infection. *Clin. Microbiol. Infect.* 21, 368 e361–369. doi: 10.1016/j.cmi.2014.11.004

Clancy, D. M., Sullivan, G. P., Moran, H. B. T., Henry, C. M., Reeves, E. P., McElvaney, N. G., et al. (2018). Extracellular Neutrophil Proteases Are Efficient Regulators of IL-1, IL-33, and IL-36 Cytokine Activity but Poor Effectors of Microbial Killing. *Cell Rep.* 22, 2937–2950. doi: 10.1016/j.celrep.2018.02.062

Cosgrove, S., Chotirmall, S. H., Greene, C. M., and McElvaney, N. G. (2011). Pulmonary proteases in the cystic fibrosis lung induce interleukin 8 expression from bronchial epithelial cells via a heme/meprin/epidermal growth factor receptor/Toll-like receptor pathway. *J. Biol. Chem.* 286, 7692–7704. doi: 10.1074/jbc.M110.183863

Dechecchi, M. C., Melotti, P., Bonizzato, A., Santacatterina, M., Chilosi, M., and Cabrini, G. (2001). Heparan sulfate glycosaminoglycans are receptors sufficient to mediate the initial binding of adenovirus types 2 and 5. *J. Virol.* 75, 8772–8780. doi: 10.1128/JVI.75.18.8772-8780.2001

Diamant, Z., Timmers, M. C., van der Veen, H., Page, C. P., van der Meer, F. J., and Sterk, P. J. (1996). Effect of inhaled heparin on allergen-induced early and late asthmatic responses in patients with atopic asthma. *Am. J. Respir. Crit. Care Med.* 153, 1790–1795. doi: 10.1164/ajrccm.153.6.8665036

Dixon, B., Schultz, M. J., Smith, R., Fink, J. B., Santamaria, J. D., and Campbell, D. J. (2010). Nebulized heparin is associated with fewer days of mechanical ventilation in critically ill patients: a randomized controlled trial. *Crit. Care* 14, R180. doi: 10.1186/cc9286

Elborn, J. S., Perrett, J., Forsman-Semb, K., Marks-Konczalik, J., Gunawardena, K., and Entwistle, N. (2012). Efficacy, safety and effect on biomarkers of AZD9668 in cystic fibrosis. *Eur. Respir. J.* 40, 969–976. doi: 10.1183/09031936.00194611

Elkins, M. R., Robinson, M., Rose, B. R., Harbour, C., Moriarty, C. P., Marks, G. B., et al. (2006). A controlled trial of long-term inhaled hypertonic saline in patients with cystic fibrosis. *N Engl. J. Med.* 354, 229–240. doi: 10.1056/NEJMoa043900

Ermund, A., Meiss, L. N., Dolan, B., Bahr, A., Klymiuk, N., and Hansson, G. C. (2018). The mucus bundles responsible for airway cleaning are retained in cystic fibrosis and by cholinergic stimulation. *Eur. Respir. J.*s 52, 1800457. doi: 10.1183/13993003.00457-2018

Farrugia, B. L., Lord, M. S., Melrose, J., and Whitelock, J. M. (2018). The Role of Heparan Sulfate in Inflammation, and the Development of Biomimetics as Anti-Inflammatory Strategies. *J. Histochem. Cytochem.* 66, 321–336. doi: 10.1369/0022155417740881

Fischer, B. M., Domowicz, D. A., Zheng, S., Carter, J. L., McElvaney, N. G., Taggart, C., et al. (2009). Neutrophil elastase increases airway epithelial nonheme iron levels. *Clin. Transl. Sci.* 2, 333–339. doi: 10.1111/j.1752-8062.2009.00151.x

Fischer, B. M., Wong, J. K., Degan, S., Kummarapurugu, A. B., Zheng, S., Haridass, P., et al. (2013). Increased expression of senescence markers in cystic fibrosis airways. *Am. J. Physiol. Lung Cell Mol. Physiol.* 304, L394–L400. doi: 10.1152/ajplung.00091.2012

Fryer, A., Huang, Y. C., Rao, G., Jacoby, D., Mancilla, E., Whorton, R., et al. (1997). Selective O-desulfation produces nonanticoagulant heparin that retains pharmacological activity in the lung. *J. Pharmacol. Exp. Ther.* 282, 208–219.

Fuchs, H. J., Borowitz, D. S., Christiansen, D. H., Morris, E. M., Nash, M. L.,

Ramsey, B. W., et al. (1994). Effect of aerosolized recombinant human DNase on exacerbations of respiratory symptoms and on pulmonary function in patients with cystic fibrosis. *N. Engl. J. Med.* 331, 637–642. doi: 10.1056/NEJM199409083311003

Gaggar, A., Chen, J., Chmiel, J. F., Dorkin, H. L., Flume, P. A., Griffin, R., et al. (2016). Inhaled alpha1-proteinase inhibitor therapy in patients with cystic fibrosis. *J. Cyst. Fibros.* 15, 227–233. doi: 10.1016/j.jcf.2015.07.009

Ghio, A. J., Roggli, V. L., Soukup, J. M., Richards, J. H., Randell, S. H., and Muhlebach, M. S. (2013). Iron accumulates in the lavage and explanted lungs of cystic fibrosis patients. *J. Cyst. Fibros.* 12, 390–398. doi: 10.1016/j.jcf.2012.10.010

Ghonim, M. A., Wang, J., Ibba, S. V., Luu, H. H., Pyakurel, K., Benslimane, I., et al. (2018). Sulfated non-anticoagulant heparin blocks Th2-induced asthma by modulating the IL-4/signal transducer and activator of transcription 6/Janus kinase 1 pathway. *J. Transl. Med.* 16, 243. doi: 10.1186/s12967-018-1621-5

Gray, R. D., McCullagh, B. N., and McCray, P. B. (2015). NETs and CF Lung Disease: Current Status and Future Prospects. *Antibiot. (Basel)* 4, 62–75. doi: 10.3390/antibiotics4010062

Gray, R. D., Hardisty, G., Regan, K. H., Smith, M., Robb, C. T., Duffin, R., et al. (2018). Delayed neutrophil apoptosis enhances NET formation in cystic fibrosis. *Thorax* 73, 134–144. doi: 10.1136/thoraxjnl-2017-210134

Griffin, K. L., Fischer, B. M., Kummarapurugu, A. B., Zheng, S., Kennedy, T. P., Rao, N. V., et al. (2014). 2-O, 3-O-desulfated heparin inhibits neutrophil elastase-induced HMGB-1 secretion and airway inflammation. *Am. J. Respir. Cell Mol. Biol.* 50, 684–689. doi: 10.1165/rcmb.2013-0338RC

Guyot, N., Butler, M. W., McNally, P., Weldon, S., Greene, C. M., Levine, R. L., et al. (2008). Elafin, an elastase-specific inhibitor, is cleaved by its cognate enzyme neutrophil elastase in sputum from individuals with cystic fibrosis. *J. Biol. Chem.* 283, 32377–32385. doi: 10.1074/jbc.M803707200

Hileman, R. E., Fromm, J. R., Weiler, J. M., and Linhardt, R. J. (1998). Glycosaminoglycan-protein interactions: definition of consensus sites in glycosaminoglycan binding proteins. *Bioessays* 20, 156–167. doi: 10.1002/(SICI)1521-1878(199802)20:2<156::AID-BIES8>3.0.CO;2-R

Horati, H., Janssens, H. M., Margaroli, C., Veltman, M., Stolarczyk, M., Kilgore, M. B., et al. (2020). Airway profile of bioactive lipids predicts early progression of lung disease in cystic fibrosis. *J. Cyst. Fibros.* doi: 10.1016/j.jcf.2020.01.010

Jackson, P. L., Xu, X., Wilson, L., Weathington, N. M., Clancy, J. P., Blalock, J. E., et al. (2010). Human neutrophil elastase-mediated cleavage sites of MMP-9 and TIMP-1: implications to cystic fibrosis proteolytic dysfunction. *Mol. Med.* 16, 159–166. doi: 10.2119/molmed.2009.00109

Jouy, F., Lohmann, N., Wandel, E., Ruiz-Gomez, G., Pisabarro, M. T., Beck-Sickinger, A. G., et al. (2017). Sulfated hyaluronan attenuates inflammatory signaling pathways in macrophages involving induction of antioxidants. *Proteomics* 17, e1700082. doi: 10.1002/pmic.201700082

Juschten, J., Tuinman, P. R., Juffermans, N. P., Dixon, B., Levi, M., and Schultz, M. J. (2017). Nebulized anticoagulants in lung injury in critically ill patients-an updated systematic review of preclinical and clinical studies. *Ann. Transl. Med.* 5, 444. doi: 10.21037/atm.2017.08.23

Karandashova, S., Kummarapurugu, A., Zheng, S., Kang, L., Sun, S., Rubin, B. K., et al. (2018). Neutrophil elastase correlates with increased sphingolipid content in cystic fibrosis sputum. *Pediatr. Pulmonol.* 53, 872–880. doi: 10.1002/ppul.24001

Kater, A., Henke, M. O., and Rubin, B. K. (2007). The role of DNA and actin polymers on the polymer structure and rheology of cystic fibrosis sputum and depolymerization by gelsolin or thymosin beta 4. *Ann. N Y Acad. Sci.* 1112, 140–153. doi: 10.1196/annals.1415.006

Khatri, I. A., Bhaskar, K. R., Lamont, J. T., Sajjan, S. U., Ho, C. K. Y., and Forstner, J. (2003). Effect of chondroitinase ABC on purulent sputum from cystic fibrosis and other patients. *Pediatr. Res.* 53, 619–627. doi: 10.1203/01.PDR.0000054780.11755.B9

Konstan, M. W., Byard, P. J., Hoppel, C. L., and Davis, P. B. (1995). Effect of high-dose ibuprofen in patients with cystic fibrosis. *N Engl. J. Med.* 332, 848–854. doi: 10.1056/NEJM199503303321303

Kummarapurugu, A. B., Afosah, D. K., Sankaranarayanan, N. V., Navaz Gangji, R., Zheng, S., Kennedy, T., et al. (2018). Molecular principles for heparin oligosaccharide-based inhibition of neutrophil elastase in cystic fibrosis. *J. Biol. Chem.* 293, 12480 12490. doi: 10.1074/jbc.RA118.002644

Lang, J., Yang, N., Deng, J., Liu, K., Yang, P., Zhang, G., et al. (2011). Inhibition of SARS pseudovirus cell entry by lactoferrin binding to heparan sulfate proteoglycans. *PloS One* 6, e23710. doi: 10.1371/journal.pone.0023710

Le Gars, M., Descamps, D., Roussel, D., Saussereau, E., Guillot, L., Ruffin, M., et al. (2013). Neutrophil elastase degrades cystic fibrosis transmembrane conductance regulator via calpains and disables channel function in vitro and in vivo. *Am. J. Respir. Crit. Care Med.* 187, 170–179. doi: 10.1164/rccm.201205-0875OC

Lima, M., Rudd, T., and Yates, E. (2017). New Applications of Heparin and Other Glycosaminoglycans. *Molecules* 22 (5), 749. doi: 10.3390/molecules22050749

Ling, Y., Yang, Z. Y., Yin, T., Li, L., Yuan, W. W., Wu, H. S., et al. (2011). Heparin changes the conformation of high-mobility group protein 1 and decreases its affinity toward receptor for advanced glycation endproducts in vitro. *Int. Immunopharmacol.* 11, 187–193. doi: 10.1016/j.intimp.2010.11.014

Liou, T. G., Adler, F. R., Keogh, R. H., Li, Y., Jensen, J. L., Walsh, W., et al. (2012). Sputum biomarkers and the prediction of clinical outcomes in patients with cystic fibrosis. *PloS One* 7, e42748. doi: 10.1371/journal.pone.0042748

Lore, N. I., Veraldi, N., Riva, C., Sipione, B., Spagnuolo, L., De Fino, I., et al. (2018). Synthesized Heparan Sulfate Competitors Attenuate Pseudomonas aeruginosa Lung Infection. *Int. J. Mol. Sci.* 19 (1), 207. doi: 10.3390/ijms19010207

Lotze, M. T., and Tracey, K. J. (2005). High-mobility group box 1 protein (HMGB1): nuclear weapon in the immune arsenal. *Nat. Rev. Immunol.* 5, 331–342. doi: 10.1038/nri1594

Markart, P., Nass, R., Ruppert, C., Hundack, L., Wygrecka, M., Korfei, M., et al. (2010). Safety and tolerability of inhaled heparin in idiopathic pulmonary fibrosis. *J. Aerosol. Med. Pulm. Drug Delivery* 23, 161–172. doi: 10.1089/jamp.2009.0780

McKelvey, M. C., Weldon, S., McAuley, D. F., Mall, M. A., and Taggart, C. C. (2019). Targeting Proteases in Cystic Fibrosis Lung Disease: Paradigms, Progress, and Potential. *Am. J. Respir. Crit. Care Med.* 201, 141–147. doi: 10.1164/rccm.201906-1190PP

Miller, A. C., Elamin, E. M., and Suffredini, A. F. (2014). Inhaled anticoagulation regimens for the treatment of smoke inhalation-associated acute lung injury: a systematic review. *Crit. Care Med.* 42, 413–419. doi: 10.1097/CCM.0b013e3182a645e5

Morla, S., Sankaranarayanan, N. V., Afosah, D. K., Kumar, M., Kummarapurugu, A. B., Voynow, J. A., et al. (2019). On the Process of Discovering Leads That Target the Heparin-Binding Site of Neutrophil Elastase in the Sputum of Cystic Fibrosis Patients. *J. Med. Chem.* 62, 5501–5511. doi: 10.1021/acs.jmedchem.9b00379

Morla, S. (2019). Glycosaminoglycans and Glycosaminoglycan Mimetics in Cancer and Inflammation. *Int. J. Mol. Sci.* 20, 5501–5511. doi: 10.3390/ijms20081963

Mulloy, B. (2019). The non-anticoagulant promise of heparin and its mimetics. *Curr. Opin. Pharmacol.* 46, 50–54. doi: 10.1016/j.coph.2019.03.009

Nadziejko, C., and Finkelstein, I. (1994). Inhibition of neutrophil elastase by mucus glycoprotein. *Am. J. Respir. Cell Mol. Biol.* 11, 103–107. doi: 10.1165/ajrcmb.11.1.7912511

Naggi, A., Casu, B., Perez, M., Torri, G., Cassinelli, G., Penco, S., et al. (2005). Modulation of the heparanase-inhibiting activity of heparin through selective desulfation, graded N-acetylation, and glycol splitting. *J. Biol. Chem.* 280, 12103–12113. doi: 10.1074/jbc.M414217200

Nelson, R. M., Cecconi, O., Roberts, W. G., Aruffo, A., Linhardt, R. J., and Bevilacqua, M. P. (1993). Heparin oligosaccharides bind L- and P-selectin and inhibit acute inflammation. *Blood* 82, 3253–3258. doi: 10.1182/blood.V82.11.3253.3253

Nichols, D. P., Odem-Davis, K., Cogen, J. D., Goss, C. H., Ren, C. L., Skalland, M., et al. (2020). Pulmonary Outcomes Associated with Long-Term Azithromycin Therapy in Cystic Fibrosis. *Am. J. Respir. Crit. Care Med.* 201, 430–437. doi: 10.1164/rccm.201906-1206OC

Ostedgaard, L. S., Moninger, T. O., McMenimen, J. D., Sawin, N. M., Parker, C. P., Thornell, I. M., et al. (2017). Gel-forming mucins form distinct morphologic structures in airways. *Proc. Natl. Acad. Sci. U.S.A.* 114, 6842–6847. doi: 10.1073/pnas.1703228114

Park, J. S., Svetkauskaite, D., He, Q., Kim, J. Y., Strassheim, D., Ishizaka, A., et al. (2004). Involvement of toll-like receptors 2 and 4 in cellular activation by high mobility group box 1 protein. *J. Biol. Chem.* 279, 7370–7377. doi: 10.1074/jbc.M306793200

Park, J. A., Sharif, A. S., Shiomi, T., Kobzik, L., Kasahara, D. I., Tschumperlin, D. J., et al. (2013). Human neutrophil elastase-mediated goblet cell metaplasia is attenuated in TACE-deficient mice. *Am. J. Physiol. Lung Cell Mol. Physiol.* 304, L701–L707. doi: 10.1152/ajplung.00259.2012

Paulsson, M., Su, Y. C., Ringwood, T., Udden, F., and Riesbeck, K. (2019). Pseudomonas aeruginosa uses multiple receptors for adherence to laminin during infection of the respiratory tract and skin wounds. *Sci. Rep.* 9, 18168. doi: 10.1038/s41598-019-54622-z

Pulsipher, A., Qin, X., Thomas, A. J., Prestwich, G. D., Oottamasathien, S., and Alt, J. A. (2017). Prevention of sinonasal inflammation by a synthetic glycosaminoglycan. *Int. Forum Allergy Rhinol.* 7, 177–184. doi: 10.1002/alr.21865

Rajarathnam KaD, U. R. (2020). Structural Insights Into How Proteoglycans Determine Chemokine-CXCR1/CXCR2 Interactions: Progress and Challenges. *Front. Immunol.* 11, 660. doi: 10.3389/fimmu.2020.00660

Raman, K., Mencio, C., Desai, U. R., and Kuberan, B. (2013). Sulfation patterns determine cellular internalization of heparin-like polysaccharides. *Mol. Pharm.* 10, 1442–1449. doi: 10.1021/mp300679a

Rao, N. V., Argyle, B., Xu, X., Reynolds, P. R., Walenga, J. M., Prechel, M., et al. (2010). Low anticoagulant heparin targets multiple sites of inflammation, suppresses heparin-induced thrombocytopenia, and inhibits interaction of RAGE with its ligands. *Am. J. Physiol. Cell Physiol.* 299, C97–110. doi: 10.1152/ajpcell.00009.2010

Reeves, E. P., Bergin, D. A., Murray, M. A., and McElvaney, N. G. (2011). The involvement of glycosaminoglycans in airway disease associated with cystic fibrosis. *ScientificWorldJournal* 11, 959–971. doi: 10.1100/tsw.2011.81

Richardson, T. P., Trinkaus-Randall, V., and Nugent, M. A. (2001). Regulation of heparan sulfate proteoglycan nuclear localization by fibronectin. *J. Cell Sci.* 114, 1613–1623.

Roesch, E. A., Nichols, D. P., and Chmiel, J. F. (2018). Inflammation in cystic fibrosis: An update. *Pediatr. Pulmonol.* 53, S30–S50. doi: 10.1002/ppul.24129

Rosen, B. H., Evans, T. I. A., Moll, S. R., Gray, J. S., Liang, B., Sun, X., et al. (2018). Infection Is Not Required for Mucoinflammatory Lung Disease in CFTR-Knockout Ferrets. *Am. J. Respir. Crit. Care Med.* 197, 1308–1318. doi: 10.1164/rccm.201708-1616OC

Rosenow, T., Mok, L. C., Turkovic, L., Berry, L. J., Sly, P. D., Ranganathan, S., et al. (2019). The cumulative effect of inflammation and infection on structural lung disease in early cystic fibrosis. *Eur. Respir. J.* 54, 1801771. doi: 10.1183/13993003.01771-2018

Rostand, K. S., and Esko, J. D. (1997). Microbial adherence to and invasion through proteoglycans. *Infect. Immun.* 65, 1–8. doi: 10.1128/IAI.65.1.1-8.1997

Sagel, S. D., Wagner, B. D., Anthony, M. M., Emmett, P., and Zemanick, E. T. (2012). Sputum biomarkers of inflammation and lung function decline in children with cystic fibrosis. *Am. J. Respir. Crit. Care Med.* 186, 857–865. doi: 10.1164/rccm.201203-0507OC

Savage, J. R., Pulsipher, A., Rao, N. V., Kennedy, T. P., Prestwich, G. D., and Ryan, M. E. (2016). Lee WY. A Modified Glycosaminoglycan, GM-0111, Inhibits Molecular Signaling Involved in Periodontitis. *PloS One* 11, e0157310.

Serisier, D. J., Shute, J. K., Hockey, P. M., Higgins, B., Conway, J., and Carroll, M. P. (2006). Inhaled heparin in cystic fibrosis. *Eur. Respir. J.* 27, 354–358. doi: 10.1183/09031936.06.00069005

Sharma, L., Wu, J., Patel, V., Sitapara, R., Rao, N. V., and Kennedy, T. P. (2014). Mantell LL. Partially-desulfated heparin improves survival in Pseudomonas pneumonia by enhancing bacterial clearance and ameliorating lung injury. *J. Immunotoxicol.* 11, 260–267. doi: 10.3109/1547691X.2013.839587

Shastri, M. D., Stewart, N., Horne, J., Zaidi, S. T., Sohal, S. S., Peterson, G. M., et al. (2015). Non-Anticoagulant Fractions of Enoxaparin Suppress Inflammatory Cytokine Release from Peripheral Blood Mononuclear Cells of Allergic Asthmatic Individuals. *PloS One* 10, e0128803. doi: 10.1371/journal.pone.0128803

Shute, J. K., Puxeddu, E., and Calzetta, L. (2018). Therapeutic use of heparin and derivatives beyond anticoagulation in patients with bronchial asthma or COPD. *Curr. Opin. Pharmacol.* 40, 39–45. doi: 10.1016/j.coph.2018.01.006

Shute, J. K., Calzetta, L., Cardaci, V., di Toro, S., Page, C. P., and Cazzola, M. (2018). Inhaled nebulised unfractionated heparin improves lung function in moderate to very severe COPD: A pilot study. *Pulm. Pharmacol. Ther.* 48, 88–96. doi: 10.1016/j.pupt.2017.10.001

Sly, P. D., Gangell, C. L., Chen, L., Ware, R. S., Ranganathan, S., Mott, L. S., et al. (2013). Risk factors for bronchiectasis in children with cystic fibrosis. *New Engl. J. Med.* 368, 1963–1970. doi: 10.1056/NEJMoa1301725

So Young Kim, W. J., Sood, A., Montgomery, D. W., Grant, O. C., Fuster, M. M., Fu, L., et al. (2020). Glycosaminoglycan binding motif at S1/S2 proteolytic cleavage site on spike glycoprotein may facilitate novel coronavirus (SARS-CoV-2) host cell entry. *PloS Pathog.* doi: 10.1101/2020.04.14.041459

Spencer, J. L., Stone, P. J., and Nugent, M. A. (2006). New insights into the inhibition of human neutrophil elastase by heparin. *Biochemistry* 45, 9104–9120. doi: 10.1021/bi060338r

Stoltz, D. A., Meyerholz, D. K., and Welsh, M. J. (2015). Origins of cystic fibrosis lung disease. *N Engl. J. Med.* 372, 351–362. doi: 10.1056/NEJMra1300109

Su, Y. C., Mattsson, E., Singh, B., Jalalvand, F., Murphy, T. F., and Riesbeck, K. (2019). The Laminin Interactome: A Multifactorial Laminin-Binding Strategy by Nontypeable Haemophilus influenzae for Effective Adherence and Colonization. *J. Infect. Dis.* 220, 1049–1060. doi: 10.1093/infdis/jiz217

Suzuki, T., Yamashita, C., Zemans, R. L., Briones, N., Van Linden, A., and Downey, G. P. (2009). Leukocyte elastase induces lung epithelial apoptosis via a PAR-1-, NF-kappaB-, and p53-dependent pathway. *Am. J. Respir. Cell Mol. Biol.* 41, 742–755. doi: 10.1165/rcmb.2008-0157OC

Thomas, A. J., Pulsipher, A., Davis, B. M., and Alt, J. A. (2017). LL-37 causes cell death of human nasal epithelial cells, which is inhibited with a synthetic glycosaminoglycan. *PloS One* 12, e0183542. doi: 10.1371/journal.pone.0183542

Truong, T. M., Li, H., Dhapare, S., Desai, U. R., Voelkel, N. F., and Sakagami, M. (2017). Sulfated dehydropolymer of caffeic acid: In vitro anti-lung cell death activity and in vivo intervention in emphysema induced by VEGF receptor blockade. *Pulm. Pharmacol. Ther.* 45, 181–190. doi: 10.1016/j.pupt.2017.06.007

Tsai, K. Y. F., Hirschi Budge, K. M., Llavina, S., Davis, T., Long, M., Bennett, A., et al. (2019). RAGE and AXL expression following secondhand smoke (SHS) exposure in mice. *Exp. Lung Res.* 45, 297–309. doi: 10.1080/01902148.2019.1684596

Tuinman, P. R., Dixon, B., Levi, M., Juffermans, N. P., and Schultz, M. J. (2012). Nebulized anticoagulants for acute lung injury - a systematic review of preclinical and clinical investigations. *Crit. Care* 16, R70. doi: 10.1186/cc11325

Twigg, M. S., Brockbank, S., Lowry, P., FitzGerald, S. P., Taggart, C., and Weldon, S. (2015). The Role of Serine Proteases and Antiproteases in the Cystic Fibrosis Lung. *Mediators Inflammation* 2015, 293053. doi: 10.1155/2015/293053

Vandivier, R. W., Fadok, V. A., Hoffmann, P. R., Bratton, D. L., Penvari, C., Brown, K. K., et al. (2002). Elastase-mediated phosphatidylserine receptor cleavage impairs apoptotic cell clearance in cystic fibrosis and bronchiectasis. *J. Clin. Invest.* 109, 661–670. doi: 10.1172/JCI0213572

Voynow, J. A., Fischer, B. M., Malarkey, D. E., Burch, L. H., Wong, T., Longphre, M., et al. (2004). Neutrophil elastase induces mucus cell metaplasia in mouse lung. *Am. J. Physiol. Lung Cell Mol. Physiol.* 287, L1293–L1302. doi: 10.1152/ajplung.00140.2004

Voynow, J. A., Fischer, B. M., and Zheng, S. (2008). Proteases and cystic fibrosis. *Int. J. Biochem. Cell Biol.* 40, 1238–1245. doi: 10.1016/j.biocel.2008.03.003

Weldon, S., McNally, P., McElvaney, N. G., Elborn, J. S., McAuley, D. F., Wartelle, J., et al. (2009). Decreased levels of secretory leucoprotease inhibitor in the Pseudomonas-infected cystic fibrosis lung are due to neutrophil elastase degradation. *J. Immunol.* 183, 8148–8156. doi: 10.4049/jimmunol.0901716

Xu, D., Young, J., Song, D., and Esko, J. D. (2011). Heparan sulfate is essential for high mobility group protein 1 (HMGB1) signaling by the receptor for advanced glycation end products (RAGE). *J. Biol. Chem.* 286, 41736–41744. doi: 10.1074/jbc.M111.299685

Xu, D., Young, J. H., Krahn, J. M., Song, D., Corbett, K. D., Chazin, W. J., et al. (2013). Stable RAGE-heparan sulfate complexes are essential for signal transduction. *ACS Chem. Biol.* 8, 1611–1620. doi: 10.1021/cb4001553

Yildiz-Pekoz, A., and Ozsoy, Y. (2017). Inhaled Heparin: Therapeutic Efficacy and Recent Formulations. *J. Aerosol. Med. Pulm. Drug Delivery* 30, 143–156. doi: 10.1089/jamp.2015.1273

Zhang, J., Xu, X., Rao, N. V., Argyle, B., McCoard, L., Rusho, W. J., et al. (2011). Novel sulfated polysaccharides disrupt cathelicidins, inhibit RAGE and reduce cutaneous inflammation in a mouse model of rosacea. *PloS One* 6, e16658. doi: 10.1371/journal.pone.0016658

Zheng, S., De, B. P., Choudhary, S., Comhair, S. A., Goggans, T., Slee, R., et al. (2003). Impaired innate host defense causes susceptibility to respiratory virus infections in cystic fibrosis. *Immunity* 18, 619–630. doi: 10.1016/S1074-7613(03)00114-6

Zheng, S., Kummarapurugu, A. B., Afosah, D. K., Sankaranarayanan, N. V., Boothello, R. S., Desai, U. R., et al. (2017). 2-O, 3-O Desulfated Heparin Blocks High Mobility Group Box 1 Release by Inhibition of p300 Acetyltransferase Activity. *Am. J. Respir. Cell Mol. Biol.* 56, 90–98. doi: 10.1165/rcmb.2016-0069OC

15

NCS 613, a Potent PDE4 Inhibitor, Displays Anti-Inflammatory and Anti-Proliferative Properties on A549 Lung Epithelial Cells and Human Lung Adenocarcinoma Explants

Issaka Yougbare[1,2], Lazare Belemnaba[2†], Caroline Morin[1], Abdurazzag Abusnina[2], Yannick F. Senouvo[1], Thérèse Keravis[2], Claire Lugnier[2,3] and Eric Rousseau[1,4]*

[1] Le Bilarium, Department of Physiology and Biophysics, Faculty of Medicine and Health Sciences, Université de Sherbrooke, Sherbrooke, QC, Canada, [2] UMR CNRS 7213, Biophotonics and Pharmacology Laboratory, Faculty of Pharmacy, University of Strasbourg, Illkirch, France, [3] Institute of Physiology, FMTS-EA 3072, Faculty of Medicine, University of Strasbourg, Strasbourg, France, [4] Department of Obstetrics and Gynecology, Faculty of Medicine and Health Sciences, Université de Sherbrooke, Sherbrooke, QC, Canada

***Correspondence:**
Eric Rousseau
Eric.Rousseau@USherbrooke.ca

†Present address:
Lazare Belemnaba, Research Institute of Health Sciences, Ouagadougou, Burkina Faso

Chronic inflammation is a deleterious process occurring in several pulmonary diseases; it is a driving force promoting tumorigenesis. By regulating local cyclic nucleotide concentration, cyclic nucleotide phosphodiesterases (PDE) govern important biological processes, including inflammation and proliferation. The aim of this study was to investigate the anti-inflammatory and anti-proliferative effects of NCS 613, a specific PDE4 inhibitor, on TNFα-treated human lung adenocarcinoma cell line (A549) and on human lung adenocarcinoma explants. PDE4 isoforms and inflammatory pathways mediated by p38 MAPK, ERK1/2, and IκBα were analyzed by Western blot and immunostainings. Proliferation were performed using [^{3}H]-thymidine incorporation under different experimental conditions. TNFα-stimulation increased p38 MAPK phosphorylation and NF-κB translocation into the nucleus, which was abolished by NCS 613 treatment. Concomitantly, NCS 613 restores IκBα detection level in human adenocarcinoma. An IC_{50} value of 8.5 μM was determined for NCS 613 on anti-proliferative properties while ERK1/2 signaling was down-regulated in A549 cells and lung adenocarcinoma explants. These findings shed light on PDE4 signaling as a key regulator of chronic inflammation and cancer epithelial cell proliferation. It suggests that PDE4 inhibition by NCS 613 represent potential and interesting strategy for therapeutic intervention in tackling chronic inflammation and cell proliferation.

Keywords: PDE4 inhibitor, cAMP signaling, inflammation, proliferation, human lung adenocarcinoma

INTRODUCTION

Chronic inflammation, which is a deleterious process occurring in inflammatory respiratory diseases, is believed to be a tumor promoter in cancer induction (Lee et al., 2009; Balkwill and Mantovani, 2010; Phillips, 2020). Evidence suggests that recurrent injury and inflammation result in genetic alterations that predispose to lung cancer (Pikarsky and Ben-Neriah, 2006). NF-κB and p38 MAPK pathways play important role in human inflammatory diseases (COPD, rheumatoid arthritis...) and cancer (Koutras et al., 2009; Wong, 2009; Luangdilok et al., 2011). NF-κB dimers binding to target promoters lead to pro-inflammatory genes transcriptions and regulation of apoptosis and proliferation (Jeon et al., 2010). NF-κB activation is prevented by IκBα, an inhibitory protein which maintains NF-κB in an inactive state in the cytoplasm (Kamata et al., 2010). Downstream of surface membrane receptor activation, cyclic nucleotide phosphodiesterases (PDE) which encompass 11 families play a pivotal role in cAMP and cGMP signaling (Lugnier, 2006; Conti and Beavo, 2007). These enzymes hydrolyze cyclic nucleotides as a feedback mechanism for rapidly returning local nucleotide concentration to basal levels (Keravis et al., 2012; Maurice et al., 2014; Baillie et al., 2019; Lugnier et al., 2020). By regulating local cyclic nucleotides levels, PDEs contribute to their compartmentalization and govern number of biological processes, including inflammation and proliferation (Growcott et al., 2006; Sosroseno and Sugiatno, 2008, Abusnina et al., 2011a; Abusnina et al., 2011b; Alhosin, et al., 2011; Keravis, et al., 2011, Yougbare et al., 2013; Li et al., 2018; Baillie et al., 2019). Specific cAMP hydrolyzing phosphodiesterases (PDE4) have been shown to be involved in the control of inflammatory responses (Houslay, 2010). Inflammation is strongly correlated to lower intracellular cAMP levels. PDE4 implication has been reported in lung diseases related to chronic inflammation such as smoking-induced lung injury, fibrosis, asthma and COPD (Dunkern et al., 2007; Udalov et al., 2010; Diamant and Spina, 2011; Yougbare et al., 2014; Phillips, 2020). Inhibition of PDE4 activity causes elevation of intracellular cAMP levels and subsequent downregulation of a variety of inflammatory cell signaling (Yougbare et al., 2011). NCS 613 is a potent PDE4 inhibitor, which is more selective for the PDE4C subtype (IC_{50} = 1.4 nM) (**Figure 1E**). Compared other PDE4 inhibitors such as pentoxifylline and denbufylline, NCS 613 was the most potent and effective molecule in inhibiting both basal and LPS-induced TNFα secretion from leucocytes of lupus patients (Keravis et al., 2012). We previously showed that *in vivo* administration of NCS 613, a new and potent PDE4 inhibitor, reduced neutrophil recruitment in LPS-treated mouse bronchi and exhibits anti-inflammatory effects by decreasing TNFα secretion in guinea pig (Boichot et al., 2000). Interestingly, NCS 613 did not stimulate gastric acid secretion suggesting that this compound may produce gastrointestinal side effects (Boichot et al., 2000). Thus, PDE4 isozymes represent attractive targets for inflammation and cancer (Keravis et al., 2012; Li et al., 2018; Baillie et al., 2019; Hsien Lai et al., 2020). The above observations prompted us to investigate whether or not cellular signaling involved in inflammation and proliferation processes may be prevented by PDE4 inhibition and local increase in cAMP concentration. This study aimed to investigate the anti-inflammatory and antiproliferative effects of NCS 613 on human lung adenocarcinoma cell line (A549) and cultured human lung adenocarcinoma explants.

MATERIAL AND METHODS

Materials

The study was approved by our institutional Ethics Committee (Protocol number CRC 05-088 S1R2). Human lung explants were obtained from 4 patients aged between 50-60 years undergoing surgery for lung carcinoma resection. Tissues samples were collected from fresh lobectomy and transported to the laboratory in physiological Krebs' solution (Sosroseno and Sugiatno, 2008). Human lung adenocarcinoma cell line (A549 cells) was from Abcam (# ab7910). NCS 613 (patent FR0601958) was given by J.J. Bourguignon and C. Lugnier (Faculty of pharmacy, Strasbourg). PDE antibodies used for Western blot analysis and immuno-staining were from FabGennix Inc. Anti-Phospho and total ERK1/2, anti-IκBα, anti-p65-NF-κB, Anti-phospho, and total p38-MAPK were from Cell Signaling Technology. $[^3H]$-thymidine (250 μCi) was obtained from New England Nuclear.

A549 Cells and Human Lung Adenocarcinoma Explants Culture

TNFα Induced Cell Responses

The adenocarcinoma human alveolar basal epithelial cells, A549 cells (1x 10^5), were allowed growth for 24 h in T-75 culture flask, as previously described (Giard et al., 1973), in RPMI culture medium supplemented with 0.3% penicillin (100 IU/ml) and streptomycin (0.1 mg/ml) in presence of 1% fetal bovine serum at 37°C under 5% CO_2. After 6 h starving period (without fetal bovine serum), cells were stimulated with TNFα to induce inflammation and treated with NCS 613 for 48 h under the following experimental conditions: control, +10 μM NCS 613, + 10 ng/ml TNFα, and +TNFα + NCS 613.

Cell Proliferation Assay

A549 cells were also cultured in 24-well plate in the presence of increasing NCS 613 concentrations of 0, 1, 2.5, 5, 7.5, 10, and 30 μM for 48 h. $[^3H]$-thymidine incorporation was performed in triplicate for a 24 h period with 1 μCi tritiated thymidine. Harvested cells were lysed with cold 20% Trichloroacetic Acid (TCA) followed by DNA precipitation with 96% ethanol on Whatman paper. Radioactivity was quantified with β-counter using 5 ml scintillation liquid. IC_{50} value for NCS 613 was determined on cell proliferation as assessed by $[^3H]$-thymidine incorporation (Denton, 1998).

Explant Proliferation Assay

After removal of connective tissues, lung adenocarcinoma explants were cultured in 6-wells culture plates containing

RPMI as previously described for pulmonary tissue culture (Guibert et al., 2005). Explants were cultured in either control condition or treated with 1, 3, or 10 μM NCS 613. Tissues and harvested cells were homogenized with a Polytron in Radio-Immuno-Precipitation Assay buffer (RIPA) and supernatant aliquots were stored at -80°C until use.

Western Blot Analysis

Proteins (25 μg) from lung adenocarcinoma and A549 cells lysates were subjected to Western blot analysis. Briefly, protein samples were electrophoresed on 10% SDS polyacrylamide gels and electro-transferred onto Polyvinylidene Difluoride (PVDF) membranes. Immunodetection was carried out with the following antibodies: anti-PDE4A, anti-PDE4B, anti-PDE4C, anti-PDE4D, anti-IκBα, anti-p38 MAPK, anti-ERK1/2 and anti-GAPDH. Immobilized antigens were detected by chemiluminescence using horseradish peroxidase-conjugated secondary antibodies, an ECL kit and autoradiography films.

Immuno-Cytochemistry

Smears were made from harvested A549 cells, delineated with Dako Pen and fixed in 4%.

Paraformaldehyde (PFA) overnight before immuno-staining. After rinsing in TBS buffered (50 mM Tris, 150 mM NaCl, pH 7.6) and permeabilization with 0.1% Triton in PBS, smears were saturated with PBS + 4% BSA for 1 h at room temperature. Immuno-stainings were performed using specific antibodies directed against PDE4B, PDE4C, and NF-κB, and subsequently revealed by secondary antibodies coupled to either Alexa-488 or Alexa-654 fluorescent probe. Cell nuclei were labeled with DAPI (1 μM). Slides were mounted using Vectashield mounting medium and observed with a Leica microscope at 40X and 60X magnifications. Images were captured at the same magnification and exposure time allowing fluorescence comparison between the various experimental conditions.

Data Analysis and Statistics

Results are expressed as means ± S.E.M. with n indicating the number of experiments.

Statistical analyses were performed using a one-way ANOVA followed by a Bonferroni post-test. Differences were considered statistically significant when $p<0.05$.

RESULTS

Effects of NCS 613 on PDE4B and PDE4C Expressions in TNFα-Treated A549 Cells

Quantitative analysis of Western blot results showed that NCS 613 prevents PDE4A 70 kDa expression in A549 cells while TNFα significantly increases it. In these cells, the specific PDE4 inhibitor overcomes the overexpression of PDE4A (**Figure 1A**). Furthermore, long term inhibition of PDE4 by NCS 613 leads to induction of PDE4B 96 kDa in adenocarcinoma A549 cell line (**Figure 1B**). PDE4B 96 kDa expression was undetectable following TNFα stimulation and its expression increased upon NCS 613 treatment (**Figure 1B**). Conversely, the PDE4B 66 kDa isoform was increased upon TNFα treatment (**Figure 1C**). The PDE4C 66 kDa isoform on the other hand was increased in presence of 10 μM NCS 613 (**Figures 1D, E**). However, we did not detect PDE4D isoforms by Western blot in A549 cell line. These results suggest that cAMP accumulation subsequent to PDE4 inhibition induces a shift in isoform transcription and biosynthesis. The data also revealed that TNFα stimulation significantly abolished PDE4B 96 kDa while it increased PDE4A 70 kDa and PDE4B 66 kDa detection in A549 cells, suggesting that these later isoforms could be involved in TNFα signaling (**Figures 1A, C**). As expected, NCS 613 treatment overcame the TNFα-induced PDE4A 70 kDa and PDE4B 66 kDa increases which return to control level, hence indicating that this compound can interfere with inflammation signaling pathways.

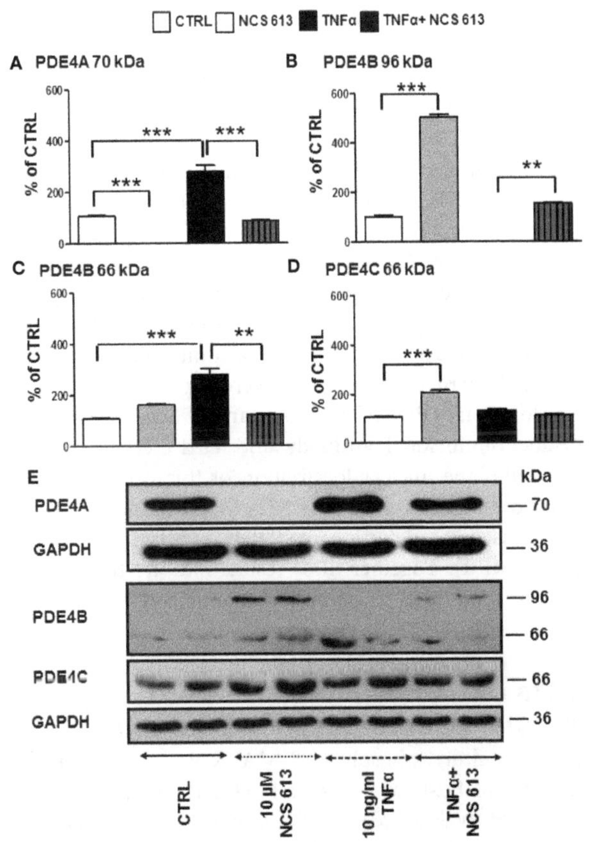

FIGURE 1 | Detection of PDE4A, PDE4B, and PDE4C expressions in control and TNFα-stimulated A549 cells following NCS 613 treatment. A549 cells were stimulated with TNFα to induce inflammation and treated with NCS 613 for 48 h under the following experimental conditions: control, +10 μM NCS 613, + 10 ng/ml TNFα, and +TNFα + NCS 613. Relative protein expression levels were calculated following digitalization and image analysis from 3 independent experiments. **(A)** NCS 613 prevents and TNFα increases PDE4A 70 kDa overexpression; **(B)** NCS 613 induces PDE4B 96 kDa expression in A549 cell line; **(C)** TNFα stimulation induces PDE4B 66 kDa upregulation which is decreased with NCS 613 treatment; **(D)** PDE4C 66 kDa increases upon NCS 613 treatment; **(E)** representative immuno-reactive bands revealed by Western blot analysis (n=3). Unpaired Student's *t*-test. Mean ± SEM. $^{**}p < 0.01$ and $^{***}p < 0.001$.

Effects of NCS 613 on PDE4B and PDE4C Locations in A549 Cells

Immuno-cytofluorescent staining confirms that NCS 613 treatment increased basal nuclear PDE4B and PDE4C expression (**Figure 2**). PDE4B 96 kDa could correspond to the nuclear isoform since this protein was only upregulated with NCS 613 treatment (**Figure 2C**). Immunostaining consistently showed that TNFα stimulation significantly increased PDE4B expression in A549 cells (**Figure 2D**). PDE4B 96 kDa was not expressed in A549 TNFα-stimulated cells (see **Figure 1B**), the 66 kDa isoform could correspond to the up-regulated cytoplasmic isoform. Interestingly, 10 μM NCS 613 treatment decreased PDE4B protein expression in TNFα-stimulated cells (**Figure 2E**). Complementary experiments were performed to delineate cellular location of PDE4C. Concomitant PDE4C detection using a specific monoclonal antibody and DAPI counter-staining demonstrates the nuclear localization of this isoform (**Figures 2F, G**). Lower panels show that NCS 613 treatments (5 and 10 μM) increased the detection of PDE4C isoform in A549 cells (**Figures 2 G–I**). Together these results indicate that NCS 613 treatment modulates the compartmentalized expression of PDE4 isoforms.

Effects of NCS 613 on p38 MAPK Phosphorylation and NF-κB Location

After 72 h culture, phospho-p38 MAPK was detected in both control and TNFα-treated A549 cells (**Figure 3A**), whereas NCS 613 treatment abolished p38 MAPK phosphorylation demonstrating a net effect of this compound. TNFα stimulation significantly increases p38 MAPK phosphorylation facilitating down-stream effectors activation. NCS 613 treatment abolishes the TNFα-induced p38 MAPK phosphorylation, while the total p38 MAPK expression level remains unchanged (**Figure 3A**). Since it has been reported that p38 MAPK phosphorylation induces NF-κB activation (Morin et al., 2008; Smith et al., 2010; Sigala et al., 2011), antibodies against the NF-κB p65-subunit were used to detect NF-κB translocation into the nucleus. NCS 613 treatment reduces NF-κB basal detection in these cells (**Figure 3B**). In contrast, TNFα stimulation enhances of NF-κB translocation into the nucleus, while NCS 613 treatment counteracted the effects of TNFα on p65-NF-κB translocation. Together, these results indicate that intracellular cAMP level, which is increased during NCS 613 treatment, modulates p38 MAPK phosphorylation and downstream nuclear translocation of p65-subunit of NF-κB.

Anti-Inflammatory Effects of NCS 613 Treatment on IκBα Expression

Increasing evidences have revealed that tissue inflammation is a recurrent component in cancer (Balkwill and Mantovani, 2010; Smith et al., 2010). To assess the putative anti-inflammatory effects of NCS 613, IκBα expression was used as a lung inflammation marker (lower detection indicates larger inflammation). IκBα was detected in fresh human lung parenchyma (positive control, **Figure 4**) whereas IκBα was undetectable in untreated (control) lung adenocarcinoma explants cultured for 72, which is correlated with an increased inflammation process. In contrast, NCS 613 (at 3 and 10 μM) rescued IκBα detection in a concentration-dependent manner, which could correlate with a lower inflammation status of the tissues.

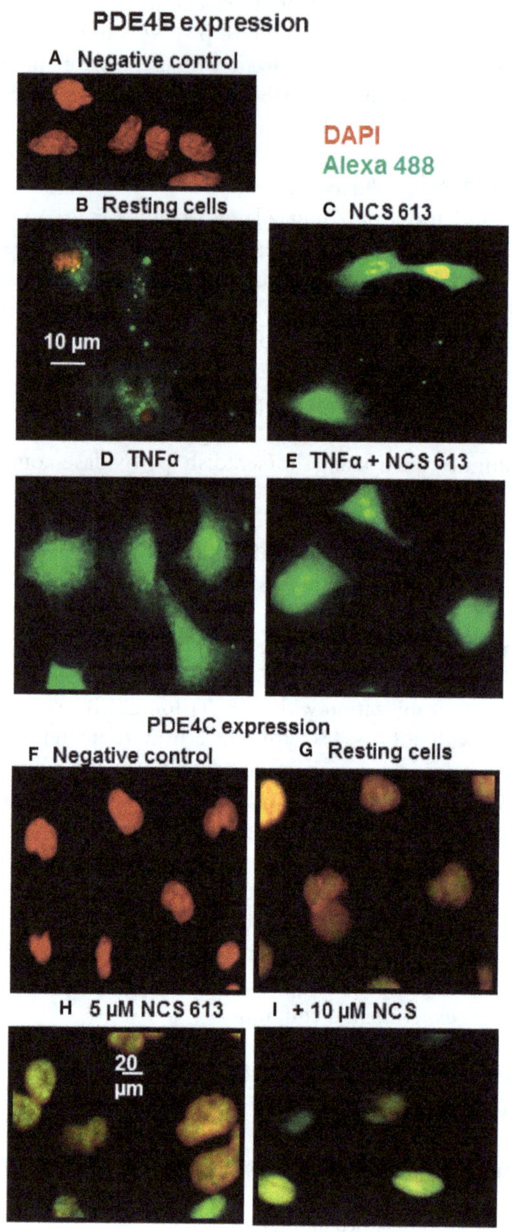

FIGURE 2 | PDE4B and PDE4C immuno-cyto-staining. **(A–E)** Detection of PDE4B isoforms in A549 cells under control and TNFα treated conditions, in the absence or presence of NCS 613. **(A)** Negative control showing anti-PDE4B specificity; **(B)** PDE4B basal level in A549 cells; **(C)** NCS 613 increases PDE4B expression; **(D)** TNFα stimulation greatly increases PDE4B expression which is reduce by NCS 613 **(E)**. **(F–I)** Detection of PDE4C in A549 cells. **(F)** Negative control and **(G)** Basal PDE4C location; **(H)** and **(I)** NCS 613 treatments increase nuclear PDE4C in A549 cells. Data are representative of 3 independent experiments. Shown are merged images [x60 **(A–E)** and x40 **(F–I)** magnification] of DAPI staining (red) and anti-rabbit-Alexa Fluor 488 (green) recognizing primary anti-PDE4B or anti-PDE4C antibody (green).

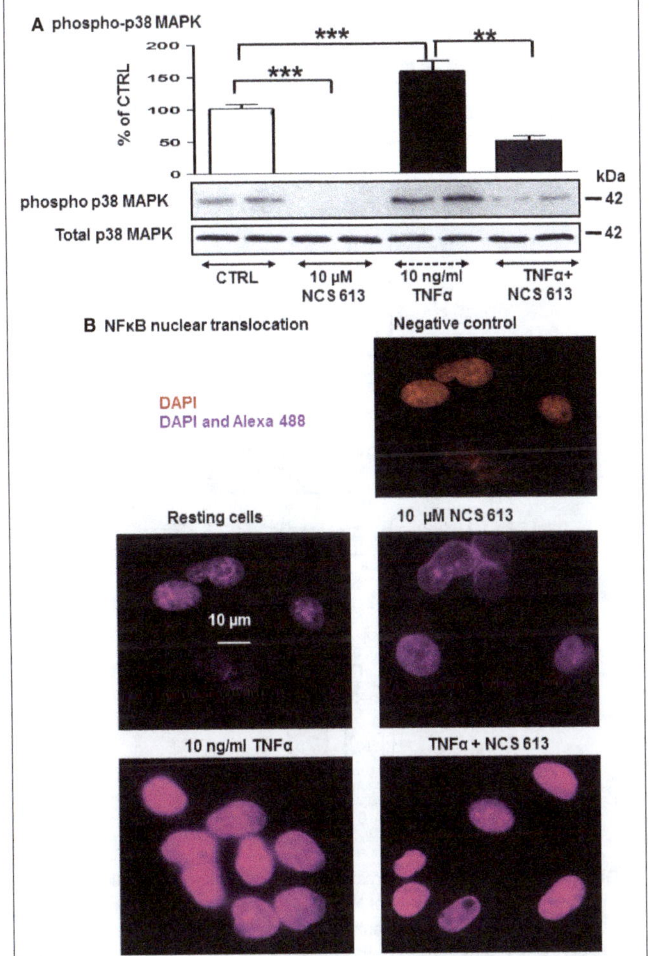

FIGURE 3 | Effect of NCS 613 on p38 MAPK phosphorylation and NF-κB nuclear translocation upon TNFα stimulation. **(A)** TNFα increases and NCS 613 reduces p38 MAPK phosphorylation in A549 cells; **(B)** NCS 613 prevents NF-κB translocation into nucleus while TNFα stimulation greatly increases NF-κB p65-subunit translocation into nucleus. Shown are merged images (60x magnification) of DAPI staining and anti-mouse Alexa 654 recognizing primary p65-NF-κB antibody (n=3). Unpaired Student's *t*-test. Mean ± SEM. $^{**}p < 0.01$ and $^{***}p < 0.001$.

NCS 613 Displays Antiproliferative Effects Through ERK1/2 Inhibition

In the absence of treatment, A549 cells proliferate and become highly confluent (**Figure 5A**). Interestingly, NCS 613 treatment opposed this effect on cells proliferation and induced cells apoptosis (**Figures 5B, C**). DMSO up to 0.3 ‰, used as vehicle did not exhibit any toxicity toward A549 cells (**Figures 4D, E**). Of note, NCS 613 (2.5–30 μM) significantly decreased [^{3}H]-thymidine incorporation, hence correlating with a lower cell proliferation rate. Moreover, inhibition curve displays an anti-proliferative effect of NCS 613 with an IC_{50} value of 8.5 μM. NCS 613 treatment reduces ERK 1/2 phosphorylation as well as total ERK 1/2 in A549 cells (**Figures 6A, B**) as well as in human lung adenocarcinoma explants (**Figures 6C, D**) attesting that this pathway is likely involved in the anti-proliferative effect of this compound. Several putative pathways involved in inflammatory responses and cell proliferation are likely modulated by NCS 613. As shown in the present results, TNFα induces PDE4B up-regulation in order to hydrolyze cAMP and activates p38 MAPK and NF-κB pathways, which in turn leads to IκBα degradation. NCS 613 on the other hand increases cAMP levels and thus prevents p38 MAPK phosphorylation. NCS 613 can also inhibit cell proliferation by a down-regulation of ERK1/2 signaling. The sustained inhibition of PDE4 by NCS 613 induces the synthesis of novel isoforms as a feedback mechanism to modulate cAMP levels.

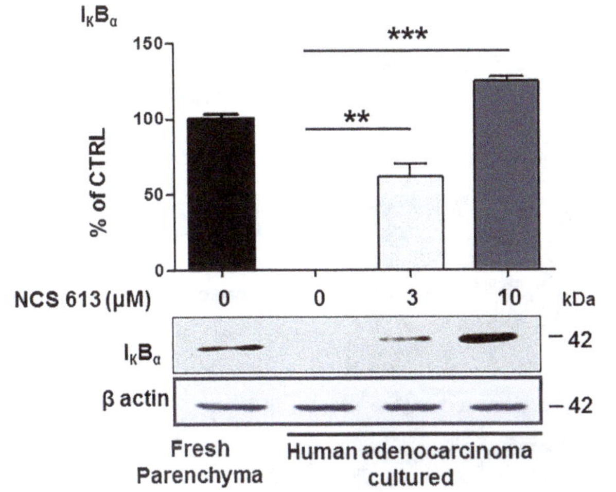

FIGURE 4 | Concentration dependent effect of NCS 613 treatment on IκBα detection in adenocarcinoma explants. IκBα was detected in fresh human lung parenchyma. After a 72 h culture period, IκBα was undetectable in control adenocarcinoma explants suggesting a high inflammation level. Three and 10 μM NCS 613 treatment reestablished IκBα detection level (n= 4). Unpaired Student's *t*-test. Mean ± SEM. $^{**}p < 0.01$ and $^{***}p < 0.001$

DISCUSSION

Chronic inflammation is a hallmark of pulmonary diseases, which can lead to emphysema and airways hyperresponsiveness. In the present study, we were able to delineate the role of PDE4 in TNFα-induced inflammation in A549 cells in which PDE4A 70 kDa and PDE4B 66 kDa were significantly up-regulated but not PDE4C and PDE4D. This upregulation of PDE4 isoforms, downstream of TNFα-receptor activation, facilitates cAMP breakdown and activation of inflammatory effectors. Under these conditions, A549 cells consistently expressed higher cytoplasmic levels of PDE4B as revealed by immuno-staining. NCS 613 treatment, which inhibits PDE4 activity, restored intracellular cAMP levels, resulting in an opposite effect on inflammatory markers. In a previous report, LPS-induced TNFα secretion was shown to be significantly reduced in macrophages from bronchi-alveolar fluid of PDE4B-deficient mice (Jin et al., 2005). Comparing the effect rolipram, NCS 613 and RP 73401, or the cell permeable analogue N6 -2'-O-dibutyryladenosine 3',5'-cyclic monophosphate (db-

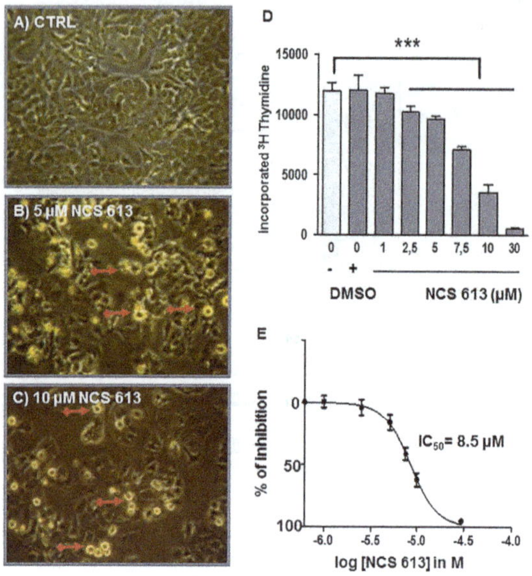

FIGURE 5 | Anti-proliferative effect of NCS 613 on A549 cells. **(A)** Control: A549 cells display rapid proliferation rate toward confluency. **(B, C)** A549 cells treated with either 5 µM or 10 µM NCS 613 for 48 h results in lower density and higher apoptosis. Plates are representative of three independent experiments; **(D)** Bar histogram showing [^{3}H]-thymidine incorporation into DNA. Gradual (2.5–30 µM) NCS 613 treatment significantly decreases A549 cells proliferation; **(E)** Concentration dependent inhibition curve displaying the antiproliferative effects of NCS 613 from which an IC_{50} value of 8.5 µM was calculated. Unpaired Student's *t*-test. Mean ± SEM. ***$p < 0.001$.

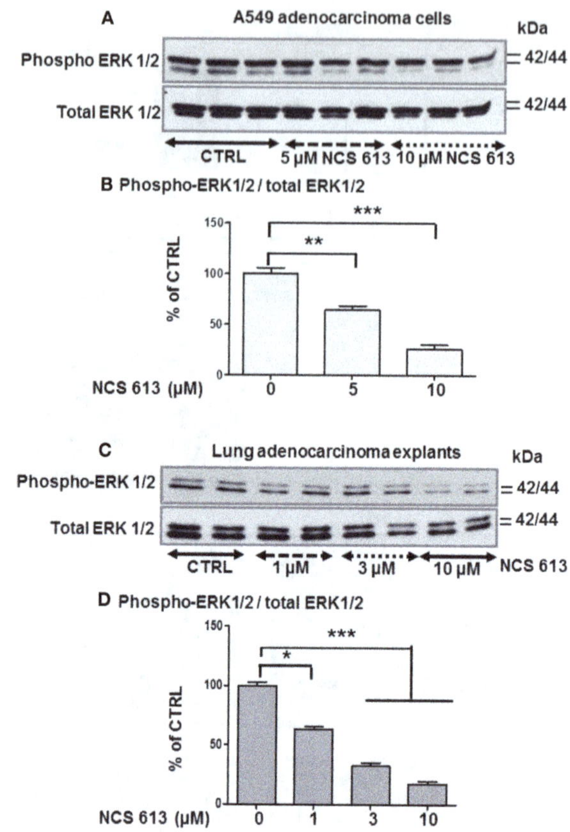

FIGURE 6 | Effect of NCS 613 treatment on ERK1/2 phosphorylation. **(A, B)** Concentration dependent effect of NCS 613 on the phosphorylation level of ERK1/2 as a function of experimental conditions (n=3); **(C, D)** Concentration dependent effect of NCS 613 on phospho-ERK1/2 detection in cultured lung adenocarcinoma explants (n=4). Unpaired Student's *t*-test. Mean ± SEM. *$p < 0.05$, **$p < 0.01$ and ***$p < 0.001$.

cAMP) on histamine release by mast cells from diabetic rats, we observed that these molecules led to a decrease of histamine secretion *in vitro* (Barreto et al., 2004). Importantly, the effectiveness of either NCS 613 or db cAMP in inhibiting antigen-induced degranulation is comparable in both normal and diabetic mast cells. Our current data suggest that the PDE4A 70 kDa and PDE4B 66 kDa isoforms are likely involved in TNFα signaling, which is consistent with the conclusion of a recent study showing that the induction of PDE4B is required for Toll-like receptor signaling in monocytes and macrophages (Jin et al., 2010).

Herein, the PDE4B 96 kDa increase in A549 cells by NCS 613 treatment, suggests that this isoform is likely involved in the regulation of cAMP metabolism. This is also supported by the upregulation of nuclear PDE4C in A549 cells. Moreover, other reports revealed that sustained increased in intracellular cAMP enhanced PDE4A/4B gene expressions in U937 cells as well as l PDE4B/4D in human myometrial cells (Dunkern et al., 2007). Interestingly, it was previously reported that PDE4B2 was upregulated by IL-1β at mRNA and protein levels from human myometrial cells through a prostaglandin E2- and cyclic adenosine 3', 5'-monophosphate-dependent pathway (Oger et al., 2002). PDE4 activity and expression in cultured pulmonary microvascular endothelial cells from rat are activated by a PKA *in situ* phosphorylation in short-term and induced in long-term *via* increases of intracellular cAMP concentrations (Zhu et al., 2004). Our work showed the specificity and functions of PDE4B and PDE4C isoforms in which 96 kDa and 66 kDa proteins respectively regulate cAMP level in A549 cells. PDE4 compartmentalization in cells tightly regulates cAMP level underpinning a complex cAMP signaling network (Houslay, 2010; Yougbare et al., 2013). Two pathways involved in the typical inflammatory response were assessed in the present study. The stress kinase p38 MAPK is thought to regulate NF-κB translocation to nuclei (Moriyuki et al., 2009; Morin et al., 2010) and TNFα stimulation increases p38 MAPK phosphorylation. In addition increasing evidence suggested that PDE4 inhibitor are negative modulator of p38 phosphorylation (Kwak et al., 2005; Yougbare et al., 2011). NCS 613 totally abolishes p38 MAPK phosphorylation and reduces NF-κB translocation to the nucleus. Consequently, the use of NCS 613 opposes to p38 MAPK activation by stress stimuli (TNFα, LPS) and its phosphorylation leading to rapid activation of NF-κB (Morin et al., 2010). Consistent with these observations, NCS 613 treatment stabilizes IκBα binding to NF-κB and prevents nuclear translocation of the latter. Under pro-inflammatory conditions, IκBα is usually phosphorylated by IκK and then ubiquitinated, leading to its degradation into proteasomes, and lower cytoplasmic detection and NF-κB translocation to the nuclei

(Houslay and Adams, 2010; Kamata et al., 2010). In cultured human lung adenocarcinoma explants IκBα was undetectable in control (untreated) conditions whereas NCS 613 was able to restore IκBα detection in a concentration-dependent manner. Thus, IκBα protection down regulates NF-κB activation which have important implications in lung cancer prevention and immunotherapy (Lin et al., 2010). Our current data suggest that NCS 613 may have potent anti-inflammatory properties in A549 cells and lung carcinoma explants.

Microscopic observation of A549 cells under specific PDE4 inhibitor treatment provides the first evidence that NCS 613 can also markedly affect cell proliferation. A549 cells death was observed with Trypan blue staining during cells count. Trypan blue, a vital stain used to selectively color dead cells in blue reveals A549 cells death mediated by NCS 613 treatment. Other compounds like CC-8075 and CC-8062 are PDE4 inhibitors that have been shown an anti-proliferative effect on various cell lines by increasing cAMP (Koutras et al., 2009; Mouratidis et al., 2009; Hsien Lai et al., 2020). The [^{3}H]-thymidine incorporation proliferation assay confirms that NCS 613 decreases cell proliferation concomitantly with lower detection of inflammatory markers suggesting the contribution of the latter in cancer progression. Several studies have used mouse cancer models and have provided direct genetic evidence for the critical role of NF-κB in carcinogenesis (Pikarsky and Ben-Neriah, 2006). With an IC50 value of 8.5 μM on cell proliferation, NCS 613 reduces cell division and likely induces apoptosis in malignant cells, which is corroborated by the downregulation of phospho- ERK1/2 in A549 cells. This observation could be correlated to a recent finding suggesting a predominant role of PDE4B in controlling molecular pathophysiological processes involved in the proliferation of human lung fibroblasts (Selige et al., 2010). The mechanism by which cAMP induced apoptosis in A549 cells remains to be established.

CONCLUSION

The present data highlight the role of PDE4B in controlling inflammatory responses and cell proliferation pathways. NCS 613 targets PDE4 and, indirectly, p38 MAPK as well as NF-κB and ERK1/2 signaling, leading to a down-regulation of inflammation in both the human A549 cell line and lung adenocarcinoma explants. NCS 613 thus represents a potent anti-inflammatory compound, which did not induce gastrointestinal side effects at 10 mg/kg i.v. (Boichot et al., 2000), which may be useful in the treatment of chronic inflammatory diseases and cancer prevention in pre-clinical studies. Further studies are needed to assess whether NCS 613 induces apoptosis in A549 and lung adenocarcinoma.

ETHICS STATEMENT

The studies involving human participants were reviewed and approved by Protocol number CRC 05-088 S1R2. The patients/participants provided their written informed consent to participate in this study.

AUTHOR CONTRIBUTIONS

IY designed and performed all the experiments, analyzed and interpreted data, and prepared and revised the manuscript. LB, AA, and YS conducted some experiments and prepared the manuscript. CM and TK provided guidance for study design and data interpretation. CL contributed to study design and data interpretation, as well as manuscript preparation. As the principle investigator, ER supervised study design, data interpretation, and manuscript preparation.

ACKNOWLEDGMENTS

The authors thank Drs Marco Sirois and Chantal Sirois for their help in patient recruitment.
The authors thank Dr. Edmond Rizcallah and the members of the pathology laboratory for their technical support.

REFERENCES

Abusnina, A., Alhosin, M., Keravis, T., Muller, C. D., Fuhrmann, G., Bronner, C., et al. (2011a). Down-regulation of cyclic nucleotide phosphodiesterase PDE1A is the key event of p73 and UHRF1 deregulation in thymoquinone-induced acute lymphoblastic leukemia cell apoptosis. *Cell Signal* 23 (1), 152–160. doi: 10.1016/j.cellsig.2010.08.015

Abusnina, A., Keravis, T., Yougbare, I., Bronner, C., and Lugnier, C. (2011b). Anti-proliferative effect of curcumin on melanoma cells is mediated by PDE1A inhibition that regulates the epigenetic integrator UHRF1. *Mol. Nutr. Food Res.* 55 (11), 1677–1689. doi: 10.1002/mnfr.201100307

Alhosin, M., Sharif, T., Mousli, M., Etienne-Selloum, N., Fuhrmann, G., Schini-Kerth, V. B., et al. (2011). Down-regulation of UHRF1, associated with re-expression of tumor suppressor genes, is a common feature of natural compounds exhibiting anti-cancer pprperties. *J. Exp. Clin. Cancer. Res.* 30 (1), 41. doi: 10.1186/1756-9966-30-41

Baillie, G. S., Tejeda, G. S., and Kelly, M. P. (2019). Therapeutic targeting of 3',5'-cyclic nucleotide phosphodiesterases: inhibition and beyond. *Nat. Rev. Drug Discovery* 18 (10), 770–796. doi: 10.1038/s41573-019-0033-4

Balkwill, F., and Mantovani, A. (2010). Cancer and inflammation: implications for pharmacology and therapeutics. *Clin. Pharmacol. Ther.* 87 (4), 401–406. doi: 10.1038/clpt.2009.312

Barreto, E. O., Carvalho, V. F., Lagente, V., Lugnier, C., Cordeiro, R. S., Martins, M. A., et al. (2004). Increased levels of cyclic adenosine monophosphate contribute to the hyporesponsiveness of mast cells in alloxan diabetes. *Int. Immunopharmacol.* 4 (6), 755–762. doi: 10.1016/j.intimp.2004.03.001

Boichot, E., Wallace, J. L., Germain, N., Corbel, M., Lugnier, C., Lagente, V., et al. (2000). Anti-inflammatory activities of a new series of selective phosphodiesterase 4 inhibitors derived from 9-benzyladenine. *J. Pharmacol. Exp. Ther.* 292 (2), 647–653.

Conti, M, and Beavo, J. (2007). Biochemistry and physiology of cyclic nucleotide phosphodiesterases: essential components in cyclic nucleotide signaling. *Annu. Rev. Biochem.* 76, 481–511. doi: 10.1146/annurev.biochem.76.060305.150444

Denton, C. P. (1998). Leucine incorporation and thymidine incorporation. *Methods Mol. Biol.* 79, 169–177. doi: 10.1385/0-89603-448-8:169

Diamant, Z., and Spina, D. (2011). PDE4-inhibitors: a novel, targeted therapy for obstructive airways disease. *Pulm. Pharmacol. Ther.* 24 (4), 353–360. doi: 10.1016/j.pupt.2010.12.011

Dunkern, T. R., Feurstein, D., Rossi, G. A., Sabatini, F., and Hatzelmann, A. (2007). Inhibition of TGF-beta induced lung fibroblast to myofibroblast conversion by phosphodiesterase inhibiting drugs and activators of soluble guanylyl cyclase. *Eur. J. Pharmacol.* 572 (1), 12–22. doi: 10.1016/j.ejphar.2007.06.036

Giard, D. J., Aaronson, S. A., Todaro, G. J., Arnstein, P., Kersey, J. H., Dosik, H., et al. (1973). In vitro cultivation of human tumors: establishment of cell lines derived from a series of solid tumors. *J. Natl. Cancer Inst.* 51 (5), 1417–1423. doi: 10.1093/jnci/51.5.1417

Growcott, E. J., Spink, K. G., Ren, X., Afzal, S., Banner, K. H., and Wharton, J. (2006). Phosphodiesterase type 4 expression and anti-proliferative effects in human pulmonary artery smooth muscle cells. *Respir. Res.* 7, 9. doi: 10.1186/1465-9921-7-9

Guibert, C., Savineau, J. P., Crevel, H., Marthan, R., and Rousseau, E. (2005). Effect of short-term organoid culture on the pharmaco-mechanical properties of rat extra- and intrapulmonary arteries. *Br. J. Pharmacol.* 146 (5), 692–701. doi: 10.1038/sj.bjp.0706379

Houslay, M. D., and Adams, D. R. (2010). Putting the lid on phosphodiesterase 4. *Nat. Biotechnol.* 28 (1), 38–40. doi: 10.1038/nbt0110-38

Houslay, M. D. (2010). Underpinning compartmentalised cAMP signalling through targeted cAMP breakdown. *Trends Biochem. Sci.* 35 (2), 91–100. doi: 10.1016/j.tibs.2009.09.007

Hsien Lai, S., Zervoudakis, G., Chou, J., Gurney, M. E., and Quesnelle, K. M. (2020). PDE4 subtypes in cancer. *Oncogene* 39 (19), 3791–3802. doi: 10.1038/s41388-020-1258-8

Jeon, K.II, Xu, X., Aizawa, T., Lim, J. H., Jono, H., Kwon, D. S., et al. (2010). Vinpocetine inhibits NF-kappaB-dependent inflammation via an IKK-dependent but PDE-independent mechanism. *Proc. Natl. Acad. Sci. U.S.A.* 107 (21), 9795–9800. doi: 10.1073/pnas.0914414107

Jin, S. L., Lan, L., Zoudilova, M., and Conti, M. (2005). Specific role of phosphodiesterase 4B in lipopolysaccharide-induced signaling in mouse macrophages. *J Immunol.* 175 (3), 1523–1531. doi: 10.4049/jimmunol.175.3.1523

Jin, S. L., Goya, S., Nakae, S., Wang, D., Bruss, M., Hou, C., et al. (2010). Phosphodiesterase 4B is essential for T(H)2-cell function and development of airway hyperresponsiveness in allergic asthma. *J. Allergy Clin. Immunol.* 126 (6), 1252–9 e12. doi: 10.1016/j.jaci.2010.08.014

Kamata, H., Tsuchiya, Y., and Asano, T. (2010). IkappaBbeta is a positive and negative regulator of NF-kappaB activity during inflammation. *Cell Res.* 20 (11), 1178–1180. doi: 10.1038/cr.2010.147

Keravis, T., Monneaux, F., Yougbare, I., Gazi, L., Bourguignon, J. J., Muller, S., et al. (2012). Disease progression in MRL/lpr lupus-prone mice is reduced by NCS 613, a specific cyclic nucleotide phosphodiesterase type 4 (PDE4) inhibitor. *PloS One* 7 (1), e28899. doi: 10.1371/journal.pone.0028899

Koutras, A., Giannopoulou, E., Kritikou, I., Antonacopoulou, A., Evans, T. R., Papavassiliou, A. G., et al. (2009). Antiproliferative effect of exemestane in lung cancer cells. *Mol. Cancer* 8, 109. doi: 10.1186/1476-4598-8-109

Kwak, H. J., Song, J. S., Heo, J. Y., Yang, S. D., Nam, J. Y., and Cheon, H. G. (2005). Roflumilast inhibits lipopolysaccharide-induced inflammatory mediators via suppression of nuclear factor-kappaB, p38 mitogen-activated protein kinase, and c-Jun NH2-terminal kinase activation. *J. Pharmacol. Exp. Ther.* 315 (3), 1188–1195. doi: 10.1124/jpet.105.092056

Lee, G., Walser, T. C., and Dubinett, S. M. (2009). Chronic inflammation, chronic obstructive pulmonary disease, and lung cancer. *Curr. Opin. Pulm. Med.* 15 (4), 303–307. doi: 10.1097/MCP.0b013e32832c975a

Li, H., Zuo, J., and Tang, W. (2018). Phosphodiesterase-4 Inhibitors for the Treatment of Inflammatory Diseases. *Front. Pharmacol.* 9, 1048. doi: 10.3389/fphar.2018.01048

Lin, Y., Bai, L., Chen, W., and Xu, S. (2010). The NF-kappaB activation pathways, emerging molecular targets for cancer prevention and therapy. *Expert Opin. Ther. Targets* 14 (1), 45–55. doi: 10.1517/14728220903431069

Luangdilok, S., Box, C., Harrington, K., Rhys-Evans, P., and Eccles, S. (2011). MAPK and PI3K signalling differentially regulate angiogenic and lymphangiogenic cytokine secretion in squamous cell carcinoma of the head and neck. *Eur. J. Cancer* 47 (4), 520–529. doi: 10.1016/j.ejca.2010.10.009

Lugnier, C. (2006). Cyclic nucleotide phosphodiesterase (PDE) superfamily: a new target for the development of specific therapeutic agents. *Pharmacol. Ther.* 109 (3), 366–398. doi: 10.1016/j.pharmthera.2005.07.003

Lugnier, C., Meyer, A., Tahla, S., and Geny, B. (2020). Cyclic nucleotide phosphodiesterases: new targets in the metabolic syndrome? *Pharmacol. Ther.* 208, 107475. doi: 10.1016/j.pharmthera.2020.107475

Maurice, D. A, Ke, H., Ahmad, F., Wang, Y., Chung, J., and Manganiello, V. (2014). Advances in targeting cyclic nucleotide phosphodiesterases. *Nat. Rev. Drug. Discov.* 13 (4), 290–314. doi: 10.1038/nrd4228

Morin, C., Sirois, M., Echave, V., Gomes, M. M., and Rousseau, E. (2008). EET displays anti-inflammatory effects in TNF-alpha stimulated human bronchi: putative role of CPI-17. *Am. J. Respir. Cell Mol. Biol.* 38 (2), 192–201. doi: 10.1165/rcmb.2007-0232OC

Morin, C., Sirois, M., Echave, V., Albadine, R., and Rousseau, E. (2010). 17,18-epoxyeicosatetraenoic acid targets PPARgamma and p38 mitogen-activated protein kinase to mediate its anti-inflammatory effects in the lung: role of soluble epoxide hydrolase. *Am. J. Respir. Cell Mol. Biol.* 43 (5), 564–575. doi: 10.1165/rcmb.2009-0155OC

Moriyuki, K., Sekiguchi, F., Matsubara, K., Nishikawa, H., and Kawabata, A. (2009). Proteinase-activated receptor-2-triggered prostaglandin E(2) release, but not cyclooxygenase-2 upregulation, requires activation of the phosphatidylinositol 3-kinase/Akt/nuclear factor-kappaB pathway in human alveolar epithelial cells. *J. Pharmacol. Sci.* 111 (3), 269–275. doi: 10.1254/jphs.09155FP

Mouratidis, P. X., Colston, K. W., Bartlett, J. B., Muller, G. W., Man, H. W., Stirling, D., et al. (2009). Antiproliferative effects of CC-8062 and CC-8075 in pancreatic cancer cells. *Pancreas* 38 (1), 78–84. doi: 10.1097/MPA.0b013e318183d72f

Oger, S., Méhats, C., Dallot, E., Cabrol, D., and Leroy, M. J. (2002). Evidence for a role of phosphodiesterase 4 in lipopolysaccharide-stimulated prostaglandin E2 production and matrix metalloproteinase-9 activity in human amniochorionic membranes. *J. Immunol.* 174 (12), 8082–8089. doi: 10.4049/jimmunol.174.12.8082

Phillips, J. E. (2020). Inhaled Phosphodiesterase 4 (PDE4) Inhibitors for Inflammatory Respiratory Diseases. *Front. Pharmacol.* 11, 259. doi: 10.3389/fphar.2020.00259

Pikarsky, E., and Ben-Neriah, Y. (2006). NF-kappaB inhibition: a double-edged sword in cancer. *Eur. J. Cancer* 42 (6), 779–784. doi: 10.1016/j.ejca.2006.01.011

Selige, J., Tenor, H., Hatzelmann, A., and Dunkern, T. (2010). Cytokine-dependent balance of mitogenic effects in primary human lung fibroblasts related to cyclic AMP signaling and phosphodiesterase 4 inhibition. *J. Cell Physiol.* 223 (2), 317–326. doi: 10.1002/jcp.22037

Sigala, I., Zacharatos, P., Toumpanakis, D., Michailidou, T., Noussia, O., Theocharis, S., et al. (2011). MAPKs and NF-kappaB differentially regulate cytokine expression in the diaphragm in response to resistive breathing: the role of oxidative stress. *Am. J. Physiol. Regul. Integr. Comp. Physiol.* 300 (5), R1152–R1162. doi: 10.1152/ajpregu.00376.2010

Smith, L. A., Paszkiewicz, G. M., Hutson, A. D., and Pauly, J. L. (2010). Inflammatory response of lung macrophages and epithelial cells to tobacco smoke: a literature review of ex vivo investigations. *Immunol. Res.* 46 (1–3), 94–126. doi: 10.1007/s12026-009-8133-6

Sosroseno, W., and Sugiatno, E. (2008). Cyclic-AMP-dependent proliferation of a human osteoblast cell line (HOS cells) induced by hydroxyapatite: effect of exogenous nitric oxide. *Acta BioMed.* 79 (2), 110–116.

Udalov, S., Dumitrascu, R., Pullamsetti, S. S., Al-tamari, H. M., Weissmann, N., Ghofrani, H. A., et al. (2010). Effects of phosphodiesterase 4 inhibition on bleomycin-induced pulmonary fibrosis in mice. *BMC Pulm. Med.* 10, 26. doi: 10.1186/1471-2466-10-26

Wong, K. K. (2009). Recent developments in anti-cancer agents targeting the Ras/ Raf/ MEK/ERK pathway. *Recent Pat. Anticancer Drug Discovery* 4 (1), 28–35. doi: 10.2174/157489209787002461

Yougbare, I., Morin, C., Senouvo, F. Y., Sirois, C., Albadine, R., Lugnier, C., et al. (2011). NCS 613, a potent and specific PDE4 inhibitor, displays anti-inflammatory effects on human lung tissues. *Am. J. Physiol. Lung Cell Mol. Physiol.* 301 (4), L441–L450. doi: 10.1152/ajplung.00407.2010

Yougbare, I., Boire, G., Roy, M., Lugnier, C., and Rouseau, E. (2013). NCS 613 exhibits anti-inflammatory effects on PBMCs from lupus patients by inhibiting p38 MAPK and NF-kappaB signalling pathways while reducing proinflammatory cytokine production. *Can. J. Physiol. Pharmacol.* 91 (5), 353–361. doi: 10.1139/cjpp-2012-0233

Yougbare, I., Keravis, T., Abusnina, A., Decossas, M., Schall, N., Muller, S., et al. (2014). Cyclic GMP catabolism up-regulation in MRL/lpr lupus-prone mice is associated with organ remodeling. *Biochim. Biophys. Acta* 1842 (7), 916–926. doi: 10.1016/j.bbadis.2014.03.001

Zhu, B., Kelly, J., Vemavarapu, L., Thompson, W. J., and Strada, S. J. (2004). Activation and induction of cyclic AMP phosphodiesterase (PDE4) in rat pulmonary microvascular endothelial cells. *Biochem. Pharmacol.* 68 (3), 479–491. doi: 10.1016/j.bcp.2004.03.039

16

Airway Epithelial Inflammation *In Vitro* Augments the Rescue of Mutant CFTR by Current CFTR Modulator Therapies

Martina Gentzsch[1,2,3], Deborah M. Cholon[1], Nancy L. Quinney[1], Mary E. B. Martino[1], John T. Minges[1], Susan E. Boyles[1], Tara N. Guhr Lee[1], Charles R. Esther Jr.[1,2] and Carla M. P. Ribeiro[1,3,4]*

[1]Marsico Lung Institute and Cystic Fibrosis Research Center, School of Medicine, University of North Carolina, Chapel Hill, NC, United States, [2]Department of Pediatrics, Division of Pediatric Pulmonology, School of Medicine, University of North Carolina School of Medicine, Chapel Hill, NC, United States, [3]Department of Cell Biology and Physiology, School of Medicine, University of North Carolina School of Medicine, Chapel Hill, NC, United States, [4]Department of Medicine, Division of Pulmonary Diseases, School of Medicine, University of North Carolina, Chapel Hill, NC, United States

***Correspondence:**
Martina Gentzsch
gentzsch@med.unc.edu

In cystic fibrosis (CF), defective biogenesis and activity of the cystic fibrosis transmembrane conductance regulator (CFTR) leads to airway dehydration and impaired mucociliary clearance, resulting in chronic airway infection and inflammation. The most common CFTR mutation, F508del, results in a processing defect in which the protein is retained in the endoplasmic reticulum and does not reach the apical surface. CFTR corrector compounds address this processing defect to promote mutant CFTR transfer to the apical membrane. When coupled with potentiators to increase CFTR channel activity, these drugs yield significant clinical benefits in CF patients carrying the F508del mutation. However, processing of CFTR and other proteins can be influenced by environmental factors such as inflammation, and the impact of airway inflammation on pharmacological activity of CFTR correctors is not established. The present study evaluated CFTR-rescuing therapies in inflamed CF airway epithelial cultures, utilizing models that mimic the inflammatory environment of CF airways. Primary bronchial epithelial cultures from F508del/F508del CF patients were inflamed by mucosal exposure to one of two inflammatory stimuli: 1) supernatant from mucopurulent material from CF airways with advanced lung disease, or 2) bronchoalveolar lavage fluid from pediatric CF patients. Cultures inflamed with either stimulus exhibited augmented F508del responses following therapy with correctors VX-809 or VX-661, and overcame the detrimental effects of chronic exposure to the CFTR potentiator VX-770. Remarkably, even the improved CFTR rescue responses resulting from a clinically effective triple therapy (VX-659/VX-661/VX-770) were enhanced by epithelial inflammation. Thus, the airway inflammatory milieu from late- and early-stage CF lung disease improves the efficacy of CFTR modulators, regardless of the combination therapy used. Our findings suggest that pre-clinical evaluation of CFTR corrector therapies should be performed under conditions mimicking the native inflammatory status of CF airways, and altering the inflammatory status of CF airways may change the efficacy of CFTR modulator therapies.

Keywords: airway inflammation, CFTR, F508del, CFTR corrector, CFTR potentiator, CFTR rescue

INTRODUCTION

The most common mutation in cystic fibrosis (CF) manifests as deletion of phenylalanine at position 508 in the cystic fibrosis transmembrane conductance regulator (F508del CFTR). F508del CFTR is retained in the endoplasmic reticulum (ER) and degraded by the proteasomal pathway, which prevents it from reaching the apical membrane. In CF airways, lack of apical functional CFTR causes airway dehydration, increases the mucus % solids, and impairs mucociliary clearance, resulting in chronic airway infection and inflammation (Ratjen and Doring 2003; Boucher 2007a).

Basic research paved the road for CFTR-targeting drugs known as CFTR modulators, e.g., correctors that enhance F508del CFTR transfer to the apical membrane, and potentiators that increase CFTR channel activity (Gentzsch and Mall 2018). However, earlier studies indicated the need for improving the efficacy of CFTR modulators. For instance, while the corrector lumacaftor (VX-809) restored F508del maturation and function to ~15% of wild-type CFTR *in vitro* (Van Goor et al., 2011; Dekkers et al., 2013; Farinha et al., 2013; He et al., 2013; Loo, Bartlett, and Clarke 2013; Okiyoneda et al., 2013; Ren et al., 2013), this drug alone did not significantly improve lung function in early phase clinical trials (Clancy et al., 2012). Adding the potentiator ivacaftor (VX-770) to VX-809, which creates the drug Orkambi, resulted in modest lung function improvements in clinical trials, but only in patients homozygous for F508del (Boyle et al., 2014; Wainwright et al., 2015). Similar outcomes were obtained with tezacaftor (VX-661) plus VX-770, which creates Symdeko (Donaldson et al., 2018). Subsequent triple combination studies adding the next generation correctors elexacaftor (VX-445) or bamocaftor (VX-659) resulted in more impressive clinical responses (Davies et al., 2018; Keating et al., 2018). In fact, the drug Trikafta (VX-445,VX-661, and VX-770) showed substantial efficacy in phase 3 clinical trials (Heijerman et al., 2019; Middleton et al., 2019) and was recently approved by the Food and Drug Administration for the treatment of CF patients aged 12 years and older who have at least one copy of the F508del mutation. While the new triple combination CFTR modulator therapy appears promising, there is still an unmet need to improve the efficacy of CFTR-targeting treatments for patients that carry one or two F508del mutations, who represent ~ 90% of the CF population. Little is known regarding the mechanisms by which CFTR modulators facilitate the rescue of F508del CFTR and whether the CF airway environment can have an impact on this process.

Because CF patients initiating CFTR modulator therapies suffer from airway inflammation, we recently evaluated the action of CFTR modulators under conditions that recapitulate the inflammatory status of human CF airways. We utilized a pre-clinical model consisting of well-differentiated primary cultures of F508del/F508del human bronchial epithelia (HBE) grown at air-liquid interface (Ribeiro et al., 2005a; Ribeiro et al., 2005b) and exposed to supernatant from mucopurulent material (SMM) harvested from the airways of excised human CF lungs (Ribeiro et al., 2005a; Ribeiro et al., 2005b; Martino et al., 2009; Ribeiro et al., 2009; Abdullah et al., 2018). SMM contains bacterial products, neutrophil factors (e.g., neutrophil elastase, MMP9, cathepsin G, BPI, lysozyme, macrophage and airway epithelial cytokines) (Abdullah et al., 2018), mucins and hundreds of peptides, and purines (Esther et al., 2008); its cytokine composition is reproducible from patient to patient (Abdullah et al., 2018). Because the airway epithelia of CF patients are exposed to multiple inflammatory mediators *in vivo*, the use of SMM is a superior approach to single inflammatory mediators for testing the impact of the CF airway inflammatory milieu on the efficacy of CFTR modulators. We found that SMM enhanced VX-809-increased F508del CFTR-mediated responses to forskolin and VX-770 (Gentzsch et al., 2018). Notably, while the immature ER-residing form of CFTR (band B) was not significantly increased in CF cultures treated with SMM or VX-809, it was significantly increased in response to the simultaneous treatment with SMM and VX-809 (Gentzsch et al., 2018). On the other hand, while the mature band C was formed in F508del cultures treated only with VX-809, SMM drastically increased VX-809-rescued band C (Gentzsch et al., 2018). SMM did not significantly affect the CFTR mRNA levels in presence or absence of VX-809 (Gentzsch et al., 2018), suggesting that its effect is not via up-regulation of F508del transcription or translation.

While these previous studies demonstrated that inflammation increases the efficacy of older-generation CFTR correctors, its impact on next-generation correctors that are components of recently approved triple combination therapy is not known. Furthermore, it is not clear how (and if) the severity of inflammation affects responses to CFTR modulator therapy. To address these key issues, we conducted studies with HBE cells from F508del homozygous CF patients exposed to SMM or bronchoalveolar lavage fluid (BALF) from pediatric CF patients. These pre-clinical models of airway epithelial inflammation were used to evaluate the efficacy of current CFTR modulator double and triple therapies on F508del rescue.

RESULTS

Airway Epithelial Inflammation Triggered by SMM or BALF Augments CFTR Correction by VX-661

We have utilized SMM as representative of the CF inflammatory airway milieu; however, since this material is isolated from patients with end-stage lung disease, it represents the airway environment from severe CF phenotypes. To explore whether functional responses of CFTR are influenced by airway inflammation from patients with less severe disease, we utilized BALF from pediatric patients with CF. Both SMM and BALF from CF patients represent the infectious/inflammatory milieu to which the airway epithelia from these patients are exposed. Because the airway epithelia of CF patients are exposed to the combination of all the factors present in SMM or BALF, as opposed to a defined inflammatory factor, the use of SMM and BALF represents a highly translational model to test

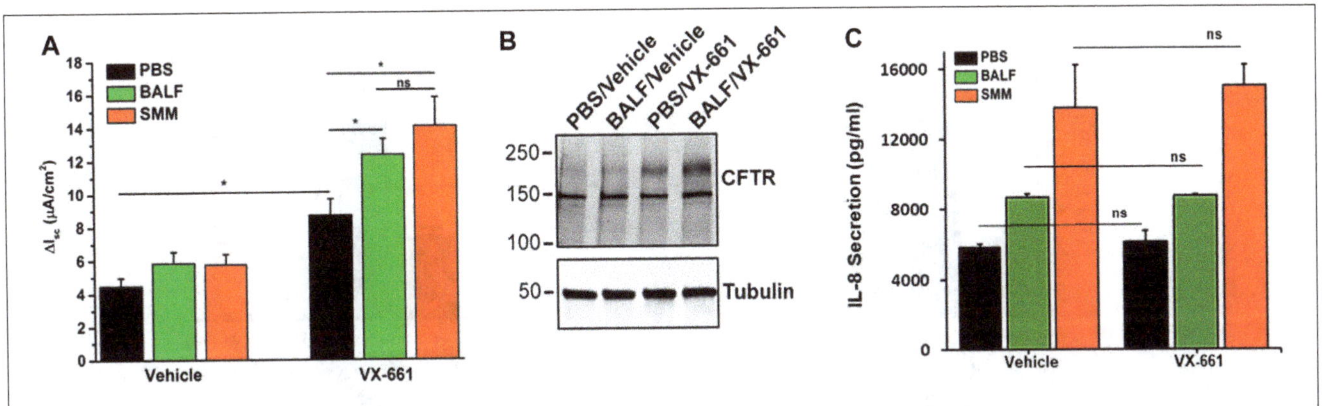

FIGURE 1 | SMM and BALF enhance F508del rescue by VX-661. **(A)** CFTR responses from F508del/F508del HBE evaluated in Ussing chambers. Cultures were exposed apically to 30 μM SMM or BALF and treated on the basolateral side with vehicle or 5 μM VX-661, as described in Methods. Data are expressed as mean ± SEM. $^{*}p < 0.05$, (t tests), ns = not significant; n = 2 donors, five to six cultures/experimental group. **(B)** Representative CFTR Western blot to analyze F508del maturation (upper band); n = 2 cultures due to limited amounts of BALF. **(C)** IL-8 secretion (pg/ml of culture media) from the F508del/F508del HBE evaluated in **(A)**. Data are expressed as mean ± SEM. Note: Because the BALF samples were diluted, they were concentrated 4-fold with Centricon centrifugal filter units.

the impact of the CF airway inflammatory milieu on the efficacy of CFTR modulators.

We evaluated Symdeko, a CF drug consisting of VX-661 combined with VX-770, which has been approved for patients homozygous for F508del as well as for other genotypes, including partial function CFTR mutations (Rowe et al., 2017; Taylor-Cousar et al., 2017; Donaldson et al., 2018). We tested whether exposure of F508del homozygous primary HBE cultures to BALF from pediatric CF patients or to SMM promoted inflammation coupled with augmentation of VX-661-induced CFTR correction. Similar to VX-809 (Gentzsch et al., 2018), VX-661-induced CFTR correction (as indicated by increased forskolin- and VX-770-induced Cl^- secretion) was enhanced by SMM (**Figure 1A**). Notably, these changes were reproduced in VX-661-rescued cultures exposed to pediatric BALF (**Figure 1A**). The augmentation of VX-661-promoted functional F508del rescue in BALF-exposed cultures correlated with an enhancement of VX-661-rescued band C levels (**Figure 1B**; upper-most band), as we have previously shown for SMM in VX-809-treated cultures (Gentzsch et al., 2018). The increased VX-661-mediated CFTR correction in cultures exposed to SMM or BALF was associated with higher levels of epithelial inflammation, based on IL-8 secretory responses (**Figure 1C**). Importantly, VX-661 did not exhibit an anti-inflammatory action, since it did not blunt the IL-8 secretory response in PBS-, BALF- or SMM-exposed cultures (**Figure 1C**).

Airway Epithelial Inflammation Overcomes Chronic VX-770 Treatment-Promoted Inhibition of F508del Rescue

We have reported that CFTR responses to chronic treatment with VX-809 or VX-661 and VX-770 are lower than when the corrector compound (VX-809 or VX-661) is applied chronically and the potentiator VX-770 is applied acutely (Cholon et al., 2014). In addition, chronic treatment (48 h) of F508de/F508del HBE with VX-770 decreased VX-809-promoted CFTR rescue in a dose-dependent manner (Cholon et al., 2014). We next tested the impact of SMM-induced inflammation regarding the inhibitory effect of chronic VX-770 treatment on VX-809- or VX-661-dependent CFTR rescue. Surprisingly, SMM exposure counteracted chronic VX-770 treatment-induced abrogation of CFTR rescue with either CFTR corrector (**Figures 2A,B**). We then evaluated the inflammatory responses of the cultures subjected to the various treatments. The baseline and SMM-increased levels of IL-8 secretion were not affected by either corrector, in the absence or presence of VX-770 (**Figures 2C,D**). Hence, these findings suggest that the increased inflammatory status of F508del HBE cultures resulting from SMM exposure is a common factor for overcoming the detrimental effects of chronic VX-770 treatment on VX-809- or VX-661-mediated CFTR rescue.

Airway Epithelial Inflammation Overcomes Chronic VX-770 Treatment-Promoted Inhibition of UTP Responses

We have also previously shown that chronic treatment with VX-809 and VX-770 inhibits UTP-induced activation of the calcium-activated chloride channel (CaCC) (Cholon et al., 2014). Therefore, we evaluated whether, similar to its protective action against the detrimental effect of chronic treatment with VX-770 on F508del CFTR, SMM would partially overcome the inhibitory effect of chronic VX-770 treatment on CaCC responses. While the UTP-induced CaCC responses were decreased by chronic treatment of F508del HBE with VX-809 or VX-661 plus VX-770, the inhibitory effect of VX-770 was reversed by exposing the cultures to SMM (**Figure 3**). Thus, chronic VX-770 treatment targets F508del CFTR and CaCC activities, and our results demonstrate that this inhibition is overcome by inflammation induced by SMM.

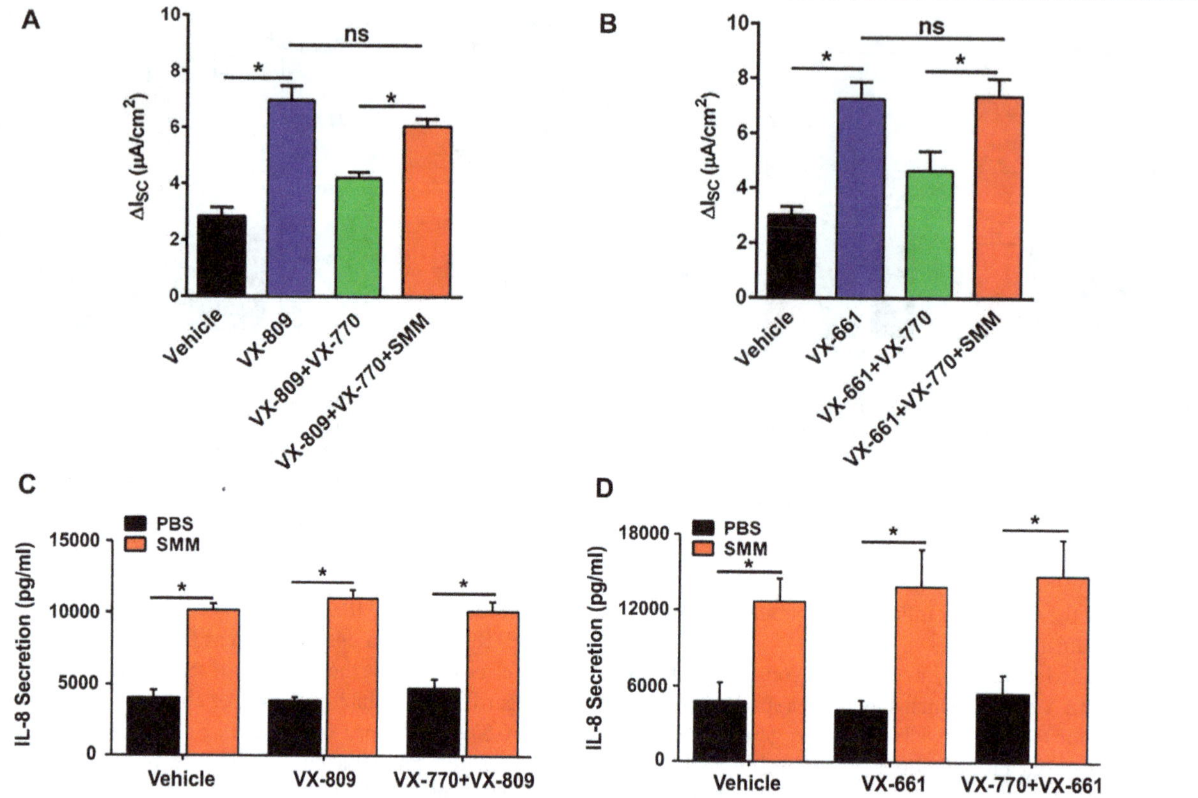

FIGURE 2 | SMM overcomes chronic VX-770 treatment-promoted inhibition of F508del rescue. F508del CFTR responses were measured in Ussing chambers. **(A)** SMM overcomes chronic VX-770 (5 μM, 48 h)-mediated abrogation of VX-809-promoted rescue. **(B)** SMM overcomes chronic VX-770 (5 μM, 48 h)-mediated abrogation of VX-661-dependent rescue. **(C),(D)** IL-8 secretion from F508del/F508del HBE cultures exposed to PBS or SMM and treated for 48 h with VX-809 **(C)** or VX-661 **(D)** ± VX-770. Data are expressed as mean ± SEM. *$p < 0.05$, ns = not significant; n = 3 CF HBE donors, three cultures/donor.

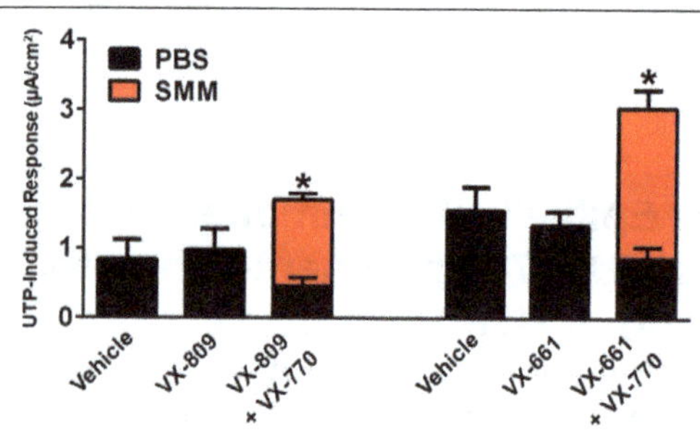

FIGURE 3 | SMM overcomes chronic VX-770 treatment-promoted inhibition of UTP-induced responses. F508del/F508del HBE cultures were exposed for 48 h to vehicle or 5 μM VX-809 or VX-661 ± 5 μM VX-770 in combination with PBS or SMM. Data are expressed as mean ± SEM. *$p < 0.05$; n = 3 F508del/F508del HBE culture donors, experiments were performed in three replicates/donor.

Airway Epithelial Inflammation Enhances Triple Combination-Promoted F508del Rescue

Because a triple combination of CFTR modulators (Trikafta consisting of VX-445, VX-661, VX-770) is currently being used in the clinic, we tested the impact of inflammation on the ability of a triple combination therapy consisting of VX-659, VX-661 and VX-770 to increase F508del CFTR rescue. VX-659 is a corrector compound with similar activity as compared to VX-445. In agreement with previous studies (Davies et al., 2018), VX-659, VX-661 and VX-770 promoted 2-fold higher F508del CFTR responses, which approached normal CFTR function, as compared with the responses resulting from the double therapy with VX-661 and VX-770 (**Figure 4A**). Remarkably, the F508del CFTR responses resulting from the triple combination were further enhanced by SMM by ~2-fold (**Figure 4A**). Similar to the findings with other combinations of CFTR modulators (**Figures 1C, 2C,D**), the triple therapy with VX-659, VX-661, and VX-770 was devoid of an effect on the inflammatory response of the F508del CFTR cultures in the absence or presence of SMM (**Figure 4B**).

DISCUSSION

The absence of functional CFTR in CF airway epithelia leads to airway surface liquid dehydration, cilia collapse, and accumulation of thickened mucus to airway surfaces. These alterations result in persistent airway infection and robust

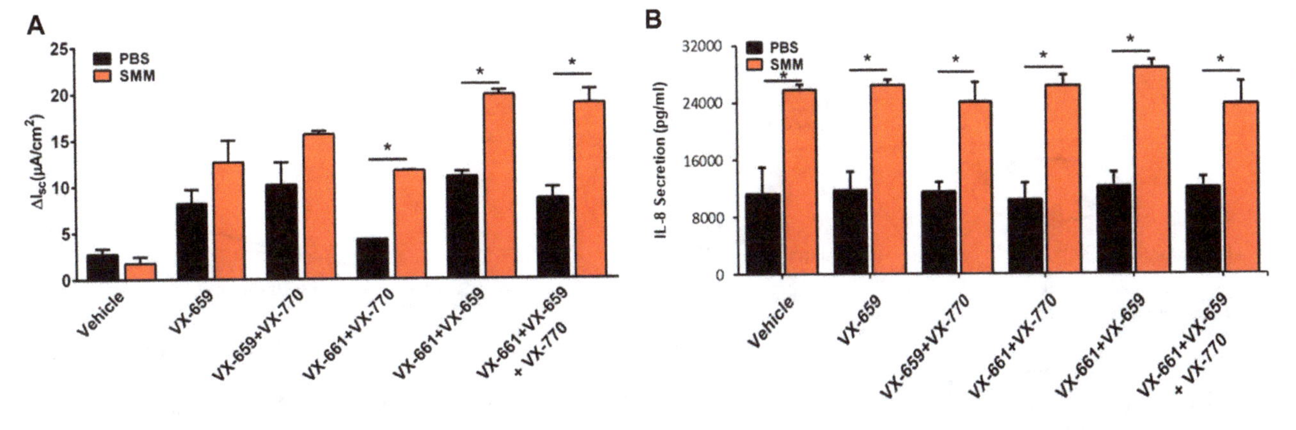

FIGURE 4 | SMM enhances triple combination-promoted F508del rescue. **(A)** CFTR responses to acute forskolin + VX-770 from F508del/F508del HBE in Ussing chambers. HBE were treated with VX-659 (1 μM), VX-661 (5 μM) and VX-770 (5 μM). **(B)** IL-8 secretion from the CF HBE cultures evaluated in **A**. Data are expressed as mean ± SEM. $^*p < 0.05$; n = 2 donors, five to six cultures/experimental group.

chronic inflammation (Doring and Worlitzsch 2000; Saiman and Siegel 2004; Boucher 2007b; Cohen-Cymberknoh et al., 2013). The chronic inflammatory status of CF airways can ultimately damage the airway walls.

Despite decades of research on the cell biology of CFTR, the mechanisms by which CFTR modulators impact rescue of F508del CFTR and the impact of the CF airway environment on this process remain unclear. Utilizing models that more accurately represent the diseased status of CF airway epithelia, our findings demonstrated that the CF airway inflammatory milieu has a major impact on the effect of newer-generation CFTR modulators concerning ion transport processes. Notably, our study has shown that the CF airway inflammatory milieu from advanced CF lung disease (SMM) improves the efficacy of various therapeutic combinations of CFTR modulators regarding their ability to increase F508del CFTR responses (**Figures 1, 2, 4**). Moreover, similar results were obtained in studies using BALF from pediatric CF patients with less severe disease (**Figure 1**). Because increased inflammation is already present early in life in CF (Esther et al., 2019), these findings suggest that inflammation-enhanced CFTR rescue is relevant to early CF lung disease. Importantly, inflammation augmented the already impressive CFTR rescue responses from the newly improved triple combination therapy (**Figure 4**). The integrity of HBE cultures and transepithelial resistance was not affected after SMM or BALF treatment under the experimental conditions utilized (data not shown).

The beneficial effects of inflammation on CFTR rescue by modulator therapy likely reflect inflammation-mediated increases of the ER protein-folding capacity, which is expected to facilitate CFTR folding and trafficking. Short-term F508del CF HBE cultures exhibit an increased expression of ER chaperones and expansion of the ER compartment as a result of their *in vivo* exposure to the CF airway inflammatory milieu; these alterations revert to normal over time in long-term cultures (Ribeiro et al., 2005a). Exposure of long-term cultures of F508del HBE to SMM reproduces the expansion of the ER compartment and its protein folding capacity observed in short-term cultures (Ribeiro et al., 2005a; Ribeiro et al., 2005b; Martino et al., 2009; Ribeiro and O'Neal 2012).

Inflammation also appears to inhibit the destabilization effect of chronic VX-770 exposure on CFTR. We and others have previously demonstrated that chronic treatment with VX-770 abrogates corrector-mediated rescue of F508del by enhancing internalization and turnover of mature CFTR proteins (Cholon et al., 2014; Veit et al., 2014). Exposure to SMM enhanced CFTR responses to chronic treatment with VX-809 or VX-661 plus VX-770 by overcoming chronic VX-770-promoted inhibition of F508del rescue (**Figure 2**). In agreement with our findings, recent studies have shown that VX-770 can also exert a similar negative effect on the stability of membrane-localized solute carriers (SLC26A3, SLC26A9, and SLC6A14), and it has been suggested that the destabilizing effect of VX-770 may be related to its lipophilicity that may impact the properties of the lipid bilayer (Chin et al., 2018). Future studies are necessary to evaluate whether inflammation of airway epithelia has a similar protective effect against VX-770-induced destabilization of solute carriers and, if so, whether such an effect is due to inflammation-promoted alterations of lipid bilayer properties.

The destabilization effect of VX-770 and the "protective" effect of airway epithelial inflammation were also observed with calcium-activated chloride secretion. UTP-induced CaCC-mediated responses were decreased by chronic treatment with VX-809 plus VX-770 (**Figure 3**), while exposure to SMM increased UTP-dependent calcium-activated secretion (**Figure 3**). These effects may further contribute to increased hydration of inflamed CF airways in patients receiving CFTR modulatr therapy. Our findings could potentially be relevant to other chronic lung diseases such as COPD in which VX-770 has been considered as a therapeutic for dysfunctional CFTR (Solomon et al., 2016), and may open new research directions toward understanding the impact of inflammation on biogenesis of other ABC proteins, which are involved in multiple diseases.

Although a recent study suggested that CFTR modulator therapy has anti-inflammatory properties (Jarosz-Griffiths et al., 2020), the experiments performed in our study did not

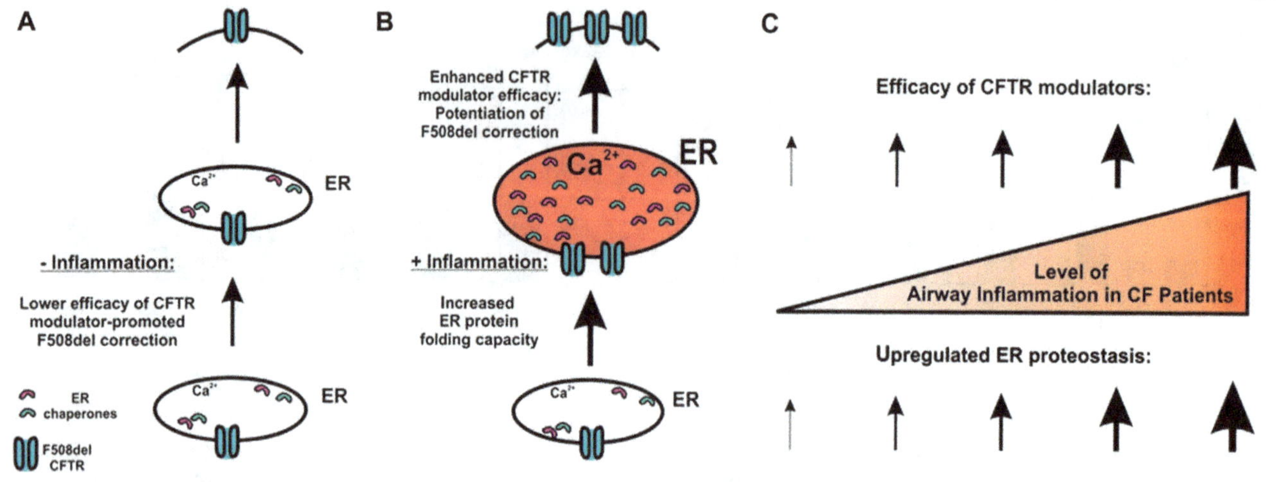

FIGURE 5 | Potential mechanism for airway inflammation-increased efficacy of F508del CFTR modulators. **(A)** In the absence of inflammation, lower expression of chaperones and lower efficacy of CFTR correctors result in a lower level of CFTR folding at the ER. **(B)** CF airway epithelial inflammation increases the ER protein folding capacity, thereby enhancing CFTR modulator efficacy. **(C)** Our model predicts that the higher the levels of airway inflammation, the higher the efficacy of CFTR modulators regarding the rescue of F508del.

demonstrate anti-inflammatory effects. None of the modulator treatments, including the triple combination, lowered SMM-induced inflammation (indicated by up-regulation of IL-8 secretion), nor lowered the baseline levels of secreted IL-8 (**Figures 1**, **2**, **4**). These findings suggest that defective CFTR function (i.e., the "intrinsic" CF defect) is not, per se, a pro-inflammatory condition in airway epithelia, in agreement with our previous studies (Ribeiro et al., 2005b). Airway inflammation in CF likely arises indirectly as a consequence of decreased mucociliary clearance and accumulation of mucus and bacteria. However, we cannot rule out the possibility that CFTR dysfunction contributes to intrinsic inflammatory responses in other cell types.

Furthermore, structural data have indicated that VX-770 directly binds to CFTR protein within membrane domains (Liu et al., 2019). To minimize interference with CFTR modulator interactions, SMM and BALF were added apically, while CFTR modulators were added basolaterally to the culture medium, which should mimic physiological conditions and limit a possible interaction.

The interplay between airway inflammation and responses to CFTR modulators has significant clinical implications. Our findings suggest that the airway inflammation that characterizes CF lung disease plays a major role in the positive clinical responses to CFTR modulator therapy, and we propose a model with a direct relationship between airway inflammation and CFTR rescue (**Figure 5**). Even the modest inflammation present early in life is likely sufficient to enhance modulator responses. This relationship could limit the clinical efficacy of modulator therapy, since treatment-related improvements in mucociliary clearance could lessen airway inflammation, which would in turn reduce treatment efficacy. Consistent with this hypothesis, two studies demonstrated that highly effective modulator therapy using the CFTR potentiator VX-770 in patients with the G551D mutation did not reduce airway inflammation despite significant improvements in other clinical parameters (Harris et al., 2020; Rowe et al., 2014), although reductions in airway inflammation were observed in a separate study (Hisert et al., 2017). Airway inflammation was not assessed in the clinical trials of the recently approved triple combination modulator therapy, and further studies will be needed to assess the relationships between inflammation and clinical efficacy with this treatment. Although clinicians would not advocate increasing airway inflammation to enhance CFTR modulator efficacy, a better understanding of the underlying mechanisms may allow development of therapies that promote the beneficial effects of inflammation on CFTR rescue without its detrimental consequences.

In summary, the airway inflammatory milieu from late- and early-stage CF lung disease improves the efficacy of CFTR modulators, including triple combination therapy with VX-659, VX-661, and VX-770. Our findings suggest that the balance between suppression of airway inflammation and enhancement of CFTR rescue should be considered in CF patients undergoing anti-inflammatory and CFTR modulator therapies. Furthermore, our findings suggest that pre-clinical evaluation of novel CFTR modulators should be performed under conditions mimicking the native inflammatory milieu found in the airways of CF patients.

MATERIALS AND METHODS

Primary Cell Culture and Drug Treatments

Primary HBE cells from explant lungs from patients homozygous for the F508del, prepared as described previously (Fulcher and Randell 2013), were obtained from Dr. Scott H. Randell (Marsico Lung Institute, The University of North Carolina at Chapel Hill, USA). The cells were obtained under protocols approved by the University of North Carolina at Chapel Hill Biomedical

Institutional Review Board. Cells were expanded in BEGM (Lonza) and then cultured at air-liquid interface on 12 mm Millicell inserts (Millipore) in a modified BEBM (Hild and Jaffe 2016) until differentiated. Well-differentiated F508del/F508del HBE cultures were exposed for 24 h to apically added PBS or pooled SMM or BALF, in combination with basolateral exposure to vehicle or CFTR modulators ivacaftor (VX-770, Selleck Chemicals; 5 μM), lumacaftor (VX-809, Selleck Chemicals; 5 μM), tezacaftor (VX-661, Selleck Chemicals; 5 μM) and bamocaftor (VX-659, a gift from Henry Danahay; 1 μM). For chronic exposure, F508del HBE cultures were treated for 48 h.

CF SMM and BALF

SMM was obtained from the airways of excised human CF lungs as previously described (Ribeiro et al., 2005b; Martino et al., 2009; Ribeiro et al., 2009; Abdullah et al., 2018) and provided by the UNC CF Center Tissue Procurement and Cell Culture Core. BALF from pediatric CF patients <18 years old, which reflect the inflammatory airway milieu of the population ultimately targeted for mutant CFTR rescue, was pooled and concentrated 4-fold.

Transepithelial Ion Transport

Changes in short-circuit current (ΔI_{sc}) were measured from CF-HBE cultures in Ussing chambers as previously described (Cholon et al., 2014; Gentzsch et al., 2016; Gentzsch et al., 2017) in a bilateral Krebs bicarbonate-Ringers solution. Amiloride (100 μM, Sigma-Aldrich) was added to the apical bath to inhibit the epithelial sodium channel, ENaC. Bilateral addition of forskolin (10 μM, Sigma-Aldrich) followed to stimulate CFTR channel activity. CFTR inhibitor-172 (10 μM, Sigma-Aldrich) was then apically introduced to inhibit CFTR. Transepithelial resistance ($\Omega\,cm^2$) was measured to assess monolayer integrity and only cultures with values larger than 100 $\Omega\,cm^2$ were utilized. UTP (100 μM, GE Healthcare) response (an index of calcium-activated chloride channel activity) was assessed as an internal control.

CFTR Western Blotting

Western blot analysis of endogenous CFTR protein was performed as described previously (Cholon et al., 2014; Gentzsch et al., 2016). Briefly, whole-cell lysates of fully differentiated CF HBE cultures were prepared and then CFTR was immunoprecipitated. Samples were separated on 4–20% gradient SDS–polyacrylamide gel electrophoresis gels (Bio-Rad) and then transferred to nitrocellulose. Blots were probed with mouse monoclonal anti-CFTR antibodies and then with IRDye–goat anti-mouse immunoglobulin G (Molecular Probes). Anti-tubulin (LI-COR) was used as a loading control. Protein bands were visualized using an Odyssey Infrared Fluorescence Imaging System (LI-COR).

SMM (or BALF)-Induced Inflammation

F508del/F508del HBE were exposed to 30 μl mucosal SMM or BALF; serosal media were collected at the end of the experimental protocol to assess IL-8 secretion (an indicator of inflammation) by ELISA, as we have reported (Ribeiro et al., 2005b; Martino et al., 2009).

Statistical Analysis

Data analysis was performed using GraphPad PRISM software. Data were subjected to ANOVA analysis. Following significant ANOVA results, statistical significance between groups was calculated using Student's t-test. $p \leq 0.05$ was considered statistically significant.

AUTHOR CONTRIBUTIONS

MG, CE, and CR developed the ideas for the study, and designed and supervised the experiments. DC, NQ, MM, and JM performed experiments and analyzed the data. SB acquired and cultured specimens. TGL was in charge of BALF biobanking. MG, CR, and CE wrote the manuscript.

ACKNOWLEDGMENTS

The authors thank Scott H. Randell and the University of North Carolina Cystic Fibrosis Center Tissue Procurement and Cell Culture Core for providing HBE cells and mucopurulent material from human CF airways. Antibodies for CFTR were provided by Tim Jensen through the UNC CFF antibody distribution program (GENTZS18XX0).

REFERENCES

Abdullah, L. H., Coakley, R., Webster, M. J., Zhu, Y., Tarran, R., Radicioni, G., et al. (2018). Mucin production and hydration responses to mucopurulent materials in normal versus cystic fibrosis airway epithelia. *Am. J. Respir. Crit. Care Med.* 197, 481–491. doi:10.1164/rccm.201706-1139OC

Boucher, R. C. (2007a). Airway surface dehydration in cystic fibrosis: pathogenesis and therapy. *Annu. Rev. Med.* 58, 157–170. doi:10.1146/annurev.med.58.071905.105316

Boucher, R. C. (2007b). Evidence for airway surface dehydration as the initiating event in CF airway disease. *J. Intern. Med.* 261, 5–16. doi:10.1111/j.1365-2796.2006.01744.x

Boyle, M. P., Bell, S. C., Konstan, M. W., McColley, S. A., Rowe, S. M., Rietschel, E., et al. (2014). A CFTR corrector (lumacaftor) and a CFTR potentiator (ivacaftor) for treatment of patients with cystic fibrosis who have a phe508del CFTR mutation: a phase 2 randomised controlled trial. *Lancet Respir. Med.* 2, 527–538. doi:10.1016/S2213-2600(14)70132-8

Chin, S., Hung, M., Won, A., Wu, Y. S., Ahmadi, S., Yang, D., et al. (2018). Lipophilicity of the Cystic Fibrosis Drug, Ivacaftor (VX-770), and Its Destabilizing Effect on the Major CF-causing Mutation: F508del. *Mol. Pharmacol.* 94, 917–925. doi:10.1124/mol.118.112177

Cholon, D. M., Quinney, N. L., Fulcher, M. L., Esther, C. R., Jr., Das, J., Dokholyan, N. V., et al. (2014). Potentiator ivacaftor abrogates pharmacological correction of DeltaF508 CFTR in cystic fibrosis. *Sci. Transl Med.* 6, 246ra96. doi:10.1126/scitranslmed.3008680

Clancy, J. P., Rowe, S. M., Accurso, F. J., Aitken, M. L., Amin, R. S., Ashlock, M. A., et al. (2012) Results of a phase IIa study of VX-809, an investigational CFTR corrector compound, in subjects with cystic fibrosis homozygous for the F508del-CFTR mutation. *Thorax* 67, 12–18. doi:10.1136/thoraxjnl-2011-200393

Cohen-Cymberknoh, M., Kerem, E., Ferkol, T., and Elizur, A. (2013). Airway inflammation in cystic fibrosis: molecular mechanisms and clinical implications. *Thorax* 68, 1157–1162. doi:10.1136/thoraxjnl-2013-203204

Davies, J. C., Moskowitz, S. M., Brown, C., Horsley, A., Mall, M. A., McKone, E. F., et al. (2018). VX-659-Tezacaftor-Ivacaftor in patients with cystic fibrosis and one or two Phe508del alleles. *N. Engl. J. Med.* 379, 1599–1611. doi:10.1056/NEJMoa1807119

Dekkers, J. F., Wiegerinck, C. L., De Jonge, H. R., Bronsveld, I., Janssens, H. M., De Winter-de Groot, K. M., et al. (2013). A functional CFTR assay using primary cystic fibrosis intestinal organoids. *Nat. Med.* 19, 939–945. doi:10.1038/nm.3201

Donaldson, S. H., Pilewski, J. M., Griese, M., Cooke, J., Viswanathan, L., Tullis, E., et al. (2018). Tezacaftor/Ivacaftor in Subjects with Cystic Fibrosis and F508del/F508del-CFTR or F508del/G551D-CFTR. *Am. J. Respir. Crit. Care Med.* 197, 214–224. doi:10.1164/rccm.201704-0717OC

Doring, G., and Worlitzsch, D. (2000). Inflammation in cystic fibrosis and its management. *Paediatr. Respir. Rev.* 1, 101–106. doi:10.1053/prrv.2000.0030

Esther, C. R., Jr., Muhlebach, M. S., Ehre, C., Hill, D. B., Wolfgang, M. C., Kesimer, M., et al. (2019). Mucus accumulation in the lungs precedes structural changes and infection in children with cystic fibrosis. *Sci. Transl Med.* 11, 486. doi:10.1126/scitranslmed.aav3488

Esther, C. R., Jr., Alexis, N. E., Clas, M. L., Lazarowski, E. R., Donaldson, S. H., Ribeiro, C. M., et al. (2008). Extracellular purines are biomarkers of neutrophilic airway inflammation. *Eur. Respir. J.* 31, 949–956. doi:10.1183/09031936.00089807

Farinha, C. M., King-Underwood, J., Sousa, M., Correia, A. R., Henriques, B. J., Roxo-Rosa, M., et al. (2013). Revertants, low temperature, and correctors reveal the mechanism of F508del-CFTR rescue by VX-809 and suggest multiple agents for full correction. *Chem. Biol.* 20, 943–955. doi:10.1016/j.chembiol.2013.06.004

Fulcher, M. L., and Randell, S. H. (2013). Human nasal and tracheo-bronchial respiratory epithelial cell culture. *Methods Mol. Biol.* 945, 109–121. doi:10.1007/978-1-62703-125-7_8

Gentzsch, M., Cholon, D. M., Quinney, N. L., Boyles, S. E., Martino, M. E. B., and Ribeiro, C. M. P. (2018). The cystic fibrosis airway milieu enhances rescue of F508del in a pre-clinical model. *Eur. Respir. J.* 52, 1801133. doi:10.1183/13993003.01133-2018

Gentzsch, M., Ren, H. Y., Houck, S. A., Quinney, N. L., Cholon, D. M., Sopha, P., et al. (2016). Restoration of R117H CFTR folding and function in human airway cells through combination treatment with VX-809 and VX-770. *Am. J. Physiol. Lung Cell Mol Physiol* 311, L550–L559. doi:10.1152/ajplung.00186.2016

Gentzsch, M., and Mall, M. A. (2018). Ion channel modulators in cystic fibrosis. *Chest* 154, 383–393. doi:10.1016/j.chest.2018.04.036

Gentzsch, M., Boyles, S. E., Cheluvaraju, C., Chaudhry, I. G., Quinney, N. L., Cho, C., et al. (2017). Pharmacological rescue of conditionally reprogrammed cystic fibrosis bronchial epithelial cells. *Am. J. Respir. Cell Mol Biol* 56, 568–574. doi:10.1165/rcmb.2016-0276MA

Harris, J. K., Wagner, B. D., Zemanick, E. T., Robertson, C. E., Stevens, M. J., Heltshe, S. L., et al. (2020). Changes in airway microbiome and inflammation with Ivacaftor treatment in patients with cystic fibrosis and the G551D mutation. *Ann. Am. Thorac. Soc.* 17, 212–20.

He, L., Kota, P., Aleksandrov, A. A., Cui, L., Jensen, T., Dokholyan, N. V., et al. (2013). Correctors of DeltaF508 CFTR restore global conformational maturation without thermally stabilizing the mutant protein. *FASEB J.* 27, 536–545. doi:10.1096/fj.12-216119

Heijerman, H. G. M., McKone, E. F., Downey, D. G., Van Braeckel, E., Rowe, S. M., Tullis, E., et al. (2019). Efficacy and safety of the elexacaftor plus tezacaftor plus ivacaftor combination regimen in people with cystic fibrosis homozygous for the F508del mutation: a double-blind, randomised, phase 3 trial. *Lancet* 394, 1940–1948. doi:10.1016/S0140-6736(19)32597-8

Hild, M., and Jaffe, A. B. (2016). Production of 3-D airway organoids from primary human airway basal cells and their use in high-throughput screening. *Curr. Protoc. Stem Cell Biol.* 37, IE91-IE915. doi:10.1002/cpsc.1

Hisert, K. B., Heltshe, S. L., Pope, C., Jorth, P., Wu, X., Edwards, R. M., et al. (2017). Restoring cystic fibrosis transmembrane conductance regulator function reduces airway bacteria and inflammation in people with cystic fibrosis and chronic lung infections. *Am J. Respir. Crit. Care Med.* 195, 1617–1628. doi:10.1164/rccm.201609-1954OC

Jarosz-Griffiths, H. H., Scambler, T., Wong, C. H., Lara-Reyna, S., Holbrook, J., Martinon, F., et al. (2020). Different CFTR modulator combinations downregulate inflammation differently in cystic fibrosis. *Elife* 9, e54556. doi:10.7554/eLife.54556

Keating, D., Marigowda, G., Burr, L., Daines, C., Mall, M. A., McKone, E. F., et al. (2018). VX-445-Tezacaftor-Ivacaftor in Patients with Cystic Fibrosis and One or Two Phe508del Alleles. *N. Engl. J. Med.* 379, 1612–1620. doi:10.1056/NEJMoa1807120

Liu, F., Zhang, Z., Levit, A., Levring, J., Touhara, K. K., Shoichet, B. K., et al. (2019). Structural identification of a hotspot on CFTR for potentiation. *Science* 364, 1184–1188. doi:10.1126/science.aaw7611

Loo, T. W., Bartlett, M. C., and Clarke, D. M. (2013). Corrector VX-809 stabilizes the first transmembrane domain of CFTR. *Biochem. Pharmacol.* 86, 612–619. doi:10.1016/j.bcp.2013.06.028

Martino, M. E., Olsen, J. C., Fulcher, N. B., Wolfgang, M. C., ONeal, W. K., and Ribeiro, C. M. (2009). Airway epithelial inflammation-induced endoplasmic reticulum Ca2+ store expansion is mediated by X-box binding protein-1. *J. Biol. Chem.* 284, 14904–14913. doi:10.1074/jbc.M809180200

Middleton, P. G., Mall, M. A., Drevinek, P., Lands, L. C., McKone, E. F., Polineni, D., et al. (2019). Elexacaftor-Tezacaftor-Ivacaftor for Cystic Fibrosis with a Single Phe508del Allele. *N. Engl. J. Med.* 381, 1809–1819. doi:10.1056/NEJMoa1908639

Okiyoneda, T., Veit, G., Dekkers, J. F., Bagdany, M., Soya, N., Xu, H., et al. (2013). Mechanism-based corrector combination restores DeltaF508-CFTR folding and function. *Nat. Chem. Biol.* 9, 444–454. doi:10.1038/nchembio.1253

Ratjen, F., and Doring, G. (2003). Cystic fibrosis. *Lancet* 361, 681–689. doi:10.1016/S0140-6736(03)12567-6

Ren, H. Y., Grove, D. E., De La Rosa, O., Houck, S. A., Sopha, P., Van Goor, F., et al. (2013). VX-809 corrects folding defects in cystic fibrosis transmembrane conductance regulator protein through action on membrane-spanning domain 1. *Mol. Biol. Cell* 24, 3016–3024. doi:10.1091/mbc.E13-05-0240

Ribeiro, C. M., Paradiso, A. M., Carew, M. A., Shears, S. B., and Boucher, R. C. (2005a). Cystic fibrosis airway epithelial Ca2+ i signaling: the mechanism for the larger agonist-mediated Ca2+ i signals in human cystic fibrosis airway epithelia. *J. Biol. Chem.* 280, 10202–10209. doi:10.1074/jbc.M410617200

Ribeiro, C. M., Paradiso, A. M., Schwab, U., Perez-Vilar, J., Jones, L., O'Neal, W., et al. (2005b). Chronic airway infection/inflammation induces a Ca2+i-dependent hyperinflammatory response in human cystic fibrosis airway epithelia. *J. Biol. Chem.* 280, 17798–17806. doi:10.1074/jbc.M410618200

Ribeiro, C. M., Hurd, H., Wu, Y., Martino, M. E., Jones, L., Brighton, B., et al. (2009). Azithromycin treatment alters gene expression in inflammatory, lipid metabolism, and cell cycle pathways in well-differentiated human airway epithelia. *PLoS One* 4, e5806. doi:10.1371/journal.pone.0005806

Ribeiro, C. M., and O'Neal, W. K. (2012). Endoplasmic reticulum stress in chronic obstructive lung diseases. *Curr. Mol. Med.* 12, 872–882. doi:10.2174/156652412801318791

Rowe, S. M., Daines, C., Ringshausen, F. C., Kerem, E., Wilson, J., Tullis, E., et al. (2017). Tezacaftor-Ivacaftor in residual-function heterozygotes with cystic fibrosis. *N. Engl. J. Med.* 377, 2024–2035. doi:10.1056/NEJMoa1709847

Rowe, S. M., Heltshe, S. L., Gonska, T., Donaldson, S. H., Borowitz, D., and Gelfond, D. and Goal Investigators of the Cystic Fibrosis Foundation Therapeutics Development Network et al. (2014). Clinical mechanism of the cystic fibrosis transmembrane conductance regulator potentiator ivacaftor in G551D-mediated cystic fibrosis. *Am J. Respir. Crit. Care Med.* 190, 175–184.

Saiman, L., and Siegel, J. (2004). Infection control in cystic fibrosis. *Clin. Microbiol. Rev.* 17, 57–71. doi:10.1128/cmr.17.1.57-71.2004

Solomon, G. M., Raju, S. V., Dransfield, M. T., and Rowe, S. M. (2016). Therapeutic approaches to acquired cystic fibrosis transmembrane conductance regulator dysfunction in chronic bronchitis. *Ann. Am. Thorac. Soc.* 13 (Suppl. 2), S169–S176. doi:10.1513/AnnalsATS.201509-601KV

Taylor-Cousar, J. L., Munck, A., McKone, E. F., Van der Ent, C. K., Moeller, A., Simard, C., et al. (2017). Tezacaftor-Ivacaftor in patients with cystic fibrosis homozygous for Phe508del. *N. Engl. J. Med.* 377, 2013–2023. doi:10.1056/NEJMoa1709846

Van Goor, F., Hadida, S., Grootenhuis, P. D., Burton, B., Stack, J. H., Straley, K. S., et al. (2011). Correction of the F508del-CFTR protein processing defect *in vitro* by the investigational drug VX-809. *Proc. Natl. Acad. Sci. U S A.* 108, 18843–18848. doi:10.1073/pnas.1105787108

Veit, G., Avramescu, R. G., Perdomo, D., Phuan, P. W., Bagdany, M., Apaja, P. M., et al. (2014). Some gating potentiators, including VX-770, diminish DeltaF508-CFTR functional expression. *Sci. Transl Med.* 6, 246ra97. doi:10.1126/scitranslmed.3008889

Wainwright, C. E., Elborn, J. S., Ramsey, B. W., Marigowda, G., Huang, X., Cipolli, M., et al. (2015). Lumacaftor-Ivacaftor in patients with cystic fibrosis homozygous for Phe508del CFTR. *N. Engl. J. Med.* 373, 220–231. doi:10.1056/NEJMoa1409547

17

Novel Anti-Inflammatory Approaches for Cystic Fibrosis Lung Disease: Identification of Molecular Targets and Design of Innovative Therapies

Christie Mitri[1], *Zhengzhong Xu*[1,2], *Pauline Bardin*[1], *Harriet Corvol*[1,3], *Lhousseine Touqui*[1,4] *and Olivier Tabary*[1*]

[1] Sorbonne Université, Inserm, Centre de Recherche Saint-Antoine, CRSA, Paris, France, [2] Yangzhou University, Yangzhou, China, [3] Département de Pédiatrie Respiratoire, Hôpital Trousseau, AP-HP, Paris, France, [4] Equipe Mucoviscidose et Bronchopathies Chroniques, Département Santé Globale, Institut Pasteur, Paris, France

***Correspondence:**
Olivier Tabary
olivier.tabary@inserm.fr

Cystic fibrosis (CF) is the most common genetic disorder among Caucasians, estimated to affect more than 70,000 people in the world. Severe and persistent bronchial inflammation and chronic bacterial infection, along with airway mucus obstruction, are hallmarks of CF lung disease and participate in its progression. Anti-inflammatory therapies are, therefore, of particular interest for CF lung disease. Furthermore, a better understanding of the molecular mechanisms involved in airway infection and inflammation in CF has led to the development of new therapeutic approaches that are currently under evaluation by clinical trials. These new strategies dedicated to CF inflammation are designed to treat different dysregulated aspects such as oxidative stress, cytokine secretion, and the targeting of dysregulated pathways. In this review, we summarize the current understanding of the cellular and molecular mechanisms that contribute to abnormal lung inflammation in CF, as well as the new anti-inflammatory strategies proposed to CF patients by exploring novel molecular targets and novel drug approaches.

Keywords: cystic fibrosis, inflammation, anti-inflammatory, mucus, antibiotic

INTRODUCTION

Cystic fibrosis (CF) is the most common lethal monogenic disorder in Caucasians estimated to affect one out of 2.500-4.000 newborns. It is caused by a *Cystic Fibrosis Transmembrane conductance Regulator* (*CFTR*) gene mutation, which encodes a chloride channel expressed at the apical membrane of the epithelial cells (Riordan et al., 1989).

CF is a multi-system disease that affects the respiratory tract, intestines, pancreas, genital tract, the hepatobiliary system, and exocrine glands, leading to diverse pathology ranges and clinical problems (Elborn, 2016). While most patients have multiple organ alterations, the leading causes of both morbidity and mortality in more than 90% of patients remain chronic progressive pulmonary disease and respiratory failure (Elborn, 2016). In CF patients, the lack of CFTR chloride channel activity leads to progressive pulmonary obstruction associated with critical and constant neutrophil-dominated endobronchial inflammation and overwhelming bacterial infection (**Figure 1**). On a pulmonary level, scientists developed many new symptomatic therapies with either anti-inflammatory properties, antibiotics, or molecules improving mucociliary clearance (mucolytics) in order to treat inflammation, infection, or mucus abnormalities (**Figure 2A**). The discovery of these new drugs was made possible by the accumulation of knowledge in these three areas. After the discovery of CFTR, researchers aimed for the development of therapies that can correct the disease's origin. Their work mainly focused on infection, rather than on anti-inflammatory drugs or mucus abnormalities. The proportion of published articles on infection is more than 70% compared to those published on inflammation or mucus. This proportion reaches more than 80% when focusing on publications on antibiotics compared to those on anti-inflammatory drugs and mucolytics (**Figures 2B, D**). In the allocation of priorities, the anti-inflammatory drugs have been, for long, the "poor relatives" in basic research compared to the modulators of CFTR activity.

These drug modulators targeting CFTR are designed to reestablish, at least partially, the CFTR expression, and improve its activity. So far, many of these treatments got through to the market, and these therapies are upgrading patients' life quality through short- and long-term improvements in clinical outcomes (Lopes-Pacheco, 2019). Despite this, the main treatments remain symptomatic, focusing on different dysregulated clinical manifestations observed in CF patients (pancreatic insufficiency, intestinal malabsorption, and lung deterioration). However, their use is limited by insufficient basic scientific knowledge (**Figure 2C**), which has reduced the number of medicinal products currently on the market (Lopes-Pacheco, 2019). A deeper understanding of the natural evolution of CF pathology brought about new treatment tactics in order to improve pulmonary functions and increase life expectancy. CFTR chloride channel is also involved in the

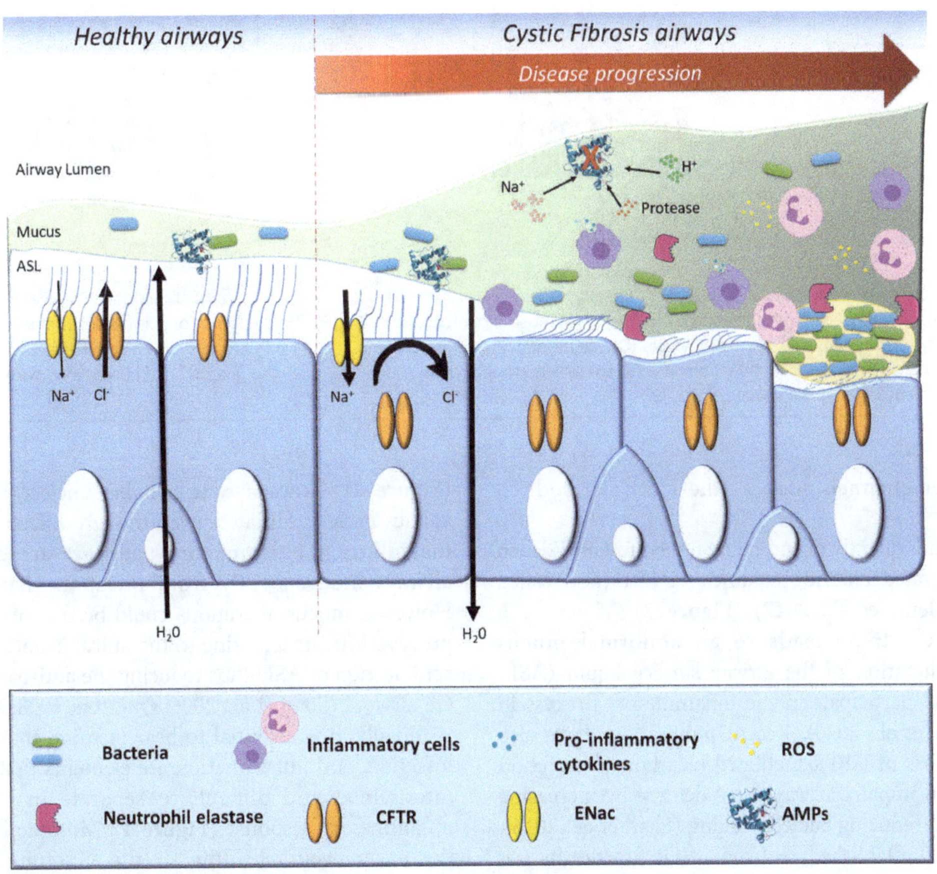

FIGURE 1 | Progression of CF pathophysiology in bronchial epithelial cells. In healthy airways, sodium (Na^+) absorption and chloride (Cl^-) secretion control hydration of the airway surface layer (ASL). In CF airways, impaired Cl^- secretion due to the CFTR absence or loss of function leads to unregulated Na^+ absorption and result in inadequate hydration of ASL, causing mucociliary clearance and bacterial killing impairment. As a result, mucus obstructs the lung airways and provides a nidus for bacterial infection and inflammation. The bacteria adhere to the surface and continue to grow, ultimately forming a biofilm. The inflammation of the CF lung is characterized by exaggerated secretion of pro-inflammatory cytokines by the airway epithelial cells, leading to the infiltration of polymorphonuclear neutrophils that release reactive oxygen species (ROS) and proteases. Neutrophil released elastase in the CF airway secretions correlates with lung function deterioration and respiratory exacerbations. The acidification of the ASL and the increase of its salt concentration, along with the increase of proteases levels, have been shown to impair the bactericidal activity of numbers of anti-microbial peptides (AMPs).

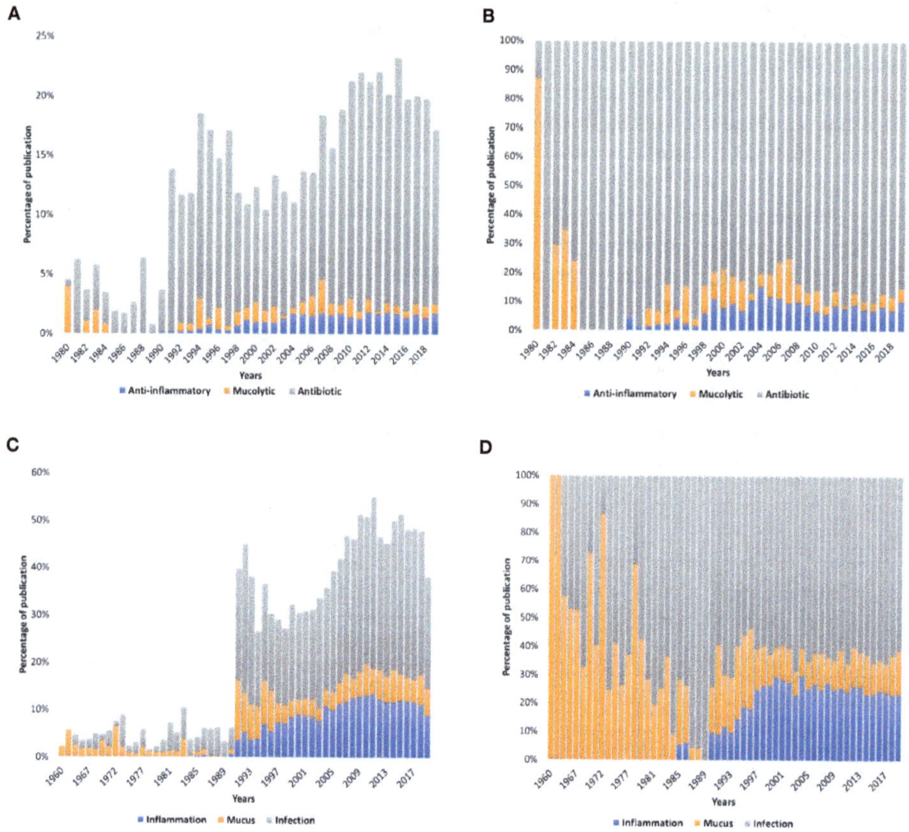

FIGURE 2 | (A) The proportion of publications published in Pubmed (https://www.ncbi.nlm.nih.gov/pubmed) by years about "anti-inflammatory," "mucolytic," and "antibiotic" in combination with "cystic fibrosis" compared to the total number of publications in CF. **(B)** The proportion of publications published in Pubmed by years about "anti-inflammatory," "mucolytic," and "antibiotic" in CF. **(C)** The proportion of publications published in Pubmed by years about "mucus," "infection," and "inflammation" in combination with "cystic fibrosis" compared to the total number of publications in CF. **(D)** The proportion of publications published in Pubmed by years about "mucus," "infection," and "inflammation" in CF.

regulation of other channels such as the epithelial sodium channel (ENaC).

Other channels are directly or indirectly linked to CFTR, such as the calcium-activated chloride channels ANO1 (also called TMEM16a) (Benedetto et al., 2017) (**Figure 3**). Therefore a deregulated CFTR activity leads to an abnormal mucus composition and alteration of the airway surface liquid (ASL) hydration that could participate in the inflammatory process in CF airways (Puthia et al., 2020). Recent publications have also highlighted that a loss of CFTR-mediated bicarbonate secretion and pH acidification impairs airways host defense by increasing mucus viscosity and reducing bacteria-killing (Shah et al., 2016). Current studies have established that the CFTR function is not restricted to ion transport regulation. Results have suggested a significant role of CFTR as a surface receptor for the internalization of *Pseudomonas aeruginosa* (*P. aeruginosa*) *via* endocytosis and consequent bacteria removal from the airway (Pier, 2000). In the CF airways, the permanent presence of bacteria might participate in the inflammatory process contributing to a vicious cycle between airway mucus obstruction, chronic infection, and exaggerated inflammation (**Figure 4**). Nowadays, it remains unclear how and why this vicious cycle is initiated, even though different elements suggest that different inflammatory pathways are deregulated in CF airways independently from infection (Bardin et al., 2019). However, mucus alterations could be one of the triggers of this process. Mucins tethering to the apical bronchial surfaces lead to acidification of ASL, thus reducing the anti-bacterial properties of CF airways (Song et al., 2006; Quinton, 2008; Adam et al., 2015).

Finally, it is essential to bear in mind that mucus alteration, infection, and inflammation are elements that are very carefully intertwined and difficult to separate in the process of an inflammatory response (**Figure 4**). Multiple hypotheses explain the early events leading to the CF lung pathophysiology progression (Jacquot et al., 2008a; Esther et al., 2019).

PATHOPHYSIOLOGY IN CF AIRWAYS

Inflammation

Although inflammation is a natural and protective process resulting from aggression, it plays a major role in CF lung

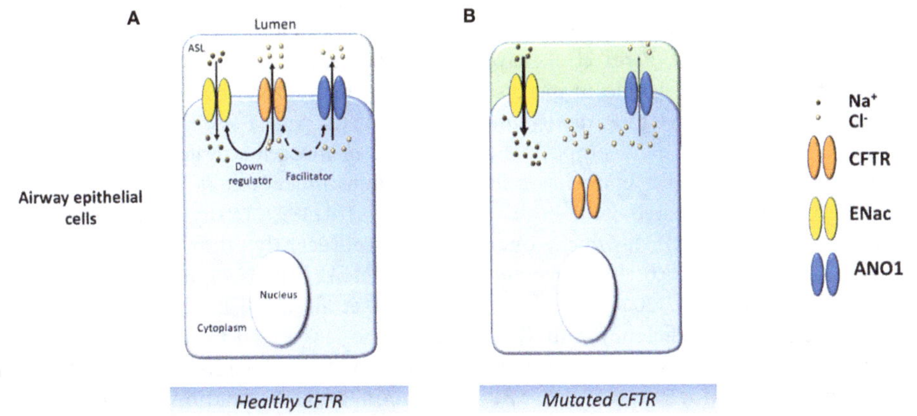

FIGURE 3 | Schematic representation of ion transports in the cystic fibrosis airway. **(A)** In healthy airways, Na^+ absorption, and CFTR and ANO1 Cl^- secretion regulate the hydration of the airway surface layer (ASL). Wild-type CFTR downregulates ENaC and participates in the activity of the ANO1 channel. **(B)** In CF airways epithelial cells, the lack of a functional CFTR channel reduces Cl^- secretion and causes Na^+ hyperabsorption leading to ASL dehydration, which favors mucostasis.

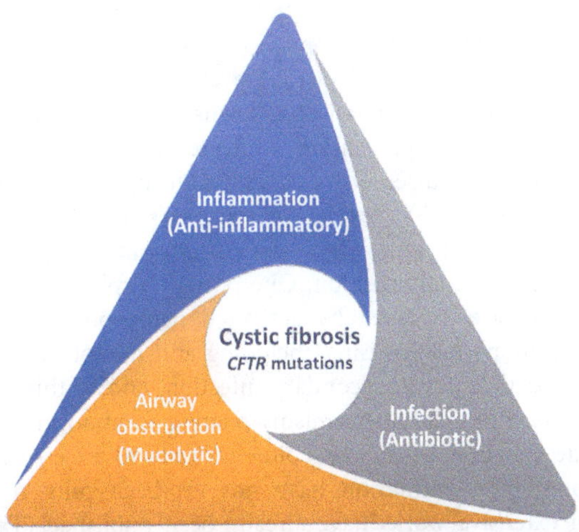

FIGURE 4 | Interrelation between the main dysregulated aspects in the airway of Cystic Fibrosis patients. *CFTR* mutations affect inflammation, mucus properties, and infection. These different aspects are very intertwined, and treating one of these elements will have consequences on the other two.

pathology and progression. Inflammation was initially recorded by the Roman encyclopedist Aulus Cornelius Celsus in the 1st century A.D. by some typical characteristic signs of inflammation as heat (calor), pain (dolor), redness (rubor), and swelling (tumor). Chronic and exaggerated inflammation in people with CF causes damages to lung tissues that can eventually lead to respiratory failure (Cantin et al., 2015). Many recent results show that bronchial epithelial cells play a significant role in the progression of the disease. In addition to being a physical barrier, epithelial cells secrete many inflammatory factors such as cytokines, eicosanoids, enzymes, and adhesion molecules (Roesch et al., 2018). This CF airway inflammation is characterized by an excessive production of interleukin (IL)-8 secreted by airway epithelial cells, and the presence of large numbers of neutrophils and macrophages among other inflammatory cells (Hubeau et al., 2001). However, it is not the only pro-inflammatory cytokine enhanced. In the airways of CF patients, TNF-α, IL-1β, IL-6, IL-8, IL-33, GM-CSF, and G-CSF are increased, also other molecules also play a major role such as the pro-inflammatory metabolites of arachidonic acid metabolism. Very recent results have highlighted the central role of other cytokines such as IL-17 (Roesch et al., 2018). In CF, the infiltration of inflammatory cells across the epithelium into the lumen can be very deleterious to epithelia and, as a consequence, requires robust regulation. Numerous works have tried to identify targets and strategies to reduce the exaggerated immune response that causes chronic inflammation without affecting the natural defenses against infection (Muhlebach and Noah, 2002). It is unclear whether the inflammation is a direct consequence of the cftr mutation or whether it is a consequence of infection and mucus accumulation. We do not know the contribution of infection to airway inflammation, but it must act as a catalyst and becomes self-perpetuating. Different studies have demonstrated the direct implication of the CFTR protein in this process mainly in the lung but also in extra-pulmonary tissues as the intestine or pancreas (Raia et al., 2000; Cohen and Prince, 2012; Stoltz et al., 2015; Bardin et al., 2019). Even before symptom onset, pulmonary inflammation and infection are often present in CF patients (Muhlebach and Noah, 2002). Although which comes first has been uncertain, this aspect is well reviewed in the article from Stoltz (Armstrong et al., 1995; Khan et al., 1995; Nixon et al., 2002; Stoltz et al., 2015). Moreover, new models lacking CFTR, including pigs, ferrets, and rat manifest inflammatory features typically observed with CF even in absence of infection (Rogers et al., 2008; Sun et al., 2010; Tuggle et al., 2014). For example, airways of CF piglets show no evidence of inflammation during the first hours after birth (Stoltz et al., 2010). Evidence has also demonstrated that non-infected human

CF airway graft is in a pro-inflammatory state (Tirouvanziam et al., 2000; Tirouvanziam et al., 2002; Perez et al., 2007; Cantin et al., 2015). These data are reinforced by *in vitro* experiments using specific CFTR inhibitor. For example, Perez et al. have shown that Inh-172 treatment conducted in significant increase in IL-8 secretion in basal but also in response to *P. aeruginosa* infection (Perez et al., 2007). All these data support the hypothesis that mutations in cftr gene make epithelial cells intrinsically more pro-inflammatory compared with healthy cells (Perez et al., 2007; Cantin et al., 2015), which, once infection is introduced, sets the stage for mucosal damage and chronic airway infection (Tirouvanziam et al., 2000).

Although the link between CFTR deficiency and host inflammatory response remains unclear, this aspect has long been recognized as a central pathological feature, and consequently, an important therapeutic target. Some have hypothesized that in CF, the unfolded proteins accumulation on the endoplasmic reticulum induced a proteinopathy responsible for inflammation, impaired trafficking, altered metabolism, cholesterol, and lipids accumulation, and impaired autophagy at the cellular level. Some have speculated that chloride dysregulation participated in a stress-inducing ionic imbalance in the airway, with the implication of calcium activation, which could induce an inflammatory state (Ribeiro et al., 2005; Tabary et al., 2006a). New hypotheses have emerged with the direct activation of NOD-, LRR-, and pyrin domain-containing protein 3 (NLRP3) inflammasome and can be a key regulator of CF inflammation and a promising target (McElvaney et al., 2019; Jarosz-Griffiths et al., 2020).

However, since the appearance of high throughput sequencing, many studies have attempted to study the deregulated mechanisms, but the heterogeneity of samples and data makes analysis difficult. A meta-analysis of the different studies has summarized all this data (Ideozu et al., 2019). To summarize, many proteins are dysregulated, including gene from signal transduction (PI3K/Akt/mTOR signaling pathway) and immune system (NFκB and MAP kinase pathways), but this method is more relevant to highlight the consequence than the cause of the inflammatory dysregulation. A very recent article has confirmed the implication of NLRP3 inflammation activation due to the alteration of electrolyte homeostasis induced by the over-activation of β-ENac channel in CF (Scambler et al., 2019).

Furthermore, different authors showed more than 15 years ago that there is a deregulation of lipid metabolism in CF with an imbalance between pro-inflammatory metabolites of arachidonic acid metabolism and pro-resolving mediators form eicosanoid pathway (Freedman et al., 2004; Karp et al., 2004; Serhan, 2017; Roesch et al., 2018). Ceramide (CER) is an airway component composed of fatty acid and sphingosine that may alter the CF inflammatory response. CER is present in the cells membrane and when in contact with a specific stimulus, like a bacterial infection, CER in transmembrane signaling processes to help regulate cellular responses to infection by activating the inflammation processes. This could be an interesting alternative to treat CF inflammatory dysregulation by inhibiting CER synthesis (Mingione et al., 2020). Although there is no consensus regarding the regulation of CER in CF cells currently, even if more recent data have demonstrated their implication on the progression of CF lung disease (Horati et al., 2020; Mingione et al., 2020). Consequently, these results have led to the proposal that upregulated inflammation is related to the molecular defect of CF with a strong implication of nuclear factor kappa B (NFκB) or mitogen-activated protein (MAP) kinase pathways with other transcription factors including NFAT, NF-IL6, AP1 and AP2 (Tabary et al., 1999; Tabary et al., 2003; Muselet-Charlier et al., 2007).

More recently, different articles have also associated microRNA (miRNA) dysregulation to CF inflammation (Fabbri et al., 2014; Bardin et al., 2018a; Bardin et al., 2019). How the lack of CFTR expression in ionocytes, ciliated, and submucosal gland epithelial cells of the respiratory tract, boosts pulmonary inflammation is still partially comprehended. Different authors have also highlighted the central role of neutrophil in CF airway inflammation, and many believed that bronchiectasis results from the proteolytic and oxidative damage induced by these cells. Longitudinal data from the Australian Respiratory Early Surveillance Team for Cystic Fibrosis demonstrated that neutrophil elastase activity at 3 months of age was a predictor of bronchiectasis at 12 months and 3 years (Wijker et al., 2020). The central role of neutrophils and its genesis has been extensively review by Nichols et al. and Perrem et al. (Nichols and Chmiel, 2015; Perrem and Ratjen, 2019).

Understanding the initial host defense defects in CF airways could suggest new prevention strategies and treatments, the means to assess disease status and efficacy of therapeutics (Stoltz et al., 2015). Several mechanisms are suggested to explain in what way CF basal inflammation promotes subsequent bacterial infection. One possible explanation is that serine protease, released by activated neutrophils, degrades innate immune mechanisms, including anti-microbial peptides (AMP), participates in secondary infection, and to this vicious cycle. The molecular mechanisms relating to abnormal CFTR chloride function in airway epithelial cells to excessive lung neutrophilic inflammation have not yet been fully clarified even if extensive works have already been published (Taggart et al., 2000; Tabary et al., 2006b). Decreased neutrophil apoptosis and the high secretion of IL-8 by epithelial cells are contributing factors. In 2016, researchers discovered the leukocyte adhesion deficiency IV (LAD-IV), which is a defect in monocyte integrin activation in CF patients. The study showed that CFTR mutations could lead to a monocyte-specific adhesion deficiency (~80%) and impairment in transmigration into the alveolar space, which could explain the extreme infiltration of neutrophil since monocytes play a crucial part in inflammation and its resolution. Thus, failing to recruit monocytes in CF patients' lungs may explain the excessive production of cytokines, the impaired inflammation resolution, and pathogen capture impairment (Sorio et al., 2016). The continuous driven recruitment of neutrophils and other immune cells and their implication in non-resolving inflammation have been already discussed in different reviews (Cantin et al., 2015; Nichols and Chmiel, 2015; Roesch et al., 2018).

Whether CFTR dysfunction causes directly or indirectly, a more important predisposition to infection and whether the inflammation occurs separately from the infection has yet to be determined. The development of new anti-inflammatory strategies in CF remains limited due to the limited researches in this area compared to infection (**Figure 2D**).

Bacterial Infection

Respiratory infections in CF occur from childhood. In progressive lung diseases like CF, typical pathogens (*P. aeruginosa, Streptococcus aureus, Burkholderia cepacia, Achromobacter xylosoxidans*) colonize the airways (Palser et al., 2019). More than 50% of children diagnosed at birth have shown positive *P. aeruginosa* cultures by five years of age (Palser et al., 2019). If *P. aeruginosa* is neither spontaneously cleared nor eradicated with antibiotic therapy, the CF lung environment facilitates the infection.

The presence of pathogens triggers inflammatory processes in the airways contributing to the destruction of the cell barrier. Since inflammation is a natural process of defense and the eradication of pathogens, limiting it too much or for a long term could be counterproductive. For this reason, antibiotics are more frequently recommended than anti-inflammatory drugs in CF lung disease treatment and could indirectly serve to diminish airway inflammation (Oermann et al., 1999). The anti-inflammatory drugs that could alter the natural defense of the lung are only prescribed during exacerbations. Constant development and ideal usage of new anti-microbial compounds are vital for improving the CF patients survival chance and quality of life (Waters and Smyth, 2015). As a result of long-term antibiotic treatment, the decrease in infection and inflammation is associated with lung function improvements and pulmonary exacerbations reduction (Waters, 2018).

In a normal situation, the airways can defend themselves by forming a physical barrier between the outside and the inside. Also, the lung is capable of secreting cytokines that will allow the recruitment of inflammatory cells, but it is also capable of secreting anti-bacterial molecules. Thus, many natural AMPs, contained in the airways, are part of the innate immune response to the airway defense (Hancock et al., 2016). AMPs exhibit microbicidal activities on a broad spectrum of microbes, but bacteria appear to be the most targeted pathogens (Scott and Hancock, 2000; Zasloff, 2002). AMPs can kill bacteria rapidly in a few minutes. If most of the AMPs kill targeted pathogens *via* an electrostatic action on their membranes, some of them kill by more sophisticated mechanisms such as the IIA secretory phospholipase A2 (sPLA2-IIA) which kills bacteria through selective hydrolysis of their membrane phospholipids (Van Hensbergen et al., 2020), or by interfering with intracellular targets in bacteria (Geitani et al., 2019; Wang et al., 2019). Except for very few examples, little is known about the specificity of AMPs toward Gram-positive *vs.* Gram-negative bacteria. The sPLA2-IIA is one of the rare AMPs that target Gram-positive bacteria that exerts its bactericidal effect at much lower concentrations than other molecules [For details, see the review (Van Hensbergen et al., 2020)].

AMPs represent an essential part of the host defenses against infections and also as a potential therapeutic tool, as has been shown in infections animal models (Morrison et al., 2002; Piris-Gimenez et al., 2005). This effect was also supported by studies in patients with infectious diseases showing that altered AMP expression and/or gene polymorphisms were associated with increased infections (Rivas-Santiago et al., 2009). On the other hand, unfavorable circumstances for AMPs actions as abnormal salt concentration or acidification, and inactivation by proteases, in ASL of CF patients (**Figure 1**), have been shown to inactivate AMPs bactericidal functions which may explain increased airway infections (Bals et al., 2001; Lecaille et al., 2016; Simonin et al., 2019). Normalizing ASL pH by inhibition of the persistent proton secretion, mediated by ATPase H^+/K^+ transporting non-gastric alpha2 subunit (ATP12A), might enhance innate airway defense in CF newborns during the onset of *S. aureus* infection. A recent study showed that the hydrophobic N-terminal domain of *Cg*-BigDef1 (a big defensin from oysters) exhibits salt-stable interactions with bacterial membranes opening the doors to eventual drug developments when physiological salt concentrations inhibit the anti-microbial activity of β-defensins such as in CF disease (Loth et al., 2019).

In parallel to their anti-microbial functions, several AMPs have been shown to play immuno-modulatory roles, in particular by interacting with the inflammatory reaction produced by host cells. Several studies have shown that AMPs can target host cells involved in innate immunity and modulated their production of inflammatory mediators, including cytokines. Although it is not always easy to dissociate these actions as most AMPs exhibit both functions, depending on their concentrations, the host cell targets, and the environments. However, AMPs have been shown to impair the inflammatory reaction induced by invading pathogens by different mechanisms (Masera et al., 1996; Finlay and Hancock, 2004; McInturff et al., 2005).

The anti-inflammatory potential of AMPs correlates with their capability of attracting and recruiting neutrophils and other inflammatory cells. They may also have direct or indirect effects on their maturation, differentiation, degranulation, or apoptosis (Lai and Gallo, 2009). AMPs also act by blocking neutrophils apoptosis, therefore prolonging their lifetime, and ultimately their phagocytic functions (Nagaoka et al., 2012). AMPs can also potentiate the effects of inflammatory cells such as macrophages while limiting other tissue damage (Brook et al., 2016).

Mucus Alteration

In healthy people, ASL is a thin liquid film covering the airways and participating in mucociliary clearance and airways desiccation (**Figure 1**). Historically, studies suggested that different secretory cells (goblet cells, submucosal glands cells, and serous cells) contribute to ASL production (Tarran et al., 2001). The recent finding of the airway "ionocyte" could similarly result in a revised understanding of ASL production (Plasschaert et al., 2018). This group has identified by RNA sequencing all the RNAs present inside airway cells and by a new method, called pulse-seq, has discovered this scarce cell type.

They created the term "ionocytes" due to the cell's likeness to ionocytes in charge of regulating ion transport and hydration in the fish gills and frog skin. In the airway, ASL consists of two main layers: 1) the apical layer consisting of a water-based polymeric mucus, and 2) a periciliary layer (PCL) that bathes the epithelium (Atanasova and Reznikov, 2019). Normal mucus is made of 97% water and 3% proteins, lipids, and salt. The mucus gel layer acts as a physical barrier to prevent most pathogens from accessing the cells (Button et al., 2012). The mucus hydration and the mucin concentration dramatically affects its viscoelastic properties, which, in turn, determines how effectively it is cleared from the distal airways toward the trachea by ciliary action and cough (Fahy and Dickey, 2010).

The commonly accepted explanation for airway disease in CF is the "low volume" hypothesis. A reduced volume of the periciliary fluid layer (PCL) causes failure of mucociliary clearance, the 'lungs' innate defense mechanism. In addition to having altered physical properties, the mucus composition is modified and will participate in the CF pathophysiology by altering host defense proteins (Henderson et al., 2014). An increase in mucin secretion and an abnormal composition of mucus are implied by the formation of endobronchial mucus plaques and plugs. Mucus present in bronchia becomes the primary site of airflow obstruction, and subsequently for chronic infection, and persistent inflammation leading to early small airways disease succeeded by bronchiectasis development. Increased mucus and airway obstruction are hallmark features of multiple respiratory diseases and contribute, especially in CF, to a complicated, inflammatory process (Puthia et al., 2020). A chronic cycle of infection and inflammation could be initiated, resulting in airways structural integrity damages and leading to bronchiectasis development (Chalmers et al., 2017). More recent studies from Esther *et al.* have shown that the increase of mucus burden and inflammatory markers without infection suggest that mucolytic therapies could serve as preventive therapy for CF lung pathology (Esther et al., 2019). More, mucus composition and properties also depend on the levels of mucin production by epithelial cells that can be increased by bacteria suggesting a complex role of inflammation, infection, and mucus, especially in CF pathology (Mohamed et al., 2012). The up-regulation of airway mucin genes by inflammatory/immune response mediators at the transcriptional and/or posttranscriptional level is one of the major contributors to mucin overproduction. The MUC5AC gene is transcriptionally up-regulated by several inflammatory mediators, including LPS, IL-9, neutrophil elastase, TNF-α, and IL-1β (Song et al., 2003). IL-8-induced binding of RNA-binding proteins to the 3-untranslated region of MUC5AC is a potential mechanism for regulating *MUC5AC* gene expression at the posttranscriptional level (Bautista et al., 2009). Several studies have shown that PMA induces a matrix metalloprotease-mediated release of transforming growth factor-(Shao et al., 2003). Eicosanoids mediate inflammation and mucus secretion in chronic pulmonary inflammatory diseases (Garcia-Verdugo et al., 2012). Some studies in the field have shown a substantial increase of eicosanoid levels, including PGE2 and LTB4 in CF airways (Bautista et al., 2009) and CF bronchial epithelial cells (BECs) stimulated by LPS from *P. aeruginosa* (Medjane et al., 2005). On the other hand, this bacterium stimulates mucus production through the induction of several mucins such as MUC5AC and MUC2 both in cultured BECs and in a mouse model of lung infection by *P. aeruginosa*. This induction mainly involves the stimulation of BECs by flagellin through the TLR5 and Naip pathways and is accompanied by the secretion of IL-8 by BECs, which amplify mucus production (Mohamed et al., 2012).

Thus, we can suggest that in CF airways, mucus abnormalities offer a niche that favors bacterial infections, which in turn amplify mucus accumulation *via* a vicious circle that can participate in the exacerbation of the severity of CF disease. This amplification can occur either directly *via* virulence factors (such as flagellin and LPS) of infecting bacteria or *via* cytokines and eicosanoids produced by CF airways during infection.

Proteases and Lipids Imbalance

Current studies on mucolytic agents therapy used in CF have been demonstrated to increase markedly neutrophil elastase (NE) activity in CF sputum. Serine proteases, including NE, cathepsin G, and proteinase 3, are the three most major proteases found in the CF lung. These proteases are not only secreted by BECs, but also by monocytes, lymphocytes, granulocytes, and, more importantly, neutrophils (Pelaia et al., 2004; Hunt et al., 2020). Different approaches have exposed their participation in intracellular and extracellular activities, including inflammation, tissue remodeling, mucin expression, bacterial killing, and neutrophil chemotaxis. NE, a significant product of neutrophils granule degranulation, is extensively studied in CF and is implicated in cleavage and inactivation of CFTR protein (Chalmers et al., 2017). Besides, NE also upregulates IL-8 and participates in activating cysteinyl cathepsins and matrix metalloproteases.

In the CF airway, different articles have described the protease and anti-protease imbalance, which could be explained by two different mechanisms (Galli et al., 2012; Causer et al., 2020). Firstly, CFTR is also a transporter of glutathione (GSH), a protease that is the main non-enzymatic antioxidant present in the ASL (Rahman and MacNee, 2000). Antioxidants are an essential protective response to tissue injury and occur mainly in an inflammatory environment. An absence of GSH in the extracellular medium disequilibrates this balance and induces an oxidative environment. This environment is intended to fight bacteria and viruses that may be present. The goal of this process is to break up and eliminate the injured tissues and, thus, promote tissue repair for the inflammatory process resolution. When this natural response arises in an uncontrolled way, the outcome is extreme tissue damage that could induce chronic inflammation, as observed in CF (**Figure 1**). During inflammation, reactive oxygen species (ROS) such as the superoxide anion are liberated by phagocytes and are thought to be the main cause of tissue damage.

In CF, the presence of numerous inflammatory cells that release many oxidants will have a significant role in the deregulation of the pro- and anti-inflammatory balance. Lung cells are vulnerable to the damaging effects of ROS and release inflammatory mediators, thereby amplifying lung inflammation. ROS are extraordinarily reactive, and when produced near the cell membranes, they diminish intracellular GSH and cause lipid peroxidation, which may harshly disrupt its function and may lead to cell death or DNA damage in alveolar epithelial cells. So, when ROS production increases, the redox balance of the airways is altered, and this can lead to bronchial hyperactivity and to further inflammation and participates in CF co-morbidity. GSH is a sulfhydryl containing tripeptide (L-γ-glutamyl-L-cysteinyl-glycine) that scavenges oxidants and could, therefore, participate in the control of the inflammatory process by reducing oxidative stress (Rahman and MacNee, 2000; Ehre et al., 2019). Therefore, a CFTR deficiency leads to an increased accumulation of intracellular GSH in the epithelial lining fluid compared with plasma. Secondly, different dysregulated parameters such as infection, inflammation, and hypoxia, increase the free radicals derived from oxygen and nitrogen. This pro-oxidative environment may directly exert its effects by activating transcription factors such as NFκB and MAP kinase pathways responsible for the coordinated expression of numerous genes involved in inflammation, cell death, proliferation, as well as cytoprotection and antioxidant defenses (Pelaia et al., 2004).

CFTR-deficient tracheal epithelial cells are characterized by high GSH levels that decrease the intracellular content of ceramide (CER). CER deficiency occurring in CF seems to be responsible for the increased activation of the pro-inflammatory transcriptional nuclear factor NFκB that, in turn, is responsible for the abnormally high inflammatory response in CF respiratory epithelial cells (Vilela et al., 2006; Aureli et al., 2016). An increasing number of studies indicate that sphingolipids play an important regulatory role in CF concerning pulmonary inflammation. In different models, it has been shown that *de novo* sphingolipid synthesis is an inflammation responsive pathway. It is enhanced by inflammatory mediators, both at transcriptional and enzyme activity level, and the accumulation of its metabolite CER potentiates inflammation in a vicious circle (Caretti et al., 2014). Sphingosine-1-phosphate (S1P), generated in the nucleus by phosphorylation of SphK2 ((Sphingosine Kinase 2), modulates HDAC (histone deacetylases) activity either by direct binding or through activation of nuclear ROS, and, regulates cell cycle and pro-inflammatory gene expression (Fu et al., 2018). The accumulation of CER causes *Cftr*$^{-}$ deficient mice to suffer from constitutive age-dependent pulmonary inflammation, death of respiratory epithelial cells, deposits of DNA in bronchi, and high susceptibility to severe *P. aeruginosa* infections (Teichgräber et al., 2008). Aggregates accrual, formed by misfolded mutant CFTR and a miscellaneous of sequestered proteins within, induces inflammation and oxidative stress, impairing proteins and lipids transport, and consequently inflammatory statement (Mingione et al., 2020).

HISTORY OF "CLASSICAL" ANTI-INFLAMMATORY DRUGS

A better understanding of the molecular mechanisms involved in inflammation has led to the development of new anti-inflammatory therapeutic strategies. In CF, the intertwining of inflammation, infection, and airway mucus obstruction complicates therapeutic approaches. Thus, anti-inflammatory treatments, combined with antibiotic therapies and airway clearance techniques, play an essential role in patient care, particularly during periods of exacerbations and hospitalization.

Steroid Anti-Inflammatory Treatments

Glucocorticoids (GC), a class of corticosteroids (CS), are potent anti-inflammatory molecules frequently applied in the treatment of "inflammatory" pulmonary diseases. GC target many of the proteins involved in inflammation, including IL-1β and IL-8 and NFκB and activator protein (AP-1) (Tabary et al., 1998; Barnes, 2006). Until recently, CS were the main anti-inflammatory CF treatments and were mainly used during exacerbations through inhaled or oral administrations (Balfour-Lynn and Welch, 2014; Lands and Stanojevic, 2019).

Since the first Prednisone clinical trials (Auerbach et al., 1985), oral CS have been shown to diminish the lung inflammation and reduce the development of the pathology in CF patients. However, the use of CS is still controversial in the CF context due to medium- and long-term use. The side effects include growth impairment, cataract formation, glucose intolerance, and osteoporosis (Balfour-Lynn and Welch, 2014). Nonetheless, oral CS are promptly used during an exacerbation to decrease inflammation in CF lungs.

Even though the use of GC in CF is common, the signaling pathways remain partially described. Interestingly, we have published that the NFκB signaling pathway was significantly involved and refractory to the action of GC in glandular epithelial cells (Tabary et al., 1998). Moreover, we have confirmed these results in airway neutrophils from CF patients (Corvol et al., 2003).

Even though inhaled CS have a better safety profile, their efficacy has not yet been demonstrated (Balfour-Lynn and Welch, 2014). The inhaled steroids withdrawal impact was established in a multicentric randomized, double-blind placebo-controlled trial, including CF children and adults (Balfour-Lynn et al., 2006). This study failed to show any beneficial effect of inhaled CS in CF patients treated for six months.

Finally, GC remain interesting molecules, especially during exacerbations, as they significantly reduce inflammation. However, their use in CF can only be limited to specific cases.

Non-Steroid Anti-Inflammatory Treatments

As GC have significant side effects, alternative molecules have been proposed. For a few years, Ibuprofen, a non-steroidal anti-inflammatory drug (NSAID), has emerged and was proposed to the CF patients as a GC alternative. Most of NSAID (such as Aspirin) are known to block cyclo-oxygenase (COX) enzymes that produce prostaglandins from free arachidonic acid (Kurumbail et al., 1996). Ibuprofen, discovered by Stewart Adams laboratory in 1961, was sold initially as Brufen to treat rheumatoid arthritis (Balfour-Lynn et al., 2006; Halford et al., 2012). In CF, Ibuprofen acts directly on neutrophil activation, inhibiting their mobility and recruitment in the airways (Konstan et al., 2003). High-dose of Ibuprofen can reduce the development of CF patients' lung disease, especially in children (Lands and Stanojevic, 2007; Lands and Stanojevic, 2019). A meta-analysis from a current update of a regular review has been published on the Cochrane database (Lands and Stanojevic, 2019). Multiple unwanted effects were a matter of concern due to the high doses usage, which has limited the Ibuprofen use in CF. Recent results have described that obvious benefits of Ibuprofen therapy outbalance the low risk of gastrointestinal bleeding, although long-term safety results are limited. In low doses, some shreds of evidence indicate that Ibuprofen may cause inflammation (Lands and Stanojevic, 2019). Nonetheless, these outcomes are still a subject of debate among scientists who suspect the inappropriate use of Ibuprofen for CF patients (Lands and Stanojevic, 2016). The association of Ibuprofen with infections is more complicated in that it confers risk in some situations but benefits in others, therefore its usage might require close monitoring (Varrassi et al., 2020).

Macrolides

Among the most exciting new anti-inflammatory drug treatments established in the last few years in the CF context the macrolides (Southern et al., 2012). Macrolides were discovered in 1952 and were initially isolated from cultures of *Streptomyces erythraea*. The frequently used macrolides have 14 (Clarithromycin, Erythromycin, and Roxithromycin) or 15 (Azithromycin) atoms attached to their macrocyclic rings and were named macrolides in regards to the presence of macrocyclic lactone ring. Macrolides are interesting original antibiotics because of their double action of not only reducing infections but also reducing inflammation. The macrolides were used as antibiotics to treat different infectious diseases, including numerous airway pathology as pneumonia, CF, bronchitis, pharyngitis (Zalewska-Kaszubska and Gorska, 2001). Surprisingly, in 1987, a Japanese group has reported a spectacular effect in panbronchiolitis patients' lifespan when treated with Erythromycin antibiotic (Kudoh et al., 1987). This pathology is a typical and representative disease of chronic respiratory tract infection in Japan, characterized by chronic inflammation localized predominantly in the respiratory bronchioles with inflammatory cells such as monocytes, macrophages, neutrophils and, T lymphocytes.

The molecule showing the most interesting effects in CF patients is Azithromycin, with an improvement of lung parameters, a decrease of *P. aeruginosa* infection, and hospitalization duration (Clement et al., 2006; Saiman et al., 2010; Nichols et al., 2020). Prolonged use of small dose Azithromycin was related to a beneficial impact on lung disease expression, well ahead of *P. aeruginosa* infection. A metanalysis of these researches proved substantial improvement or maintenance of the forced expiratory volume in one second (FEV1, a measure of lung function) and forced vital capacity (FVC) in treated patients *vs.* controls after 12 months of therapy. Even though there was no decline in the intravenous antibiotic therapy necessity or the hospitalization duration of any of these studies, a positive effect on the restoration of Cl^- efflux in CF has also been shown (Saint-Criq et al., 2011).

Moreover, some scientists demonstrated that macrolides operate by limiting pro-inflammatory cytokines and provoking direct alterations in the neutrophils function (Equi et al., 2002; Southern and Barker, 2004; Haydar et al., 2019). However, they failed to reduce the inflammation in BECs in CF patients (Saint-Criq et al., 2012). One recently published article has demonstrated that Azithromycin could modify the M2 phenotype macrophage and, therefore, indirectly modify the inflammatory process by inhibiting NFκB activation by increasing IKKβ expression in J774 murine macrophages (Haydar et al., 2019).

However, some macrolides, such as Clarithromycin, can induce neutrophil extracellular trap (NET) generation, a mechanism implicated in innate immunity and some inflammatory processes. NETosis is a mechanism by which neutrophils extrude their DNA and protein contents to form NET, including AMPs. The physiology and the formation of the NET have been extensively described in the review from Ravindran et al. (2019). In the fetal stage and early childhood, neutrophilic inflammation in the peri-bronchial regions is present in CF patients who have mucus excess and obstructive secretions but no persistent bacterial infections. Various microbial components like inflammatory cytokines, lipid mediators, and extracellular DNA found in CF patients induce NET formation (Henke and Ratjen, 2007). In CF airways, neutrophils are recruited to the airway upon infection and exacerbate the disease by producing NETs, which can increase mucus viscosity and consequently participate in the airway obstruction. The excess of NETs and their cytotoxic components, associated with hypervisquous mucus, exacerbate CF NET produced by Clarithromycin and inhibit *Acinetobacter baumannii* infection by acting on its growth and biofilm formation in an LL-37-dependent manner (Konstantinidis et al., 2016; Khan et al., 2019). Clarithromycin also enhances the antibacterial defense of fibroblasts and improves their wound healing capacity through the upregulation of LL-37 on NET structures (Arampatzioglou et al., 2018). Although Azithromycin and Chloramphenicol show that neutrophils pretreatment with these macrolides decreases the NETs release. Moreover, Azithromycin showed a concentration-dependent effect on respiratory burst in neutrophils, whereas Chloramphenicol did not affect degranulation, apoptosis or respiratory burst. So, these antibiotics modulate the ability of neutrophils to release NETs influencing human innate immunity (Bystrzycka et al., 2017). The macrolide immunomodulatory role depends on the macrolide used and the pathology involved.

As a final point, conventional anti-inflammatory treatments for CF are limited and have not been explicitly developed for this pathology, and could induce counterproductive effects. Research in this field is still limited compared to antibiotics, but despite this, new molecules or strategies are being evaluated.

NOVEL ANTI-INFLAMMATORY APPROACHES

Better insight into the pathways involved has led to the development of new therapeutic approaches that are currently being evaluated under cell experiments or clinical trials. These new strategies aiming at the CF inflammation are designed to treat different dysregulated aspects such as channel modulators, oxidative stress, cytokines secretion, lung remodeling, and the regulation of dysregulated pathways.

New Channel Modulators

CFTR Channel

The discovery of the *CFTR* gene in 1989 resulted in insights on how CFTR mutations induce CF pathology and encouraged many researchers to develop new drugs or strategies to correct the mutation or increase the protein activity (Riordan et al., 1989). Genetic therapy using adeno-associated virus (AAV) or other strategies aiming to correct the CFTR gene was very promising because CF is a monogenic disease. Nonetheless, the subsequent realization tempered expectations because the airways are well defended and are not absorptive surfaces. The natural barrier of mucus considerably impairs gene transfer into the lungs, and the epithelium renewing necessitates numerous administrations. For these reasons, only one study has demonstrated a significant but moderate effect on CF patients. Thus, further optimizations or other strategies are needed and in progress (Alton et al., 2015; Alton et al., 2017).

These data provided the grounds for pharmacologic modulations of chloride transport, by targeting mutant CFTR and/or alternative ion channels as anoctamin-1 (ANO1) that can compensate for CFTR malfunction. This excitement has now proven to be warranted because numerous new therapies approved by the FDA or EMA are now either in the pipeline or available for CF patients (**Figure 5**). This finding contributes to the innovation of genetic disease pharmacotherapy with *Vertex Pharmaceuticals* as a leader in the CF research field. Fundamental CF research has set the stage for a better molecular understanding of *CFTR* mutations by supplying structural pieces of information to design new approaches for the pharmacology dynamic even if the different drugs proposed were obtained by high-throughput screening (Callebaut et al., 2017). Till date, two CFTR-directed molecule classes have been developed: "potentiator" compounds increasing mutated CFTR activity at the cell surface and, "corrector" drugs improving altered protein processing and trafficking to the cell surface (Wainwright et al., 2015; Rowe et al., 2017; Davies et al., 2018) (**Figure 6**). The first generation of the compounds has either been limited to a few patients with specific mutations (Ivacaftor) or was addressed to a larger group (Orkambi) and demonstrated moderate effects in CF (Mayer, 2016). For this reason, the U.K. National Institute for Health and Care Excellence (NICE) issued a draft guidance against recommending Orkambi. Recently, the FDA has approved an auspicious combination of molecules (Elexacaftor–Tezacaftor–Ivacaftor called Trikafta) to restore the function of p.Phe508del CFTR protein in CF patients even if patients had a single p.Phe508del allele. The combination of drugs relative to the control resulted in a percentage of predicted FEV1 that was more than 14 points higher and a rate of pulmonary exacerbations that was 60% lower through 24 weeks of treatment (Keating et al., 2018; Middleton et al., 2019). Unfortunately, a few pieces of information are available for the inflammatory aspects of these treatments. Although, recent evidence showed that the inflammation and lung status hampers these medications and can hinder their effects. Only one article has demonstrated that CFTR modulators can reduce excessive pro-inflammatory response following LPS (lipopolysaccharide) stimulation of CF monocytes (Jarosz-Griffiths et al., 2020). Moreover, in this article, the authors have also demonstrated that IL-8, IL-1β, and TNF-α (Tumor necrosis factor-α) decreased significantly in the serum of CF patients treated with Ivacaftor and Tezacaftor treatment. It is not known whether the observed effects are due to the restoration of Cl^- efflux, GSH (glutathione), or CFTR protein interactions present at the membrane.

Other new classes of mutation are in development, such as CFTR amplifiers, CFTR stabilizers, and read-through agents

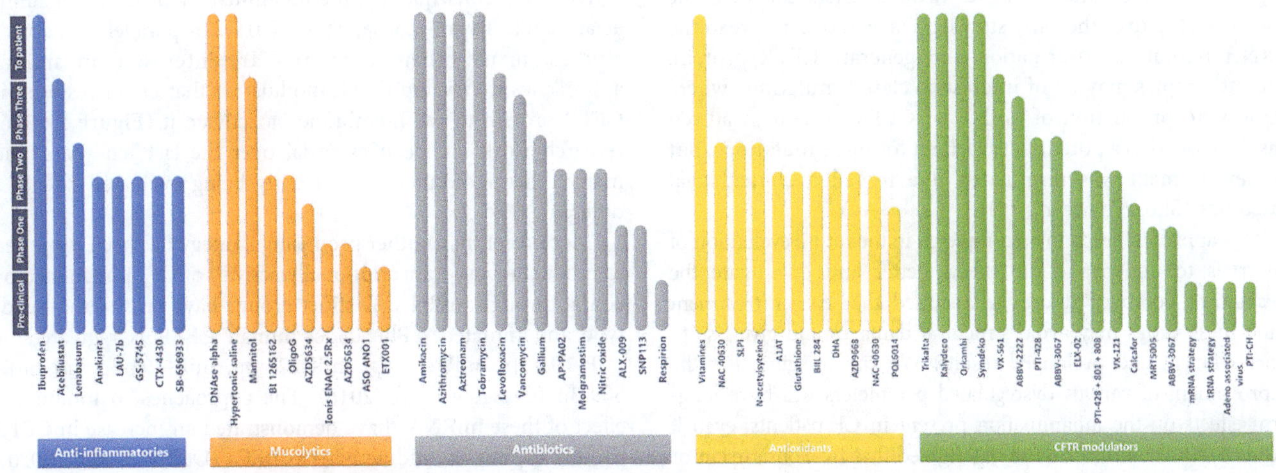

FIGURE 5 | List of the different categories of drugs under development or clinical trials in the context of CF.

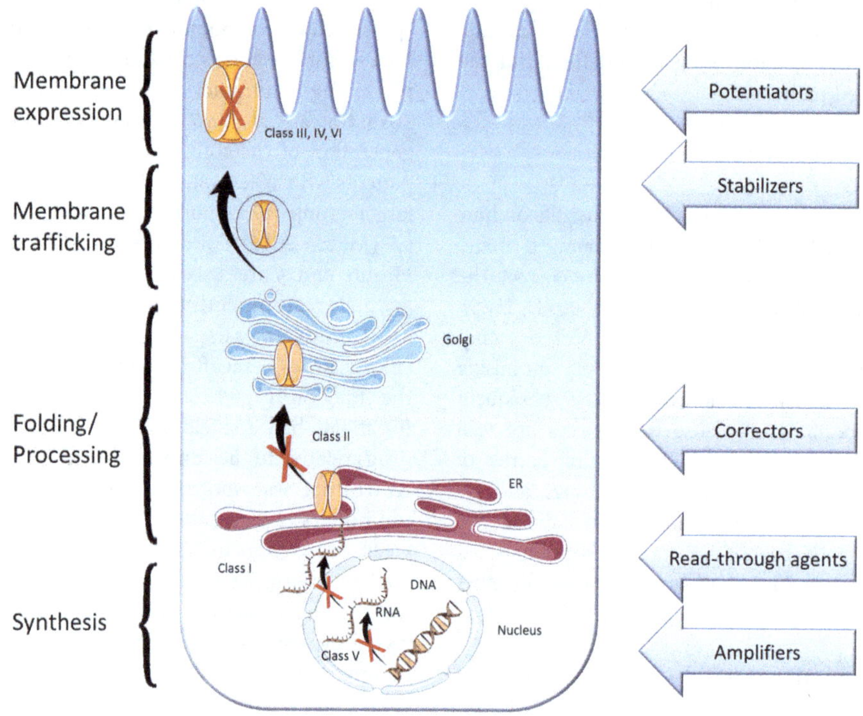

FIGURE 6 | Description of the different classes of CFTR mutations related to the different therapeutic proposed in the literature. I—ynthesis defect, II—processing defect, III—channel gating defect, IV—channel conductance defect, V—reduced CFTR production, VI—defect of stability; ER, endoplasmic reticulum.

(**Figure 6**). CFTR amplifiers upregulate the expression, and indirectly, the activity of mutant CFTR. PTI-428 and PTI-CH are the two amplifiers who seem promising in pre-clinical and clinical studies. PTI-428 can enhance lung function in CF patients receiving Orkambi with no significant adverse effects. CFTR stabilizer as Cavosonstat inhibits the enzyme that is involved in regulating how much CFTR protein is present at the cell surface (Donaldson et al., 2017). It could potentially increase the benefits of other medications that target the CFTR function. Read-through drugs can help the ribosome skip over the early stop sequence in order to read the mRNA remaining information and generate CFTR protein. These therapies may be of interest to class I mutations where there is no production of mRNA or CFTR protein. Ataluren was developed as a potential treatment for these mutations, but its development was terminated due to failed clinical trial outcomes (Shoseyov et al., 2016).

This approach needs to be completed in the future evaluation of CF trials to understand the effects better and investigate the mechanism complex. It can be assumed that earlier treatment using these drugs may avoid structural damages and give rise to more efficient and prolonged results. We can imagine that the improvement of various dysregulated parameters will have long-term effects on the inflammation present in CF patients, even if indirectly. A recent article has highlighted that by Tobramycin or the AMP, 6K-F17 could restore the effects of Orkambi on p.Phe508del-CFTR protein, suggesting a significant role of infection in the CF pathology (Laselva et al., 2020). Furthermore, using this approach, they have demonstrated that the active AMP can down-regulate the expression of pro-inflammatory cytokines like IL-8, IL-6, and TNF-α in p.Phe508del-CFTR human BECs (Laselva et al., 2020).

Some exciting improvements in chloride efflux have been demonstrated using Sildenafil, a phosphodiesterase type 5 (PDE5) inhibitor. This drug recues p.Phe508del-CFTR trafficking *in vitro* experiments and decreases sputum elastase activity and, consequently, the inflammatory process (Lubamba et al., 2011; Taylor-Cousar et al., 2015). In parallel to Vertex's studies, many other companies are interested in similar approaches to develop CFTR modulators that either restore the CFTR protein to the membrane or activate it (**Figure 5**). This research work has been essential over the last ten years, and many other molecules are currently being evaluated and at a different stage.

More recently, another promising strategy has been proposed to modulate post-transcriptionally activity of CFTR regulated by acting through miRNA. Distinct groups have proved that wild-type and mutated p.Phe508del human CFTR is regulated by miR-101-3p, miR-145-5p, miR-223-3p, miR-494-3p,and miR-509-3p (Glasgow et al., 2018). The approaches to inhibit the effect of these miRNAs have demonstrated an increase in CFTR protein expression and activity in BECs (De Santi et al., 2020). This approach is exciting, but further researches are needed to understand the subtility of this regulation better.

ENaC Channel

Since CFTR negatively regulates the activity of the ENaC sodium channel, different strategies have been proposed to decrease its activity. The first proposed molecule was Amiloride, which acts as a potassium-sparing diuretic, showing some benefit in both animal studies and clinical trials. Unfortunately, its efficacy was limited due to its short half-life (Zhou et al., 2008). This approach was repeated with the use of a new ENaC blocker called AZD5634 from AstraZeneca and BI1265162 from Boehringer Ingelheim. A phase Ib study and a phase II study to test, respectively, the safety and effectiveness of AZD5634 and BI 1265162 are underway in CF adults. Nowadays, a more recent and exciting approach, using aerosol antisense oligonucleotide (ASO) targeting ENaC mRNA (Ionis ENAC 2.5Rx), has demonstrated some interesting and impressive results on mice by restoring inflammation and inhibiting ENaC activity (Crosby et al., 2017). A first clinical study with this therapy is currently ongoing.

In the same way, Arrowhead asks to open a phase I/II trial into inhaled small interference RNA (iRNA) therapy. The drug, called ARO-ENaC, is an investigational RNA therapy designed to lower the production of the epithelial sodium channel alpha subunit (αENaC) in the lungs of CF patients. ARO-ENaC is an iRNA molecule intending to block the production of ENaC channels. It works by targeting and destroying the αENaC mRNA molecules, which are genetic messengers that carry the necessary information for making αENaC proteins and consequently ENaC activity.

ANO1 Channel

Since functional CFTR rescue remains limited, with mutation-dependent effects, alternative strategies have been suggested to compensate for the CFTR deficiency and were proposed as a potential CF therapeutic target. Such a strategy was the stimulation of calcium-activated chloride channels (CaCCs) such as the Anoctamin 1 channel (ANO1) (**Figure 3**). In the nineties, Knowles *et al.* have discovered that adenosine '5'-triphosphate and uridine-5'-triphosphate stimulated Cl^- secretion in both standards and CF respiratory epithelial, offering a potential by-pass mechanism for defective CFTR (Knowles et al., 1991). These activators transduce a signal through P2Y2 receptors that lead to the release of intracellular calcium and activate the CaCCs. An analog called Denufosol was developed. Different studies have demonstrated that this drug can increase Cl^- secretion through a CaCC, inhibit sodium absorption *via* the epithelial sodium channel called ENaC, and stimulate epithelial ciliary beat frequency (Accurso et al., 2011). Based on these data, 'Denufosol' clinical trials begun in 2001 using a wet nebulization direct airway delivery approach. Unfortunately, the last phase III had failed to demonstrate any benefit, and the project was dropped, but the idea of developing this approach remained (Moss, 2013). At the time of this study, CaCCs were poorly known. Their identity remained elusive for over 20 years until 2008 (Nilius and Droogmans, 2003; Caputo et al., 2008; Schroeder et al., 2008; Yang et al., 2008). When ANO1, the principal CaCC present in the airways, was identified in 2008, it allowed for more targeted approaches. Attractively, ANO1 channel has, at the apical membrane of epithelial cells, the same expression pattern as CFTR channels, and this protein was shown to be essential in the activity of CFTR as a chloride channel (Benedetto et al., 2017; Benedetto et al., 2019). Besides, ANO1 is implicated in HCO_3 different permeability, proliferation, wound healing, inflammation, and its expression decreased in CF patients (Veit et al., 2012; Jung et al., 2013; Ruffin et al., 2013). Moreover, a recent article highlighted that ANO1 inhibition decreased ASL height. The authors have also demonstrated that ANO1 is not required for MUC5AC expression, the main protein of the mucus (Simoes et al., 2019). For this reason, a novel ANO1 potentiator was developed (ETX001), and airway epithelial function and mucus transport were evaluated in the human cells and animal models. This approach confirmed previous results and demonstrated that this drug could increase epithelial fluid secretion and enhance mucus clearance (Danahay et al., 2020).

Recently, our group has proposed a particular strategy using an ASO specific to ANO1 to reestablish ANO1 expression in the context of CF. This strategy "hijacks" the miRNA regulatory system and allows highly targeted effects. We have demonstrated that ASO-ANO1 could be used to inhibit the fixation of miR-9 on ANO1 mRNA by a target site blocker, and consequently to activate the alternative chloride channel to compensate CFTR Cl^- deficiency regardless of the mutation (Sonneville et al., 2017). We have also shown that with this strategy, we can improve tissue repair on cell lines but also on CF primary patient cells. We have likewise demonstrated that with this approach, we can activate mucociliary clearance on primary cells but also CF mice. Although we have not studied the effects of ANO1 modulation of inflammation, preliminary studies have already shown that activating ANO1 limits the secretion of IL-8 (Veit et al., 2012).

Novel Anti-Cytokines Approaches

A pathophysiology pulmonary characteristic of CF is a severe neutrophil accumulation, which is correlated with high levels of pro-inflammatory cytokines (IL-8, IL-6, TNF-α), and low levels of anti-inflammatory mediators like IL-10 (Jacquot et al., 2008b). For numerous years, different approaches, as curcumin or vitamin D, have been proposed to limit IL-8 secretion and neutrophils influx (Gaggar et al., 2011; Olszowiec-Chlebna et al., 2019). Some pre-clinical data have demonstrated that using antibodies, like antibodies directed against intercellular adhesion molecule (ICAM)-1 and IL-8, could be a promising target. The most advanced therapy using SB-656933, an oral CXCR2 antagonist, was already tested in CF patients and has demonstrated along with safety some exciting results in the modulation of airway inflammation (Moss et al., 2013). However, another study using SCH527123 (MK-7123, Navarixin), a CXCR1/2 antagonist, was also attempted in chronic obstructive pulmonary disease (COPD) but was abandoned because of a severe decline in neutrophil number (Rennard et al., 2015). By contrast, a phase II clinical trial has already been carried out in patients with ulcerative colitis and demonstrated inhibition of ozone-induced airway inflammation in humans (Lazaar et al., 2011). Numerous other modulators of cytokines in the context of CF have been proposed, but only *in vitro* experiments have been performed (Lampronti et al., 2017; De Fenza et al., 2019). Cytokine modulation shows that cytokines have a significant role in limiting infections, although these approaches are confusing. A recent publication has highlighted the role of an IL-1 signaling pathway in sterile neutrophilic inflammation and mucus hypersecretion and has suggested that treatment with IL-1 receptor antagonist as Anakinra could be promising to prevent lung inflammation (Balazs and Mall, 2019).

The possibility of increasing gene expression and protein activity by the use of ASO has become more and more promising in the last years. However, long-term efficacy, safe delivery, and side effects of long-term treatment must be evaluated in order to be applied in patients with CF (Bardin et al., 2018b; Vencken et al., 2019). Fabbri *et al.* have developed this original concept by modulating the IL-8 expression by increasing miR-93 in BECs during *P. aeruginosa* infection (Fabbri et al., 2014). More recent results have highlighted that other miRNA involved in CF pathology, like miR-199a-3p or miR-636, could be targeted to control the CF lung inflammatory process (Bardin et al., 2018a; Bardin et al., 2019). Other interesting approaches have been performed to modulate the cascade of inflammation targeting NFκB activity by using, for example, Angelicin derived from different angiosperms or Sulindac, an NSAID (Rocca et al., 2016). Unfortunately, these approaches are not specific, and the risk of side effects remains high.

New Development in Antibiotic Approaches

"Synthetic" Antibiotics

In CF, antibiotics are utilized for various applications, such as initial infection prevention, eradication (for early infection), control (for chronic infection), and finally, pulmonary exacerbations treatment. The antibiotics are given in three different primary ways: oral, inhalation, or intravenous. The choice of antibiotics depends on the nature of the pathogen to be eliminated, the age of the patient, and the nature of other pathogens present such as *H. influenza*, *S. aureus*, or *P. aeruginosa* infections.

P. aeruginosa is an opportunistic Gram-negative pathogen and is one of the main reasons for morbidity and mortality in CF and immunosuppressed patients. In order to eradicate new *P. aeruginosa* infections, antibiotic regimens are now a care standard around the world. Different groups assessed the effectiveness of inhaled Tobramycin, Aztreonam, and Colistin as well as oral Ciprofloxacin in eradicating new *P. aeruginosa* infection (Waters, 2018; Pang et al., 2019), although *P. aeruginosa* eradication is now much more challenging as a result of its impressive capability to resist antibiotics. These organisms become embedded in an exopolysaccharide biofilm, which protects the organism from phagocytosis and reduces the efficacy of anti-microbial drugs (Doring, 2010). Once this change has occurred, the mucoid *P. aeruginosa* could acquire multi-drug resistance, and this bacterium is virtually impossible to eradicate (Southern et al., 2012). If the *P. aeruginosa* infection cannot be cleared, the affected person is faced with an increased treatment burden, accelerated decline in lung function, increased symptom severity, and increased mortality (Nixon et al., 2002).

Recently, there has been a growing number of "new" antibiotics, of different classes and formulations, for pulmonary infection treatments in CF patients (Waters and Smyth, 2015). In order to limit toxicity and reduce side effects while directly targeting the lungs, many studies took an interest in using aerosols as a method of administration. In this frame of mind, Levofloxacin was developed for CF patients to target *P. aeruginosa* infections (Chirgwin et al., 2019; Epps et al., 2019). This drug, derived from the fluoroquinolone family, inhibits topoisomerases, which is essential for the synthesis of bacterial DNA. In the same way, inhaled Zitreonam is now available to treat *P. aeruginosa* infections in CF patients. Although its aerosolized formulation was proven to be beneficial, the formulation for intravenous injections induces significant lung inflammation, which has limited its use. Another example of the existing improvement of drugs is Tobramycin, presented as a dry powder. Inhaled tobramycin provides, in less than 5 minutes, a rapid action directly at the site of the lung infection.

In order to increase the efficacy of *P. aeruginosa* eradication and have a less often resistance development in comparison to the existing "classical" antibiotics, recent *P. aeruginosa* suggested treatment is the use of a combination of antibiotics and the development of new ones. Also, they can be associated with an alternative strategy such as EDTA (Respirion) or inhaled glycopolymer (SNP113).

Thus, a new carbapenem antibiotic called Doripenem has been developed with wide spectrum activity against bacteria through bacterial cell wall synthesis inhibition. Different authors have shown *in vitro* that this molecule has more significant activity than other antibiotics of the same family on strains isolated from CF patients (Traczewski and Brown, 2006; Riera et al., 2011). A clinical phase III study showed that patients infected with *P. aeruginosa* and treated with Doripenem had higher recovery rates in comparison to Imipenem-treated patients but, no clinical trial with CF patients is in progress (Chastre et al., 2008). In the same way, Plazomicin (a semisynthetic aminoglycoside) and POL7001 (a protein epitope mimetic) came out as an interesting strategy against *P. aeruginosa* (Cigana et al., 2016). These drugs have demonstrated *in vitro* some exciting effects on the multidrug-resistant *P. aeruginosa* isolated from CF patients (Cigana et al., 2016).

"Natural" Approaches

For many years an original approach using bacteriophages has been advanced. Bacteriophages were discovered in 1915 and can kill bacteria by causing lysis (Summers, 2001). Bacteriophage therapy was applied extensively in the 1930s and 1940s before antibiotics, and it is still being used in Eastern Europe. Nevertheless, after antibiotics became broadly accessible, phage therapy was renounced in Western countries. Many phages can target *P. aeruginosa* and have demonstrated some exciting effects on mice by decreasing the bacteria burden in the lungs or preventing infection (Morello et al., 2011). Even if clinical studies have shown relative effectiveness, treatments using phages remain negligible so far. Various reasons have limited the treatments with bacteriophages. The idea of introducing a living organism into the body is difficult to accept and remains an important psychological barrier. Moreover, early tests showed that the preparation generated impurities and that these preparations were not very stable (Morello et al., 2011). Although the use of phages in combination with quorum sensing inhibitors seems interesting, this approach remains marginal (Pang et al., 2019), and only a phase Ib/II trial is planned to test the safety and tolerability of AP-PA02 in adults with CF. AP-PA02 is a type of phage intended to control *P. aeruginosa* infections in CF patients. In *in vitro* studies, AP-PA02 can kill more than 80% of *P. aeruginosa* strains from CF people, and some first results are encouraging (Law et al., 2019).

Another "natural strategy" is inhaled nitric oxide (NO) for which an initial phase II study is underway. NO is a gas derived from nitrogen with anti-microbial properties. Some *in vivo* studies have validated this approach to eradicate the infection and to decrease mucus viscoelastic (Rouillard et al., 2020).

In the late 1970s, various studies showed that iron played an essential role in bacterial growth and was involved in particular in DNA replication, energy production, and pathogen-host interaction (Payne and Finkelstein, 1978). Recent results demonstrated that the iron content of human sputum is considerably high in CF, which facilitates chronic infections in the lungs of CF patients (Reid et al., 2007). These observations resulted in the development of novel therapeutic strategies in order to limit the amount of iron present in the airways. Gallium is a compound that shares the same properties with iron. It has demonstrated *in vitro* and *in vivo* anti-Pseudomonas properties (Tovar-García et al., 2020). The FDA has already approved the intravenous administration of Gallium. Clinical studies, in phase II for intravenous and a phase I for an inhaled strategy, are ongoing to evaluate its efficiency in treating *P. aeruginosa* infections in CF patients (Tovar-García et al., 2020).

During the last decades, AMPs naturally emerged as a potential therapy to cure infections with antibiotic resistance, in CF included. Treatments of bacterial infections by antibiotics result in a worldwide spread of dissemination of antibiotic resistance, both in the community and clinical settings. Besides, the development of new antibiotics is costly and time-consuming. It is hence of great importance to note that AMPs can treat methicillin-resistant *S. aureus* and multidrug-resistant *P. aeruginosa* that are resistant to conventional antibiotics (Geitani et al., 2019). Studies showed that treatments of antibiotic-resistant bacterial strains with AMPs were associated with almost no induced resistance to AMPs, which may encourage their use as potential replacement therapy for antibiotics. AMPs can exert anti-inflammatory actions either by suppressing the production of pro-inflammatory cytokines or by stimulating that of anti-inflammatory cytokines by host cells (**Figure 7**). Cathelicidin LL-37 (one of the most studied AMPs) enhances the production of the anti-inflammatory cytokine IL-1R by the human peripheral blood-derived mononuclear cells and macrophages (Choi et al., 2014), and similar results were observed with LL-37 and beta-defensin-3 (hBD-3) (Mookherjee et al., 2009; Smithrithee et al., 2015). Besides their direct actions on host cells involved in the initiation/modulation of inflammation, a number of AMPs, such as LL-37, Magainin-2, and bactericidal-permeability-increasing (BPI), can neutralize the activity of bacterial toxins such as LPS, thus participating in maintaining a balance between pro- and anti-inflammatory cytokines (Sun and Shang, 2015; Skovbakke and Franzyk, 2017).

Most of the reported studies in the field have focused on the roles of AMPs in the modulation of cytokine production. However, cytokines are only the tip of the iceberg in the inflammatory process, and other mediators of inflammation, such as eicosanoids, deserve to be investigated to identify their relative role in the modulation of inflammation by AMPs. Indeed, studies have reported that AMPs such as LL-37 modulates the production of eicosanoids, including leukotriene B4 (LTB4) and thromboxane A2 (TXA2) by macrophages (Agier et al., 2015). TXB2 and LTB4 are metabolites of arachidonic acid conversion by COX and lipoxygenase (LOX), respectively, and known to induce platelet aggregation and neutrophils recruitment at the site of infection (Yeung and Holinstat, 2011). It has been shown that LL-37 AMP blocks the expression of pro-inflammatory pathways involved, such as NF-κB in the presence of LPS (Agier et al., 2015). However, further studies are awaited to decipher the importance of the AMPs/eicosanoids network in the inflammatory reaction and potential implication in inflammatory diseases such as COPD, asthma, and CF. Similar anti-inflammatory effects were observed with WALK11.3 (an AMP with amphipathic helical conformation) in the mouse alveolar macrophage cell line RAW264.7 (Shim et al., 2015). They revealed the ability of this peptide to inhibit the expression of several inflammatory mediators, including NO, COX-derived metabolites, IL-1β, IL-6, interferon (IFN)-β, and TNF-α (**Figure 7**). The chicken cathelicidin-2 (CATH-2), the known ortholog of the human LL-37, has been shown to reduce inflammation in parallel to its anti-microbial activity against *P. aeruginosa*-resistant strains from CF patients (Banaschewski et al., 2017). The ability of CATH-2 to downregulate inflammation occurred through the anti-microbial-independent process, as this down-regulation was observed by silencing the inflammatory response that arises from killed bacteria. It is now clear that AMPs play a key role in host defense toward infectious by invading pathogens and represent a potential therapeutic tool to control infections by antibiotic-resistant bacterial strains. They also have the potential to protect the host from harmful inflammation that may result from these infections. Drug design and structure-relationship studies will greatly improve our knowledge of AMPs and the relative importance of their bactericidal *vs* anti-inflammatory functions, which will be of great help to optimize their potential therapeutic use in disease characterized by both chronic infection and inflammation such as CF.

All these data suggested that AMPs could be useful for clinical applications in the view of the protective function against pathogens. A series of clinical trials have started mostly in the pediatric population, and some compounds have been used as topical treatments but not known in the CF context. Different

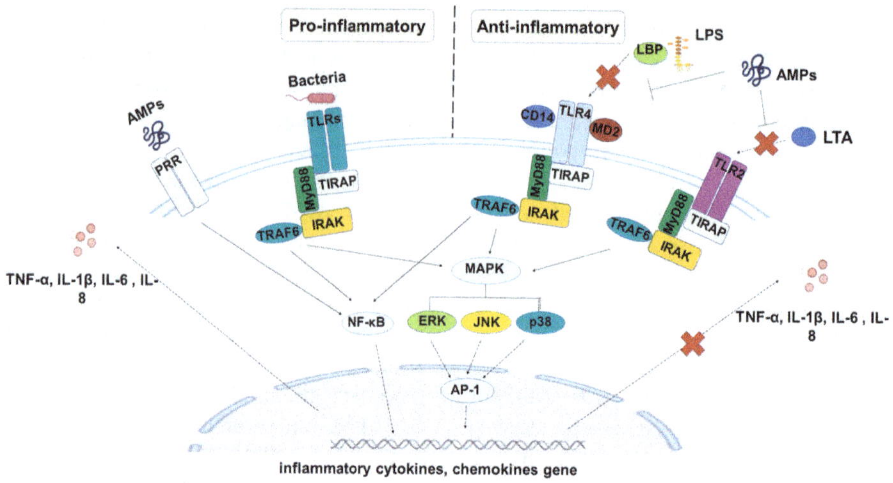

FIGURE 7 | General mechanisms by which AMPs exert anti-inflammatory actions on host cells. AMPs can bind to bacterial virulence factors such as LPS or LTA and prevent their interactions with host cells. AMPs are also able to interfere with host cell signaling pathways involved in the inflammatory reaction. The overall consequence is that AMPs reduce the production of inflammatory mediators by these cells that may help in the resolution of inflammation.

AMPs are under evaluation for the treatment of acute skin infection as Bralicidin, Omiganan, LTC109 (phase II clinical trial), or Pexiganam (phase III clinical trial). Other strategies and applications are currently under study. For example, in sepsis, Talactoferrin was tested by systemic injection in phase II clinical study (Guntupalli et al., 2013). Initial results showed a significant decrease in mortality after 28 days of treatment. However, phase II/III oral Talactoferrin was stopped for problems of safety and efficacy (Vincent et al., 2015). In the case of meningococcemia, rBPI21 pre-clinical trial has demonstrated some anti-bacterial and anti-LPS effects. Encouraging results led to the initiation of a phase III study in children with severe meningococcal sepsis (Giroir et al., 2001). The study outcome showed a reduction in complications with a shorter hospitalization also suggests the possibility to treat with rBPI21 other patients, including CF. The therapeutic applications of *P. aeruginosa* have been summarized in a recent publication (Magrone et al., 2018). An alternative therapeutic pathway for the use of AMPs has been envisaged by indirectly promoting their expression through the use of natural compounds. Several compounds have been identified as the use of Apigenin to enhance the expression and activity of β-3 defensin and cathelicidin in mice (Hou et al., 2013). Similar effects have been observed with vitamin D on *in vitro* studies to increase β-2 defensins and LL-37 on keratinocytes (Kim et al., 2009).

The use of natural or synthetic antibiotics can have a significant influence on the emergence of new pathogens. It is well established now that microbiota composition and dynamic impact the host immunity, health, and diseases (Belkaid and Hand, 2014). However, a new concept is now progressively emerging, suggesting that the innate immune response of the host can also modulate, at least in part *via* AMPs, the microbiota composition. For example, recent studies reported the involvement of sPLA2-IIA in the selection of species in pathologies characterized by polymicrobial infections such as CF. *P. aeruginosa* is known to progressively colonize CF airways to become the dominant pathogen at later stages of CF. This pathogen induces the production by CF airways of sPLA2-IIA, which in turn eradicate *S. aureus*, therefore helping in its gradual elimination from CF airways and its substitution by *P. aeruginosa* (Pernet et al., 2014). This effect is mostly due to the intrinsic resistance of *P. aeruginosa* and high susceptibility of *S. aureus* to sPLA2-IIA, respectively. Finally, it emerges that AMPs represent valid substitutes of antibiotics when a condition of antibiotic resistance is established.

Alternative Strategies

Anti-Proteases

CF "anti-protease therapies" can be separated into two separate groups of drugs: some to increase anti-protease and some to inhibit protease expression. CFTR is an essential apical GSH transporter in the lung, and can indirectly participate in the inflammatory process by reducing oxidative stress. Evidence supporting the occurrence of oxidative stress in CF is established and extensively described (Galli et al., 2012; Causer et al., 2020). Some interesting works have demonstrated that oxidative stress could suppress CFTR expression (Cantin et al., 2006). Oxidative stress has a major role in the development of lung pathology in CF children and will, in addition to having a role in lung remodeling, have a role in the pulmonary microbiota (Shi et al., 2019). A recent metanalysis has positively correlated the expression of antioxidants with body mass index and lung function in CF (Causer et al., 2020). The malabsorption of nutrients with antioxidants properties in CF, participate in the imbalance in favor of oxidative stress and disrupt redox signaling, and, finally, molecular damages even if some data appears to be conflicting (Shamseer et al., 2010; Siwamogsatham et al., 2014). Therefore, multiple studies have been carried out to check the anti-protease supplementation in CF (Galli et al., 2012). Some studies have focused on especially serine proteases *via* two distinct administration routes: aerosolized and intravenously (McKelvey et al., 2020). In CF, exocrine pancreatic insufficiency and reduced bile acids induce critical antioxidants malabsorption, including carotenoids (β-carotene), tocopherols (vitamin E), coenzyme Q10, and selenium. Supplementation of antioxidant micronutrients (vitamin E, C, D, β-carotene, and selenium) may, therefore, potentially help maintain an oxidant-antioxidant balance, and this aspect has been extensively reviewed (Sagel et al., 2011; Ciofu et al., 2019). In the same approach, LAU-7b, an oral drug, is a derived form related to vitamin A. This compound can reduce the lung inflammatory response of CF people. In parallel, a phase II clinical study to test the effectiveness and safety of LAU-7b in CF patients is underway (Lands and Stanojevic, 2016). LAU-7b, also called, Fenretidine, work to increase docosahexaenoic acid (DHA) and consequently CER concentration. Some authors supported that the decrease of CER concentration contributes to the persistent bacterial infection and the constitutive MAP kinases and NFκB activation (Guilbault et al., 2008; Guilbault et al., 2009).

Human α-1 antitrypsin (A1AT) is still the most studied drug by far. Different clinical trials were already achieved. An inhaled α1-proteinase inhibitor is known to reduce NE burden in some patients with CF. A phase I in non-CF bronchiectasis and an IIa clinical study with purified A1AT products given through inhalation in CF subjects were just finalized and have demonstrated safety and efficacy (Gaggar et al., 2016; Watz et al., 2019). In the conclusion of the second study, the daily α-1 hydrophobic chromatography process delivered for three weeks was safe, well-tolerated, and effective in raising the α1-PI levels in the sputum of subjects with CF. However, the effects were transient and difficult to predict due to the proteases' variability in CF patients' lungs. The administration by airway routeway effectively increased the concentration of A1AT in sputum. The current study was not powered to assess changes in FEV1 or biomarkers in sputum, and further clinical are needed.

In parallel, A1AT gene therapy is emerging. Some recent data have demonstrated encouraging results in the inhibition of miRNA, which targets the A1AT gene called SERPINA1 (Hunt et al., 2020). This strategy aims to by-pass protein regulation systems of the most abundant inhibitor of NE in the airways. It is an alternative to the delivery of recombinant by using miRNA-targeted therapies. It was found that dual miRNA and adeno-associated viral (AAV)-based therapy engendered the long-term knockdown of circulating Z-A1AT and could be a new strategy in CF (Mueller et al., 2012). This approach was fully described in a review published (Hunt et al., 2020). The other approach is to directly activate SERPINA1 using gene therapy by using viral vectors like retrovirus or adenovirus, but numerous side effects have been observed (Gregory et al., 2011). Their use remains challenging, especially in the CF field.

Another strategy proposed is to use serine protease inhibitors such as secretory leukoprotease inhibitor (SLPI) which act locally to maintain a protease/anti-protease balance, thereby preventing protease-mediated tissue destruction. SLPI is a well-characterized member of the trapping gene family of proteins and is produced by respiratory tract epithelial cells and phagocytic neutrophils. Different approaches have been proposed to increase the anti-protease activity by nebulizing SLPI, but the efficacy is currently being evaluated alone or in association with other strategies (McElvaney et al., 1993; Quabius et al., 2017). Currently, novel protease inhibitor drugs, which have promising interest in the CF context, are in development (DX-890, AZD9668, POL6014, Grifols T6006-201) in order to improve their resistance against inactivation.

Promoting tissue repair represents another strategy by focusing on the proteins involved. Matrix metalloproteinases (MMP) are a group of distinct metalloendopeptidase enzymes that regulate various inflammatory and repair processes. They are either secreted or anchored to the cell surface, and therefore their activity is directed against membrane proteins or extracellular proteins, including inflammatory mediators. In CF patients, different articles have demonstrated that MMP is upregulated in the sputum of patients and is related to tissue damage (Delacourt et al., 1995; Gaggar et al., 2011). Various pro-inflammatory cytokines induce them at the transcription level. They might include the activation of a diverse group of intracellular signaling pathways (such as p38 MAPK or ERK 1/2 MAPK), causing the activation of nuclear signaling factors like AP1, NFκB, and STAT (signal transducer and activator of transcription). Activation of MMP can be induced by proteases or oxidants and are controlled by tissue inhibitor of metalloproteases (TIMP). There have been increasing interests in modulating MMP activity to enhance disease outcomes, and different clinical studies are in progress with promising effects in CF. A phase II study with Andecaliximab/GS-5745 in CF adults is in progress and was tolerated in patients with ulcerative colitis or Crohn's disease, and could be an exciting approach to control pulmonary degradation.

The approaches using protease inhibitors are very varied, and many studies are still in progress. Although these therapies have been shown to improve patients' health outcomes, they can only be considered in combination with other therapeutic targets.

Eicosanoids Pathway

Alterations in the metabolism of fatty acids present in membrane lipids may have an essential role in the inflammatory CF pulmonary disease. The arachidonic acid (AA): docosahexaenoic acid (DHA) ratio in blood serum, pulmonary airways, and rectal biopsies are increased in CF patients with either pancreatic sufficiency or pancreatic insufficiency, as compared with healthy control subjects (Freedman et al., 2004). AA is stored in cell membranes and is released from membrane lipids by various PLA2 proteins. Some interesting studies have highlighted the implication of sPLA2 in the pathogenicity of CF mice showing that reduced CFTR expression increased cytosolic PLA2α (cPLA2α) activity. A review has summarized the state of the art of fatty acid metabolism in CF (Strandvik, 2010). These effects improved mucus secretion and accumulation in airway epithelia independent of CFTR chloride transport function (Medjane et al., 2005; Dif et al., 2010). Therefore, cPLA2α has been proposed as an appropriate new target for therapeutic intervention in CF (Dif et al., 2010). Small lipid mediators were produced in the course of inflammation resolution and generated varied responses, which are cell types and tissue specific. A large number of these molecules modulate inflammation processes and provide essential functions in chemoattraction, aggregation, and degranulation of inflammatory cells. They are also implicated in tissue and vascular permeability, bronchoconstriction, and mucus production. Some of the lipid mediators include lipoxins (LX), resolvins, protectins, and maresins, which are generated by the activity of lipoxygenases lipoxin A4 (LXA4).

Interestingly, inhibitors of the 12R-lipoxygenase have demonstrated an essential role in mucin expression. The inhibitors decreased MUC5AC mucin expression by the inhibition of the ERK/SP1 dependent mechanism (Garcia-Verdugo et al., 2012). LXA4 has been described as a significant signal for the inflammation resolution and is generated at a low level in the CF patients' lungs. LXA4 and RvD1 activate a GPCR termed ALX/FPR2.

This pro-resolving receptor is recognized by annexin A1, an endogenous anti-inflammatory peptide. A recent article provides evidence that the miR-181b, overexpressed in CF cells, may be considered as a new strategy to decrease the anti-inflammatory process in CF *via* the normalization of the expression receptor-dependent LXA4 (Pierdomenico et al., 2017). The LXA4 inhalation consequences have been examined in a pilot study of asthmatic and healthy adult subjects. The drug was well-tolerated, and no harmful effect was observed (Christie et al., 1992). Some impressive results were observed in the topical treatment of infantile eczema (Wu et al., 2013). Together with data showing beneficial actions of LXA4 in the CF context, these results highlight additional studies to check whether the upregulation of the lipidic mediators' pathway can be considered as an appropriate tactic to fight inflammation in CF patients (Higgins et al., 2015).

Similarly, the LTB4 produced by resting BECs has been proposed as a target. Inflammatory stimuli increase the production of LTB4 and might also contribute to progressive pulmonary destruction in CF. Bronchial epithelial LTB4 acts as a potent chemoattractant for neutrophils *via* the cell surface integrins upregulation. When these cells are activated and present at the site of inflammation, they can also participate in the secretion of LTB4. LTB4 synthesis includes lipid peroxidation by 5-lipoxygenase, and produce numerous ROS, and consequently, pro-inflammatory activation. A clinical trial with Montelukast (BIIL 284), a leukotriene receptor agonist, counting a small number of patients, has provided contentious results in CF patients. This therapy has demonstrated a notable decrease in serum eosinophil cationic protein levels and eosinophils without any significant improvement in FEV1, and FEF25–75%. Also, this strategy has shown a significant decrease in cough, serum, and sputum levels of eosinophil cationic protein and IL-8 chemokine. Moreover, an increase in serum and sputum levels of IL-10 has been observed. The trial was stopped early due to a significant increase in the risk of severe pulmonary events in patients receiving the active drug (Schmitt-Grohe and Zielen, 2005). A more recent drug, Acebilustat (CTX-4430), has been evaluated in CF patients. This drug has shown anti-inflammatory activity *via* the LTA4 hydrolase inhibition and LTB4 modulation. In two-phase I clinical trials, Acebilustat decreased the production of LTB4 and pro-inflammatory cytokines in healthy volunteers and CF patients, and in phase II, optimal dose and duration were identified for future studies (Elborn et al., 2017; Elborn et al., 2018).

Cannabinoid-Derived Drug

Ajulemic acid (JBT-101, Lenabasum) is a cannabinoid-derived molecule that preferably binds to the active CB2 receptor and is non-psychoactive. In some pre-clinical trials done on human lung cells obtained from CF patients, it was shown that Lenabasum stopped the production of both TNF-α and IL-6, two crucial pro-inflammatory cytokines that trigger inflammation. In phase I and II clinical trials, this drug demonstrated favorable safety and tolerability. Recently, a group has also shown significant efficacy in mice models of inflammation and fibrosis (Burstein, 2018). Therefore, phase II was initiated. It will be used to test safety, tolerability, pharmacokinetics, and efficacy of JBT-101 in 70 subjects ≥ 18 and < 65 years of age with documented CF. Treatment of CF patients with Lenabasum twice daily has been able to decrease the number of acute lung exacerbations as well as a reduction of inflammatory cells and mediators present in the sputum. A new clinical trial is undergoing and seeks to enroll more than 400 CF patients over numerous clinical sites.

Mucus Therapies

In the lungs, the abnormal production of mucus has been assumed to participate actively in the early CF pathogenesis (Ehre et al., 2014). For many years, researchers and clinicians have been trying to understand the origin of mucus abnormalities and found mucoactive drugs molecules to control CF bronchial obstruction. Mucoactive drugs are regularly used as a therapeutic option and are defined by their activity as mucolytics, expectorants, and cough facilitating drug. The expectorants, such as hypertonic solution (HSS), increase the ASL layer and decrease mucus adhesiveness. Mucolytics, such as both N-acetylcysteine (NAC) and recombinant human DNase (rhDNase), reduce sputum viscosity. Medications such as inhaled mannitol, rhDNase (Dornase), and hypertonic HSS have proven efficacy in CF and indirectly reduced inflammation in airways of CF patients (Tarrant et al., 2017). The low volume hypothesis would estimate that approaches increasing the ASL height will increase mucociliary clearance, and consequently reduce lung infection. In order to increase the ASL height and fluidity, an HSS (3 to 7% NaCl) has been proposed to treat CFTR deficiency for better mucociliary clearance. Recently, Wark &

McDonald have performed a meta-analysis of 17 different clinical trials of HSS and concluded that, after four weeks, a small enhancement in the lung function was observed but was not sustained at 48 weeks. HSS might also have a little impact on improving life quality in adults (Wark and McDonald, 2018). New clinical trials are in progress in order to establish who may benefit most and whether this benefit is sustained in the longer term (https://www.cff.org/Trials/Finder).

In the same manner, a meta-analysis was performed with mannitol, which is a naturally occurring sugar alcohol. When inhaled mannitol creates a change in the osmotic gradient. It leads to water movement into the CF airway hydrating the ASL, and enhancing mucociliary clearance. In the different studies, there was no evidence showing that the mannitol treatment for over six months is related to an enhancement of lung function in CF patients compared to control (Nevitt et al., 2018). Recently, different groups have observed expression, biochemical and biophysical alterations of the mucous present in the airways of CF patients (Rhim et al., 2001). More, they observed that abnormal glycosylation of the airway mucins is associated with bacterial infection and inflammation. The effects of altered host mucin glycosylation affect *P. aeruginosa* adhesion and so pathogenicity. A review from Ventalakrishan et al. has extensively described this feature (Venkatakrishnan et al., 2013). Different therapeutic approaches have been proposed to correct this observation by using, for example, mannose-biding lectin, which recognizes bacterial glycoconjugates and participates in an effective defense against pathogens (Moller-Kristensen et al., 2006).

Another strategy used in CF is to disrupt the high DNA content present in the airway mucus of CF patients. DNA is a polyanion compound responsible for the viscosity and adhesiveness of the pulmonary secretions. DNA release and accumulation in ASL occur as a result of tissue destruction caused by inflammatory cells on bacteria and epithelial cells. The strategy is to use a recombinant human deoxyribonuclease I (rhDNase), an enzyme that selectively cleaves DNA, hence decreasing mucus viscosity (Puchelle et al., 1995). Nebulized rhDNase hydrolyzes extracellular DNA within the mucus and transforms it from an adhesive gel into a liquid form of fluid through dilution within minutes. In contrast to mannitol or HSS, rhDNase has shown some significant effects on the improvement of lung function of CF patients and is considered as an effective treatment for the liquefaction of viscous mucus in CF. However, individual responses are unpredictable (Yang and Montgomery, 2018).

The only approved reducing agent for human use is N-acetylcysteine (NAC), a well-known antioxidant GSH drug. This drug ameliorates the redox imbalance in neutrophils present in the blood and inhibits their recruitment in the airways of CF patients (Tirouvanziam et al., 2006). NAC is also used in CF as an aerosolized mucus solution to break down disulfide bonds between mucin proteins in order to fluidify mucus (Duijvestijn and Brand, 1999). Some evidence demonstrated that NAC has excellent anti-bacterial properties, the capacity to intervene with biofilm formation and, to disturb the adherence of respiratory pathogens to respiratory epithelial cells (Blasi et al., 2016). In CF patients, NAC has been proven to be safe at large doses with negligible interaction with other drugs. NAC was investigated in CF despite its partial effectiveness as an inhaled mucolytic agent because the extremely oxidizing CF airway environment consumes aerosolized antioxidants quickly (Tirouvanziam et al., 2006; Cantin et al., 2007). Finally, inhaled NAC is being used as a mucolytic drug in CF for several decades, although the positive results remain limited. Newer agents targeting other components of CF mucus are currently in development or clinical trials (NAC 40630) and exhibit an exciting effect on mucus (Blasi et al., 2016).

Another original approach is undergoing with OligoG CF-5/20. OligoG is an alginate oligosaccharide derived from natural seaweed. It is administrated using a dry powder inhaler and also developed as a liquid to use with a nebulizer. Studies have shown that this dry power drug is capable of reducing the mucus thickness in the lungs. In addition, this drug enhances the efficiency of antibiotics and may facilitate mucus clearance in CF patients. The drug could detach CF mucus by calcium chelation (Ermund et al., 2017). Initiated in 2018, phase II includes more than 120 patients from European and Australian sites. It aims to determine the optimal dose of OligoG and to describe long-term safety and efficacy, with FEV1 as a primary endpoint.

Recently, numerous articles have been published to describe new regulation mechanisms of the different proteins present in the mucus and especially on mucins expressed in the airways. The epigenetic regulation role of MUC5AC and MUC5B, the main mucins expressed in the airways, has been thoroughly researched in COPD and have highlighted the implication of methylation and miRNA. Different specific therapies are in progress to modulate the miRNA, and new treatment ways are in progress in CF (Bardin et al., 2018b).

CONCLUSION

Although current anti-inflammatory drugs (corticosteroids and Ibuprofen) in CF patients have shown little effectiveness, the creation and improvement of new anti-inflammatory drugs for CF lungs has been overlooked for a long time. In the last decade, most of the research fields in CF therapy, have focused mainly on the discovery of new CFTR activators. Despite this, basic researches that are now in the evaluation phase have shown that new approaches could be very promising in resolving efficiently the CF lungs' ongoing inflammatory vicious cycle. However, treatment complexity is challenging. Currently available treatments offered to CF patients certainly help reduce inflammation, but in indirect and non-specific pathways, by targeting the viscosity of the mucus, reducing infection, or activating Cl^- efflux. As the traditional approaches have shown their limitations, it seems essential to us that original work should continue in order to identify innovative approaches that would be more specific. The identification of critical druggable molecular targets to decrease inflammation is still an unsatisfied demand that needs numerous additional researches.

AUTHOR CONTRIBUTIONS

All authors: CM, PB, ZX, HC, LT, and OT have written and reviewed the manuscript.

REFERENCES

Accurso, F. J., Moss, R. B., Wilmott, R. W., Anbar, R. D., Schaberg, A. E., Durham, T. A., et al. (2011). Denufosol tetrasodium in patients with cystic fibrosis and normal to mildly impaired lung function. *Am. J. Respir. Crit. Care Med.* 183, 627–634. doi: 10.1164/rccm.201008-1267OC

Adam, D., Roux-Delrieu, J., Luczka, E., Bonnomet, A., Lesage, J., Merol, J. C., et al. (2015). Cystic fibrosis airway epithelium remodelling: involvement of inflammation. *J. Pathol.* 235, 408–419. doi: 10.1002/path.4471

Agier, J., Efenberger, M., and Brzezińska-Błaszczyk, E. (2015). Review paper Cathelicidin impact on inflammatory cells. *Cent. Eur. J. Immunol.* 2, 225–235. doi: 10.5114/ceji.2015.51359

Alton, E. W. F. W., Armstrong, D. K., Ashby, D., Bayfield, K. J., Bilton, D., Bloomfield, E. V., et al. (2015). Repeated nebulisation of non-viral CFTR gene therapy in patients with cystic fibrosis: a randomised, double-blind, placebo-controlled, phase 2b trial. *Lancet Respirat. Med.* 3, 684–691. doi: 10.1016/S2213-2600(15)00245-3

Alton, E. W., Beekman, J. M., Boyd, A. C., Brand, J., Carlon, M. S., Connolly, M. M., et al. (2017). Preparation for a first-in-man lentivirus trial in patients with cystic fibrosis. *Thorax.*

Arampatzioglou, A., Papazoglou, D., Konstantinidis, T., Chrysanthopoulou, A., Mitsios, A., Angelidou, I., et al. (2018). Clarithromycin Enhances the Antibacterial Activity and Wound Healing Capacity in Type 2 Diabetes Mellitus by Increasing LL-37 Load on Neutrophil Extracellular Traps. *Front. Immunol.* 9, 2064. doi: 10.3389/fimmu.2018.02064

Armstrong, D. S., Grimwood, K., Carzino, R., Carlin, J. B., Olinsky, A., and Phelan, P. D. (1995). Lower respiratory infection and inflammation in infants with newly diagnosed cystic fibrosis. *BMJ* 310, 1571–1572. doi: 10.1136/bmj.310.6994.1571

Atanasova, K. R., and Reznikov, L. R. (2019). Strategies for measuring airway mucus and mucins. *Respir. Res.* 20, 261. doi: 10.1186/s12931-019-1239-z

Auerbach, H. S., Williams, M., Kirkpatrick, J. A., and Colten, H. R. (1985). Alternate-day prednisone reduces morbidity and improves pulmonary function in cystic fibrosis. *Lancet* 2, 686–688. doi: 10.1016/S0140-6736(85)92929-0

Aureli, M., Schiumarini, D., Loberto, N., Bassi, R., Tamanini, A., Mancini, G., et al. (2016). Unravelling the role of sphingolipids in cystic fibrosis lung disease. *Chem. Phys. Lipids* 200, 94–103. doi: 10.1016/j.chemphyslip.2016.08.002

Balazs, A., and Mall, M. A. (2019). Mucus obstruction and inflammation in early cystic fibrosis lung disease: Emerging role of the IL-1 signaling pathway. *Pediatr. Pulmonol.* 54 Suppl 3, S5–S12. doi: 10.1002/ppul.24462

Balfour-Lynn, I. M., and Welch, K. (2014). Inhaled corticosteroids for cystic fibrosis. *Cochrane Database Syst. Rev.* 10, CD001915. doi: 10.1002/14651858.CD001915.pub4

Balfour-Lynn, I. M., Lees, B., Hall, P., Phillips, G., Khan, M., Flather, M., et al. (2006). Multicenter randomized controlled trial of withdrawal of inhaled corticosteroids in cystic fibrosis. *Am. J. Respir. Crit. Care Med.* 173, 1356–1362. doi: 10.1164/rccm.200511-1808OC

Bals, R., Weiner, D. J., Meegalla, R. L., Accurso, F., and Wilson, J. M. (2001). Salt-Independent Abnormality of Antimicrobial Activity in Cystic Fibrosis Airway Surface Fluid. *Am. J. Respir. Cell Mol. Biol.* 25, 21–25. doi: 10.1165/ajrcmb.25.1.4436

Banaschewski, B. J. H., Baer, B., Arsenault, C., Jazey, T., Veldhuizen, E. J. A., Delport, J., et al. (2017). The Antibacterial and Anti-inflammatory Activity of Chicken Cathelicidin-2 combined with Exogenous Surfactant for the Treatment of Cystic Fibrosis-Associated Pathogens. *Sci. Rep.* 7, 15545. doi: 10.1038/s41598-017-15558-4

Bardin, P., Marchal-Duval, E., Sonneville, F., Blouquit-Laye, S., Rousselet, N., Le Rouzic, P., et al. (2018a). Small RNA and transcriptome sequencing reveal the role of miR-199a-3p in inflammatory processes in cystic fibrosis airways. *J. Pathol.* 245, 410–420. doi: 10.1002/path.5095

Bardin, P., Sonneville, F., Corvol, H., and Tabary, O. (2018b). Emerging microRNA Therapeutic Approaches for Cystic Fibrosis. *Front. Pharmacol.* 9, 1113. doi: 10.3389/fphar.2018.01113

Bardin, P., Foussignière, T., Rousselet, N., Rebeyrol, C., Porter, J. C., Corvol, H., et al. (2019). miR-636: A Newly-Identified Actor for the Regulation of Pulmonary Inflammation in Cystic Fibrosis. *Front. Immunol.* 10, 2643. doi: 10.3389/fimmu.2019.02643

Barnes, P. J. (2006). Transcription factors in airway diseases. *Lab. Invest.* 86, 867–872. doi: 10.1038/labinvest.3700456

Bautista, M. V., Chen, Y., Ivanova, V. S., Rahimi, M. K., Watson, A. M., and Rose, M. C. (2009). IL-8 Regulates Mucin Gene Expression at the Posttranscriptional Level in Lung Epithelial Cells. *J. Immunol.* 183, 2159–2166. doi: 10.4049/jimmunol.0803022

Belkaid, Y., and Hand, T. W. (2014). Role of the Microbiota in Immunity and Inflammation. *Cell* 157, 121–141. doi: 10.1016/j.cell.2014.03.011

Benedetto, R., Ousingsawat, J., Wanitchakool, P., Zhang, Y., Holtzman, M. J., Amaral, M., et al. (2017). Epithelial Chloride Transport by CFTR Requires TMEM16A. *Sci. Rep.* 7, 12397. doi: 10.1038/s41598-017-10910-0

Benedetto, R., Ousingsawat, J., Cabrita, I., Pinto, M., Lerias, J. R., Wanitchakool, P., et al. (2019). Plasma membrane-localized TMEM16 proteins are indispensable for expression of CFTR. *J. Mol. Med. (Berl.)* 97, 711–722. doi: 10.1007/s00109-019-01770-4

Blasi, F., Page, C., Rossolini, G. M., Pallecchi, L., Matera, M. G., Rogliani, P., et al. (2016). The effect of N-acetylcysteine on biofilms: Implications for the treatment of respiratory tract infections. *Respir. Med.* 117, 190–197. doi: 10.1016/j.rmed.2016.06.015

Brook, M., Tomlinson, G. H., Miles, K., Smith, R. W. P., Rossi, A. G., Hiemstra, P. S., et al. (2016). Neutrophil-derived alpha defensins control inflammation by inhibiting macrophage mRNA translation. *Proc. Natl. Acad. Sci.* 113, 4350–4355. doi: 10.1073/pnas.1601831113

Burstein, S. H. (2018). Ajulemic acid: potential treatment for chronic inflammation. *Pharmacol. Res. Perspect.* 6, e00394. doi: 10.1002/prp2.394

Button, B., Cai, L. H., Ehre, C., Kesimer, M., Hill, D. B., Sheehan, J. K., et al. (2012). A periciliary brush promotes the lung health by separating the mucus layer from airway epithelia. *Science* 337, 937–941. doi: 10.1126/science.1223012

Bystrzycka, W., Manda-Handzlik, A., Sieczkowska, S., Moskalik, A., Demkow, U., and Ciepiela, O. (2017). Azithromycin and Chloramphenicol Diminish Neutrophil Extracellular Traps (NETs) Release. *Int. J. Mol. Sci.* 18, 2666. doi: 10.3390/ijms18122666

Callebaut, I., Hoffmann, B., Lehn, P., and Mornon, J. P. (2017). Molecular modelling and molecular dynamics of CFTR. *Cell Mol. Life Sci.* 74, 3–22. doi: 10.1007/s00018-016-2385-9

Cantin, A. M., Bilodeau, G., Ouellet, C., Liao, J., and Hanrahan, J. W. (2006). Oxidant stress suppresses CFTR expression. *Am. J. Physiol. Cell Physiol.* 290, C262–C270. doi: 10.1152/ajpcell.00070.2005

Cantin, A. M., White, T. B., Cross, C. E., Forman, H. J., Sokol, R. J., and Borowitz, D. (2007). Antioxidants in cystic fibrosis. Conclusions from the CF antioxidant workshop, Bethesda, Maryland, November 11-12, 2003. *Free Radic. Biol. Med.* 4, 15–31. doi: 10.1016/j.freeradbiomed.2006.09.022

Cantin, A. M., Hartl, D., Konstan, M. W., and Chmiel, J. F. (2015). Inflammation in cystic fibrosis lung disease: Pathogenesis and therapy. *J. Cyst. Fibros* 14, 419–430. doi: 10.1016/j.jcf.2015.03.003

Caputo, A., Caci, E., Ferrera, L., Pedemonte, N., Barsanti, C., Sondo, E., et al. (2008). TMEM16A, a membrane protein associated with calcium-dependent chloride channel activity. *Science* 322, 590–594. doi: 10.1126/science.1163518

Caretti, A., Bragonzi, A., Facchini, M., De Fino, I., Riva, C., Gasco, P., et al. (2014). Anti-inflammatory action of lipid nanocarrier-delivered myriocin: therapeutic potential in cystic fibrosis. *Biochim. Biophys. Acta* 1840, 586–594. doi: 10.1016/j.bbagen.2013.10.018

Causer, A. J., Shute, J. K., Cummings, M. H., Shepherd, A. I., Gruet, M., Costello, J. T., et al. (2020). Circulating biomarkers of antioxidant status and oxidative stress in people with cystic fibrosis: A systematic review and meta-analysis. *Redox Biol.* 32, 101436. doi: 10.1016/j.redox.2020.101436

Chalmers, J. D., Moffitt, K. L., Suarez-Cuartin, G., Sibila, O., Finch, S., Furrie, E., et al. (2017). Neutrophil Elastase Activity Is Associated with Exacerbations and Lung Function Decline in Bronchiectasis. *Am. J. Respir. Crit. Care Med.* 195, 1384–1393. doi: 10.1164/rccm.201605-1027OC

Chastre, J., Wunderink, R., Prokocimer, P., Lee, M., Kaniga, K., and Friedland, I. (2008). Efficacy and safety of intravenous infusion of doripenem versus imipenem in ventilator-associated pneumonia: a multicenter, randomized study. *Crit. Care Med.* 36, 1089–1096. doi: 10.1097/CCM.0b013e3181691b99

Chirgwin, M. E., Dedloff, M. R., Holban, A. M., and Gestal, M. C. (2019). Novel Therapeutic Strategies Applied to Pseudomonas aeruginosa Infections in Cystic Fibrosis. *Materials* 12, 4093. doi: 10.3390/ma12244093

Choi, K.-Y. G., Napper, S., and Mookherjee, N. (2014). Human cathelicidin LL-37 and its derivative IG-19 regulate interleukin-32-induced inflammation. *Immunology* 143, 68–80. doi: 10.1111/imm.12291

Christie, P. E., Spur, B. W., and Lee, T. H. (1992). The effects of lipoxin A4 on airway responses in asthmatic subjects. *Am. Rev. Respir. Dis.* 145, 1281–1284. doi: 10.1164/ajrccm/145.6.1281

Cigana, C., Bernardini, F., Facchini, M., Alcalá-Franco, B., Riva, C., De Fino, I., et al. (2016). Efficacy of the Novel Antibiotic POL7001 in Preclinical Models of Pseudomonas aeruginosa Pneumonia. *Antimicrob. Agents Chemother.* 60, 4991–5000. doi: 10.1128/AAC.00390-16

Ciofu, O., Smith, S., and Lykkesfeldt, J. (2019). Antioxidant supplementation for lung disease in cystic fibrosis. *Cochrane Database Syst. Rev.* 10, CD007020. doi: 10.1002/14651858.CD007020.pub4

Clement, A., Tamalet, A., Leroux, E., Ravilly, S., Fauroux, B., and Jais, J. P. (2006). Long term effects of azithromycin in patients with cystic fibrosis: A double blind, placebo controlled trial. *Thorax* 61, 895–902. doi: 10.1136/thx.2005.057950

Cohen, T. S., and Prince, A. (2012). Cystic fibrosis: a mucosal immunodeficiency syndrome. *Nat. Med.* 18, 509–519. doi: 10.1038/nm.2715

Corvol, H., Fitting, C., Chadelat, K., Jacquot, J., Tabary, O., Boule, M., et al. (2003). Distinct cytokine production by lung and blood neutrophils from children with cystic fibrosis. *Am. J. Physiol. Lung Cell Mol. Physiol.* 284, L997–1003. doi: 10.1152/ajplung.00156.2002

Crosby, J. R., Zhao, C., Jiang, C., Bai, D., Katz, M., Greenlee, S., et al. (2017). Inhaled ENaC antisense oligonucleotide ameliorates cystic fibrosis-like lung disease in mice. *J. Cyst. Fibros.* 16, 671–680. doi: 10.1016/j.jcf.2017.05.003

Danahay, H. L., Lilley, S., Fox, R., Charlton, H., Sabater, J., Button, B., et al. (2020). TMEM16A Potentiation: A Novel Therapeutic Approach for the Treatment of Cystic Fibrosis. *Am. J. Respir. Crit. Care Med.* 201 (8), 946–954. doi: 10.1164/rccm.201908-1641OC

Davies, J. C., Moskowitz, S. M., Brown, C., Horsley, A., Mall, M. A., McKone, E. F., et al. (2018). VX-659-Tezacaftor-Ivacaftor in Patients with Cystic Fibrosis and One or Two Phe508del Alleles. *N. Engl. J. Med.* 379, 1599–1611. doi: 10.1056/NEJMoa1807119

De Fenza, M., D'Alonzo, D., Esposito, A., Munari, S., Loberto, N., Santangelo, A., et al. (2019). Exploring the effect of chirality on the therapeutic potential of N-alkyl-deoxyiminosugars: anti-inflammatory response to Pseudomonas aeruginosa infections for application in CF lung disease. *Eur. J. Med. Chem.* 175, 63–71. doi: 10.1016/j.ejmech.2019.04.061

De Santi, C., Fernandez Fernandez, E., Gaul, R., Vencken, S., Glasgow, A., Oglesby, I. K., et al. (2020). Precise Targeting of miRNA Sites Restores CFTR Activity in CF Bronchial Epithelial Cells. *Mol. Ther.* 28 (4), 1190–1199. doi: 10.1016/j.ymthe.2020.02.001

Delacourt, C., Le Bourgeois, M., D'Ortho, M. P., Doit, C., Scheinmann, P., Navarro, J., et al. (1995). Imbalance between 95 kDa type IV collagenase and tissue inhibitor of metalloproteinases in sputum of patients with cystic fibrosis. *Am. J. Respir. Crit. Care Med.* 152, 765–774. doi: 10.1164/ajrccm.152.2.7633740

Dif, F., Wu, Y. Z., Burgel, P. R., Ollero, M., Leduc, D., Aarbiou, J., et al. (2010). Critical role of cytosolic phospholipase A2{alpha} in bronchial mucus hypersecretion in CFTR-deficient mice. *Eur. Respir. J.* 36, 1120–1130. doi: 10.1183/09031936.00183409

Donaldson, S. H., Solomon, G. M., Zeitlin, P. L., Flume, P. A., Casey, A., McCoy, K., et al. (2017). Pharmacokinetics and safety of cavosonstat (N91115) in healthy and cystic fibrosis adults homozygous for F508DEL-CFTR. *J. Cystic Fibrosis* 16, 371–379. doi: 10.1016/j.jcf.2017.01.009

Doring, G. (2010). Prevention of Pseudomonas aeruginosa infection in cystic fibrosis patients. *Int. J. Med. Microbiol.* 300, 573–577. doi: 10.1016/j.ijmm.2010.08.010

Duijvestijn, Y. C., and Brand, P. L. (1999). Systematic review of N-acetylcysteine in cystic fibrosis. *Acta Paediatr.* 88, 38–41. doi: 10.1111/j.1651-2227.1999.tb01265.x

Ehre, C., Ridley, C., and Thornton, D. J. (2014). Cystic fibrosis: an inherited disease affecting mucin-producing organs. *Int. J. Biochem. Cell Biol.* 52, 136–145. doi: 10.1016/j.biocel.2014.03.011

Ehre, C., Rushton, Z. L., Wang, B., Hothem, L. N., Morrison, C. B., Fontana, N. C., et al. (2019). An Improved Inhaled Mucolytic to Treat Airway Muco-obstructive Diseases. *Am. J. Respir. Crit. Care Med.* 199, 171–180. doi: 10.1164/rccm.201802-0245OC

Elborn, J. S., Horsley, A., MacGregor, G., Bilton, D., Grosswald, R., Ahuja, S., et al. (2017). Phase I Studies of Acebilustat: Biomarker Response and Safety in Patients with Cystic Fibrosis. *Clin. Transl. Sci.* 10, 28–34. doi: 10.1111/cts.12428

Elborn, J. S., Ahuja, S., Springman, E., Mershon, J., Grosswald, R., and Rowe, S. M. (2018). EMPIRE-CF: A phase II randomized placebo-controlled trial of once-daily, oral acebilustat in adult patients with cystic fibrosis - Study design and patient demographics. *Contemp. Clin. Trials* 72, 86–94. doi: 10.1016/j.cct.2018.07.014

Elborn, J. S. (2016). Cystic fibrosis. *Lancet* 388 (10059), 2519–2531. doi: 10.1016/S0140-6736(16)00576-6

Epps, Q. J., Epps, K. L., Young, D. C., and Zobell, J. T. (2019). State of the art in cystic fibrosis pharmacology—Optimization of antimicrobials in the treatment of cystic fibrosis pulmonary exacerbations: I. Anti-methicillin-resistant Staphylococcus aureus (MRSA) antibiotics. *Pediatr. Pulmonol.* 55 (1), 35–57. doi: 10.1002/ppul.24537

Equi, A., Balfour-Lynn, I. M., Bush, A., and Rosenthal, M. (2002). Long term azithromycin in children with cystic fibrosis: a randomised, placebo-controlled crossover trial. *Lancet* 360, 978–984. doi: 10.1016/S0140-6736(02)11081-6

Ermund, A., Recktenwald, C. V., Skjåk-Braek, G., Meiss, L. N., Onsøyen, E., Rye, P. D., et al. (2017). OligoG CF-5/20 normalizes cystic fibrosis mucus by chelating calcium. *Clin. Exp. Pharmacol. Physiol.* 44, 639–647. doi: 10.1111/1440-1681.12744

Esther, C. R. Jr., Muhlebach, M. S., Ehre, C., Hill, D. B., Wolfgang, M. C., Kesimer, M., et al. (2019). Mucus accumulation in the lungs precedes structural changes and infection in children with cystic fibrosis. *Sci. Transl. Med.* 11, eaav3488. doi: 10.1126/scitranslmed.aav3488

Fabbri, E., Borgatti, M., Montagner, G., Bianchi, N., Finotti, A., Lampronti, I., et al. (2014). Expression of miR-93 and IL-8 During Pseudomonas aeruginosa Mediated Induction of Pro-Inflammatory Responses. *Am. J. Respir. Cell Mol. Biol.* 50 (6), 1144–1155. doi: 10.1165/rcmb.2013-0160OC

Fahy, J. V., and Dickey, B. F. (2010). Airway mucus function and dysfunction. *N. Engl. J. Med.* 363, 2233–2247. doi: 10.1056/NEJMra0910061

Finlay, B. B., and Hancock, R. E. (2004). Can innate immunity be enhanced to treat microbial infections? *Nat. Rev. Microbiol.* 2, 497–504. doi: 10.1038/nrmicro908

Freedman, S. D., Blanco, P. G., Zaman, M. M., Shea, J. C., Ollero, M., Hopper, I. K., et al. (2004). Association of cystic fibrosis with abnormalities in fatty acid metabolism. *N. Engl. J. Med.* 350, 560–569. doi: 10.1056/NEJMoa021218

Fu, P., Ebenezer, D. L., Ha, A. W., Suryadevara, V., Harijith, A., and Natarajan, V. (2018). Nuclear lipid mediators: Role of nuclear sphingolipids and sphingosine-1-phosphate signaling in epigenetic regulation of inflammation and gene expression. *J. Cell. Biochem.* 119 (8), 6337–6353. doi: 10.1002/jcb.26707

Gaggar, A., Hector, A., Bratcher, P. E., Mall, M. A., Griese, M., and Hartl, D. (2011). The role of matrix metalloproteinases in cystic fibrosis lung disease. *Eur. Respir. J.* 38, 721–727. doi: 10.1183/09031936.00173210

Gaggar, A., Chen, J., Chmiel, J. F., Dorkin, H. L., Flume, P. A., Griffin, R., et al. (2016). Inhaled alpha1-proteinase inhibitor therapy in patients with cystic fibrosis. *J. Cyst. Fibros* 15, 227–233. doi: 10.1016/j.jcf.2015.07.009

Galli, F., Battistoni, A., Gambari, R., Pompella, A., Bragonzi, A., Pilolli, F., et al. (2012). Fibrosis, Oxidative stress and antioxidant therapy in cystic fibrosis. *Biochim. Biophys. Acta* 1822, 690–713. doi: 10.1016/j.bbadis.2011.12.012

Garcia-Verdugo, I., Benmohamed, F., Tattermusch, S., Leduc, D., Charpigny, G., Chignard, M., et al. (2012). A role for 12R-lipoxygenase in MUC5AC expression by respiratory epithelial cells. *Eur. Respirat. J.* 40, 714–723. doi: 10.1183/09031936.00023111

Geitani, R., Ayoub Moubareck, C., Touqui, L., and Karam Sarkis, D. (2019). Cationic antimicrobial peptides: alternatives and/or adjuvants to antibiotics active against methicillin-resistant Staphylococcus aureus and multidrug-resistant Pseudomonas aeruginosa. *BMC Microbiol.* 19, 54. doi: 10.1186/s12866-019-1416-8

Giroir, B. P., Scannon, P. J., and Levin, M. (2001). Bactericidal/permeability-increasing protein–lessons learned from the phase III, randomized, clinical trial of rBPI21 for adjunctive treatment of children with severe meningococcemia. *Crit. Care Med.* 29, S130–S135. doi: 10.1097/00003246-200107001-00039

Glasgow, A. M. A., De Santi, C., and Greene, C. M. (2018). Non-coding RNA in cystic fibrosis. *Biochem. Soc. Trans.* 46 (3), 619–630. doi: 10.1042/BST20170469

Gregory, S. M., Nazir, S. A., and Metcalf, J. P. (2011). Implications of the innate immune response to adenovirus and adenoviral vectors. *Future Virol.* 6, 357–374. doi: 10.2217/fvl.11.6

Guilbault, C., De Sanctis, J. B., Wojewodka, G., Saeed, Z., Lachance, C., Skinner, T. A., et al. (2008). Fenretinide corrects newly found ceramide deficiency in cystic fibrosis. *Am. J. Respir. Cell Mol. Biol.* 38, 47–56. doi: 10.1165/rcmb.2007-0036OC

Guilbault, C., Wojewodka, G., Saeed, Z., Hajduch, M., Matouk, E., De Sanctis, J. B., et al. (2009). Cystic fibrosis fatty acid imbalance is linked to ceramide deficiency and corrected by fenretinide. *Am. J. Respir. Cell Mol. Biol.* 41, 100–106. doi: 10.1165/rcmb.2008-0279OC

Guntupalli, K., Dean, N., Morris, P. E., Bandi, V., Margolis, B., Rivers, E., et al. (2013). A phase 2 randomized, double-blind, placebo-controlled study of the safety and efficacy of talactoferrin in patients with severe sepsis. *Crit. Care Med.* 41, 706–716. doi: 10.1097/CCM.0b013e3182741551

Halford, G. M., Lordkipanidzé, M., and Watson, S. P. (2012). 50th anniversary of the discovery of ibuprofen: an interview with Dr Stewart Adams. *Platelets* 23, 415–422. doi: 10.3109/09537104.2011.632032

Hancock, R. E. W., Haney, E. F., and Gill, E. E. (2016). The immunology of host defence peptides: beyond antimicrobial activity. *Nat. Rev. Immunol.* 16, 321–334. doi: 10.1038/nri.2016.29

Haydar, D., Cory, T. J., Birket, S. E., Murphy, B. S., Pennypacker, K. R., Sinai, A. P., et al. (2019). Azithromycin Polarizes Macrophages to an M2 Phenotype via Inhibition of the STAT1 and NF-κB Signaling Pathways. *J. Immunol.* 203, 1021–1030. doi: 10.4049/jimmunol.1801228

Henderson, A. G., Ehre, C., Button, B., Abdullah, L. H., Cai, L. H., Leigh, M. W., et al. (2014). Cystic fibrosis airway secretions exhibit mucin hyperconcentration and increased osmotic pressure. *J. Clin. Invest.* 124, 3047–3060. doi: 10.1172/JCI73469

Henke, M. O., and Ratjen, F. (2007). Mucolytics in cystic fibrosis. *Paediatric Respirat. Rev.* 8, 24–29. doi: 10.1016/j.prrv.2007.02.009

Higgins, G., Ringholz, F., Buchanan, P., McNally, P., and Urbach, V. (2015). Physiological impact of abnormal lipoxin A(4) production on cystic fibrosis airway epithelium and therapeutic potential. *BioMed. Res. Int.* 2015, 781087. doi: 10.1155/2015/781087

Horati, H., Janssens, H. M., Margaroli, C., Veltman, M., Stolarczyk, M., Kilgore, M. B., et al. (2020). Airway profile of bioactive lipids predicts early progression of lung disease in cystic fibrosis. *J. Cystic Fibrosis.* 46 (3), 619–630. doi: 10.1016/j.jcf.2020.01.010

Hou, M., Sun, R., Hupe, M., Kim, P. L., Park, K., Crumrine, D., et al. (2013). Topical apigenin improves epidermal permeability barrier homoeostasis in normal murine skin by divergent mechanisms. *Exp. Dermatol.* 22, 210–215. doi: 10.1111/exd.12102

Hubeau, C., Lorenzato, M., Couetil, J. P., Hubert, D., Dusser, D., Puchelle, E., et al. (2001). Quantitative analysis of inflammatory cells infiltrating the cystic fibrosis airway mucosa. *Clin. Exp. Immunol.* 124, 69–76. doi: 10.1046/j.1365-2249.2001.01456.x

Hunt, A. M. D., Glasgow, A. M. A., Humphreys, H., and Greene, C. M. (2020). Alpha-1 Antitrypsin-A Target for MicroRNA-Based Therapeutic Development for Cystic Fibrosis. *Int. J. Mol. Sci.* 21, 836. doi: 10.3390/ijms21030836

Ideozu, J. E., Zhang, X., McColley, S., and Levy, H. (2019). Transcriptome Profiling and Molecular Therapeutic Advances in Cystic Fibrosis: Recent Insights. *Genes (Basel)* 10, 180. doi: 10.3390/genes10030180

Jacquot, J., Tabary, O., Le Rouzic, P., and Clement, A. (2008a). Airway epithelial cell inflammatory signalling in cystic fibrosis. *Int. J. Biochem. Cell Biol.* 40, 1703–1715. doi: 10.1016/j.biocel.2008.02.002

Jacquot, J., Tabary, O., and Clement, A. (2008b). Hyperinflammation in airways of cystic fibrosis patients: what's new? *Expert Rev. Mol. Diagn.* 8, 359–363. doi: 10.1586/14737159.8.4.359

Jarosz-Griffiths, H. H., Scambler, T., Wong, C. H., Lara-Reyna, S., Holbrook, J., Martinon, F., et al. (2020). Different CFTR modulator combinations downregulate inflammation differently in cystic fibrosis. *Elife* 9. doi: 10.7554/eLife.54556

Jung, J., Nam, J. H., Park, H. W., Oh, U., Yoon, J. H., and Lee, M. G. (2013). Dynamic modulation of ANO1/TMEM16A HCO3(-) permeability by Ca2+/calmodulin. *Proc. Natl. Acad. Sci. U.S.A.* 110, 360–365. doi: 10.1073/pnas.1211594110

Karp, C. L., Flick, L. M., Park, K. W., Softic, S., Greer, T. M., Keledjian, R., et al. (2004). Defective lipoxin-mediated anti-inflammatory activity in the cystic fibrosis airway. *Nat. Immunol.* 5, 388–392. doi: 10.1038/ni1056

Keating, D., Marigowda, G., Burr, L., Daines, C., Mall, M. A., McKone, E. F., et al. (2018). VX-445-Tezacaftor-Ivacaftor in Patients with Cystic Fibrosis and One or Two Phe508del Alleles. *N. Engl. J. Med.* 379, 1612–1620. doi: 10.1056/NEJMoa1807120

Khan, T. Z., Wagener, J. S., Bost, T., Martinez, J., Accurso, F. J., and Riches, D. W. (1995). Early pulmonary inflammation in infants with cystic fibrosis. *Am. J. Respir. Crit. Care Med.* 151, 1075–1082. doi: 10.1164/ajrccm/151.4.1075

Khan, M. A., Ali, Z. S., Sweezey, N., Grasemann, H., and Palaniyar, N. (2019). Progression of Cystic Fibrosis Lung Disease from Childhood to Adulthood: Neutrophils, Neutrophil Extracellular Trap (NET) Formation, and NET Degradation. *Genes* 10, 183. doi: 10.3390/genes10030183

Kim, B. J., Rho, Y. K., Lee, H. I., Jeong, M. S., Li, K., Seo, S. J., et al. (2009). The effect of calcipotriol on the expression of human beta defensin-2 and LL-37 in cultured human keratinocytes. *Clin. Dev. Immunol.* 2009, 645898. doi: 10.1155/2009/645898

Knowles, M. R., Clarke, L. L., and Boucher, R. C. (1991). Activation by extracellular nucleotides of chloride secretion in the airway epithelia of patients with cystic fibrosis. *N. Engl. J. Med.* 325, 533–538. doi: 10.1056/NEJM199108223250802

Konstan, M. W., Krenicky, J. E., Finney, M. R., Kirchner, H. L., Hilliard, K. A., Hilliard, J. B., et al. (2003). Effect of ibuprofen on neutrophil migration in vivo in cystic fibrosis and healthy subjects. *J. Pharmacol. Exp. Ther.* 306, 1086–1091. doi: 10.1124/jpet.103.052449

Konstantinidis, T., Kambas, K., Mitsios, A., Panopoulou, M., Tsironidou, V., Dellaporta, E., et al. (2016). Immunomodulatory Role of Clarithromycin in Acinetobacter baumannii Infection via Formation of Neutrophil Extracellular Traps. *Antimicrobial. Agents Chemother.* 60, 1040–1048. doi: 10.1128/AAC.02063-15

Kudoh, S., Uetake, T., Hagiwara, K., Hirayama, M., Hus, L. H., Kimura, H., et al. (1987). Clinical effects of low-dose long-term erythromycin chemotherapy on diffuse panbronchiolitis. *Nihon Kyobu Shikkan Gakkai zasshi* 25, 632–642.

Kurumbail, R. G., Stevens, A. M., Gierse, J. K., McDonald, J. J., Stegeman, R. A., Pak, J. Y., et al. (1996). Structural basis for selective inhibition of cyclooxygenase-2 by anti-inflammatory agents. *Nature* 384, 644–648. doi: 10.1038/384644a0

Lai, Y., and Gallo, R. L. (2009). AMPed up immunity: how antimicrobial peptides have multiple roles in immune defense. *Trends Immunol.* 30, 131–141. doi: 10.1016/j.it.2008.12.003

Lampronti, I., Dechecchi, M. C., Rimessi, A., Bezzerri, V., Nicolis, E., Guerrini, A., et al. (2017). beta-Sitosterol Reduces the Expression of Chemotactic Cytokine Genes in Cystic Fibrosis Bronchial Epithelial Cells. *Front. Pharmacol.* 8, 236. doi: 10.3389/fphar.2017.00236

Lands, L. C., and Stanojevic, S. (2007). Oral non-steroidal anti-inflammatory drug therapy for cystic fibrosis. *Cochrane Database Syst. Rev.* 4, CD001505. doi: 10.1002/14651858.CD001505.pub2

Lands, L. C., and Stanojevic, S. (2016). Oral non-steroidal anti-inflammatory drug therapy for lung disease in cystic fibrosis. *Cochrane Database Syst. Rev.* 4, CD001505. doi: 10.1002/14651858.CD001505.pub4

Lands, L. C., and Stanojevic, S. (2019). Oral non-steroidal anti-inflammatory drug therapy for lung disease in cystic fibrosis. *Cochrane Database Syst. Rev.* doi: 10.1002/14651858.CD001505.pub5

Laselva, O., Stone, T. A., Bear, C. E., and Deber, C. M. (2020). Anti-Infectives Restore ORKAMBI((R)) Rescue of F508del-CFTR Function in Human Bronchial Epithelial Cells Infected with Clinical Strains of P. aeruginosa. *Biomolecules* 10, 334. doi: 10.3390/biom10020334

Law, N., Logan, C., Yung, G., Furr, C. L., Lehman, S. M., Morales, S., et al. (2019). Successful adjunctive use of bacteriophage therapy for treatment of multidrug-resistant Pseudomonas aeruginosa infection in a cystic fibrosis patient. *Infection* 47, 665–668. doi: 10.1007/s15010-019-01319-0

Lazaar, A. L., Sweeney, L. E., MacDonald, A. J., Alexis, N. E., Chen, C., and Tal-Singer, R. (2011). SB-656933, a novel CXCR2 selective antagonist, inhibits ex vivo neutrophil activation and ozone-induced airway inflammation in humans. *Br. J. Clin. Pharmacol.* 72, 282–293. doi: 10.1111/j.1365-2125.2011.03968.x

Lecaille, F., Lalmanach, G., and Andrault, P. M. (2016). Antimicrobial proteins and peptides in human lung diseases: A friend and foe partnership with host proteases. *Biochimie* 122, 151–168. doi: 10.1016/j.biochi.2015.08.014

Lopes-Pacheco, M. (2019). CFTR Modulators: The Changing Face of Cystic Fibrosis in the Era of Precision Medicine. *Front. Pharmacol.* 10, 1662. doi: 10.3389/fphar.2019.01662

Loth, K., Vergnes, A., Barreto, C., Voisin, S. N., Meudal, H., Da Silva, J., et al. (2019). The Ancestral N-Terminal Domain of Big Defensins Drives Bacterially Triggered Assembly into Antimicrobial Nanonets. *mBio* 10, e01821-19. doi: 10.1128/mBio.01821-19

Lubamba, B., Lebacq, J., Reychler, G., Marbaix, E., Wallemacq, P., Lebecque, P., et al. (2011). Inhaled phosphodiesterase type 5 inhibitors restore chloride transport in cystic fibrosis mice. *Eur. Respir. J.* 37, 72–78. doi: 10.1183/09031936.00013510

Magrone, T., Russo, M. A., and Jirillo, E. (2018). Antimicrobial Peptides in Human Disease: Therapeutic Approaches. Second of Two Parts. *Curr. Pharm. Des.* 24, 1148–1156. doi: 10.2174/1381612824666180327155230

Masera, R. G., Bateman, A., Muscettola, M., Solomon, S., and Angeli, A. (1996). Corticostatins/defensins inhibit in vitro NK activity and cytokine production by human peripheral blood mononuclear cells. *Regul. Pept.* 62, 13–21. doi: 10.1016/0167-0115(95)00150-6

Mayer, M. (2016). Lumacaftor-ivacaftor (Orkambi) for cystic fibrosis: behind the 'breakthrough'. *Evid. Based. Med.* 21, 83–86. doi: 10.1136/ebmed-2015-110325

McElvaney, N. G., Doujaiji, B., Moan, M. J., Burnham, M. R., Wu, M. C., and Crystal, R. G. (1993). Pharmacokinetics of recombinant secretory leukoprotease inhibitor aerosolized to normals and individuals with cystic fibrosis. *Am. Rev. Respir. Dis.* 148, 1056–1060. doi: 10.1164/ajrccm/148.4_Pt_1.1056

McElvaney, O. J., Zaslona, Z., Becker-Flegler, K., Palsson-McDermott, E. M., Boland, F., Gunaratnam, C., et al. (2019). Specific Inhibition of the NLRP3 Inflammasome as an Antiinflammatory Strategy in Cystic Fibrosis. *Am. J. Respir. Crit. Care Med.* 200, 1381–1391. doi: 10.1164/rccm.201905-1013OC

McInturff, J. E., Wang, S. J., Machleidt, T., Lin, T. R., Oren, A., Hertz, C. J., et al. (2005). Granulysin-derived peptides demonstrate antimicrobial and anti-inflammatory effects against Propionibacterium acnes. *J. Invest. Dermatol.* 125, 256–263. doi: 10.1111/j.0022-202X.2005.23805.x

McKelvey, M. C., Weldon, S., McAuley, D. F., Mall, M. A., and Taggart, C. C. (2020). Targeting Proteases in Cystic Fibrosis Lung Disease. Paradigms, Progress, and Potential. *Am. J. Respir. Crit. Care Med.* 201, 141–147. doi: 10.1164/rccm.201906-1190PP

Medjane, S., Raymond, B., Wu, Y., and Touqui, L. (2005). Impact of CFTR DeltaF508 mutation on prostaglandin E2 production and type IIA phospholipase A2 expression by pulmonary epithelial cells. *Am. J. Physiol. Lung Cell Mol. Physiol.* 289, L816–L824. doi: 10.1152/ajplung.00466.2004

Middleton, P. G., Mall, M. A., Dřevínek, P., Lands, L. C., McKone, E. F., Polineni, D., et al. (2019). Elexacaftor–Tezacaftor–Ivacaftor for Cystic Fibrosis with a Single Phe508del Allele. *New Engl. J. Med.* 381, 1809–1819. doi: 10.1056/NEJMoa1908639

Mingione, A., Dei Cas, M., Bonezzi, F., Caretti, A., Piccoli, M., Anastasia, L., et al. (2020). Inhibition of Sphingolipid Synthesis as a Phenotype-Modifying Therapy in Cystic Fibrosis. *Cell Physiol. Biochem.* 54, 110–125. doi: 10.33594/000000208

Mohamed, F. B., Garcia-Verdugo, I., Medina, M., Balloy, V., Chignard, M., Ramphal, R., et al. (2012). A Crucial Role of Flagellin in the Induction of Airway Mucus Production by Pseudomonas aeruginosa. *PloS One* 7, e39888. doi: 10.1371/journal.pone.0039888

Moller-Kristensen, M., Ip, W. K. E., Shi, L., Gowda, L. D., Hamblin, M. R., Thiel, S., et al. (2006). Deficiency of Mannose-Binding Lectin Greatly Increases Susceptibility to Postburn Infection with Pseudomonas aeruginosa. *J. Immunol.* 176, 1769–1775. doi: 10.4049/jimmunol.176.3.1769

Mookherjee, N., Hamill, P., Gardy, J., Blimkie, D., Falsafi, R., Chikatamarla, A., et al. (2009). Systems biology evaluation of immune responses induced by human host defence peptide LL-37 in mononuclear cells. *Mol. Biosyst.* 5, 483–496. doi: 10.1039/b813787k

Morello, E., Saussereau, E., Maura, D., Huerre, M., Touqui, L., and Debarbieux, L. (2011). Pulmonary Bacteriophage Therapy on Pseudomonas aeruginosa Cystic Fibrosis Strains: First Steps Towards Treatment and Prevention. *PloS One* 6, e16963. doi: 10.1371/journal.pone.0016963

Morrison, G., Kilanowski, F., Davidson, D., and Dorin, J. (2002). Characterization of the Mouse Beta Defensin 1, Defb1. *Mutant Mouse Model. Infection Immun.* 70, 3053–3060. doi: 10.1128/IAI.70.6.3053-3060.2002

Moss, R. B., Mistry, S. J., Konstan, M. W., Pilewski, J. M., Kerem, E., Tal-Singer, R., et al. (2013). Safety and early treatment effects of the CXCR2 antagonist SB-656933 in patients with cystic fibrosis. *J. Cyst. Fibros* 12, 241–248. doi: 10.1016/j.jcf.2012.08.016

Moss, R. B. (2013). Pitfalls of drug development: lessons learned from trials of denufosol in cystic fibrosis. *J. Pediatr.* 162, 676–680. doi: 10.1016/j.jpeds.2012.11.034

Mueller, C., Tang, Q., Gruntman, A., Blomenkamp, K., Teckman, J., Song, L., et al. (2012). Sustained miRNA-mediated knockdown of mutant AAT with simultaneous augmentation of wild-type AAT has minimal effect on global liver miRNA profiles. *Mol. Ther.* 20, 590–600. doi: 10.1038/mt.2011.292

Muhlebach, M. S., and Noah, T. L. (2002). Endotoxin activity and inflammatory markers in the airways of young patients with cystic fibrosis. *Am. J. Respir. Crit. Care Med.* 165, 911–915. doi: 10.1164/ajrccm.165.7.2107114

Muselet-Charlier, C., Roque, T., Boncoeur, E., Chadelat, K., Clement, A., Jacquot, J., et al. (2007). Enhanced IL-1beta-induced IL-8 production in cystic fibrosis lung epithelial cells is dependent of both mitogen-activated protein kinases and NF-kappaB signaling. *Biochem. Biophys. Res. Commun.* 357, 402–407. doi: 10.1016/j.bbrc.2007.03.141

Nagaoka, I., Suzuki, K., Niyonsaba, F., Tamura, H., and Hirata, M. (2012). Modulation of Neutrophil Apoptosis by Antimicrobial Peptides. *ISRN Microbiol.* 2012, 1–12. doi: 10.5402/2012/345791

Nevitt, S. J., Thornton, J., Murray, C. S., and Dwyer, T. (2018). Inhaled mannitol for cystic fibrosis. *Cochrane Database Syst. Rev.* 2, CD008649. doi: 10.1002/14651858.CD008649.pub3

Nichols, D. P., and Chmiel, J. F. (2015). Inflammation and its genesis in cystic fibrosis. *Pediatr. Pulmonol.* 50 Suppl 40, S39–S56. doi: 10.1002/ppul.23242

Nichols, D. P., Odem-Davis, K., Cogen, J. D., Goss, C. H., Ren, C. L., Skalland, M., et al. (2020). Pulmonary Outcomes Associated with Long-Term Azithromycin Therapy in Cystic Fibrosis. *Am. J. Respir. Crit. Care Med.* 201, 430–437. doi: 10.1164/rccm.201906-1206OC

Nilius, B., and Droogmans, G. (2003). Amazing chloride channels: an overview. *Acta Physiol. Scand.* 177, 119–147. doi: 10.1046/j.1365-201X.2003.01060.x

Nixon, G. M., Armstrong, D. S., Carzino, R., Carlin, J. B., Olinsky, A., Robertson, C. F., et al. (2002). Early airway infection, inflammation, and lung function in cystic fibrosis. *Arch. Dis. Child* 87, 306–311. doi: 10.1136/adc.87.4.306

Oermann, C. M., Sockrider, M. M., and Konstan, M. W. (1999). The use of anti-inflammatory medications in cystic fibrosis: trends and physician attitudes. *Chest* 115, 1053–1058. doi: 10.1378/chest.115.4.1053

Olszowiec-Chlebna, M., Koniarek-Maniecka, A., Brzozowska, A., Blauz, A., Rychlik, B., and Stelmach, I. (2019). Vitamin D inhibits pro-inflammatory cytokines in the airways of cystic fibrosis patients infected by Pseudomonas aeruginosa- pilot study. *Ital. J. Pediatr.* 45, 41. doi: 10.1186/s13052-019-0634-x

Palser, S., Smith, S., Nash, E. F., Agarwal, A., and Smyth, A. R. (2019). Treatments for preventing recurrence of infection with Pseudomonas aeruginosa in people with cystic fibrosis. *Cochrane Database Syst. Rev.* 12, CD012300. doi: 10.1002/14651858.CD012300.pub2

Pang, Z., Raudonis, R., Glick, B. R., Lin, T.-J., and Cheng, Z. (2019). Antibiotic resistance in Pseudomonas aeruginosa: mechanisms and alternative therapeutic strategies. *Biotechnol. Adv.* 37, 177–192. doi: 10.1016/j.biotechadv.2018.11.013

Payne, S. M., and Finkelstein, R. A. (1978). The critical role of iron in host-bacterial interactions. *J. Clin. Invest.* 61, 1428–1440. doi: 10.1172/JCI109062

Pelaia, G., Cuda, G., Vatrella, A., Gallelli, L., Fratto, D., Gioffre, V., et al. (2004). Effects of hydrogen peroxide on MAPK activation, IL-8 production and cell viability in primary cultures of human bronchial epithelial cells. *J. Cell Biochem.* 93, 142–152. doi: 10.1002/jcb.20124

Perez, A., Issler, A. C., Cotton, C. U., Kelley, T. J., Verkman, A. S., and Davis, P. B. (2007). CFTR inhibition mimics the cystic fibrosis inflammatory profile. *Am. J. Physiol. Lung Cell Mol. Physiol.* 292, L383–L395. doi: 10.1152/ajplung.00403.2005

Pernet, E., Guillemot, L., Burgel, P.-R., Martin, C., Lambeau, G., Sermet-Gaudelus, I., et al. (2014). Pseudomonas aeruginosa eradicates Staphylococcus aureus by manipulating the host immunity. *Nat. Commun.* 5, 5105. doi: 10.1038/ncomms6105

Perrem, L., and Ratjen, F. (2019). Anti-inflammatories and mucociliary clearance therapies in the age of CFTR modulators. *Pediatr. Pulmonol.* 54 Suppl 3, S46–S55. doi: 10.1002/ppul.24364

Pier, G. B. (2000). Role of the cystic fibrosis transmembrane conductance regulator in innate immunity to Pseudomonas aeruginosa infections. *Proc. Natl. Acad. Sci. U.S.A.* 97, 8822–8828. doi: 10.1073/pnas.97.16.8822

Pierdomenico, A. M., Patruno, S., Codagnone, M., Simiele, F., Mari, V. C., Plebani, R., et al. (2017). microRNA-181b is increased in cystic fibrosis cells and impairs lipoxin A4 receptor-dependent mechanisms of inflammation resolution and antimicrobial defense. *Sci. Rep.* 7, 13519. doi: 10.1038/s41598-017-14055-y

Piris-Gimenez, A., Paya, M., Lambeau, G., Chignard, M., Mock, M., Touqui, L., et al. (2005). In Vivo Protective Role of Human Group IIA Phospholipase A2 against Experimental Anthrax. *J. Immunol.* 175, 6786–6791. doi: 10.4049/jimmunol.175.10.6786

Plasschaert, L. W., Zilionis, R., Choo-Wing, R., Savova, V., Knehr, J., Roma, G., et al. (2018). A single-cell atlas of the airway epithelium reveals the CFTR-rich pulmonary ionocyte. *Nature* 560, 377–381. doi: 10.1038/s41586-018-0394-6

Puchelle, E., de Bentzmann, S., and Zahm, J. M. (1995). Physical and functional properties of airway secretions in cystic fibrosis–therapeutic approaches. *Respiration* 62 Suppl 1, 2–12. doi: 10.1159/000196486

Puthia, M., Butrym, M., Petrlova, J., Stromdahl, A. C., Andersson, M. A., Kjellstrom, S., et al. (2020). A dual-action peptide-containing hydrogel targets wound infection and inflammation. *Sci. Transl. Med.* 12, eaax6601. doi: 10.1126/scitranslmed.aax6601

Quabius, E. S., Bogershausen, B., Getzin, L., Gorogh, T., Gebhard, M. P., Hoffmann, A. S., et al. (2017). SLPI and AnxA2 expression in neoplasm-free palatine tonsils is associated with smoking habit of individuals. *Mol. Clin. Oncol.* 7, 427–434. doi: 10.3892/mco.2017.1343

Quinton, P. M. (2008). Cystic fibrosis: impaired bicarbonate secretion and mucoviscidosis. *Lancet* 372, 415–417. doi: 10.1016/S0140-6736(08)61162-9

Rahman, I., and MacNee, W. (2000). Oxidative stress and regulation of glutathione in lung inflammation. *Eur. Respir. J.* 16, 534–554. doi: 10.1034/j.1399-3003.2000.016003534.x

Raia, V., Maiuri, L., De Ritis, G., De Vizia, B., Vacca, L., Conte, R., et al. (2000). Evidence of Chronic Inflammation in Morphologically Normal Small Intestine of Cystic Fibrosis Patients. *Pediatr. Res.* 47, 344–350. doi: 10.1203/00006450-200003000-00010

Ravindran, M., Khan, M. A., and Palaniyar, N. (2019). Neutrophil Extracellular Trap Formation: Physiology, Pathology, and Pharmacology. *Biomolecules* 9, 365. doi: 10.3390/biom9080365

Reid, D. W., Carroll, V., O'May, C., Champion, A., and Kirov, S. M. (2007). Increased airway iron as a potential factor in the persistence of Pseudomonas aeruginosa infection in cystic fibrosis. *Eur. Respir. J.* 30, 286–292. doi: 10.1183/09031936.00154006

Rennard, S. I., Dale, D. C., Donohue, J. F., Kanniess, F., Magnussen, H., Sutherland, E. R., et al. (2015). CXCR2 Antagonist MK-7123. A Phase 2 Proof-of-Concept Trial for Chronic Obstructive Pulmonary Disease. *Am. J. Respir. Crit. Care Med.* 191, 1001–1011. doi: 10.1164/rccm.201405-0992OC

Rhim, A. D., Stoykova, L., Glick, M. C., and Scanlin, T. F. (2001). Terminal glycosylation in cystic fibrosis (CF): a review emphasizing the airway epithelial cell. *Glycoconj J.* 18, 649–659. doi: 10.1023/A:1020815205022

Ribeiro, C. M., Paradiso, A. M., Carew, M. A., Shears, S. B., and Boucher, R. C. (2005). Cystic fibrosis airway epithelial Ca2+ i signaling: the mechanism for the larger agonist-mediated Ca2+ i signals in human cystic fibrosis airway epithelia. *J. Biol. Chem.* 280, 10202–10209. doi: 10.1074/jbc.M410617200

Riera, E., Cabot, G., Mulet, X., Garcia-Castillo, M., Del Campo, R., Juan, C., et al. (2011). Pseudomonas aeruginosa carbapenem resistance mechanisms in Spain: impact on the activity of imipenem, meropenem and doripenem. *J. Antimicrobial. Chemother.* 66, 2022–2027. doi: 10.1093/jac/dkr232

Riordan, J. R., Rommens, J. M., Kerem, B., Alon, N., Rozmahel, R., Grzelczak, Z., et al. (1989). Identification of the cystic fibrosis gene: cloning and characterization of complementary DNA. *Science* 245, 1066–1073. doi: 10.1126/science.2475911

Rivas-Santiago, B., Serrano, C. J., and Enciso-Moreno, J. A. (2009). Susceptibility to Infectious Diseases Based on Antimicrobial Peptide Production. *Infection Immun.* 77, 4690–4695. doi: 10.1128/IAI.01515-08

Rocca, J., Manin, S., Hulin, A., Aissat, A., Verbecq-Morlot, W., Pruliere-Escabasse, V., et al. (2016). New use for an old drug: COX-independent anti-inflammatory effects of sulindac in models of cystic fibrosis. *Br. J. Pharmacol.* 173, 1728–1741. doi: 10.1111/bph.13464

Roesch, E. A., Nichols, D. P., and Chmiel, J. F. (2018). Inflammation in cystic fibrosis: An update. *Pediatr. Pulmonol.* 53, S30–S50. doi: 10.1002/ppul.24129

Rogers, C. S., Stoltz, D. A., Meyerholz, D. K., Ostedgaard, L. S., Rokhlina, T., Taft, P. J., et al. (2008). Disruption of the CFTR Gene Produces a Model of Cystic Fibrosis in Newborn Pigs. *Science* 321, 1837–1841. doi: 10.1126/science.1163600

Rouillard, K. R., Hill, D. B., and Schoenfisch, M. H. (2020). Antibiofilm and mucolytic action of nitric oxide delivered via gas or macromolecular donor using in vitro and ex vivo models. *J. Cystic Fibrosis* 20, 30075–30078. doi: 10.1016/j.jcf.2020.03.004

Rowe, S. M., Daines, C., Ringshausen, F. C., Kerem, E., Wilson, J., Tullis, E., et al. (2017). Tezacaftor-Ivacaftor in Residual-Function Heterozygotes with Cystic Fibrosis. *N. Engl. J. Med.* 377, 2024–2035. doi: 10.1056/NEJMoa1709847

Ruffin, M., Voland, M., Marie, S., Bonora, M., Blanchard, E., Blouquit-Laye, S., et al. (2013). Anoctamin 1 dysregulation alters bronchial epithelial repair in cystic fibrosis. *Biochim. Biophys. Acta* 1832, 2340–2351. doi: 10.1016/j.bbadis.2013.09.012

Sagel, S. D., Sontag, M. K., Anthony, M. M., Emmett, P., and Papas, K. A. (2011). Effect of an antioxidant-rich multivitamin supplement in cystic fibrosis. *J. Cyst. Fibros* 10, 31–36. doi: 10.1016/j.jcf.2010.09.005

Saiman, L., Anstead, M., Mayer-Hamblett, N., Lands, L. C., Kloster, M., Hocevar-Trnka, J., et al. (2010). Effect of azithromycin on pulmonary function in patients with cystic fibrosis uninfected with Pseudomonas aeruginosa: a randomized controlled trial. *Jama* 303, 1707–1715. doi: 10.1001/jama.2010.563

Saint-Criq, V., Rebeyrol, C., Ruffin, M., Roque, T., Guillot, L., Jacquot, J., et al. (2011). Restoration of chloride efflux by azithromycin in airway epithelial cells of cystic fibrosis patients. *Antimicrob. Agents Chemother.* 55, 1792–1793. doi: 10.1128/AAC.01403-10

Saint-Criq, V., Ruffin, M., Rebeyrol, C., Guillot, L., Jacquot, J., Clement, A., et al. (2012). Azithromycin fails to reduce inflammation in cystic fibrosis airway epithelial cells. *Eur. J. Pharmacol.* 674, 1–6. doi: 10.1016/j.ejphar.2011.10.027

Scambler, T., Jarosz-Griffiths, H. H., Lara-Reyna, S., Pathak, S., Wong, C., Holbrook, J., et al. (2019). ENaC-mediated sodium influx exacerbates NLRP3-dependent inflammation in cystic fibrosis. *eLife* 8, e49248. doi: 10.7554/eLife.49248

Schmitt-Grohe, S., and Zielen, S. (2005). Leukotriene receptor antagonists in children with cystic fibrosis lung disease : anti-inflammatory and clinical effects. *Paediatr. Drugs* 7, 353–363. doi: 10.2165/00148581-200507060-00004

Schroeder, B. C., Cheng, T., Jan, Y. N., and Jan, L. Y. (2008). Expression cloning of TMEM16A as a calcium-activated chloride channel subunit. *Cell* 134, 1019–1029. doi: 10.1016/j.cell.2008.09.003

Scott, M. G., and Hancock, R. E. (2000). Cationic antimicrobial peptides and their multifunctional role in the immune system. *Crit. Rev. Immunol.* 20, 407–431. doi: 10.1615/CritRevImmunol.v20.i5.40

Serhan, C. N. (2017). Treating inflammation and infection in the 21st century: new hints from decoding resolution mediators and mechanisms. *FASEB J.* 31, 1273–1288. doi: 10.1096/fj.201601222R

Shah, V. S., Meyerholz, D. K., Tang, X. X., Reznikov, L., Abou Alaiwa, M., Ernst, S. E., et al. (2016). Airway acidification initiates host defense abnormalities in cystic fibrosis mice. *Science* 351, 503–507. doi: 10.1126/science.aad5589

Shamseer, L., Adams, D., Brown, N., Johnson, J. A., and Vohra, S. (2010). Antioxidant micronutrients for lung disease in cystic fibrosis. *Cochrane Database Syst. Rev.* 12, CD007020. doi: 10.1002/14651858.CD007020.pub2

Shao, M. X. G., Ueki, I. F., and Nadel, J. A. (2003). Tumor necrosis factor -converting enzyme mediates MUC5AC mucin expression in cultured human airway epithelial cells. *Proc. Natl. Acad. Sci.* 100, 11618–11623. doi: 10.1073/pnas.1534804100

Shi, X., Gao, Z., Lin, Q., Zhao, L., Ma, Q., Kang, Y., et al. (2019). Meta-analysis Reveals Potential Influence of Oxidative Stress on the Airway Microbiomes of Cystic Fibrosis Patients. *Genom. Proteomics Bioinf.* 17, 590–602. doi: 10.1016/j.gpb.2018.03.009

Shim, D.-W., Heo, K.-H., Kim, Y.-K., Sim, E.-J., Kang, T.-B., Choi, J.-W., et al. (2015). Anti-Inflammatory Action of an Antimicrobial Model Peptide That Suppresses the TRIF-Dependent Signaling Pathway via Inhibition of Toll-Like Receptor 4 Endocytosis in Lipopolysaccharide-Stimulated Macrophages. *PloS One* 10, e0126871. doi: 10.1371/journal.pone.0126871

Shoseyov, D., Cohen-Cymberknoh, M., and Wilschanski, M. (2016). Ataluren for the treatment of cystic fibrosis. *Expert Rev. Respir. Med.* 10, 387–391. doi: 10.1586/17476348.2016.1150181

Simoes, F. B., Quaresma, M. C., Clarke, L. A., Silva, I. A., Pankonien, I., Railean, V., et al. (2019). TMEM16A chloride channel does not drive mucus production. *Life Sci. Alliance* 2, e201900462. doi: 10.26508/lsa.201900462

Simonin, J., Bille, E., Crambert, G., Noel, S., Dreano, E., Edwards, A., et al. (2019). Airway surface liquid acidification initiates host defense abnormalities in Cystic Fibrosis. *Sci. Rep.* 9, 6516. doi: 10.1038/s41598-019-42751-4

Siwamogsatham, O., Dong, W., Binongo, J. N., Chowdhury, R., Alvarez, J. A., Feinman, S. J., et al. (2014). Relationship Between Fat-Soluble Vitamin Supplementation and Blood Concentrations in Adolescent and Adult Patients With Cystic Fibrosis. *Nutr. Clin. Pract.* 29, 491–497. doi: 10.1177/0884533614530170

Skovbakke, S. L., and Franzyk, H. (2017). Anti-inflammatory Properties of Antimicrobial Peptides and Peptidomimetics: LPS and LTA Neutralization. *Methods Mol. Biol.* 1548, 369–386. doi: 10.1007/978-1-4939-6737-7_27

Smithrithee, R., Niyonsaba, F., Kiatsurayanon, C., Ushio, H., Ikeda, S., Okumura, K., et al. (2015). Human β-defensin-3 increases the expression of interleukin-37 through CCR6 in human keratinocytes. *J. Dermatol. Sci.* 77, 46–53. doi: 10.1016/j.jdermsci.2014.12.001

Song, K. S., Lee, W.-J., Chung, K. C., Koo, J. S., Yang, E. J., Choi, J. Y., et al. (2003). Interleukin-1β and Tumor Necrosis Factor-α InduceMUC5ACOverexpression through a Mechanism Involving ERK/p38 Mitogen-activated Protein Kinases-MSK1-CREB Activation in Human Airway Epithelial Cells. *J. Biol. Chem.* 278, 23243–23250. doi: 10.1074/jbc.M300096200

Song, Y., Salinas, D., Nielson, D. W., and Verkman, A. S. (2006). Hyperacidity of secreted fluid from submucosal glands in early cystic fibrosis. *Am. J. Physiol. Cell Physiol.* 290, C741–C749. doi: 10.1152/ajpcell.00379.2005

Sonneville, F., Ruffin, M., Coraux, C., Rousselet, N., Rouzic, P. L., Blouquit-Laye, S., et al. (2017). MicroRNA-9 downregulates the ANO1 chloride channel and contributes to cystic fibrosis lung pathology. *Nat. Commun.* 8, 710. doi: 10.1038/s41467-017-00813-z

Sorio, C., Montresor, A., Bolomini-Vittori, M., Caldrer, S., Rossi, B., Dusi, S., et al. (2016). Mutations of Cystic Fibrosis Transmembrane Conductance Regulator Gene Cause a Monocyte-Selective Adhesion Deficiency. *Am. J. Respiratory Crit. Care Med.* 193, 1123–1133. doi: 10.1164/rccm.201510-1922OC

Southern, K. W., and Barker, P. M. (2004). Azithromycin for cystic fibrosis. *Eur. Respiratory J.* 24, 834–838. doi: 10.1183/09031936.04.00084304

Southern, K. W., Barker, P. M., Solis-Moya, A., and Patel, L. (2012). Macrolide antibiotics for cystic fibrosis. *Cochrane Database Syst. Rev.* 11, CD002203. doi: 10.1002/14651858.CD002203.pub4

Stoltz, D. A., Meyerholz, D. K., Pezzulo, A. A., Ramachandran, S., Rogan, M. P., Davis, G. J., et al. (2010). Cystic fibrosis pigs develop lung disease and exhibit defective bacterial eradication at birth. *Sci. Trans. Med.* 2, 29ra31–29ra31. doi: 10.1126/scitranslmed.3000928

Stoltz, D. A., Meyerholz, D. K., and Welsh, M. J. (2015). Origins of cystic fibrosis lung disease. *New Engl. J. Med.* 372, 351–362. doi: 10.1056/NEJMra1300109

Strandvik, B. (2010). Fatty acid metabolism in cystic fibrosis. *Prostaglandins Leukot. Essent. Fatty Acids* 83, 121–129. doi: 10.1016/j.plefa.2010.07.002

Summers, W. C. (2001). Bacteriophage Therapy. *Annu. Rev. Microbiol.* 55, 437–451. doi: 10.1146/annurev.micro.55.1.437

Sun, Y., and Shang, D. (2015). Inhibitory Effects of Antimicrobial Peptides on Lipopolysaccharide-Induced Inflammation. *Mediators Inflammation* 2015, 1–8. doi: 10.1155/2015/167572

Sun, X., Sui, H., Fisher, J. T., Yan, Z., Liu, X., Cho, H.-J., et al. (2010). Disease phenotype of a ferret CFTR-knockout model of cystic fibrosis. *J. Clin. Invest.* 120, 3149–3160. doi: 10.1172/JCI43052

Tabary, O., Zahm, J. M., Hinnrasky, J., Couetil, J. P., Cornillet, P., Guenounou, M., et al. (1998). Selective up-regulation of chemokine IL-8 expression in cystic fibrosis bronchial gland cells in vivo and in vitro. *Am. J. Pathol.* 153, 921–930. doi: 10.1016/S0002-9440(10)65633-7

Tabary, O., Escotte, S., Couetil, J. P., Hubert, D., Dusser, D., Puchelle, E., et al. (1999). Genistein inhibits constitutive and inducible NFkappaB activation and decreases IL-8 production by human cystic fibrosis bronchial gland cells. *Am. J. Pathol.* 155, 473–481. doi: 10.1016/S0002-9440(10)65143-7

Tabary, O., Muselet, C., Escotte, S., Antonicelli, F., Hubert, D., Dusser, D., et al. (2003). Interleukin-10 Inhibits Elevated Chemokine Interleukin-8 and Regulated on Activation Normal T Cell Expressed and Secreted Production in Cystic Fibrosis Bronchial Epithelial Cells by Targeting the I(k)B Kinase alpha/beta Complex. *Am. J. Pathol.* 162, 293–302. doi: 10.1016/S0002-9440(10)63820-5

Tabary, O., Boncoeur, E., de Martin, R., Pepperkok, R., Clement, A., Schultz, C., et al. (2006a). Calcium-dependent regulation of NF-(kappa)B activation in cystic fibrosis airway epithelial cells. *Cell Signal* 18, 652–660. doi: 10.1016/j.cellsig.2005.06.004

Tabary, O., Corvol, H., Boncoeur, E., Chadelat, K., Fitting, C., Cavaillon, J. M., et al. (2006b). Adherence of airway neutrophils and inflammatory response are increased in CF airway epithelial cell-neutrophil interactions. *Am. J. Physiol. Lung Cell Mol. Physiol.* 290, L588–L596. doi: 10.1152/ajplung.00013.2005

Taggart, C., Coakley, R. J., Greally, P., Canny, G., O'Neill, S. J., and McElvaney, N. G. (2000). Increased elastase release by CF neutrophils is mediated by tumor necrosis factor-alpha and interleukin-8. *Am. J. Physiol. Lung Cell Mol. Physiol.* 278, L33–L41. doi: 10.1152/ajplung.2000.278.1.L33

Tarran, R., Grubb, B. R., Parsons, D., Picher, M., Hirsh, A. J., Davis, C. W., et al. (2001). The CF salt controversy: in vivo observations and therapeutic approaches. *Mol. Cell* 8, 149–158. doi: 10.1016/S1097-2765(01)00286-6

Tarrant, B. J., Le Maitre, C., Romero, L., Steward, R., Button, B. M., Thompson, B. R., et al. (2017). Mucoactive agents for chronic, non-cystic fibrosis lung disease: A systematic review and meta-analysis. *Respirology* 22, 1084–1092. doi: 10.1111/resp.13047

Taylor-Cousar, J. L., Wiley, C., Felton, L. A., St Clair, C., Jones, M., Curran-Everett, D., et al. (2015). Pharmacokinetics and tolerability of oral sildenafil in adults with cystic fibrosis lung disease. *J. Cyst. Fibros* 14, 228–236. doi: 10.1016/j.jcf.2014.10.006

Teichgräber, V., Ulrich, M., Endlich, N., Riethmüller, J., Wilker, B., De Oliveira-Munding, C. C., et al. (2008). Ceramide accumulation mediates inflammation, cell death and infection susceptibility in cystic fibrosis. *Nat. Med.* 14, 382–391. doi: 10.1038/nm1748

Tirouvanziam, R., de Bentzmann, S., Hubeau, C., Hinnrasky, J., Jacquot, J., Peault, B., et al. (2000). Inflammation and infection in naive human cystic fibrosis airway grafts. *Am. J. Respir. Cell Mol. Biol.* 23, 121–127. doi: 10.1165/ajrcmb.23.2.4214

Tirouvanziam, R., Khazaal, I., and Peault, B. (2002). Primary inflammation in human cystic fibrosis small airways. *Am. J. Physiol. Lung Cell Mol. Physiol.* 283, L445–L451. doi: 10.1152/ajplung.00419.2001

Tirouvanziam, R., Conrad, C. K., Bottiglieri, T., Herzenberg, L. A., and Moss, R. B. (2006). High-dose oral N-acetylcysteine, a glutathione prodrug, modulates inflammation in cystic fibrosis. *Proc. Natl. Acad. Sci. U.S.A.* 103, 4628–4633. doi: 10.1073/pnas.0511304103

Tovar-García, A., Angarita-Zapata, V., Cazares, A., Jasso-Chávez, R., Belmont-Díaz, J., Sanchez-Torres, V., et al. (2020). Characterization of gallium resistance induced in a Pseudomonas aeruginosa cystic fibrosis isolate. *Arch. Microbiol.* 202, 617–622. doi: 10.1007/s00203-019-01777-y

Traczewski, M. M., and Brown, S. D. (2006). In Vitro Activity of Doripenem against Pseudomonas aeruginosa and Burkholderia cepacia Isolates from both Cystic Fibrosis and Non-Cystic Fibrosis Patients. *Antimicrobial. Agents Chemother.* 50, 819–821. doi: 10.1128/AAC.50.2.819-821.2006

Tuggle, K. L., Birket, S. E., Cui, X., Hong, J., Warren, J., Reid, L., et al. (2014). Characterization of Defects in Ion Transport and Tissue Development in Cystic Fibrosis Transmembrane Conductance Regulator (CFTR)-Knockout Rats. *PloS One* 9, e91253. doi: 10.1371/journal.pone.0091253

Van Hensbergen, V. P., Wu, Y., Van Sorge, N. M., and Touqui, L. (2020). Type IIA Secreted Phospholipase A2 in Host Defense against Bacterial Infections. *Trends Immunol.* 41, 313–326. doi: 10.1016/j.it.2020.02.003

Varrassi, G., Pergolizzi, J. V., Dowling, P., and Paladini, A. (2020). Ibuprofen Safety at the Golden Anniversary: Are all NSAIDs the Same? A Narrative Review. *Adv. Ther.* 37, 61–82. doi: 10.1007/s12325-019-01144-9

Veit, G., Bossard, F., Goepp, J., Verkman, A. S., Galietta, L. J., Hanrahan, J. W., et al. (2012). Proinflammatory cytokine secretion is suppressed by TMEM16A or CFTR channel activity in human cystic fibrosis bronchial epithelia. *Mol. Biol. Cell* 23, 4188–4202. doi: 10.1091/mbc.e12-06-0424

Vencken, S., Foged, C., Ramsey, J. M., Sweeney, L., Cryan, S. A., MacLoughlin, R. J., et al. (2019). Nebulised lipid-polymer hybrid nanoparticles for the delivery of a therapeutic anti-inflammatory microRNA to bronchial epithelial cells. *ERJ Open Res.* 5, 00161–2018. doi: 10.1183/23120541.00161-2018

Venkatakrishnan, V., Packer, N. H., and Thaysen-Andersen, M. (2013). Host mucin glycosylation plays a role in bacterial adhesion in lungs of individuals with cystic fibrosis. *Expert Rev. Respir. Med.* 7, 553–576. doi: 10.1586/17476348.2013.837752

Vilela, R. M., Lands, L. C., Meehan, B., and Kubow, S. (2006). Inhibition of IL-8 release from CFTR-deficient lung epithelial cells following pre-treatment with fenretinide. *Int. Immunopharmacol.* 6, 1651–1664. doi: 10.1016/j.intimp.2006.06.012

Vincent, J. L., Marshall, J. C., Dellinger, R. P., Simonson, S. G., Guntupalli, K., Levy, M. M., et al. (2015). Talactoferrin in Severe Sepsis: Results From the Phase II/III Oral tAlactoferrin in Severe sepsIS Trial. *Crit. Care Med.* 43, 1832–1838. doi: 10.1097/CCM.0000000000001090

Wainwright, C. E., Elborn, J. S., Ramsey, B. W., Marigowda, G., Huang, X., Cipolli, M., et al. (2015). Lumacaftor-Ivacaftor in Patients with Cystic Fibrosis Homozygous for Phe508del CFTR. *N. Engl. J. Med.* 373 (3), 220–231. doi: 10.1056/NEJMoa1409547

Wang, J., Dou, X., Song, J., Lyu, Y., Zhu, X., Xu, L., et al. (2019). Antimicrobial peptides: Promising alternatives in the post feeding antibiotic era. *Med. Res. Rev.* 39, 831–859. doi: 10.1002/med.21542

Wark, P., and McDonald, V. M. (2018). Nebulised hypertonic saline for cystic fibrosis. *Cochrane Database Syst. Rev.* 9, CD001506. doi: 10.1002/14651858.CD001506.pub4

Waters, V., and Smyth, A. (2015). Cystic fibrosis microbiology: Advances in antimicrobial therapy. *J. Cyst. Fibros.* 14, 551–560. doi: 10.1016/j.jcf.2015.02.005

Waters, V. (2018). Chronic Antibiotic Use in Cystic Fibrosis: A Fine Balance. *Ann. Am. Thoracic Soc.* 15, 667–668. doi: 10.1513/AnnalsATS.201803-172ED

Watz, H., Nagelschmitz, J., Kirsten, A., Pedersen, F., van der Mey, D., Schwers, S., et al. (2019). Safety and efficacy of the human neutrophil elastase inhibitor BAY 85-8501 for the treatment of non-cystic fibrosis bronchiectasis: A randomized controlled trial. *Pulm. Pharmacol. Ther.* 56, 86–93. doi: 10.1016/j.pupt.2019.03.009

Wijker, N. E., Vidmar, S., Grimwood, K., Sly, P. D., Byrnes, C. A., Carlin, J. B., et al. (2020). Early markers of cystic fibrosis structural lung disease: follow-up of the ACFBAL cohort. *Eur. Respirat. J.* 55, 1901694. doi: 10.1183/13993003.01694-2019

Wu, S. H., Chen, X. Q., Liu, B., Wu, H. J., and Dong, L. (2013). Efficacy and safety of 15(R/S)-methyl-lipoxin A(4) in topical treatment of infantile eczema. *Br. J. Dermatol.* 168, 172–178. doi: 10.1111/j.1365-2133.2012.11177.x

Yang, C., and Montgomery, M. (2018). Dornase alfa for cystic fibrosis. *Cochrane Database Syst. Rev.* 9, CD001127. doi: 10.1002/14651858.CD001127.pub4

Yang, Y. D., Cho, H., Koo, J. Y., Tak, M. H., Cho, Y., Shim, W. S., et al. (2008). TMEM16A confers receptor-activated calcium-dependent chloride conductance. *Nature* 455, 1210–1215. doi: 10.1038/nature07313

Yeung, J., and Holinstat, M. (2011). 12-lipoxygenase: a potential target for novel anti-platelet therapeutics. *Cardiovasc. Hematol. Agents Med. Chem.* 9, 154–164. doi: 10.2174/187152511797037619

Zalewska-Kaszubska, J., and Gorska, D. (2001). Anti-inflammatory capabilities of macrolides. *Pharmacol. Res.* 44, 451–454. doi: 10.1006/phrs.2001.0884

Zasloff, M. (2002). Antimicrobial peptides of multicellular organisms. *Nature* 415, 389–395. doi: 10.1038/415389a

Zhou, Z., Treis, D., Schubert, S. C., Harm, M., Schatterny, J., Hirtz, S., et al. (2008). Preventive but not late amiloride therapy reduces morbidity and mortality of lung disease in betaENaC-overexpressing mice. *Am. J. Respir. Crit. Care Med.* 178, 1245–1256. doi: 10.1164/rccm.200803-442OC

Permissions

All chapters in this book were first published by Frontiers; hereby published with permission under the Creative Commons Attribution License or equivalent. Every chapter published in this book has been scrutinized by our experts. Their significance has been extensively debated. The topics covered herein carry significant findings which will fuel the growth of the discipline. They may even be implemented as practical applications or may be referred to as a beginning point for another development.

The contributors of this book come from diverse backgrounds, making this book a truly international effort. This book will bring forth new frontiers with its revolutionizing research information and detailed analysis of the nascent developments around the world.

We would like to thank all the contributing authors for lending their expertise to make the book truly unique. They have played a crucial role in the development of this book. Without their invaluable contributions this book wouldn't have been possible. They have made vital efforts to compile up to date information on the varied aspects of this subject to make this book a valuable addition to the collection of many professionals and students.

This book was conceptualized with the vision of imparting up-to-date information and advanced data in this field. To ensure the same, a matchless editorial board was set up. Every individual on the board went through rigorous rounds of assessment to prove their worth. After which they invested a large part of their time researching and compiling the most relevant data for our readers.

The editorial board has been involved in producing this book since its inception. They have spent rigorous hours researching and exploring the diverse topics which have resulted in the successful publishing of this book. They have passed on their knowledge of decades through this book. To expedite this challenging task, the publisher supported the team at every step. A small team of assistant editors was also appointed to further simplify the editing procedure and attain best results for the readers.

Apart from the editorial board, the designing team has also invested a significant amount of their time in understanding the subject and creating the most relevant covers. They scrutinized every image to scout for the most suitable representation of the subject and create an appropriate cover for the book.

The publishing team has been an ardent support to the editorial, designing and production team. Their endless efforts to recruit the best for this project, has resulted in the accomplishment of this book. They are a veteran in the field of academics and their pool of knowledge is as vast as their experience in printing. Their expertise and guidance has proved useful at every step. Their uncompromising quality standards have made this book an exceptional effort. Their encouragement from time to time has been an inspiration for everyone.

The publisher and the editorial board hope that this book will prove to be a valuable piece of knowledge for researchers, students, practitioners and scholars across the globe.

List of Contributors

Maelle Briottet, Mickael Shum and Valerie Urbach
Institut national de la santé et de la recherche médicale (Inserm) U955, Institut Mondor de Recherche Biomédicale (IMRB), Créteil, France

Caterina Di Pietro, Hasan H. Öz, Thomas S. Murray and Emanuela M. Bruscia
Department of Pediatrics, Yale University School of Medicine, New Haven, CT, United States

Hua Jin, Zuguo Zhao, Qian Lan, Haotong Zhou, Zesen Mai, Yuan Wang, Xiaowen Ding, Wenting Zhang and Xinguang Liu
College of Pharmacy, Guangdong Provincial Key Laboratory of Medical Molecular Diagnostics, Guangdong Medical University, Dongguan, China

Jiang Pi
Department of Microbiology and Immunology, University of Illinois at Chicago, Chicago, IL, United States

Colin E. Evans
Feinberg School of Medicine, Northwestern University, Chicago, IL, United States

Lisa Künzi
Division of Pulmonary, Allergy and Critical Care Medicine, University of Alabama at Birmingham, Birmingham, AL, United States
Epidemiology, Biostatistics and Prevention Institute, Department of Public and Global Health, University of Zürich, Zürich, Switzerland

Molly Easter and Meghan June Hirsch
Division of Pulmonary, Allergy and Critical Care Medicine, University of Alabama at Birmingham, Birmingham, AL, United States

Stefanie Krick
Division of Pulmonary, Allergy and Critical Care Medicine, University of Alabama at Birmingham, Birmingham, AL, United States
Gregory Fleming Cystic Fibrosis Research Center, University of Alabama at Birmingham, Birmingham, AL, United States
Comprehensive Center for Healthy Aging, University of Alabama at Birmingham, Birmingham, AL, United States

Antonio Recchiuti, Sara Patruno, Roberto Plebani and Mario Romano
Laboratory of Molecular Medicine, Center on Advanced Studies and Technology (CAST), Department of Medical, Oral e Biotechnological Sciences, "G. d'Annunzio" University of Chieti-Pescara, Chieti, Italy

Lucy Perrem and Felix Ratjen
Division of Respiratory Medicine, The Hospital for Sick Children, Toronto, ON, Canada
Department of Paediatrics, University of Toronto, Toronto, ON, Canada
Translational Medicine Program, SickKids Research Institute, Toronto, ON, Canada

Yong Zhang, Zhen Han, Aimin Jiang, Di Wu, Shuangqiu Li, Ziyi Liu and Changming Guo
College of Veterinary Medicine, Jilin University, Changchun, China

Zhengkai Wei and Zhengtao Yang
College of Life Sciences and Engineering, Foshan University, Foshan, China

Anna M. van Heeckeren
Pediatrics, Case Western Reserve University School of Medicine, Cleveland, OH, United States

Morgan T. Sutton
Pediatrics, Case Western Reserve University School of Medicine, Cleveland, OH, United States
Department of Biology, Case Western Reserve University School of Medicine, Cleveland, OH, United States
Skeletal Research Center, Case Western Reserve University School of Medicine, Cleveland, OH, United States
National Center for Regenerative Medicine, Case Western Reserve University School of Medicine, Cleveland, OH, United States
Departments of Genetics and Genome Sciences, Case Western Reserve University School of Medicine, Cleveland, OH, United States
St. Jude Children's Research Hospital Graduate School of Biomedical Sciences, Memphis, TN, United States

David R. Fletcher
Pediatrics, Case Western Reserve University School of Medicine, Cleveland, OH, United States
National Center for Regenerative Medicine, Case Western Reserve University School of Medicine, Cleveland, OH, United States
Departments of Genetics and Genome Sciences, Case Western Reserve University School of Medicine, Cleveland, OH, United States

Craig A. Hodges
Pediatrics, Case Western Reserve University School of Medicine, Cleveland, OH, United States
Departments of Genetics and Genome Sciences, Case Western Reserve University School of Medicine, Cleveland, OH, United States

Arnold I. Caplan
Department of Biology, Case Western Reserve University School of Medicine, Cleveland, OH, United States
Skeletal Research Center, Case Western Reserve University School of Medicine, Cleveland, OH, United States
National Center for Regenerative Medicine, Case Western Reserve University School of Medicine, Cleveland, OH, United States

Tracey L. Bonfield
Pediatrics, Case Western Reserve University School of Medicine, Cleveland, OH, United States
Department of Biology, Case Western Reserve University School of Medicine, Cleveland, OH, United States
Skeletal Research Center, Case Western Reserve University School of Medicine, Cleveland, OH, United States
National Center for Regenerative Medicine, Case Western Reserve University School of Medicine, Cleveland, OH, United States
Departments of Genetics and Genome Sciences, Case Western Reserve University School of Medicine, Cleveland, OH, United States

Karen McQuillan, Fatma Gargoum, Mark P. Murphy, Oliver J. McElvaney, Noel G. McElvaney and Emer P. Reeves
Irish Centre for Genetic Lung Disease, Department of Medicine, Royal College of Surgeons in Ireland, Education and Research Centre, Beaumont Hospital, Dublin, Ireland

Zsolt Bene
Department of Laboratory Medicine, Faculty of Medicine, University of Debrecen, Debrecen, Hungary
Department of Pediatrics, Faculty of Medicine, University of Debrecen, Debrecen, Hungary
Kálmán Laki Doctoral School of Biomedical and Clinical Sciences, Faculty of Medicine, University of Debrecen, Debrecen, Hungary

Zsolt Fejes and Béla Nagy Jr.
Department of Laboratory Medicine, Faculty of Medicine, University of Debrecen, Debrecen, Hungary
Kálmán Laki Doctoral School of Biomedical and Clinical Sciences, Faculty of Medicine, University of Debrecen, Debrecen, Hungary

Tibor Gabor Szanto and Gyorgy Panyi
Department of Biophysics and Cell Biology, Faculty of Medicine, University of Debrecen, Debrecen, Hungary

Ferenc Fenyvesi and Judit Váradi
Department of Pharmaceutical Technology, Faculty of Pharmacy, University of Debrecen, Debrecen, Hungary

Luka A. Clarke and Margarida D. Amaral
Faculty of Sciences, BioISI-Biosystems and Integrative Sciences Institute, University of Lisboa, Lisboa, Portugal

Milan Macek Jr.
Department of Biology and Medical Genetics, Charles University—2nd Faculty of Medicine and Motol University Hospital, Prague, Czech

István Balogh
Department of Laboratory Medicine, Faculty of Medicine, University of Debrecen, Debrecen, Hungary
Division of Clinical Genetics, Department of Laboratory Medicine, Faculty of Medicine, University of Debrecen, Debrecen, Hungary

Katherine B. Hisert
Division of Pulmonary, Critical Care, and Sleep Medicine, Department of Medicine, National Jewish Health, Denver, CO, United States
Center for Lung Biology, Division of Pulmonary, Critical Care, and Sleep Medicine, Department of Medicine, University of Washington, Seattle, WA, United States

Timothy P. Birkland, Matthew E. Long, W. Conrad Liles, Anne M. Manicone and Sina A. Gharib
Center for Lung Biology, Division of Pulmonary, Critical Care, and Sleep Medicine, Department of Medicine, University of Washington, Seattle, WA, United States

Kelly Q. Schoenfelt and Lev Becker
Ben May Department for Cancer Research, University of Chicago, Chicago, IL, United States

Brenda Grogan, Suzanne Carter and Edward F. McKone
Department of Medicine, St. Vincent's University Hospital, Dublin, Ireland

Simone Patergnani and Veronica A.M. Vitto
Department of Medical Sciences and Laboratory for Technologies of Advanced Therapies (LTTA), University of Ferrara, Ferrara, Italy

Paolo Pinton and Alessandro Rimessi
Department of Medical Sciences and Laboratory for Technologies of Advanced Therapies (LTTA), University of Ferrara, Ferrara, Italy
Center of Research for Innovative Therapies in Cystic Fibrosis, University of Ferrara, Ferrara, Italy

Judith A. Voynow, Shuo Zheng and Apparao B. Kummarapurugu
Department of Pediatric Pulmonology, Children's Hospital of Richmond at VCU, Richmond, VA, United States

Issaka Yougbare
Le Bilarium, Department of Physiology and Biophysics, Faculty of Medicine and Health Sciences, Université de Sherbrooke, Sherbrooke, QC, Canada
UMR CNRS 7213, Biophotonics and Pharmacology Laboratory, Faculty of Pharmacy, University of Strasbourg, Illkirch, France

Caroline Morin and Yannick F. Senouvo
Le Bilarium, Department of Physiology and Biophysics, Faculty of Medicine and Health Sciences, Université de Sherbrooke, Sherbrooke, QC, Canada

Lazare Belemnaba, Abdurazzag Abusnina and Thérèse Keravis
UMR CNRS 7213, Biophotonics and Pharmacology Laboratory, Faculty of Pharmacy, University of Strasbourg, Illkirch, France

Claire Lugnier
UMR CNRS 7213, Biophotonics and Pharmacology Laboratory, Faculty of Pharmacy, University of Strasbourg, Illkirch, France
Institute of Physiology, FMTS-EA 3072, Faculty of Medicine, University of Strasbourg, Strasbourg, France

Eric Rousseau
Le Bilarium, Department of Physiology and Biophysics, Faculty of Medicine and Health Sciences, Université de Sherbrooke, Sherbrooke, QC, Canada
Department of Obstetrics and Gynecology, Faculty of Medicine and Health Sciences, Université de Sherbrooke, Sherbrooke, QC, Canada

Martina Gentzsch
Marsico Lung Institute and Cystic Fibrosis Research Center, School of Medicine, University of North Carolina, Chapel Hill, NC, United States
Department of Pediatrics, Division of Pediatric Pulmonology, School of Medicine, University of North Carolina School of Medicine, Chapel Hill, NC, United States
Department of Cell Biology and Physiology, School of Medicine, University of North Carolina School of Medicine, Chapel Hill, NC, United States

Deborah M. Cholon, Nancy L. Quinney, Mary E. B. Martino, John T. Minges, Susan E. Boyles and Tara N. Guhr Lee
Marsico Lung Institute and Cystic Fibrosis Research Center, School of Medicine, University of North Carolina, Chapel Hill, NC, United States

Charles R. Esther Jr.
Marsico Lung Institute and Cystic Fibrosis Research Center, School of Medicine, University of North Carolina, Chapel Hill, NC, United States
Department of Pediatrics, Division of Pediatric Pulmonology, School of Medicine, University of North Carolina School of Medicine, Chapel Hill, NC, United States

Carla M. P. Ribeiro
Marsico Lung Institute and Cystic Fibrosis Research Center, School of Medicine, University of North Carolina, Chapel Hill, NC, United States
Department of Cell Biology and Physiology, School of Medicine, University of North Carolina School of Medicine, Chapel Hill, NC, United States
Department of Medicine, Division of Pulmonary Diseases, School of Medicine, University of North Carolina, Chapel Hill, NC, United States

Christie Mitri, Pauline Bardin and Olivier Tabary
Sorbonne Université, Inserm, Centre de Recherche Saint-Antoine, CRSA, Paris, France

Zhengzhong Xu
Sorbonne Université, Inserm, Centre de Recherche Saint-Antoine, CRSA, Paris, France
Yangzhou University, Yangzhou, China

Harriet Corvol
Sorbonne Université, Inserm, Centre de Recherche Saint-Antoine, CRSA, Paris, France
Département de Pédiatrie Respiratoire, Hôpital Trousseau, AP-HP, Paris, France

Lhousseine Touqui
Sorbonne Université, Inserm, Centre de Recherche Saint-Antoine, CRSA, Paris, France
Equipe Mucoviscidose et Bronchopathies Chroniques, Département Santé Globale, Institut Pasteur, Paris, France

Index

www.ingramcontent.com/pod-product-compliance
Lightning Source LLC
LaVergne TN
LVHW082130200926
848484LV00008B/2032
* 9 7 9 8 8 8 7 4 0 5 8 3 4 *